D1451848

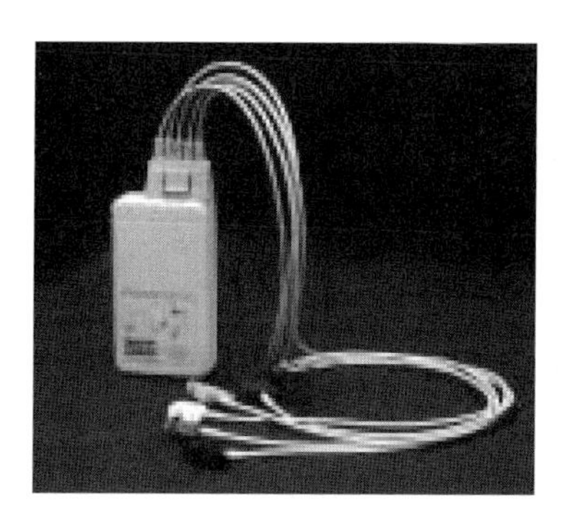

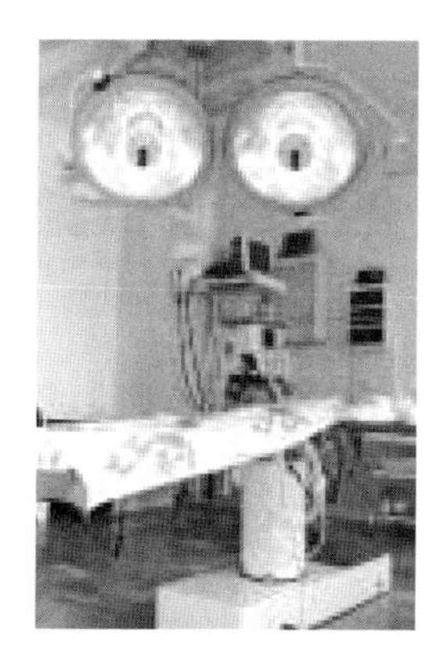

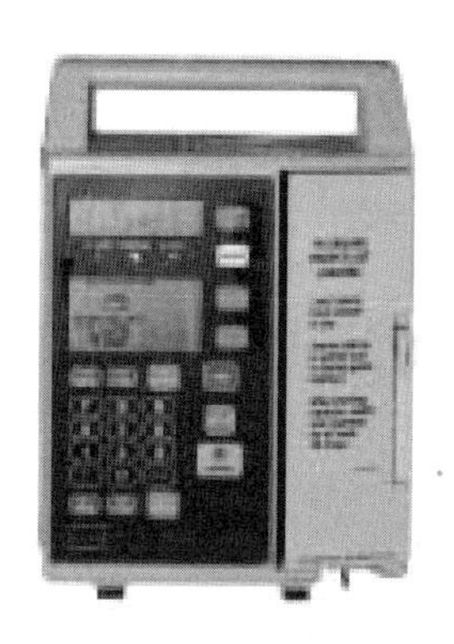

Biomedical Instrumentation Systems

■ Shakti Chatterjee, Ph.D.

Senior Professor
DeVry University
Columbus, Ohio

■ Aubert Miller, B.S., M.B.A.

Senior Director, Biomedical Engineering
Baton Rouge General Medical Center
Baton Rouge, Louisiana

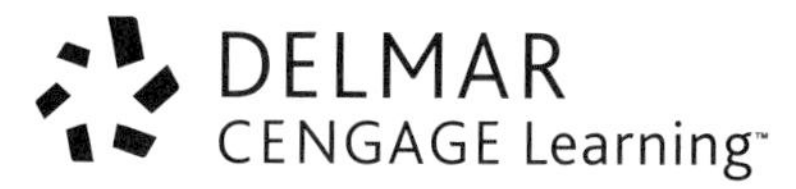

Australia Canada Mexico Singapore Spain United Kingdom United States

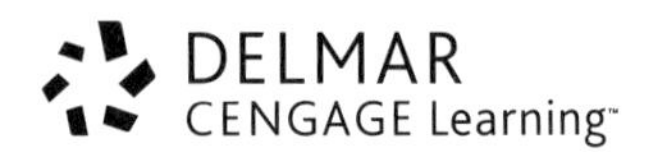

Biomedical Instrumentation Systems
Shakti Chatterjee and Aubert Miller

Vice President, Career and Professional Editorial: Dave Garza

Director of Learning Solutions: Sandy Clark

Acquisitions Editor: Stacy Masucci

Managing Editor: Larry Main

Senior Production Manager: Michelle Ruelos Cannistraci

Senior Editorial Assistant: Dawn Daugherty

Vice President, Career and Professional Marketing: Jennifer McAvey

Executive Marketing Manager: Deborah S. Yarnell

Senior Marketing Manager: Erin Coffin

Marketing Coordinator: Mark Pierro

Production Director: Wendy Troeger

Production Manager: Mark Bernard

Content Project Manager: Christopher Chien

Senior Art Director: David Arsenault

Technology Project Manager: Christopher Catalina

Production Technology Analyst: Thomas Stover

Production and Project Management: MPS Content Services, a Macmillan Company

For product information and technology assistance, contact us at
Professional Group Cengage Learning Customer & Sales Support, 1-800-354-9706
For permission to use material from this text or product, submit all requests online at **cengage.com/permissions**.
Further permissions questions can be e-mailed to
permissionrequest@cengage.com.

Library of Congress Control Number: 2008935167

ISBN-13: 978-1-4180-1866-5
ISBN-10: 1-4180-1866-X

Delmar
5 Maxwell Drive
Clifton Park, NY 12065-2919
USA

Cengage Learning is a leading provider of customized learning solutions with office locations around the globe, including Singapore, the United Kingdom, Australia, Mexico, Brazil, and Japan. Locate your local office at: **international.cengage.com/region**

Cengage Learning products are represented in Canada by Nelson Education, Ltd.

For your lifelong learning solutions, visit **delmar.cengage.com**
Visit our corporate website at **cengage.com**

Notice to the Reader
Publisher does not warrant or guarantee any of the products described herein or perform any independent analysis in connection with any of the product information contained herein. Publisher does not assume, and expressly disclaims, any obligation to obtain and include information other than that provided to it by the manufacturer. The reader is expressly warned to consider and adopt all safety precautions that might be indicated by the activities described herein and to avoid all potential hazards. By following the instructions contained herein, the reader willingly assumes all risks in connection with such instructions. The publisher makes no representations or warranties of any kind, including but not limited to, the warranties of fitness for particular purpose or merchantability, nor are any such representations implied with respect to the material set forth herein, and the publisher takes no responsibility with respect to such material. The publisher shall not be liable for any special, consequential, or exemplary damages resulting, in whole or part, from the readers' use of, or reliance upon, this material.

Printed in the United States of America
2 3 4 5 6 17 16 15 14 13

DEDICATION

This book is dedicated to my father, the late Rabindra Nath Chatterjee, who always encouraged me to achieve higher goals in life. For me, writing a book is one of the higher goals of achievement.

Contents

Foreword

Biomedical Engineering Technology is without a doubt one of the most exciting and rewarding areas of study available to students in the twenty-first century. This field integrates the graduate's knowledge of biology, chemistry, anatomy, physiology, physics, mathematics, electronics, computers, and networks into a coherent background that provides the basis for employment in a clinical setting such as a hospital or employment with a biomedical equipment manufacturer. A major component of any Biomedical Engineering Technology program is biomedical instrumentation.

Dr. Shakti Chatterjee's textbook, *Biomedical Instrumentation Systems*, is the product of a distinguished and lengthy career in teaching, research, and experience in the field of Biomedical Engineering and Engineering Technology. Dr. Chatterjee's textbook provides in-depth, comprehensive coverage of this fundamental element of a Biomedical Engineering Technology curriculum. The text starts with an overview of the field, followed by the fundamental concepts from electronics upon which all biomedical instrumentation is based. The text then logically addresses a wide range of instruments, integrating science, mathematics, clinical, safety, and regulatory concepts as appropriate. The text is written from a practitioner's point of view rather than from a researcher's vantage point. This approach is exactly what is required for Biomedical Engineering Technology programs.

In addition to its value as a resource in an educational environment, *Biomedical Instrumentation Systems* will serve to enhance the knowledge of an individual working in either a clinical setting or in industry with up-to-date and in-depth coverage of the field. The textbook also would well serve an individual wishing to simply enhance his or her knowledge of the field.

Please consider this outstanding textbook if you have any interest in the field of biomedical instrumentation. I can assure you that it was written with care and devotion to excellence by a very dedicated faculty member who is truly loved by the many students whom he has influenced over the years.

Edward A. Wilson, Ph.D.
Associate Dean, Engineering
College of Engineering and Information Sciences
DeVry University

Preface

Biomedical engineering has only recently (within the last few decades) emerged as its own discipline, in contrast to many other engineering fields such as electrical engineering, mechanical engineering, and civil engineering, which have existed for over one hundred years. Biomedical engineering combines the design and problem-solving skills of engineering with the sciences of medicine and biology to improve health care diagnosis and treatment. Biomedical Equipment Technicians (BMETs), Biomedical Engineers, and Clinical Engineers interact every day with patients, staff, and the technology that supports and sustains life.

Biomedical Instrumentation Systems introduces biomedical technicians, technologists, and engineers to a variety of hospital equipment. Even though the Internet has become an invaluable tool for gathering information on hospital equipment, as well as for transferring patient data through wired and wireless communication links, understanding how a piece of hospital equipment works still depends on a sound knowledge of basic electronics. The purpose of this book is to combine hands-on knowledge of electronics with the use of the Internet to acquire a complete understanding of the hospital equipment covered in the book.

The early chapters of the book present the reader with general information on the field of biomedical engineering, the various departments in a hospital, different types of medical equipment, and the companies and organizations involved in health care. In the later chapters the author includes descriptions of various medical devices and provides the reader with a review of anatomy, physiology, and basic analog and digital electronics.

The book is easy to read. The information on electronic circuits and devices includes simple mathematical equations, and the reader is encouraged to use the Internet for research in working on the problems at the end of each chapter (the author intentionally did not provide all the necessary information for solving these). Discussion of medical device regulations, standards, and medical safety features enhances the knowledge of hospital equipment. The use of software simulation packages like MATLAB and MultiSIM emphasizes a better understanding of electronics concepts related to hospital equipment.

Each chapter includes a list of appropriate Internet Web sites, examples, lists of medical or technical terms, quizzes, end-of-chapter problems, case studies, and research problems. Throughout the book, equipment is described using block diagrams, and the use of elaborate electronic circuits is minimized.

INTENDED AUDIENCE

This book is designed to support a twelve- to fifteen-week course in either the third year of a four-year biomedical engineering technology or biomedical engineering program, or the second year of an associate degree program for Biomedical Equipment Technicians. This book may be used in more than one course of a university curriculum. The text should be considered as an introduction to biomedical instrumentation.

CHAPTER DESCRIPTIONS

Chapter 1: Introduction to Biomedical Instrumentation Systems

This chapter provides the reader with a general introduction to the field of biomedical instrumentation. Several examples of medical instrumentation in the various departments of a hospital are presented in this chapter. It also includes information on the activities of biomedical organizations, products made by various medical device manufacturers, and a simple block diagram of a medical device.

Chapter 2: Anatomy and Physiology

This chapter provides a review of anatomy and physiology. It includes coverage of the cardiovascular, circulatory, respiratory, nervous, digestive, and renal systems. The main internal organs such as the heart, lungs, brain, and kidneys are discussed.

Chapter 3: Biosignals and Noise

This chapter discusses biosignals and types of noise. The process of digitizing biosignals is also explained. The parameters of noise, such as noise temperature, noise figure, and signal-to-noise ratio are included in the discussion. Noisy biosignals are shown in this chapter.

Chapter 4: Biomedical Electronics: Analog

This chapter reviews basic analog electronics. Starting with simple RLC circuits, the chapter discusses op-amp amplifiers, filters, differentiators, integrators, diodes, and transistors. The loading problem and the maximum power transfer concepts are explained in this chapter. The chapter emphasizes the application of analog electronic circuits to medical equipment.

Chapter 5: Biomedical Electronics: Digital

This chapter reviews digital electronics. It includes the concepts of R/2R ladder networks, successive approximation registers, flip-flops, microprocessors, and computers. The chapter illustrates the application of digital circuits in medical equipment.

Chapter 6: Biomedical Electrodes, Sensors, and Transducers

This chapter establishes the differences among electrodes, sensors, and transducers. The chapter presents and explains a model of a biomedical electrode, and includes discussion of transducers such as those used to measure pressure, displacement, and flow.

Chapter 7: Instrumentation in Diagnostic Cardiology

This chapter discusses normal and abnormal ECG signals, ECG leads, and ECG machines, including coverage of the Holter monitor and ECG simulators.

Chapter 8: Defibrillators and Pacemakers

This chapter presents the electronic circuits of defibrillators and pacemakers and describes their operation through the use of simple mathematical equations. In addition, the chapter provides block diagrams of a biphasic defibrillator and pacemaker.

Chapter 9: Instrumentation in Blood Circulation

This chapter discusses a variety of biomedical instruments such as blood pressure and cardiac output monitors, infusion pumps, and plethysmographs. In addition, the chapter also covers the topic of catheterization and presents the mathematical equations of fluid dynamics.

Chapter 10: Instrumentation in Extracorporeal Circulation and Cardiac Assist Devices

This chapter covers the concepts and block diagrams of hemodialysis systems, apheresis systems, heart-lung machines, extracorporeal membrane oxygenation (ECMO), ventricular assist devices, and intra-aortic balloon pumps.

Chapter 11: Instrumentation in Respiration

This chapter presents some of the important instruments used in hospitals for patients with respiratory disorders. In addition to reviewing the human respiratory system and pulmonary circulation, the chapter provides the mathematical relationships for pulmonary volumes and capacities.

Chapter 12: Electroencephalography and EMG Instrumentation

This chapter explains the bioelectric function of the brain and the skeletal muscles using EEG and EMG instrumentation, respectively. It includes discussions of EEG electrodes, EEG lead systems, and nerve conduction studies.

Chapter 13: Artifacts and Noise in Medical Instrumentation

This chapter presents the types and sources of noises that affect biomedical signals. The chapter also discusses digital signal processing techniques for reducing noise.

Chapter 14: Instrumentation in Diagnostic Ultrasound

This chapter discusses ultrasound physics and the associated mathematical equations before introducing concepts of ultrasound transducers and techniques of ultrasound diagnostic imaging. The chapter also includes a block diagram of an ultrasound system and covers the theory of Doppler ultrasound.

Chapter 15: Instrumentation in Medical Imaging

This chapter introduces the theory and instrumentation of radiological systems such as X-ray, CT, MRI, and nuclear medicine. The chapter also presents simple mathematical equations used to determine intensity of radiation, material densities, and radiation exposure.

Chapter 16: Fiber Optics and Lasers in Bioinstrumentation

This chapter describes the physics of fiber optics and laser technologies and their applications in health care. It also discusses various endoscopic techniques such as sigmoidoscopy and colonoscopy.

Chapter 17: Instrumentation in Intensive Care Units

This chapter discusses various bioinstrumentation devices such as bedside monitors, patient monitors, intravenous lines, and telemetry units used in hospital intensive care units.

Chapter 18: Instrumentation in the Operating Room

This chapter familiarizes the reader with the environment of a hospital operating room, and includes coverage of the electrosurgical machine, anesthesia machine, and sterilization practices.

Chapter 19: Biomedical Laboratory Instrumentation

This chapter introduces the various laboratories found in a hospital and discusses the types of equipment (specifically, the hemacytometer, urine analyzer, centrifuges, incubators, and po_2 and pco_2 electrodes) used in these laboratories.

Chapter 20: Medical Safety

This chapter describes hospital safety issues such as electrical safety, radiation safety, chemical safety, and biological safety. It identifies the federal and state agencies (such as NFPA and OSHA) that regulate hospital safety, and describes and explains the purpose of Material Safety Data Sheets (MSDS), which are required in all hospitals.

Chapter 21: Regulation and Standards

This chapter presents information on the various agencies that regulate the medical device industry, as well as on the management of equipment in a hospital. The chapter also identifies organizations that set standards for medical equipment used in hospitals.

Chapter 22: Preventive Maintenance

This chapter familiarizes the reader with the issue of scheduled maintenance of hospital medical equipment and includes an example of the calibration process for a specific piece of medical equipment.

Chapter 23: Computers and Telemedicine

This chapter identifies the components of a digital hospital. It discusses computer infrastructure inside and outside the hospital, particularly picture archiving and communication systems, and it includes coverage of the network concepts of subnets and routing.

Chapter 24: New Technologies and Advances in Medical Instrumentation

This chapter introduces the emerging concepts of nanotechnology and tissue engineering in medical instrumentation. The chapter also includes a list of organizations in the fields of nanotechnology and tissue engineering.

FEATURES OF THE TEXT

The book includes the following features to help ensure a successful learning experience:

- **Chapter Outline:** Each chapter opens up with a list of main topics.
- **Objectives:** A list of learning objectives sets the stage for the lessons to be learned in the text.
- **Internet Web Sites:** References to medical Web sites enhance the reader's understanding of chapter topics.
- **Examples:** Examples provide opportunities for immediate practice and for applying theory.
- **Summary:** This bulleted list of concise statements summarizes the major points of the chapter.
- **Medical/Technical Terminology:** A list of terms and definitions reinforces the content in each chapter. Medical terminology at the end of each chapter provides valuable learning resources.
- **Quiz:** Readers can test their understanding of each chapter with this set of review questions.
- **Research Topics:** Research topics stimulate reader interest and motivation.
- **Case Studies:** Realistic case studies test the reader's understanding of challenging medical and technical concepts.
- **Problems:** Problem assignments at the end of each chapter check the reader's knowledge of electronics concepts.

ACKNOWLEDGMENTS

The author would like to thank the following health care providers who educated him in several ways in the preparation of the book:

Thomas Baidoo, BMET, Field Service Engineer, Phillips Healthcare, Lansing, Michigan

Atindra Nath Chatterji, M.D., Gastroenterologist, Internal Medicine and Liver Diseases; Clinical Assistant Professor, Department of Internal Medicine, Wright State University, Dayton, Ohio

Richard Davis, Ph.D., Associate Executive Director, Ross Heart Hospital, The Ohio State University Medical Center, Columbus, Ohio

Duane L. Hart, B.S., CBET, Imaging Engineering Service Manager, Clinical Engineering Services, The Ohio State University Medical Center, Columbus, Ohio

Felix M. Lake Jr., BMET, Biomedical Equipment Specialist, GS-11 Engineering Services, Alvin C. York Veterans Administration Medical Center, Murfreesboro, Tennessee

Anthony McCabe, BMET, The Ohio State University Health System, Columbus, Ohio

Ashok Mukherjee, M.D., Cardiologist, Rouge Valley Health System, Toronto, Canada

Alexander Price, BSCET, Technical Program Manager, Fresenius Medical Care North America, Columbus, Ohio

Allison Bednarski Spiwak, Ph.D., Director Circulation Technology, School of Allied Medical Professions, The Ohio State University, Columbus, Ohio

The author and Cengage Learning would like to thank the following reviewers:

Barbara Christe, Indiana University Purdue University Indianapolis, Indianapolis, IN
Myron D. Hartman, Pennsylvania State University, New Kensington, PA
Ron Lundak, DeVry University, Fremont, CA
Paul Svatik, Owens Community College, Toledo, OH
Ron Tinckham, Santa Fe Community College, Gainesville, FL
Mohammad Zakai, DeVry University, Atlanta, GA

There is no question that the author is grateful to the very talented team of Delmar, Cengage Learning. A very special thank-you goes to **Steve Helba** for his confidence in me and for his continuous encouragement throughout the preparation of the manuscript. I am indebted to **Michelle Ruelos Cannistraci** for her continuing support and guidance, her immense patience, and her involvement in the preparation of the manuscript; to **Christopher Chien** for our numerous discussions and his thorough content editing in each and every chapter; and finally to **Stacy Masucci** for her patience and unique ability to smooth out the waves during the production of the book.

The author also owes much appreciation to **Shanin Dockrey** for copyediting the original manuscript; to **Monica Ohlinger** and **Erin Curtis** for their tremendous help in contacting medical companies in acquiring photos of medical equipment for the book; and to **Martha Wetherill** and **Nincis Asencio** for many helpful discussions and organizing the page proofs and the design efforts.

I am greatly appreciative of my good friends of many years, **Amin Karim** and **Edward Wilson** of DeVry University; Amin had involved me in several biomedical and electronics engineering projects and Edward was kind enough to write a wonderful foreword for this book.

My thank-you to **Bob Miller**, my co-author, for providing access to numerous service manuals from the Children's Hospital, and for contributing to the text and providing equipment photos.

I am especially indebted to my friend **Michael Shumway** for helping me throughout the preparation of the book by generating hundreds of circuit diagrams using various software applications, and for help with typing the manuscript.

To my students, who over the years have helped me to discover the joy of teaching.

Finally, of course, I would like to thank my wife **Padma**, and my children, **Sujeet** and **Monica**, for their patience, continuous encouragement, and support for me during this massive project.

Shakti Chatterjee

CHAPTER 1

Introduction to Biomedical Instrumentation Systems

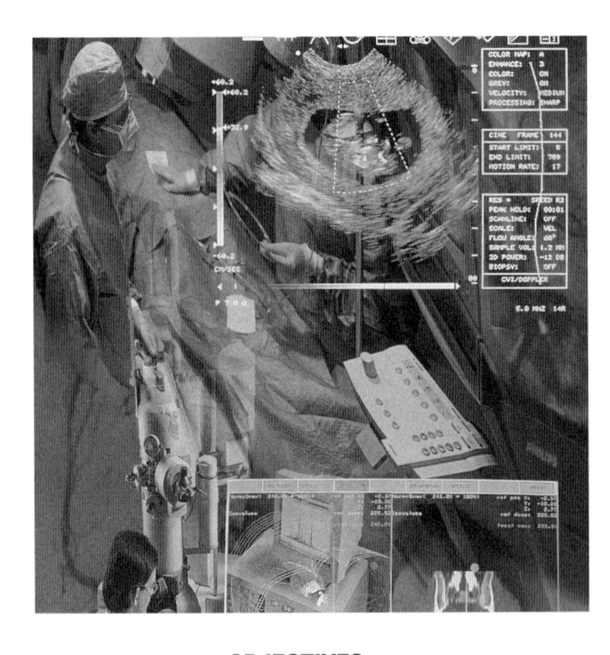

■ CHAPTER OUTLINE

■ OBJECTIVES

The objective of this chapter is to familiarize the reader with the organizational structure of the biomedical field in the industry, at universities, in hospitals, and on the Internet prior to learning the scope, theory, and practice of biomedical instrumentation systems.

Upon completion of this chapter, the reader will be able to:

- Define biomedical engineering and discuss areas of the biomedical field.
- Name the major medical instruments in a hospital.
- Name the components of a medical instrument.
- Name the biomedical organizations and companies and their perspectives.
- Name medical equipment regulatory organizations and their functions.

INTERNET WEB SITES

http://www.aami.org (Association for the Advancement of Medical Instrumentation)
http://www.bmes.org (Biomedical Engineering Society)
http://www.embs.org (Institute of Electrical and Electronics Engineers [IEEE] Engineering in Medicine and Biology Society)
http://www.medicalengineer.co.uk (Medical Engineer)
http://www.mymeta.org (Medical Equipment and Technology Association)
http://www.bmenet.org (Biomedical Engineering Network [The Whitaker Foundation])
http://www.amia.org (American Medical Informatics Association)
http://www.ieee.org (Institute of Electrical and Electronics Engineering)
http://www.aimbe.org (American Institute for Medical and Biological Engineering)

INTRODUCTION

As the health care field continues to expand and technology plays a growing role in analytical, diagnostic, therapeutic, and research activities, the domain of biomedical instrumentation systems is also rapidly growing in biomaterials, nanotechnology, telemedicine, tissue engineering, hospital safety, and regulatory methodology. The Internet has added another dimension of patient health care involving various hospital instruments, telecommunication links, and biomedical databases. This is an exciting era of medical inventions and high-tech patient care.

Every major hospital has a separate department for biomedical engineering and employs biomedical engineers, Biomedical Engineering Technologists or Biomedical Equipment Technicians (BMETs), for the maintenance of hospital equipment, machines, and the computer networks. The Institute of Electrical and Electronics Engineers (IEEE) Engineering in Medicine and Biology Society (EMBS) defines the field of biomedical engineering as "the application of concepts and methods of the physical and engineering sciences in biology and medicine. This covers a broad spectrum ranging from formalized mathematical theory through experimental science and technological development to practical clinical applications." Universities and colleges worldwide have biomedical engineering programs that attract a wide range of students to the biomedical disciplines every year.

The profession of biomedical engineering has grown in recent years. In hospitals, biomedical engineers typically supervise the maintenance of medical equipment, assist in acquisition of new equipment, and train the medical staff to use this new equipment. In the medical device industry, these professionals are involved with the design and development of new products. They may also be involved in medical research projects in universities and governmental regulatory agencies enforcing hospital and medical device regulations. In contrast, BMETs have different goals and perspectives. Generally, these professionals are the technicians in the forefront of maintaining the medical equipment in a hospital.

In the twenty-first century, we are witnessing extraordinary changes in patient care at hospitals and clinics around the world. Some hospitals are even accommodating patients with environments that compare to five-star hotels with Internet access, better patient relations, family accommodations, advanced medical equipment, and even valet parking!

Today's digital hospital gives doctors, engineers, and technicians alike the opportunity to work with personal digital assistants (PDAs) for database searches. With this technology, they can check any status record with real-time access to the various pieces of medical equipment. Because today's technology allows electronic transfer, retrieval, and storage of information, the historical need for a long paper trail is rapidly becoming extinct!

This introductory chapter provides a survey of the medical instrumentation in hospitals and explains the components of a simple medical instrument. We will discuss also the role of various regulatory organizations and the competitive field of the manufacturing companies in health care.

■

1.1 OVERVIEW OF BIOINSTRUMENTATION IN HOSPITALS

Nearly every hospital or clinic houses a wide array of medical instruments and other pieces of equipment that must be maintained properly. Preventive maintenance is important and should be conducted regularly throughout the year to ensure minimal risk and to repair any equipment as needed. As you explore this book, keep in mind the medical equipment discussed; this will give you insight to the biomedical instrumentation theory and the design practices covered in later chapters.

Figure 1-1 shows a list of important hospital equipment housed in different areas of the hospital. The list shows diagnostic (D) and therapeutic (T) equipment. Hospital equipment is classified further according to which specific organs and systems of the human body it is used to study (for example, cardiology equipment is used to study the heart and respiratory equipment is used to study the respiratory system). Notice the equipment in each category.

Cardiology equipment is used to study the structure, function, and diseases related to the normal and abnormal heart.

Vascular equipment studies the blood vessels in terms of blood pressure, flow, and volume in the vessels.

Respiratory equipment detects the gaseous exchanges that occur in the various parts of the respiratory system—nasopharynx, nose, larynx, trachea, bronchi, and lungs.

Sensory equipment monitors brain waves and records them as electroencephalogram (EEG) signals. Moreover, sensory equipment may also record electric impulses from the surface of muscles as electromyogram (EMG) signals.

Imaging equipment is also called radiological and nuclear medicine imaging equipment. Machines using X-ray, computer tomography (CT), magnetic resonance imaging (MRI), and positron emission tomography (PET) technologies generate images of the body's organs and systems. These are primarily diagnostic machines used by radiologists to detect any abnormalities.

Fiber optics and *laser equipment* are used in endoscopic examinations and in surgery.

Intensive care equipment and *operating equipment* are used in the intensive care unit (ICU) and the operating room (OR). The ICU uses highly specialized therapeutic and resuscitation equipment and monitoring systems, while the OR uses anesthesia machines to anesthetize patients and electrosurgical equipment to treat deformities and injuries. Responsibility for the anesthesia and electrosurgical machines lies with the anesthesiologists and surgeons, respectively.

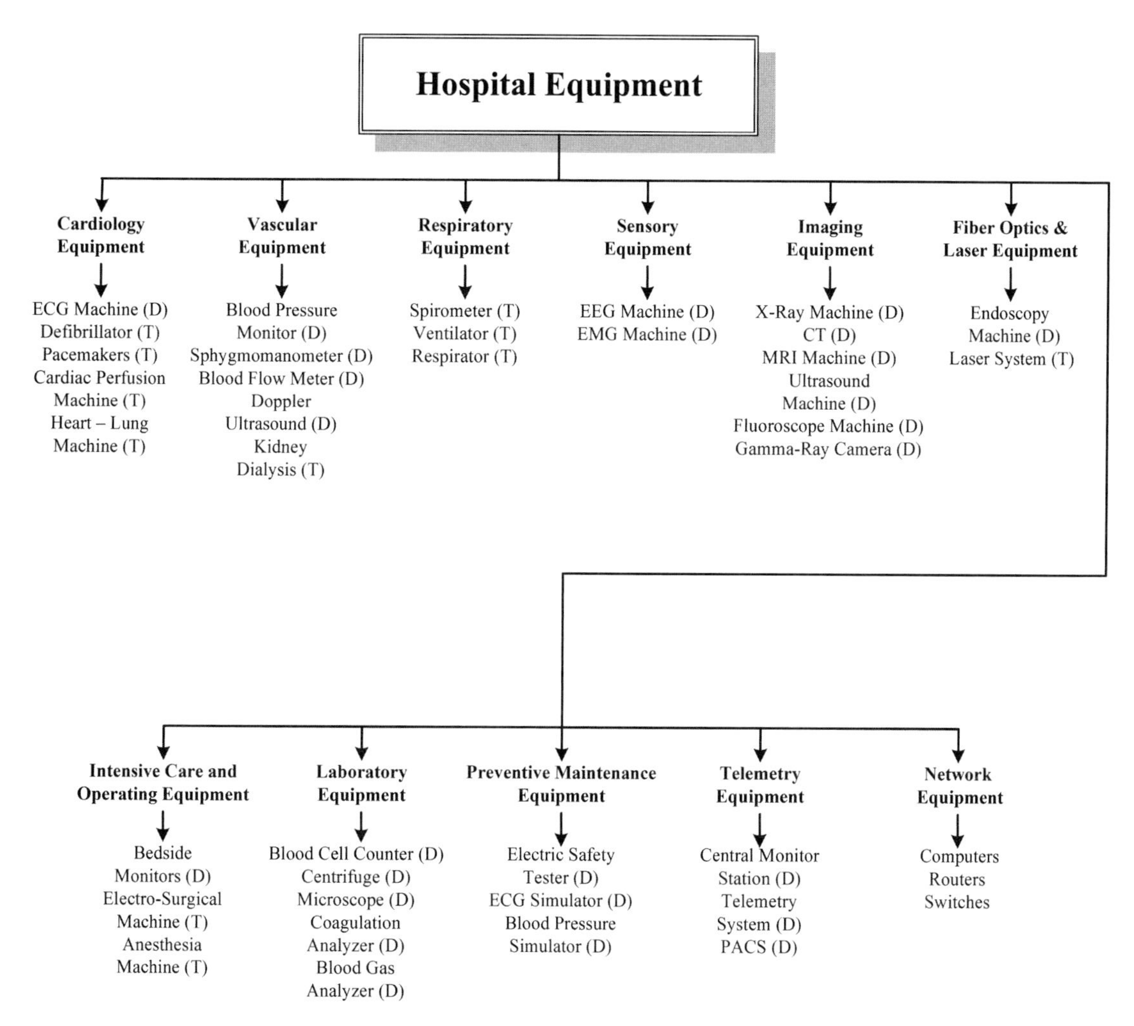

FIGURE 1-1 A list of hospital equipment with respective departments.

Laboratory equipment is used for blood, urine, and other lab tests such as fluid analysis for sodium, potassium, chlorides, and blood gas. Other lab equipment is also assigned in chemistry, hematology, microbiology, virology, or histology labs.

Preventive maintenance equipment is used by hospitals in effective preventive maintenance programs to ensure a high degree of patient safety from electrical and mechanical hazards, reduce equipment repairs, and extend equipment life, thus improving the quality of health care.

Telemetry equipment is used to remotely monitor the patient's vital signs such as blood pressure or the ECG or it is used in the patient's room in real time via radio frequency.

Network equipment includes the sophisticated hubs, switches, and routers the hospital network uses to communicate with the outside world on fast-speed, packet-switched wide area networks. The hospital intranet is called a Local Area Network (LAN); the Internet is called a Wide Area Network (WAN).

1.2 BLOCK DIAGRAM OF A MEDICAL INSTRUMENT

Figure 1-2 shows the human-machine interface and explains the input and output relationships to the machine. This simple example is a block diagram typical of any biomedical instrument. The medical machine consists of signal conditioning, a monitor, and data storage. As shown, the input to the medical machine is the electrode or a transducer output. The output of the machine is then displayed as a biosignal such as an electrocardiogram (ECG), arterial blood pressure, or oxygen saturation in blood. In some cases, the machine sends a stimulus signal to the human body to control a particular physiological process.

Generally, the input or output of an electrode is an electrical signal; however, the input or output of a transducer is not necessarily an electrical signal. For example, the transducer may convert pressure or sound to an electrical signal. The human-machine interface has the following components:

The *patient* is the person who receives medical care. Electrodes are connected to the patient's arms, legs, or chest.

The *electrodes, sensors,* and *transducers* are devices used to detect electrical and biomedical signals. An electrode detects electrical signals mainly from the surface of the body, and a variety of sensors detect biomedical signals, such as pressure, flow, or temperature. At times, a sensor may itself be called a transducer, or it may be a part of the transducer unit or circuit. Typically, the sensor output is an electrical signal that the transducer may change into other types of signals such as pressure, flow, temperature, or light.

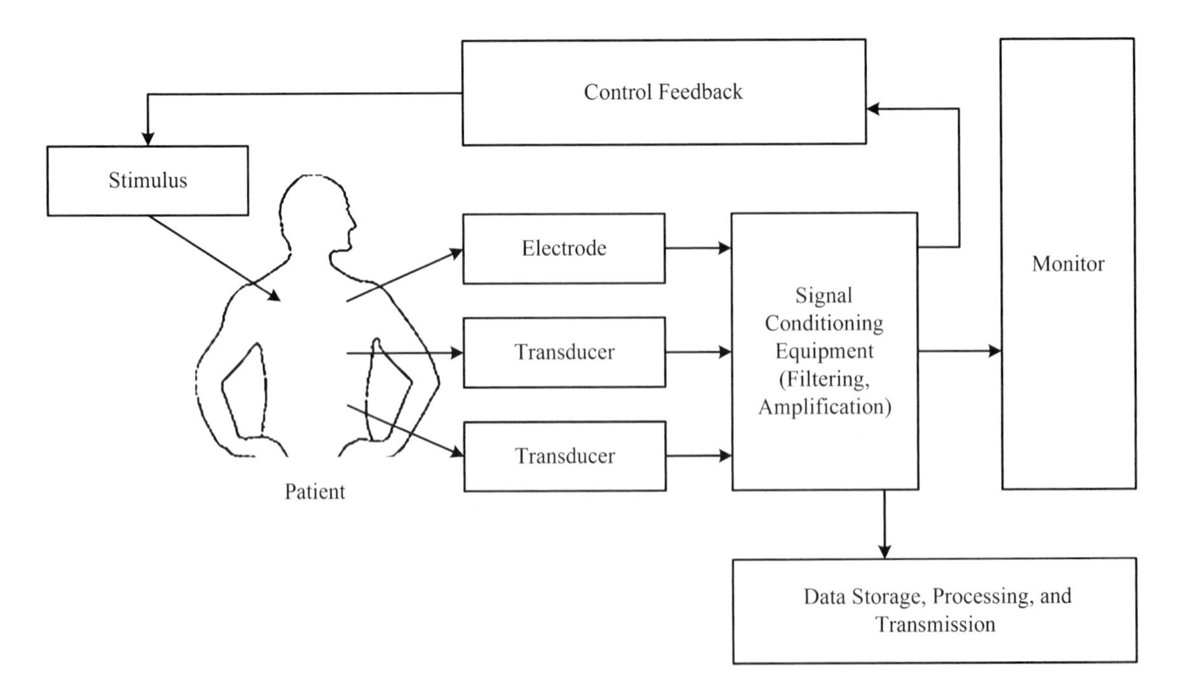

FIGURE 1-2 A simple block diagram of human-machine interface.

Signal conditioners are devices used to filter and amplify biomedical signals. These signals are generally weak and "noisy," so they must be amplified and filtered of unwanted frequencies. This process is called signal conditioning and uses special electronic devices and circuits called signal conditioner circuits.

Displays are devices used to display biomedical signals. These devices include monitors, video screens, and scopes (cathode ray tubes, or CRT).

Feedback stimulus concerns muscle and organ stimulation. Once the biomedical signals are signal conditioned and interpreted, some of the electronic circuits can be activated to generate signals that in return can stimulate the muscles or organs as feedback stimuli. At times, this external stimulus is required to determine the patient's response.

1.3 BIOMEDICAL SIMULATORS FOR TRAINING

Just as airline flight simulators help to train pilots, medical simulators are used to teach medical professionals new skill sets prior to treating patients. This reduces the medical errors in real situations and improves patient safety in hospitals.

These simulators allow the health care provider to review and practice the procedures as often as necessary until he or she achieves proper proficiency, thereby reducing risk to the patient's health. There are several types of medical simulation tools (usually computer based). They replicate the clinical situations, provide training, save money, and improve the overall quality of patient care.

Companies like the Pinnacle Technology Group manufacture patient simulators such as the arrhythmia training simulator shown in **Figure 1-3.** Its display waveforms use 3- to 12-lead ECG data. Using actual patient data, students receive proper training prior to working with patients. Other companies such as National Instruments' iWorx, BioPAC Systems' BioPAC Student Lab, and CleveMed's CleveLabs create integrated hardware and software products that are designed to teach physiology and biomedical electronics to students and researchers who plan to join the health care field.

iWorx develops, manufactures, and distributes electronic systems and components for physiology teaching and research. BioPAC laboratories exercises provide detailed procedures to demonstrate the principles of biophysics and biological measurements. The data can be exported to MATLAB and LabView as well as to a Microsoft Word document or an Excel spreadsheet. **Figure 1-4** shows a BioPAC simulator. The simulator has input channels from transducers that can be connected to an actual patient.

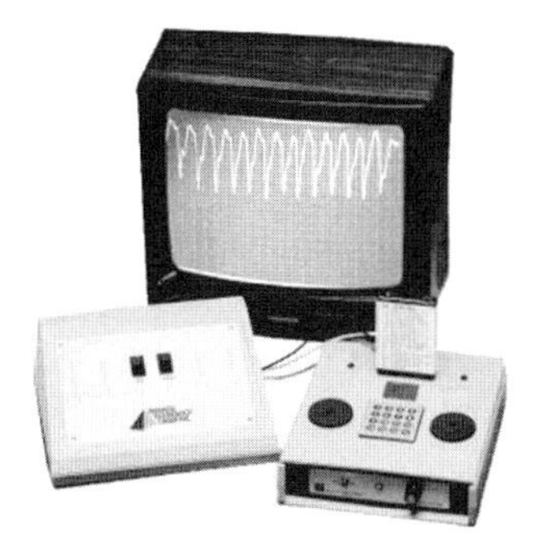

FIGURE 1-3 An arrhythmia training simulator. (*Courtesy of Pinnacle Technology Group*)

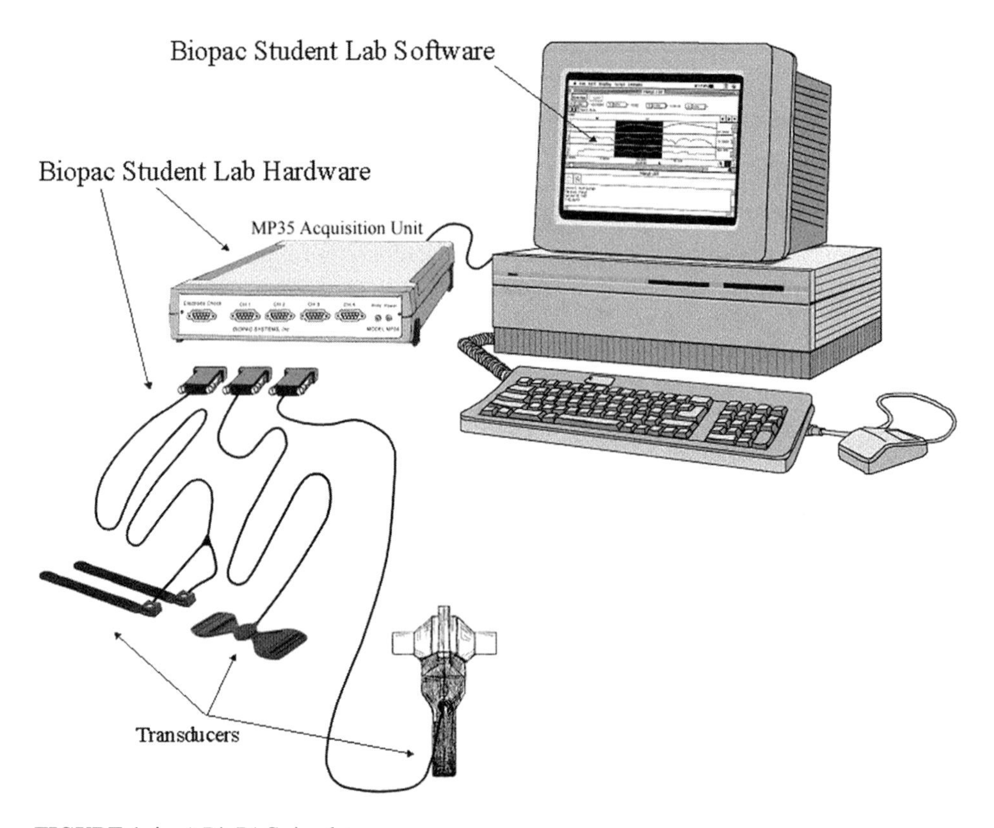

FIGURE 1-4 A BioPAC simulator.

The CleveLabs laboratory course includes disposable electrodes, sensors, transducers, and oral/nasal airflow cannulas for physiology signal acquisition. Wireless hardware that is lightweight and programmable allows these devices to monitor and record physiological signals.

The human patient simulator allows medical students to gain appropriate experience before they treat actual patients. These simulators are lifelike computerized mannequins. Medical centers such as the University of Louisville School of Medicine are creating new simulation centers that teach students a variety of medical scenarios using these types of simulators.

Patient simulators are used in hospitals to generate normal and abnormal blood pressure or ECG signals when testing blood pressure or ECG equipment for any necessary repair. Simulators such as that shown in **Figure 1-5** are used for blood pressure, ECG, respiration, and temperature testing.

1.4 A PERSPECTIVE OF BIOMEDICAL ENGINEERING

Medical instrumentation has been prevalent for centuries. During the past century, however, the invention of new instruments for patient care has been a particularly competitive field for both large and small companies in the United States and Europe. Throughout the 1900s, from the invention of x-ray equipment to that of the newest large-size MRI equipment,

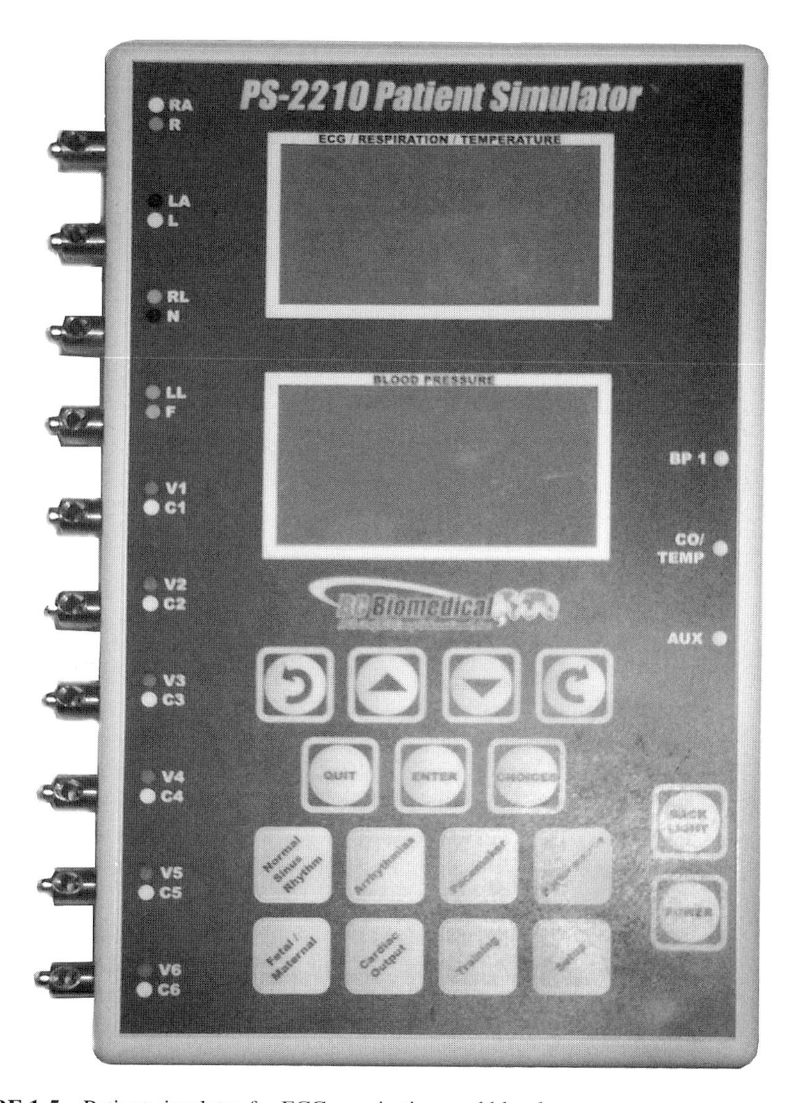

FIGURE 1-5 Patient simulator for ECG, respiration, and blood pressure.

humankind has gained great insight into diseases and their control. We can prolong human life with the help of new kinds of treatments and procedures using sophisticated instruments. Today, many diseases that were once usually terminal, such as many cancers, AIDS, and heart disease, are under increasingly greater control.

From the invention of the stethoscope in 1816 to the most recent innovations in modern cardiac pacemakers, technology has made great strides in diagnostic and imaging techniques; every year, new medical machines are being developed and introduced in hospitals.

For example, there has been tremendous change in the design and applications of manufacturing pacemakers in the last few decades. The clinical use of cardiac pacing started in 1952 and today, with more advanced technology, small, lightweight pacemakers are implanted into thousands of patients each year.

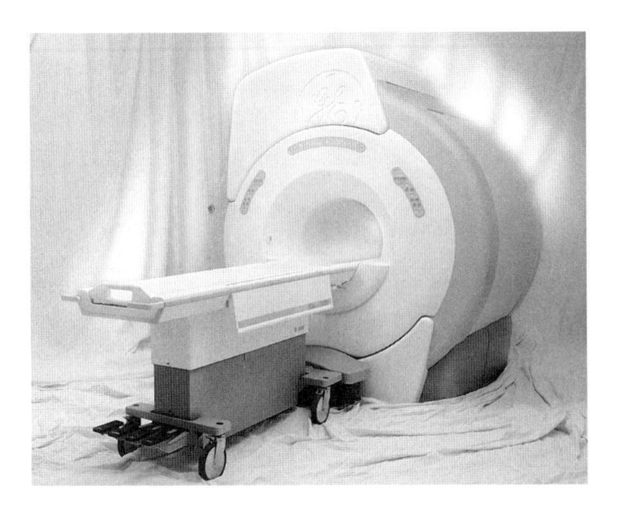

FIGURE 1-6 MRI unit with movable patient table and stationary magnet.

Similarly, in recent years, high-field MRI scanners, powerful CT machines, and many other expensive devices have come to the forefront of diagnostic equipment. The MRI unit consists of a stationary magnet with a strong magnetic field, radio frequency (RF) coils, a table for the patient, and a sophisticated computer for processing the resulting images. A typical MRI unit is shown in **Figure 1-6.** The CT monitor shown in **Figure 1-7** displays a wide range of features that assist in the diagnosis of patient images.

Today, most noninvasive patient examinations—from neurological, musculoskeletal, and abdominal imaging to cardiac studies, contrast-enhanced angiography, and spectroscopic imaging—can be performed quickly. These MR and CT scanners produce high-resolution and clear images in little time, freeing the scanner for use on other patients as soon as the scan is completed.

The following figures show examples of medical equipment. A portable ECG machine is shown in **Figure 1-8** and the Parks Medical ultrasonic Doppler flow detector is shown in **Figure 1-9.** The blood flow is detected when the ultrasound probe is

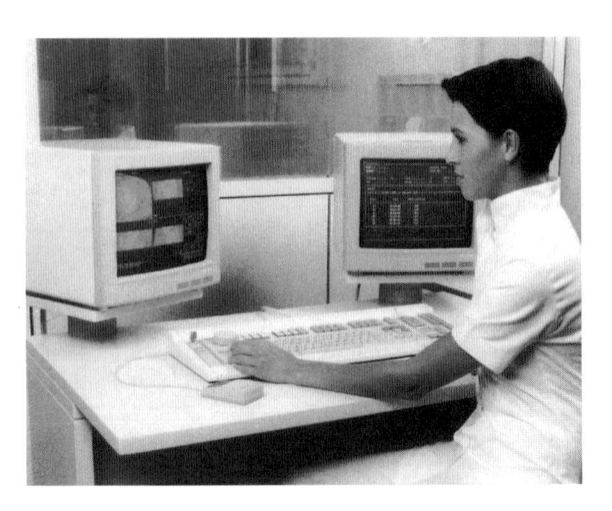

FIGURE 1-7 CT monitor with CRT display.

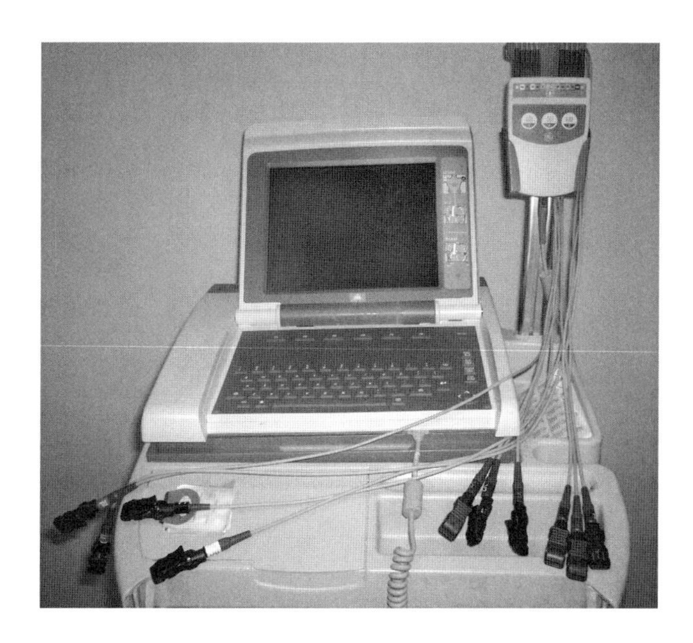

FIGURE 1-8 ECG machine.

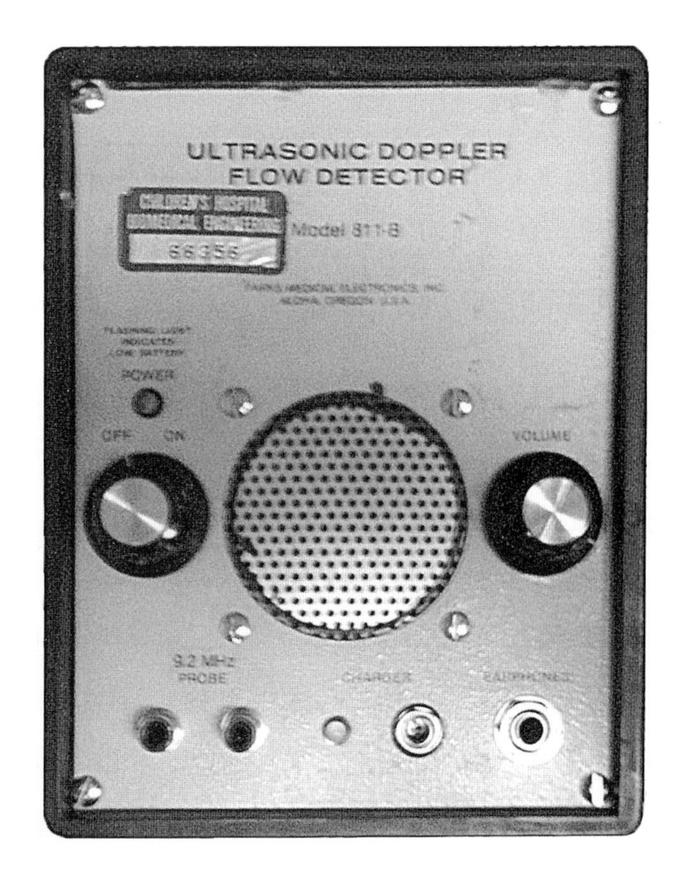

FIGURE 1-9 Ultrasound Doppler flow detector.

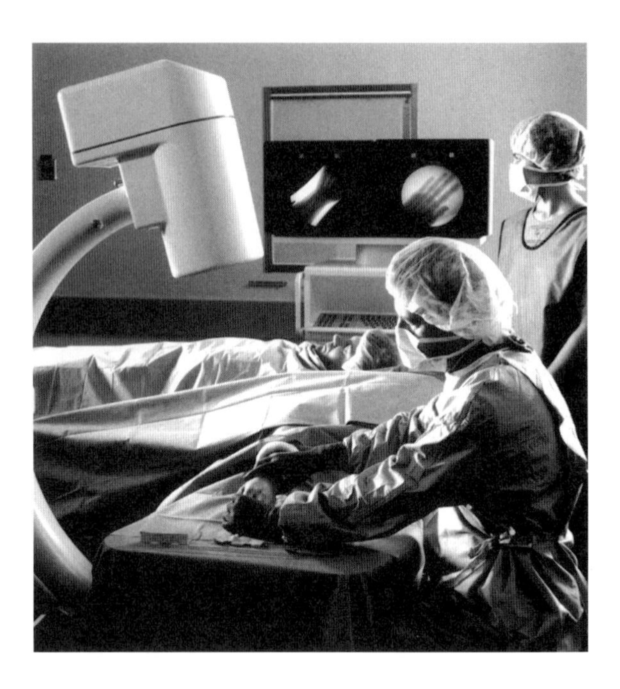

FIGURE 1-10 A mobile C-arm fluoroscopic unit.

placed over the patient's artery or vein. **Figure 1-10** shows a fluoroscopy system with a mobile C-arm.

Advanced telemetry equipment and computer networks using various databases now connect central nursing stations, as shown in **Figure 1-11**.

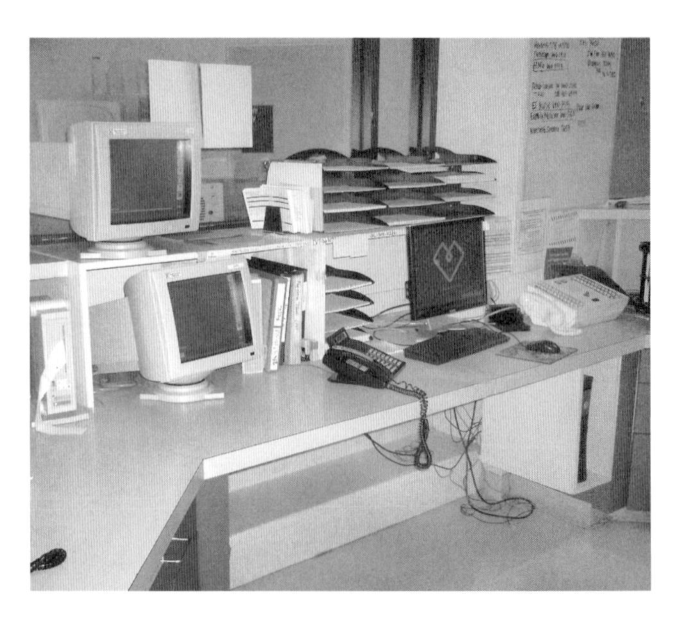

FIGURE 1-11 Nursing station.

1.5 BIOMEDICAL ORGANIZATIONS

There are several professional biomedical and regulatory organizations in the country (**Figure 1-12** lists a few of these organizations). These organizations hold conferences every year and research papers are presented on the various topics of bioinstrumentation.

The Association of Advancement of Medical Instrumentation (AAMI) is dedicated to the understanding, safety, and efficacy of medical instrumentation and is considered an important national and international standards organization for medical devices. Founded in 1967, the AAMI builds consensus among members on medical device information, policy, and technology.

The IEEE Engineering in Medicine and Biology Society (EMBS) is one of the largest international societies of biomedical engineers with more than 8,000 members. It publishes several IEEE transactions and magazines each year. The publications cover topics in information technology in biomedicine, neural systems, rehabilitation engineering, nanobioscience, medical imaging, bioinstrumentation, practical clinical applications, and several other areas.

Name	Type	Web site	Activities
Whitaker Foundation	Foundation	www.whitaker.org	Supports Medical Research
AHRQ (Agency for Health Care Research and Quality)	Government Agency	www.ahrq.gov	Health Care Improvement
IEEE EMBS (Engineering in Medicine and Biology Society)	Engineering Society	www.embs.org	Publishes Magazines and IEEE Transactions
NIH (National Institutes of Health)	Institute	www.nih.gov	Funding Agency
FDA (Food and Drug Administration)	Government Agency	www.fda.gov	Regulates Medicines and Medical Development
AIMBE (American Institute for Medical and Biological Engineering)	Engineering Society	www.aimbe.org	Promotes Awareness
BMES (Biomedical Engineering Society)	Engineering Society	www.bmes.org	Public Education
CDRH (Center for Devices and Radiological Health)	Government Agency	www.fda.gov/cdrh	Regulates Biomedical Devices

FIGURE 1-12 A list of biomedical organizations.

The Whitaker Foundation was established in 1975 to support the interdisciplinary medical research primarily focusing on biomedical engineering. By the year 2004, the foundation had awarded more than $720 million to universities and medical schools for faculty research, graduate students, and for the construction of facilities.

The Biomedical Engineering Society (BMES) and the American Institute for Medical and Biological Engineering (AIMBE) are two other organizations promoting awareness of medical and biological engineering and its utilization. The BMES was started in 1968 and is headquartered in Landover, Maryland. The AIMBE is a leading advocate in Washington, D.C. Each organization sets goals to educate the public and government policy makers about the value of biomedical technology. In the last decade, the National Institute for Bioimaging and Bioengineering Establishment Act and the Biomaterials Access Assurance Act were created with the help of the AIMBE.

1.6 REGULATORY AND NONREGULATORY (STANDARDS) ORGANIZATIONS

The Food and Drug Administration (FDA) is a public health agency that regulates not only medicine, but also medical devices for safe use in homes and in hospitals. The FDA monitors the manufacture, import, transport, storage, and sale of approximately $1 trillion in products each year. One of the most important responsibilities of the FDA is to ensure proper product labeling and patient information so that the devices are used appropriately with minimal risk.

The FDA also classifies medical devices and establishes the registration and device listings. It creates the performance and effectiveness requirements on devices and checks the clinical data for accuracy. Under the FDA, the Center for Devices and Radiological Health (CDRH) evaluates the medical devices and works closely with the Office of Compliance and the Office of Health and Industry Programs.

The FDA initiatives include instructions on filing the Investigational Device Exemption (IDE)'s 510K and Premarket Notification Approvals (PMAs) with a checklist for all required components. The IDE allows an investigational device to be used in a clinical study to collect safety and effectiveness data required to support a PMA.

The Joint Commission (JC) is an independent, nonprofit organization that sets standards in health care. The JC's evaluation and accreditation services are provided for general hospitals, health care networks, home care organizations, and nursing homes. One of their Web sites, **http://www.qualitycheck.org**, includes each accredited organization's name, address, accreditation decision, status, and quality report.

The Association for the Advancement of Medical Instrumentation (AAMI) is another primary resource for the industry, government, and the hospitals for national and international standards on medical instrumentation and technology. Even though the AAMI is not a regulatory organization, it provides a unique forum for health professionals with an interest in medical devices. The membership in this organization includes biomedical engineers, physicians, nurses, hospital administrators, educators, manufacturers, government representatives, and other health care providers.

1.7 BIOMEDICAL COMPANIES

There are several major biomedical companies in the United States that manufacture hospital equipment used for radiology, cardiac care, blood testing, drug therapy, telemedicine and monitoring systems, and other types of medical systems. The following lists a few of these companies.

Datascope

Datascope products include patient monitoring equipment, anesthesia units, and intra-aortic balloon pumps.

GE Healthcare

GE Healthcare provides products mostly in computer tomography (CT), MRI, X-ray, ultrasound, and diagnostic ECG.

Hitachi Medical

Hitachi Medical is located in Twinsburg, Ohio, and is a major provider of permanent-magnet MRI systems. It also distributes the positron emission tomography (PET) imaging systems and a line of ultrasound products.

Philips Medical

Philips Medical is a leading company in diagnostic imaging. The products it manufactures include CT, X-ray systems for radiography, fluoroscopy, molecular imaging, magnetic resonance, and the nuclear medicine gamma cameras as well as patient monitoring equipment.

Medtronics

Medtronics was founded in 1949 in Minneapolis, Minnesota, and provides a wide range of products in the treatment of chronic heart diseases. Under Cardiac Rhythm Management, it develops cardiac resynchronization devices, implantable pacemakers, automated external defibrillators, cardiac ablation catheters, and monitoring and diagnostic devices. A line of heart valve products is marketed under Medtronic Cardiac Surgery, while Medtronic Vascular markets balloon angioplasty catheters and other related accessories. Other Medtronic products include infusion and neurostimulation systems, shunts, surgical tools, and spinal and ENT systems.

Parks Medical

Parks Medical is the world's oldest manufacturer of Doppler ultrasound systems. The manufacturing facilities are located in Aloha, Oregon, and the products include more than thirty different Doppler devices, such as directional and nondirectional Dopplers and combined vascular and obstetrical Dopplers.

Siemens Medical

Siemens Medical provides a broad spectrum of picture archiving communication system (PACS) software for computer tomography, magnetic resonance, ultrasound, and nuclear medicine.

Tyco Healthcare

Tyco Healthcare produces electrosurgical units, pulse oximeters, ventilators, and feeding pumps.

Zoll Medical Corporation

Zoll Medical Corporation markets noninvasive cardiac resuscitation devices, disposable electrodes, mobile ECG systems, and other products related to defibrillation. Dr. Paul Zoll started the company in 1952. The first clinical use of cardiac pacing was achieved that same year with the first successful use of external defibrillation following in 1956. By 1999, Zoll had introduced the biphasic waveform technology in their defibrillators, improving outcomes in cardioversion while lowering the energy requirements.

1.8 FACT SHEET OF A HOSPITAL

Every hospital in the country provides information about their operations to the public nearly every year. For example, the following is an example of a fact sheet for The Ohio State University Medical Center, Columbus. It is acquired with the courtesy of **http://www.Hospital-Data.com** for the year 2008.

Number of beds 971
Number of physicians 369
Number of resident physicians 380
Number of registered nurses 803
Number of registered pharmacists 38
Number of occupational therapists 21
Number of other personnel 2,452
Number of certified anesthetists 13
Number of dieticians 17
Number of psychiatric unit beds 94

Figure 1-13 shows an alphabetical list of various departments, their functions, and the health care providers. The list covers the main areas of patient care not only in The Ohio State University, but also in most hospitals around the United States.

~ Department ~	~ Function ~	~ Healthcare Provider ~
Anesthesia	Administer/adjust anesthetics to prevent patients from feeling pain	Anesthesiologist
Audiology	Habilitation/rehabilitation of patients with hearing impairment	Audiologist
Biomedical	Responsible for applying engineering technology for the improvement/delivery of health services	Biomedical engineer, clinical engineer, BMET technician
Cardiology	Diagnosis and treatment of heart disorders	Cardiologist
Dermatology	Diagnosis, treatment and prevention of diseases of skin, hair, nails, oral cavity, and genitals	Dermatologist
Digestive Health	Diagnostic and therapeutic services for gastrointestinal disease and disorders	Gastroenterologist
Dietetics	Clinical advice on specific diets to help treat certain medical conditions	Dietician
Endoscopy	Procedures using endoscopes to diagnose or treat conditions of upper GI	Gastroenterologist
ENT	Diagnosis and treatment of the head and neck (ears, nose and throat)	ENT physician, Otolaryngologist
Endocrinology	Treatment of endocrine glands, hormones and related disorders (such as diabetes)	Endocrinologist
Family Medicine	Comprehensive healthcare for individuals and family	Family Physician, General Practitioner
Emergency	Immediate evaluation, diagnosis, stability and treatment of patients with acute injuries and illnesses	ER Specialist
ICU	Life support or organ support in patients (Intensive Care Medicine or Critical Care Medicine)	Intensivists
Imaging	Provide diagnostic imaging in radiographic procedures, CT, MRI or ultrasound	Radiologist

FIGURE 1-13 A list of departments in a hospital with their functions and provider specialties. (*continued*)

Laboratory	Study of chemical and cellular laboratory work for patient's blood, urine and fluids (hematology, immunology, microbiology, virology)	Pathologist, Lab Assistant
Kidney Disorders	Diagnosis and treatment of kidney and urinary tract diseases	Nephrologist
Neurology	Diagnosis and treatment of disorders of the nervous system	Neurologist
Nephrology	Related to kidney diseases	Nephrologist
Orthopedics	Prevention or correction of injuries of the skeletal system and associated muscles, joints and ligaments	Orthopedic Surgeon
Ophthalmology	Deals with the diagnosis and treatment of the diseases of the eye	Ophthalmologist
Optometry	Diagnosis and non-surgical treatment of disorders of the eye, and vision care (glaucoma and cataracts)	Optometrist
Oncology	Diagnosis, treatment and prevention of tumors and cancer	Oncologist
Pulmonary Services	Diagnosis and treatment of problems relating to the lungs, and cardiopulmonary system	Pulmonary Specialist, Pulmonologist
Podiatry	Diagnosis and treatment of disorders of the feet	Podiatrist
Plastic/Cosmetic Surgery	Specializing in reducing scarring or disfigurement or to change a body part to look better	Plastic Surgeon
Pharmacy	Preparation, dispensing and appropriate use of medicines	Pharmacist
Psychiatry	Specializing in mental health, diagnosis and treatment of mental illness	Psychiatrist
Occupational Medicine	Concerned with injuries and illnesses in the workplace (occupation), environmental illnesses	Clinical Occupational Health Specialist

FIGURE 1-13 *(continued)*

Medical Records	Historical and current patient files containing records and bills of the patient	Medical Record Director or Manager
Radiology	Imaging services	Radiologist
Rehabilitation	Acute care and long term rehabilitation	Rehabilitation Director
Respiratory Care	Patients requiring respiration and cardiopulmonary care	Respiratory Therapist RCP Practitioner
Rheumatology	Diagnosis and non-surgical treatment of diseases and disorders of the joints, bones and tendons (arthritis and degenerative joint diseases)	Rheumatologist
Surgery/OR	Treat disease or injury by operative procedures	Surgeon OR Doctor
Sleep Disorders	Diagnosis of the disorder that affects, disrupts or involves sleep	Sleep Specialist Sleep Physician
Sports Medicine	Prevention, diagnosis and treatment of the injuries sustained in sports and athletic activities	Sports Therapists Orthopedic Surgeon
Thoracic	Diagnosis and treatment pertaining to the chest including heart and lungs	Thoracic Surgeon
Urology	Concerned with the urinary tract and the genital tract diseases	Urologist
Vascular	Diagnosis and treatment of vascular (blood vessels) diseases	Vascular Surgeon Vascular Physician
Women's Health	Management of pregnancy, labor, breast cancer, heart and women's sexual health	Obstetrician Gynecologist

FIGURE 1-13 *(concluded)*

1.9 THE RICHARD M. ROSS HEART HOSPITAL, OHIO STATE UNIVERSITY MEDICAL CENTER

Many major hospitals are developing heart centers. The Ross Heart Hospital at The Ohio State University in Columbus, shown in **Figure 1-14a,** is a good example of such a center. This hospital is a 100-bed, high-tech hospital with complete care for patients with cardiovascular diseases including heart or peripheral vascular disorders. The care includes catheterization, surgical bypass, pacemaker implants, and mechanical heart pumps. It also has six operating rooms, six cardiology suites, an outpatient clinic with twenty examination rooms, and ten consultation rooms.

The Ross Heart Hospital is unique in that it has several new laser-guided robots working around the clock to assist the nurses in a variety of tasks, such as transporting various pieces of medical equipment, boxes that might need to be relocated, and even transporting laundry to the laundry facilities!

These robots, as shown in **Figure 1-14b,** can move with normal traffic around the hospital and use special elevators to move to a different floor.

1.10 FLOWCHART OF A MEDICAL CENTER

Figure 1-15 shows a simple medical center flowchart. As you can see, a medical center is not only a hospital, but also a vast complex with various departments, all with the common goal of patient care. A typical American medical center has numerous buildings housing not only medical research institutes, but the hospital itself and patient care centers as well.

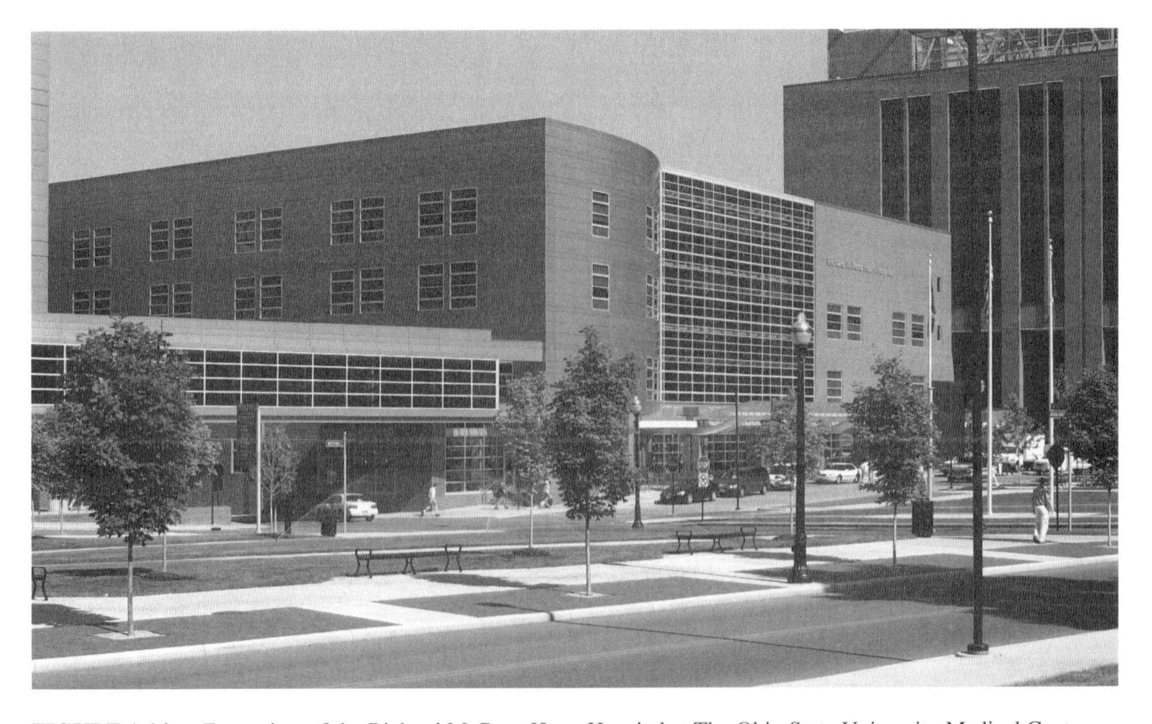

FIGURE 1-14a Front view of the Richard M. Ross Heart Hospital at The Ohio State University Medical Center.

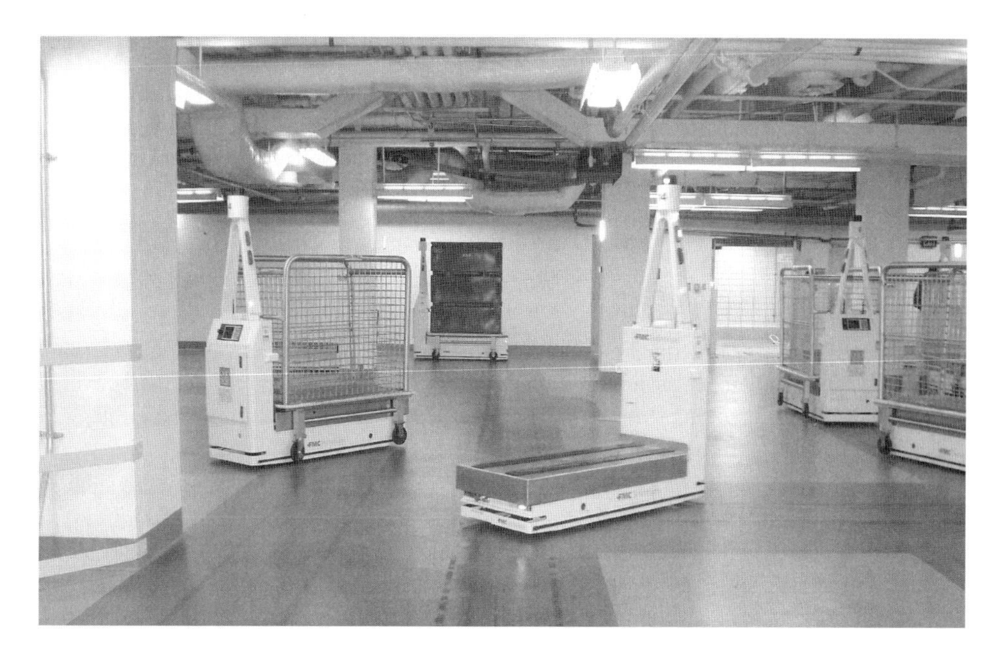

FIGURE 1-14b Laser-guided robots in the Richard M. Ross Heart Hospital.

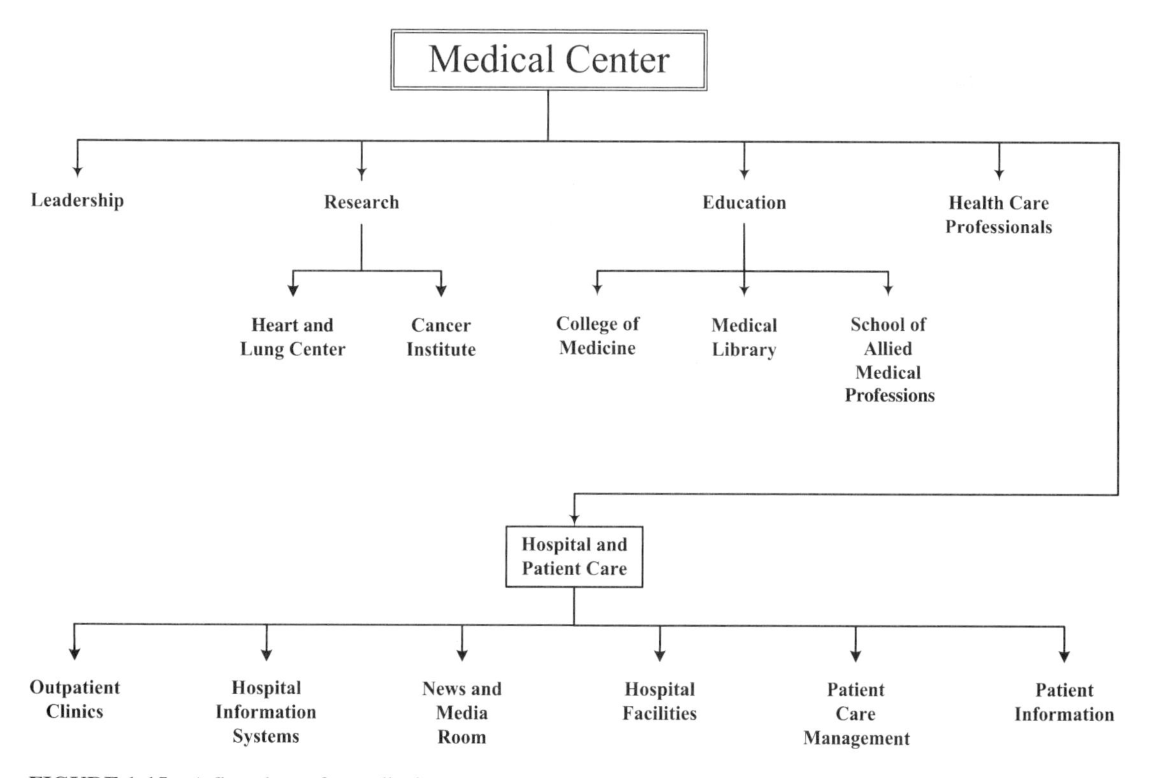

FIGURE 1-15 A flowchart of a medical center.

1.11 PERSPECTIVE OF BIOMEDICAL WEB SITES

There are several Internet Web sites for the biomedical field that provide information on medical instrumentation, organizational activities, company products in health care, and research papers under various forums. These Web sites encourage readers to become members (some for a fee), attend Web seminars in real time, enroll in courses on the Internet, and take certification examinations.

SUMMARY

- Biomedical engineering is the application of concepts and methods of the physical and engineering sciences in biology and medicine. This field covers a broad spectrum ranging from formalized mathematical theory through experimental science and technological development to practical clinical applications.
- In hospitals, biomedical engineers typically supervise the maintenance, acquisition, and staff training for medical equipment. In the medical device industry, these professionals may be involved with the design, development, and research of new products.
- Biomedical Engineering Technologists or Biomedical Equipment Technicians (BMETs) are the technicians in the forefront of maintaining the medical equipment in a hospital.
- There are various types of biomedical equipment used in hospitals for patient diagnosis, testing, and treatment. The most common devices used by health care providers are used in cardiology, imaging, intensive care units, operating rooms, and laboratories.
- The typical biomedical machine is a human-machine interface using input and output relationships. This interface includes components such as the patient, electrodes, sensors, transducers, signal conditioners, displays, and feedback stimulus.
- Defibrillators, ECG, CT, MRI, and X-ray machines are all types of biomedical devices.
- Biomedical devices may also be simulators. Simulators allow the health care provider to review and practice procedures prior to treating patients, thus reducing risk to the patient's health.
- There are many types of companies and organizations in the biomedical field, including those involved in manufacturing, research and development, and regulation.

MEDICAL TERMINOLOGY

The following is a list of medical terms mentioned in this chapter.

Angiography: a display of the blood vessels or organs by X-ray after a dye is injected into the body.

Biomedical Engineering Technologist or **Biomedical Equipment Technician (BMET):** a highly skilled technician in a hospital responsible for repairing, calibrating, and installing medical equipment.

Cannula: a small tube for insertion into a body cavity or into a duct or vessel.

Computer tomography (CT): a computer technique used to display an image of thin layers of the body as opposed to an image of the whole body in one scan.

Fluoroscopy: a display of the movement of the body structure on a fluorescent screen.

Magnetic resonance imaging (MRI): a computerized technique to image patients without the use of X-rays. The technique uses strong magnetic field and a radiofrequency signal to detect the magnetization of the hydrogen protons.

Nanotechnology: a field of science that studies the manipulation of atoms and molecules to create computer chips and microscopic devices that better deliver drugs to specific cells in the human body or to detect and treat diseases.

Picture archiving communication system (PACS): a standard of archiving, processing, and sending radiological images over computer networks.

Positron emission tomography (PET): a nuclear medicine imaging technique that uses a special type of camera and a radioactive tracer to look at the organs in the body.

Spectroscopic imaging: imaging based on a signal breaking down in several frequencies and wavelengths.

Telemedicine: a transfer of medical images through a wireless medium or through computer networks.

QUIZ

1. An electroencephalogram is the medical recording of:

a) X-ray electromagnetic waves. b) Brain waves.
c) Ultrasound waves. d) None of the above.

2. A defibrillator uses electrical current discharge to defibrillate the:

a) Lungs. b) Heart. c) Kidneys. d) Patient.

3. The most important feature incorporated into clinical (hospital) medical equipment (as opposed to research or industrial medical equipment) is:

a) Compact size. b) Sterile. c) Safety. d) Better display.

4. True or False: A transducer can be a sensor.

a) True b) False

5. Typically, the first task a nurse performs is:

a) Taking the patient's pulse. b) Taking the patient's blood pressure.
c) Performing an ECG. d) Asking the patient a series of questions.

6. True or False: X-ray and ultrasound are radiation-type imaging techniques.

a) True b) False

7. Radiologists work with:

a) ECG graphs. b) CT scans. c) Laser therapy. d) Surgery.

8. PET stands for:

a) Positive electrode terminal. b) Positron emission tomography.
c) Pulse transmission. d) None of the above.

9. The main responsibility of a Respiratory Therapist is:

____

10. The main responsibility of a Circulation Technologist is:

____

PROBLEMS

1. Research a professional biomedical engineering society on the Internet and list its analysis of a major hospital machine. The analysis should include safety features, calibration methodology, quality, cost, and comparison with other machines.

Use the Internet or visit a hospital to complete Problems 2 through 7.

2. Provide information on a working day in the life of a Respiratory Technologist in a hospital.
3. Provide information on a working day in the life of a Biomedical Engineer or a Biomedical Equipment Technician (BMET) in a hospital.
4. Collect information about the type of equipment a Registered Nurse (RN) uses during a typical workday in a hospital or a clinic. Write a few paragraphs describing these pieces of equipment.
5. Write an essay on the regulations on biohazards in hospitals as recommended by the regulatory agencies.
6. View a homepage of a biomedical engineering society. Discuss the society and provide a list of society's activities.
7. List the three government agencies that regulate the medical equipment in a hospital and discuss their instructions, warnings, and penalties. You may use the Internet in your research.
8. Discuss the ways in which doctors, biomedical engineers, or BMETs use PDAs and how the PDA connectivity works in a hospital network.
9. Match the professional responsibility with the appropriate health care provider in the following columns:

____ diagnosis of eye diseases	a) radiologist
____ women's sexual health	b) pulmonologist
____ treatment of urinary diseases	c) ophthalmologist
____ diagnosis of cancer	d) orthopedic surgeon
____ reading CT scans	e) podiatrist
____ treatment of lung problems	f) gynecologist
____ treatment of arthritis	g) oncologist
____ diagnosis of feet disorders	h) rheumatologist
____ cardiopulmonary care	i) nephrologist
____ correction of joints	j) respiratory therapist

10. Match the following health care providers with their appropriate responsibility in the following columns:

____ dermatologist	a) diagnosis of upper GI
____ occupational specialist	b) treatment of head or neck diseases
____ gastroenterologist	c) treatment of workplace illnesses
____ otolaryngologist	d) treatment of gland diseases
____ endocrinologist	e) prevention of skin diseases

CASE STUDIES

1. A patient with slight chest pain arrives at the urgent care facility (not a hospital) in his neighborhood. An ECG is performed and nothing abnormal is found. The patient's heart rate, blood pressure, and temperature are all normal. However, the doctor does not suggest that the patient return home, but instead calls an ambulance to take him to a nearby heart hospital. Why does the doctor send the patient directly to the specialty hospital?
2. On a cold winter night, a 30-year-old man feels severe lower back pain while in his home. The patient has previously played a long game of table tennis and now feels very tired from the exercise. He has no history of back pain. This patient's medical insurance will cover a visit to a specialist. He prefers to go to a specialist for this issue, but does not know which specialist to choose. Select the specialist this man should visit for consultation and discuss the reasons for this selection.

RESEARCH TOPICS

1. Provide examples of nanotechnology and explain how a biomedical engineer or technologist can best work in this new area of medicine.
2. Provide examples of the job responsibilities for biomedical engineers in pharmaceutical companies.

CHAPTER 2

Anatomy and Physiology

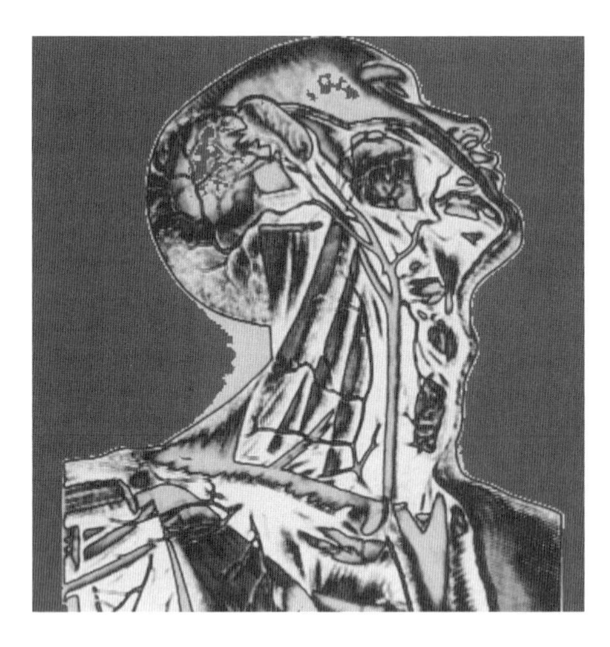

CHAPTER OUTLINE

OBJECTIVES

The objective of this chapter is to review the anatomy and physiology of the human cardiovascular system, circulatory system, respiratory system, nervous system, digestive system, and renal system.

Upon completion of this chapter, the reader will be able to:

- Identify the muscles and bones in the skeletomuscular structure.
- Identify major organs in the human body.
- Discuss the simple physiology of circulation.
- Discuss action potential and its communication aspects.
- Discuss the function of the brain.
- Identify the respiratory circuit components.
- Discuss the process of respiration.
- Discuss the diseases of the heart, lungs, and brain.
- Discuss the structure of gastrointestinal tract.
- Identify the functions of the kidneys.

INTERNET WEB SITES

http://www.anatomy.org (American Association of Anatomists)
http://www.physiology.org (American Physiological Society)
http://www.ama-assn.org/ama/pub/category (American Medical Association)

INTRODUCTION

The human body is a complex functional system. It is comprised of several internal subsystems that constantly "communicate" with each other in order to respond to and regulate the body's environment. This physiological control system is without parallel to any of the known systems in the universe.

In this chapter, we review the basics of anatomy and the several physiological processes of the human body. The functional system of the body is divided into six separate subsystems: cardiovascular, circulatory, respiratory, nervous, digestive, and renal. We begin this chapter reviewing anatomy and then follow with a discussion of the physiology of each subsystem.

2.1 HUMAN ANATOMY

The human body can be viewed in three sections: anterior (forward or frontal), posterior (backward or back), and lateral (sideways or side). The internal organization of the body is divided into six subsystems: the cardiovascular system, circulatory system, respiratory system, nervous system, digestive system, and renal system. The main internal organs in these systems are the heart, lungs, brain, and kidneys. **Figure 2-1** through **Figure 2-4** show the anatomical line drawings of the human organs, the skeleton system, and the muscles of the body.

Figure 2-1 illustrates the human torso with the major organs and **Figure 2-2** illustrates the skeletal system and the locations of the major bones and joints. The skeletal system is comprised of two structures: the axial skeleton (the skull, ribs, sternum, and spinal column) and the appendicular skeleton (the shoulder girdles, arms, wrists, hands, hip girdles, legs, ankles, and feet).

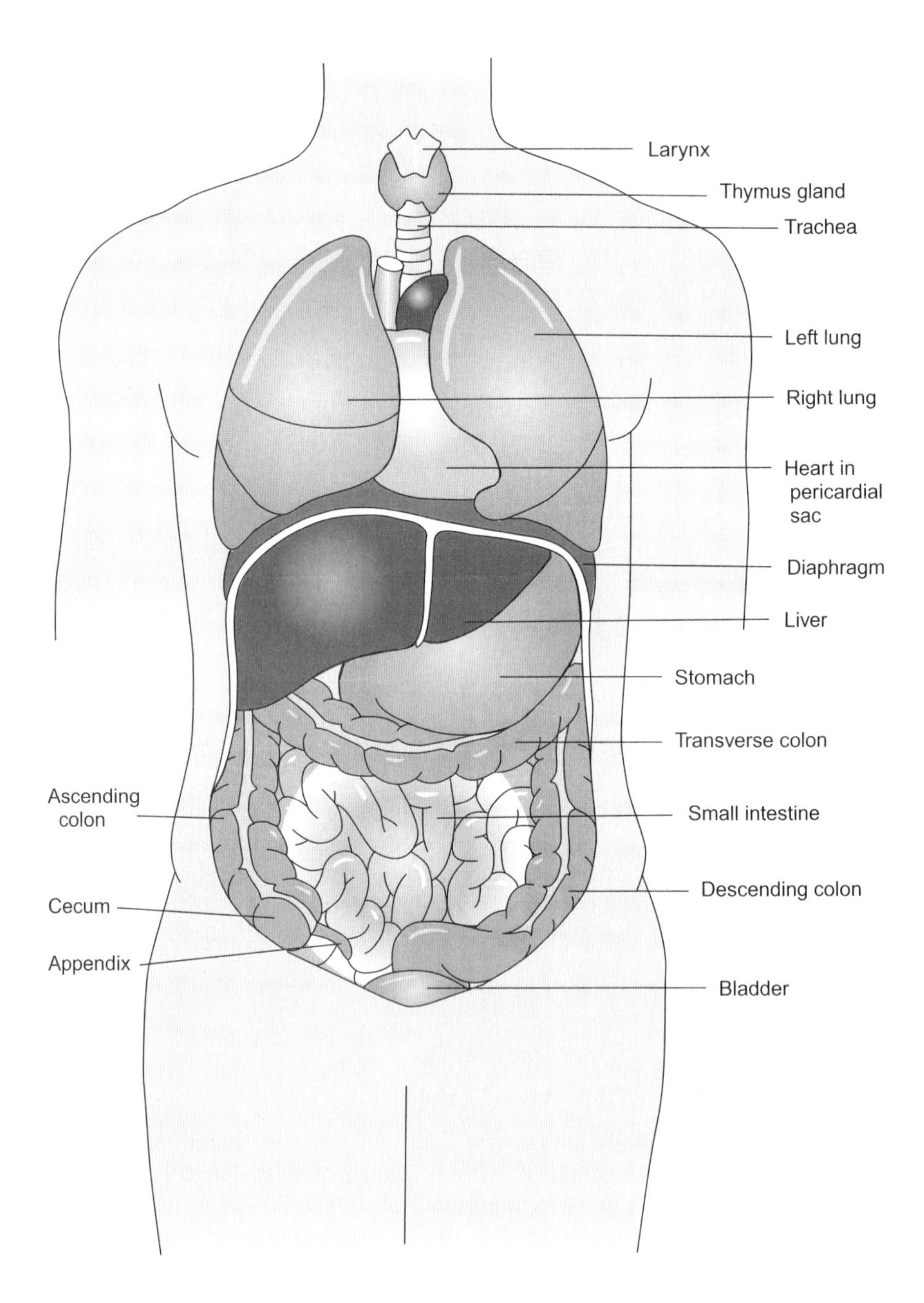

FIGURE 2-1 Organs in thoracic and abdominopelvic cavities of the body.

Figure 2-3 and **Figure 2-4** are the front and back views of the muscle system. The muscle system maintains the body movement, posture, and the body temperature. The types of muscles include skeletal muscles, smooth muscles, and the cardiac muscle (the heart muscle). The skeletal muscles are attached to bones and

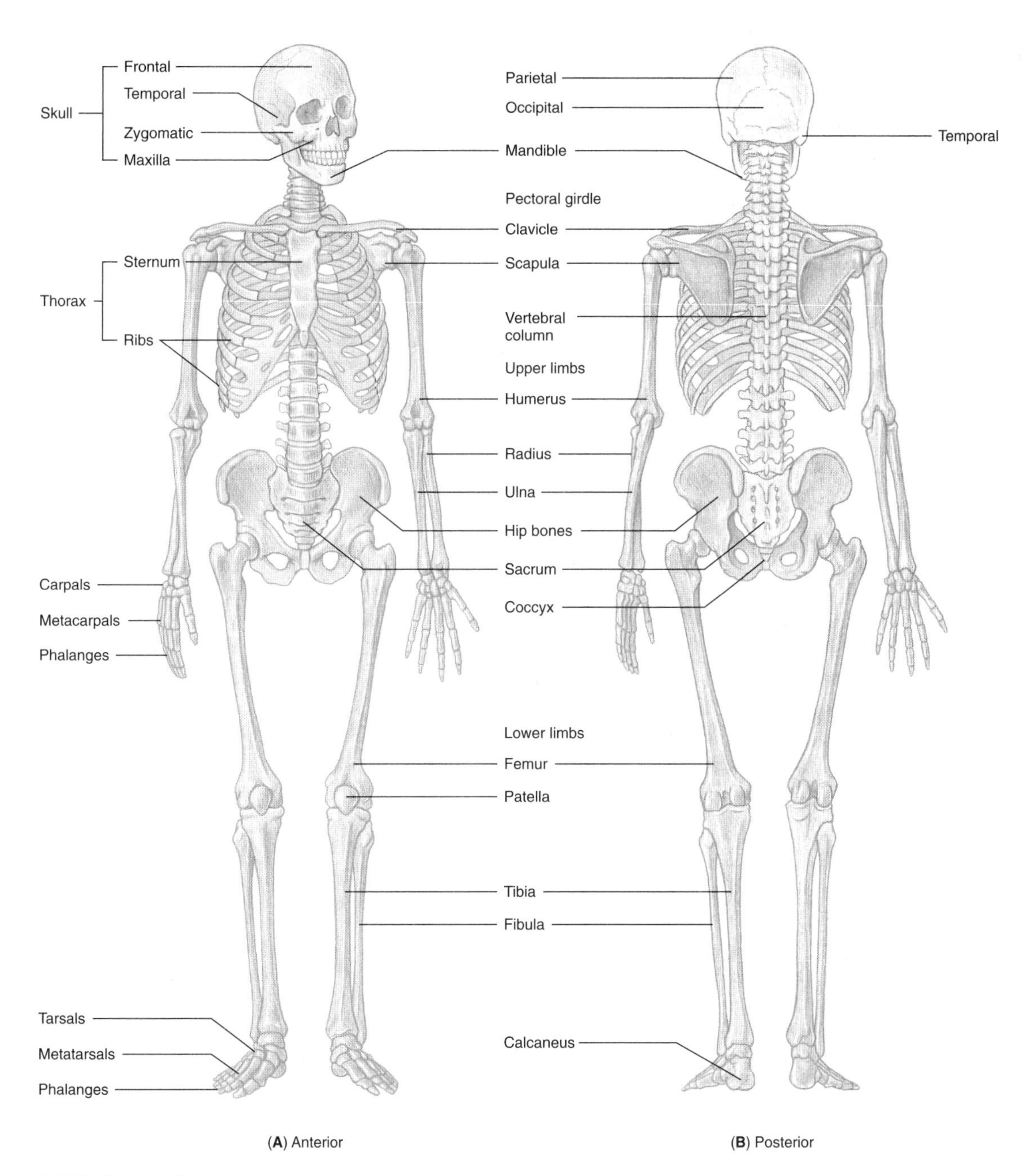

FIGURE 2-2 Skeletal system: anterior and posterior views.

are called "striated muscles" (muscle tissue that is marked by transverse dark and light bands and made up of elongated fibers). Smooth muscles are muscles that lack cross striations and are found in organs and structures such as the small intestine and bladder.

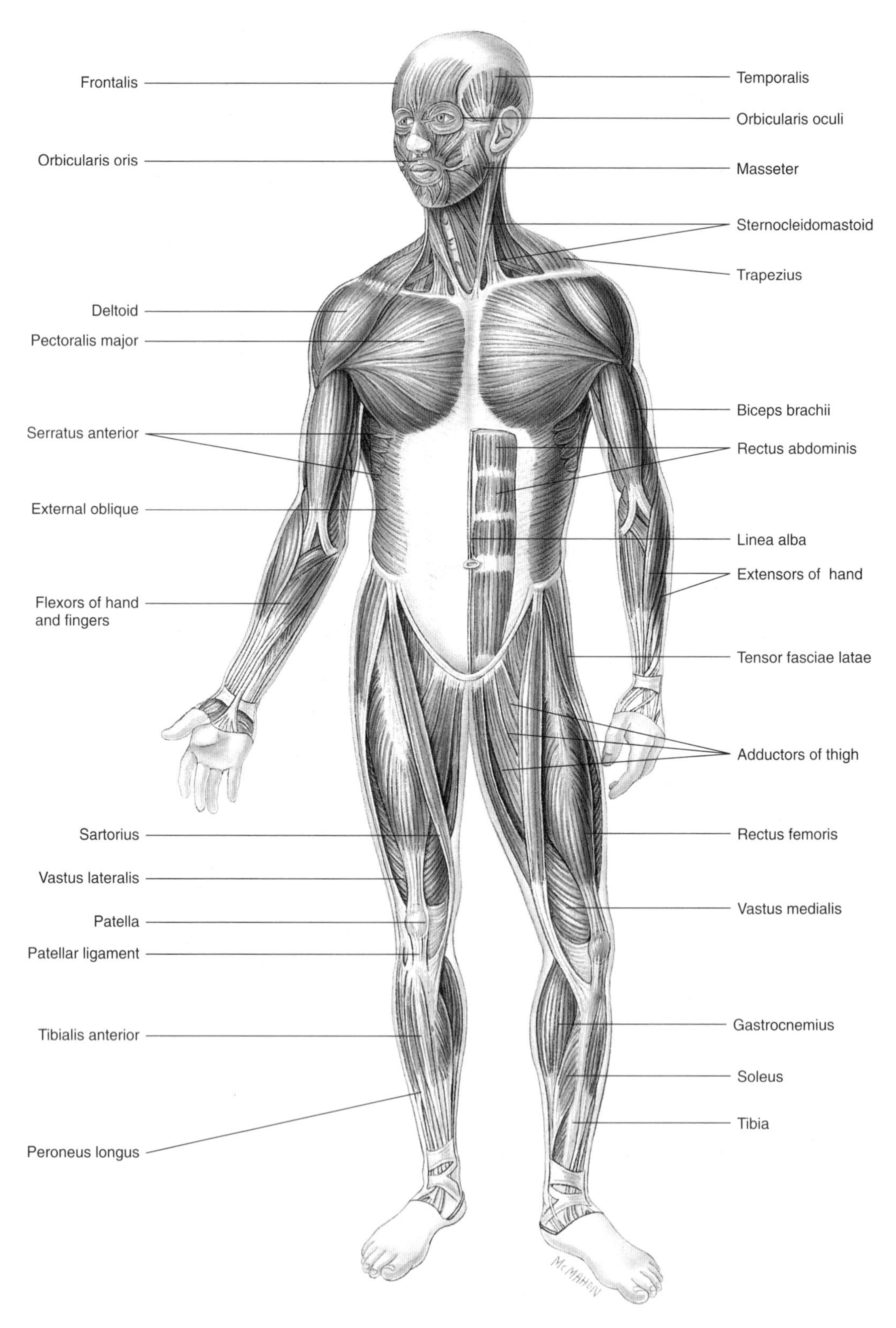

FIGURE 2-3 Muscles of the body: anterior view.

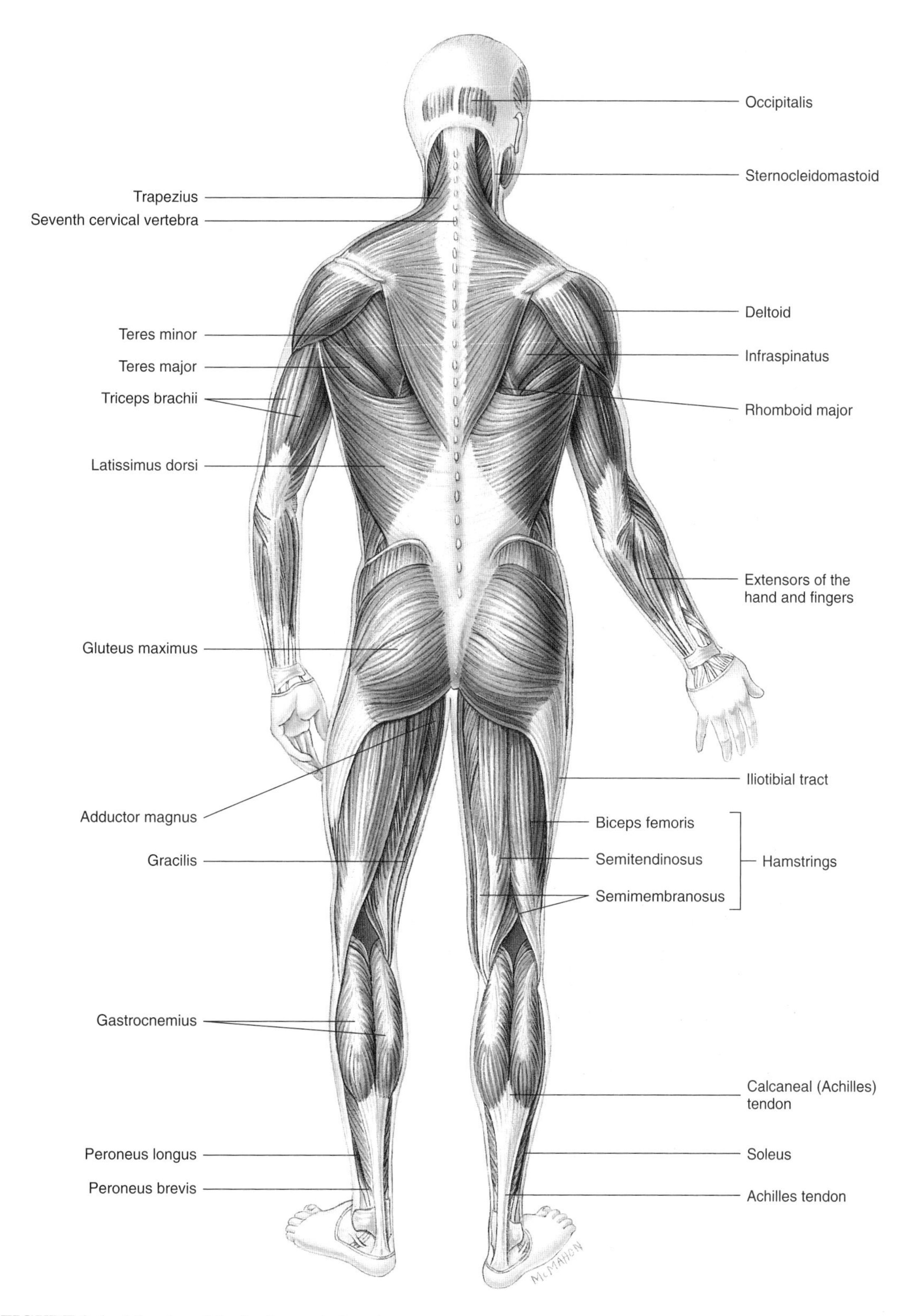

FIGURE 2-4 Muscles of the body: posterior view.

2.2 HUMAN PHYSIOLOGY

Can you see the relation between engineering mechanics and human physiology? The skeleton, muscles, arteries, veins, and nerves are very similar to engineering structures. We can even apply engineering terms to human physiology! Think of the following:

Hydraulic System (Cardiovascular System)

The body's "hydraulic" system, or **cardiovascular** system, has a four-chamber heart pump and it is connected to flexible blood vessel tubing. The tubing branches out into small arteries and veins, regroups, then connects back to the heart pump to complete a closed-loop system. The four-chamber heart pump is really two synchronized, but functionally isolated, two-stage pumps. The fluidic blood flows smoothly and orderly (without any turbulence) in the tubes and faces resistance to its flow due to diameter changes in the tubing. Typically, the blood flow overcomes the resistance by changing its pressure in the tube.

Pneumatic System (Respiratory System)

The human respiratory system is a pneumatic system. With a pump and tubing similar to the hydraulic system, air is pumped by the diaphragm. This pumping creates negative and positive pressures in the sealed thoracic cavity causing air to be sucked in and out of the two elastic lung bags. These lung bags are connected to the outside of the body through the tubing of nasal cavities, pharynx, larynx, trachea, and bronchi.

Chemical System (Biochemical System)

The body is a chemical factory that receives fluid (such as water) and fuel (such as food and oxygen). Fluids and food are consumed through the mouth and oxygen is breathed in through the mouth or nose. This produces chemical reactions required to carry out efficient bodily functions. The cells in the body constantly perform metabolic functions by maintaining the concentration of various ions, such as sodium, potassium, and calcium in their intracellular and extracellular fluid and thus numerous chemical reactions then produce energy for the activity of the body.

Computer System (Central Nervous System)

A computer system requires a certain amount of memory and a central processing unit (CPU). The human body has a supercomputer—the brain. The human brain contains over 100 billion cells! It is so dynamic that its processing capabilities have yet to be understood fully by humankind. Like a computer, the brain has inputs and outputs. It interfaces with several sensors such as the eyes, nose, ears, and numerous internal glands. The output of the brain controls internal body functions and the external movements of the limbs. This computer is capable of not only serial processing, but also parallel processing just like supercomputers.

Communication System and Networking (Nervous System)

The amazing network of nerves carries information on millions of communication lines and links. The information is the coded action potential moving very rapidly from the central brain computer, or server, to their destinations. The brain computer integrates input information from all parts of the body, makes decisions, and then coordinates output information for the body activity.

Mechanical System (Biomechanical System)

The human body incorporates mechanical properties such as strength, elasticity, hardness, and brittleness of muscle fibers, bones, and organ systems. Abnormal conditions of force and pressure may cause deformation or damage of these living tissues.

Robotics (Hand-eye Coordination)

The hand-eye coordination is controlled by the central processor in the brain. The robotics of the body control the system of movement while coordinating the optical sensing. The hand-eye coordination may also help in the movement of legs and the neck.

Fluid Mechanics (Circulatory System)

Blood flow is the fluid in the arteries and veins and is affected by the principles of pressure, volume, and temperature. Blood viscosity affects blood flow. If the blood thickens for whatever reason, blood flow through the vessels is restricted.

2.3 CELLULAR STRUCTURE AND ITS PHYSIOLOGY

To understand the organs of the human body, it is essential to explore the structure and physiology of cells. This is because the organs are actually cells held together by intercellular supporting structures. There are various types of cells in the body; however, they do have common characteristics. Did you know, for example, that cells require nutrients and that they reproduce whenever some of them are destroyed? Cells also use oxygen and discard the products of their chemical reactions into surrounding fluids. There are trillions of cells in the body. **Figure 2-5a** shows a single cell as viewed through a microscope. Notice that the nucleus is surrounded by smooth and rough endoplasmic reticulum, mitochondria, and centrioles. They are then separated from the surrounding fluid by the cell membrane.

The main substances of a cell are water, electrolytes, proteins, carbohydrates, and lipids. The intracellular fluid contains potassium, magnesium, and phosphate ions. The extracellular fluid contains a large amount of sodium and chloride ions. The mechanism of transporting ions between intracellular and extracellular fluid through the cell membrane is due to diffusion and active processes.

Figure 2-5b shows the composition of the fluids inside and outside the cell. The extracellular fluid circulates in the spaces between the cells and provides the cells the nutrients needed for cellular function.

Diffusion is the continual movement of ions, molecules, and nutrients in fluid or gas. Several factors affect the rate of diffusion from one area to another area. Some of these factors include:

1. The net rate of diffusion from the area of high concentration to low concentration is directly proportional to the difference of these two concentrations. A greater rate of concentration creates a greater rate of diffusion.

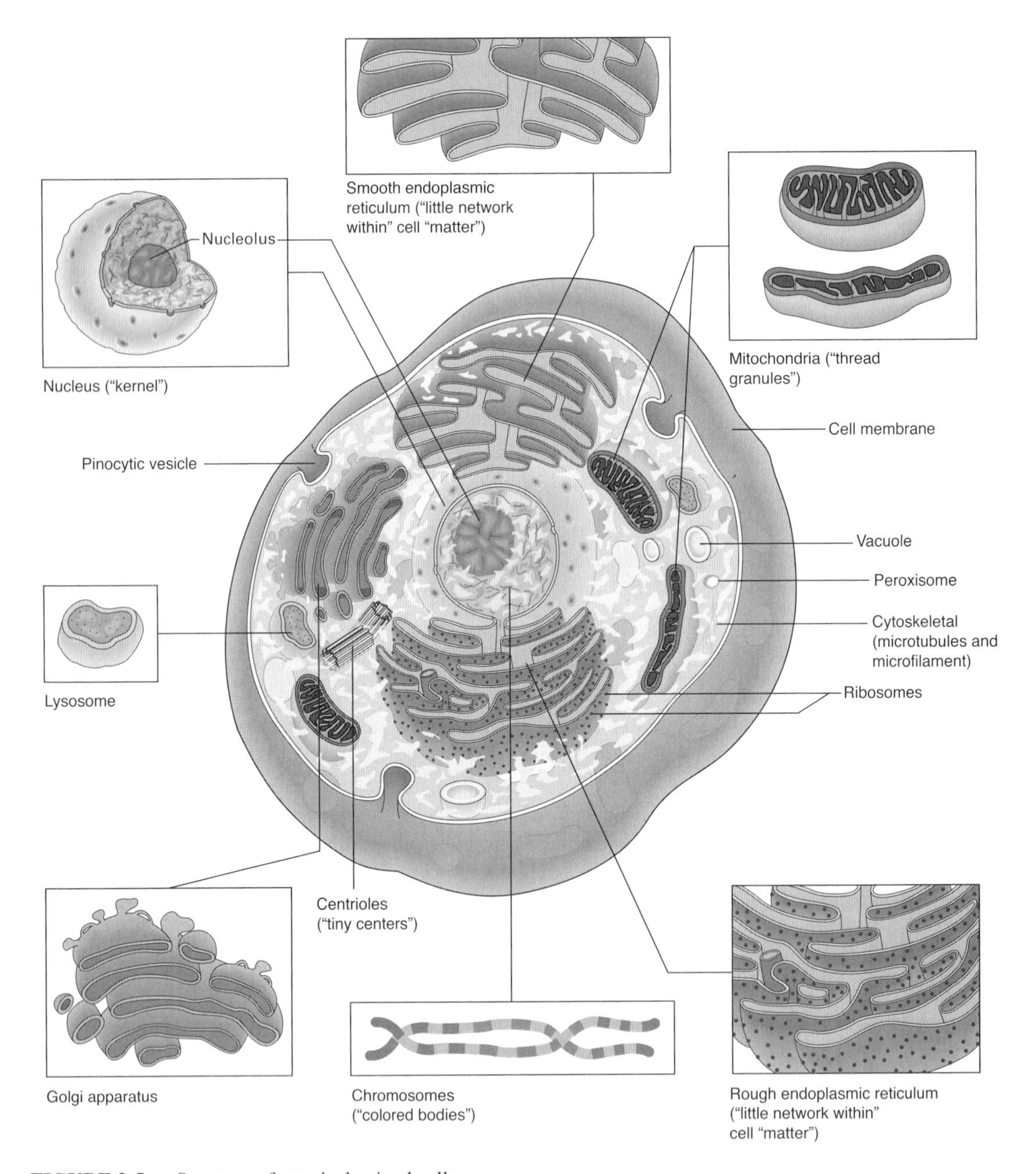

FIGURE 2-5a Structure of a typical animal cell.

2. If the cross-section area where the diffusion occurs is large, the diffusion rate is greater.
3. If the molecular weight of the molecules involved is less, the diffusion rate is greater.

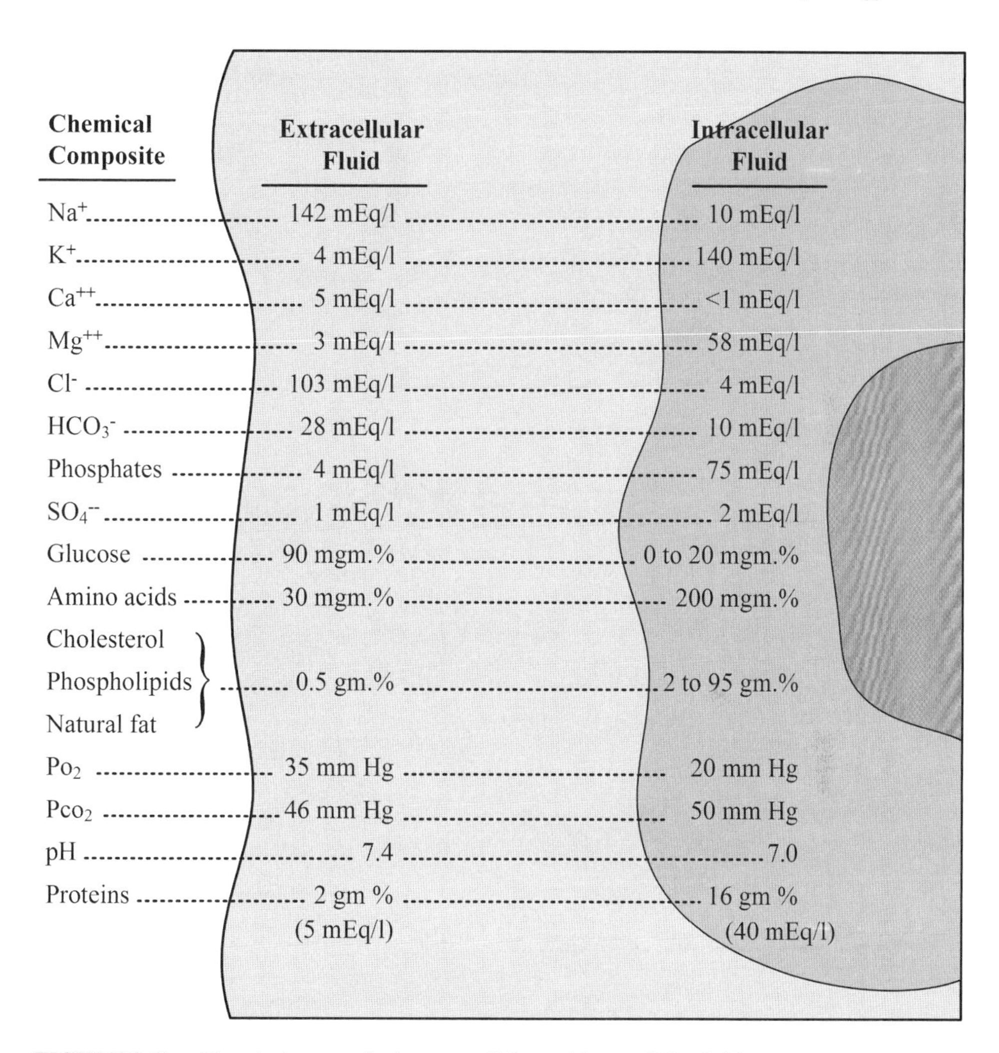

Chemical Composite	Extracellular Fluid	Intracellular Fluid
Na^+	142 mEq/l	10 mEq/l
K^+	4 mEq/l	140 mEq/l
Ca^{++}	5 mEq/l	<1 mEq/l
Mg^{++}	3 mEq/l	58 mEq/l
Cl^-	103 mEq/l	4 mEq/l
HCO_3^-	28 mEq/l	10 mEq/l
Phosphates	4 mEq/l	75 mEq/l
SO_4^{--}	1 mEq/l	2 mEq/l
Glucose	90 mgm.%	0 to 20 mgm.%
Amino acids	30 mgm.%	200 mgm.%
Cholesterol, Phospholipids, Natural fat	0.5 gm.%	2 to 95 gm.%
Po_2	35 mm Hg	20 mm Hg
Pco_2	46 mm Hg	50 mm Hg
pH	7.4	7.0
Proteins	2 gm % (5 mEq/l)	16 gm % (40 mEq/l)

FIGURE 2-5b Chemical composite in extracellular and intracellular fluids.

4. The temperature of the fluid is important also. The diffusion rate is greater with increased temperature. Molecular motion increases with increased temperature.
5. The diffusion rate will increase in shorter distances as well.

The following is an equation of the diffusion rate:

$$\text{Diffusion Rate} = \frac{(\text{Concentration Difference}) \times (\text{Cross-sectional Area}) \times \text{Temperature}}{\text{Distance} \times \text{Square Root of Molecular Weight}}$$

Diffusion through the cell membrane is due to the nutrients dissolving in the lipid matrix of the cell membrane and then diffusing through it to the other side. **Figure 2-6** shows the structure of the cell membrane that consists of a lipid bilayer and the interspersed proteins in the lipid film.

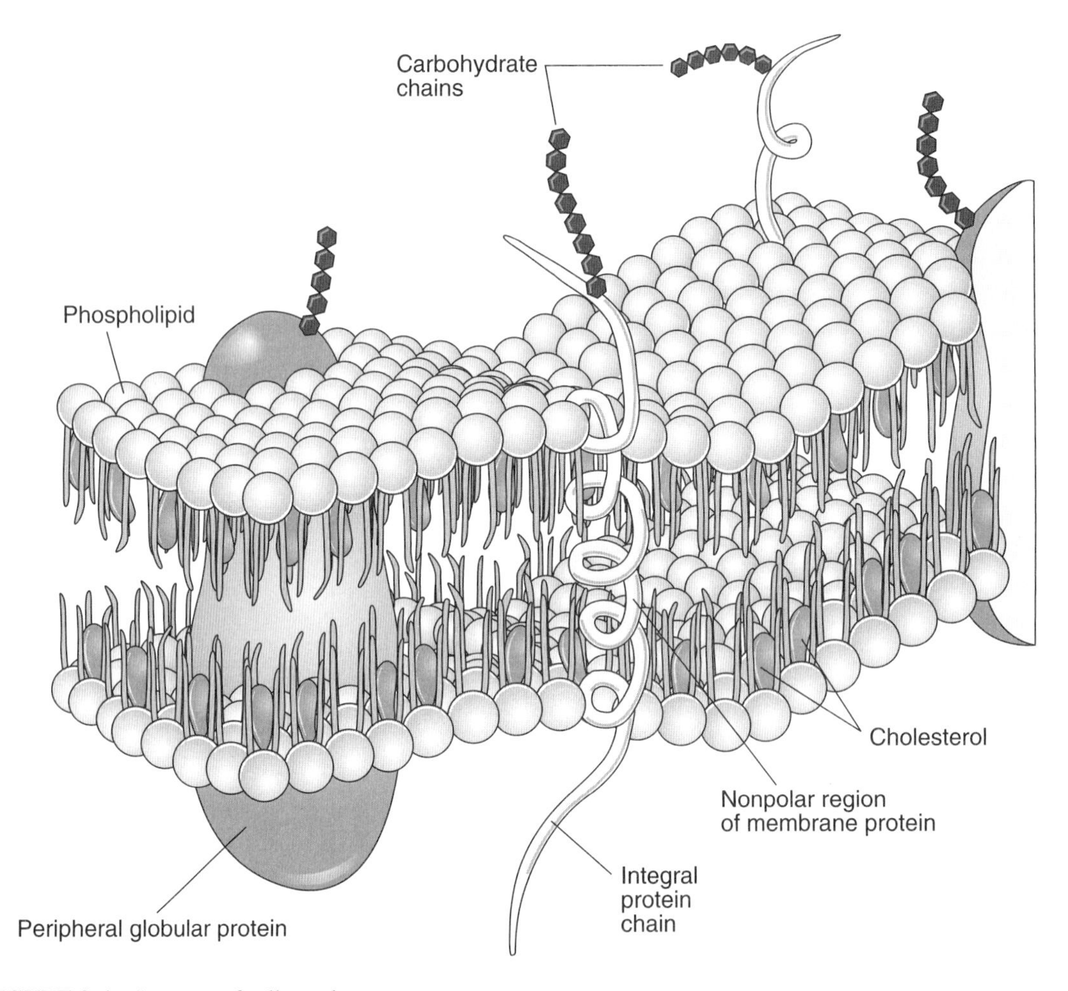

FIGURE 2-6 Structure of cell membrane.

Active transport involves sodium ions, potassium ions, calcium ions, sugars, and amino acids. These substances are transported through the cell membrane. The cell membrane moves these ions against the concentration gradient (meaning the difference in concentration) in a process called active transport. These active transport ions receive energy from adenosine triphosphate (ATP) or the proton motive force (PMF) and pump against the concentration gradient.

2.4 ANATOMY AND PHYSIOLOGY OF THE CIRCULATORY SYSTEM

The two major subdivisions of blood circulation in the human body are pulmonary circulation and systemic circulation. The heart pumps blood through an adult body (at rest) typically at a volume of about 5,000 ml per minute. **Figure 2-7a** and **Figure 2-7b** show this

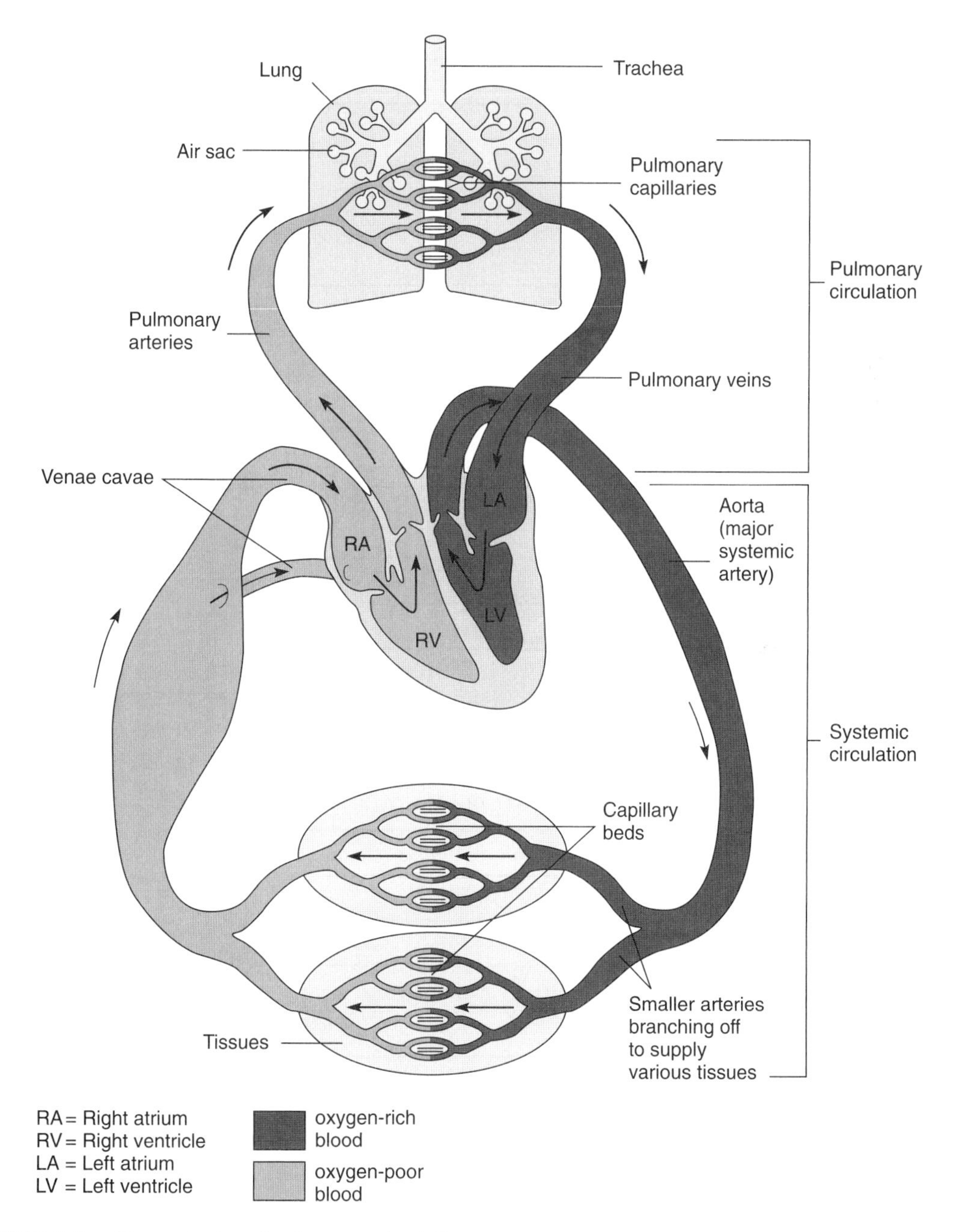

FIGURE 2-7a The systemic and pulmonary circulation.

relationship of the circulation in arteries, veins, and different organs. **Figure 2-7a** shows that veins are more distensible than arteries, but that arterioles and capillaries are not distensible and are quite resistive to the blood flow. As shown in **Figure 2-7b,** kidneys normally receive about one-fourth of the cardiac output.

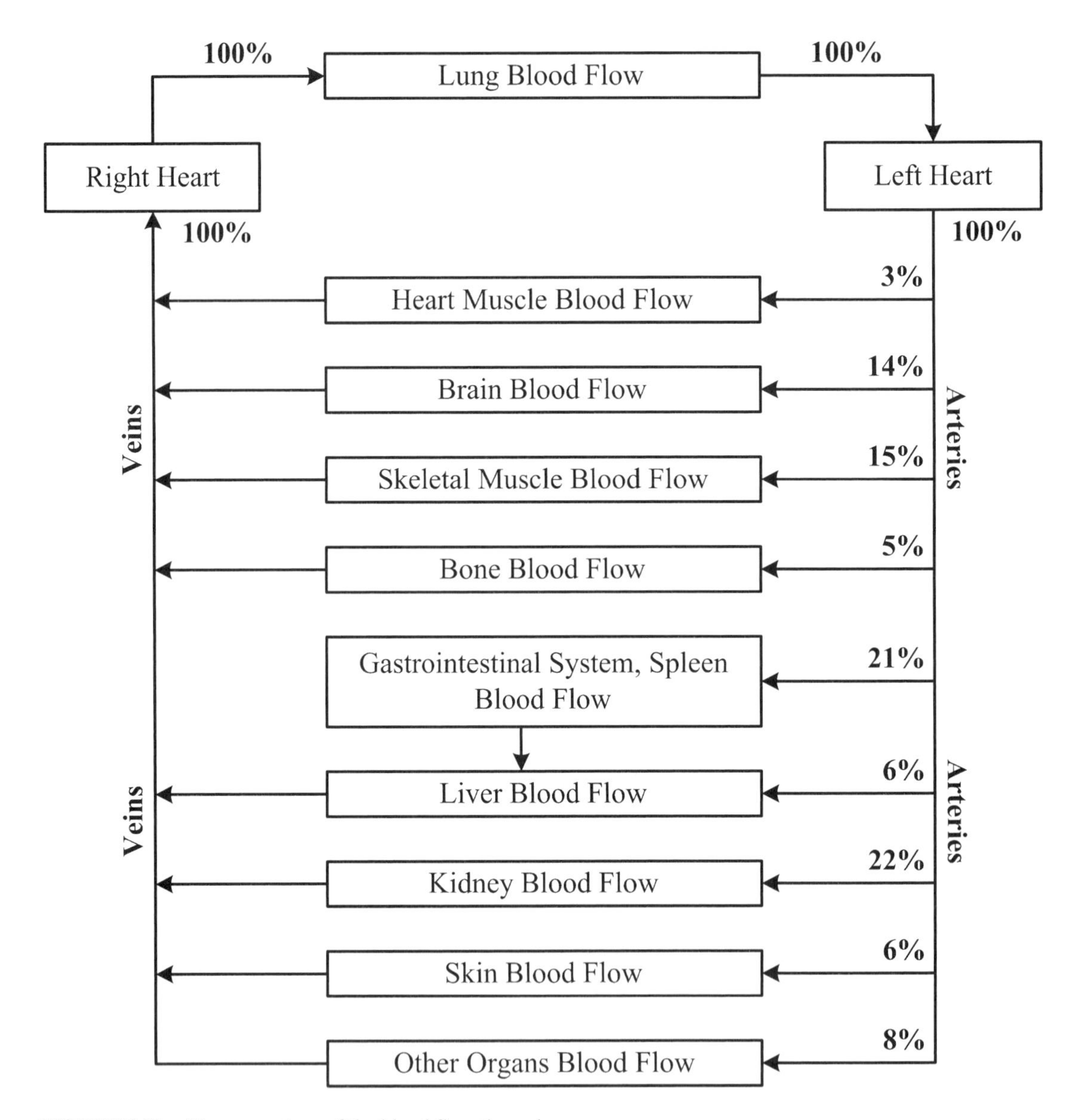

FIGURE 2-7b The percentage of the blood flow through organs.

2.5 ANATOMY AND PHYSIOLOGY OF THE HEART

In **Figure 2-8,** notice that the heart is located in the chest between the right lung and the left lung, just behind the sternum and above the diaphragm. Pericardium surrounds the heart and the walls of the heart are composed of cardiac muscle, called myocardium. The lining of the heart is called endocardium. The heart has four compartments: the right atrium, left atrium, right ventricle, and left ventricle. It has four valves: the tricuspid valve, the mitral valve, the pulmonary valve, and the aortic valve, as shown in **Figure 2-9.**

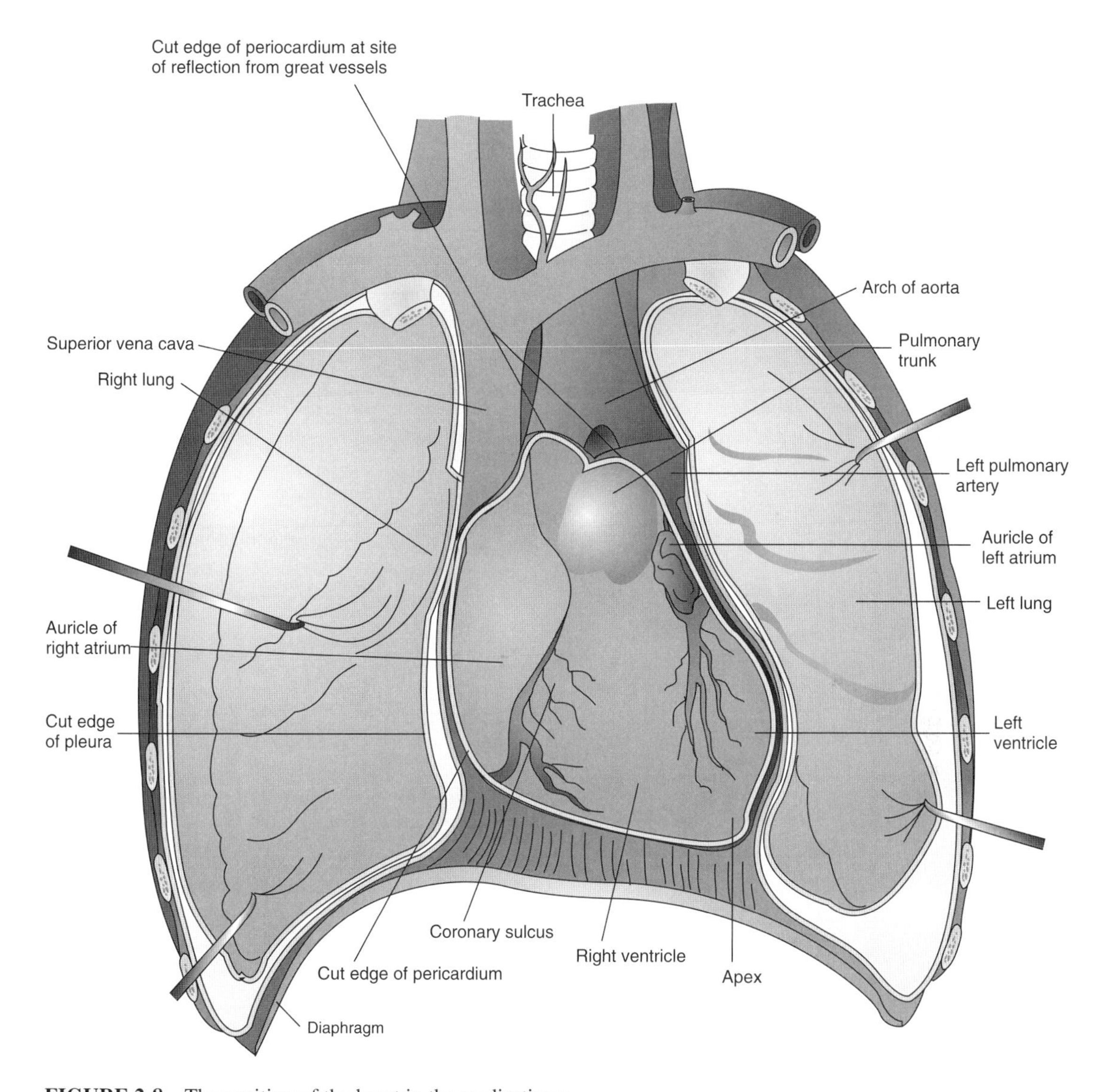

FIGURE 2-8 The position of the heart in the mediastinum.

The blood flows from the systemic circulation of the body into the right atrium. It then flows through the tricuspid valve into the right ventricle. Next, the blood is pumped from the right ventricle through the pulmonary valve into the lungs, where it is oxygenated. Oxygenated blood then returns from the lungs into the left atrium, through the mitral valve, and into the left ventricle. Finally, blood is pumped through the aortic valve and the aorta and then back into the systemic circulation.

The inflow of sodium ions across the heart muscle cells activates the electric action potential. The amplitude of this action potential can reach close to a value of 100 mV. This phase of electric conduction is called depolarization. On the outflow of the potassium ions in the cells, the repolarization takes place, with the action potential reaching a normal rest-

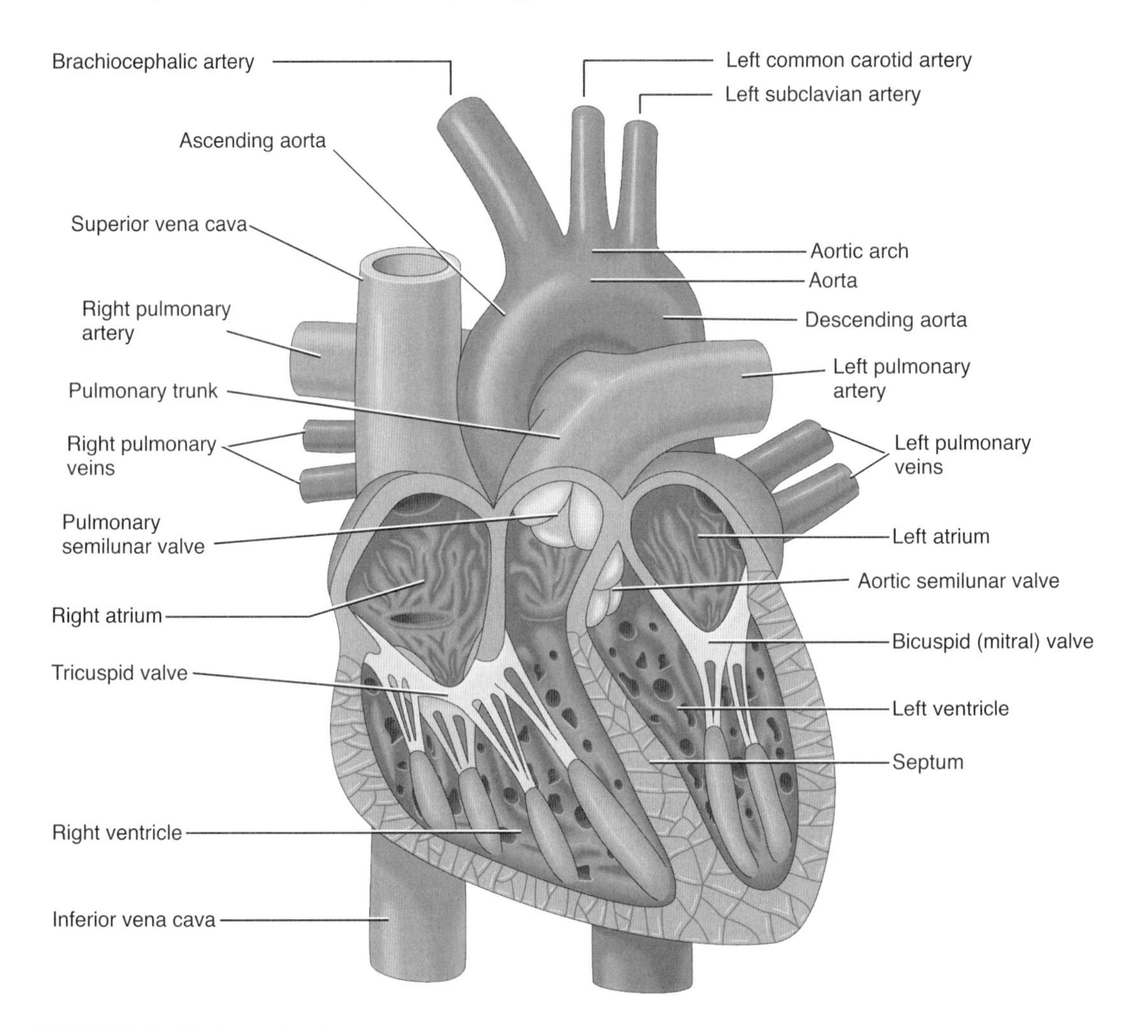

FIGURE 2-9 The heart chamber.

ing value of approximately −80 mV. **Figure 2-10** illustrates this process. In phase 1, the peak portion of the action potential is characterized by the abrupt decrease in sodium permeability. Phases 2 and 3 are early and late stages of repolarization, respectively. In phase 4, the cell is permeable to the sodium ions and slowly develops a more positive membrane potential.

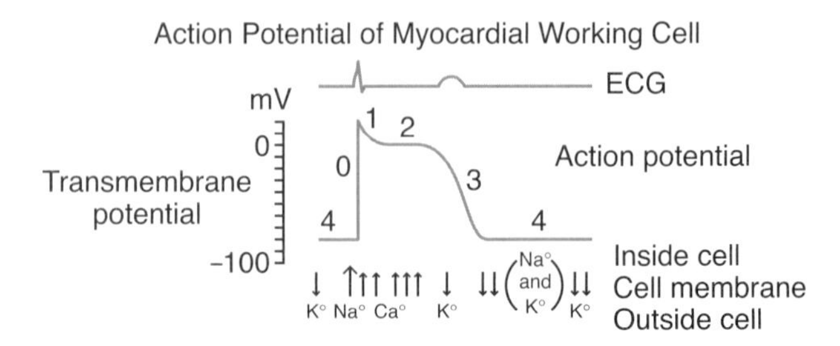

FIGURE 2-10 Action potential of a myocardial cell.

The sinoatrial (SA) node located at the superior vena cava is the pacemaker of the action potential and it triggers the action potential with about 70 pulses per minute. **Figure 2-9** shows the action potentials at various points in the heart. From the SA node, the action potential spreads throughout the atria, and through the AV (atrioventricular) node located at the boundary of atria and ventricles. The bundle of His and Purkinje fibers then spread the action potential from cell to cell within the ventricular region. **Figure 2-10** shows the process of this action potential at the cellular level, the different waveforms at the specialized heart cells, and the cumulative effect in creating an ECG signal. The sequence of times in generating a QRS complex is shown also in the figure. The total time of depolarization to repolarization is about 600 msec for the normal heart.

2.6 DISEASES OF THE HEART

Heart disease is a term used to describe several abnormal conditions that affect the heart and the blood vessels in the heart. In an effort to find cures for heart disease, hospitals are creating sophisticated heart centers for research and treatment. Following is a brief list of some of the diseases of the heart:

Aneurysm refers to the localized dilation of the artery or chamber of the heart.

Angina refers to a temporary reduction of oxygen supply to the muscle of the heart.

Arrhythmia is a disturbance in the electrical conduction of the heart. The heartbeats can become irregular and the symptoms result in fainting, shortness of breath, chest discomfort, and palpitations.

Cardiomyopathy is the disease of the heart muscle that impairs the heart to fill or eject blood. It causes symptoms of heart failure.

Myocardial infarction is caused by an occluded coronary artery. Arteries can become clogged by blood clotting on the surface due to buildup of plaque, resulting in a heart attack.

Aortic valve stenosis occurs when an aortic valve is unable to open fully. The causes of this condition are buildup of excessive calcium on the valve. It can also be caused by congenital conditions.

2.7 ANATOMY AND PHYSIOLOGY OF RESPIRATORY SYSTEM

The main function of the respiratory system is to deliver oxygen to the blood and remove carbon dioxide from the blood. This exchange occurs in the lungs. The components of the respiratory system can be grouped into two tracts. The upper respiratory tract includes the nose, mouth, larynx, and trachea. The lower respiratory tract includes the lungs, bronchi, and alveoli.

Figure 2-11 shows the anatomy of the respiratory system. The two major respiratory organs are the lungs. The word pulmonary means "pertaining to the lungs" and pulmonary circulation indicates the blood circulation between the lungs and the heart. Deoxygenated

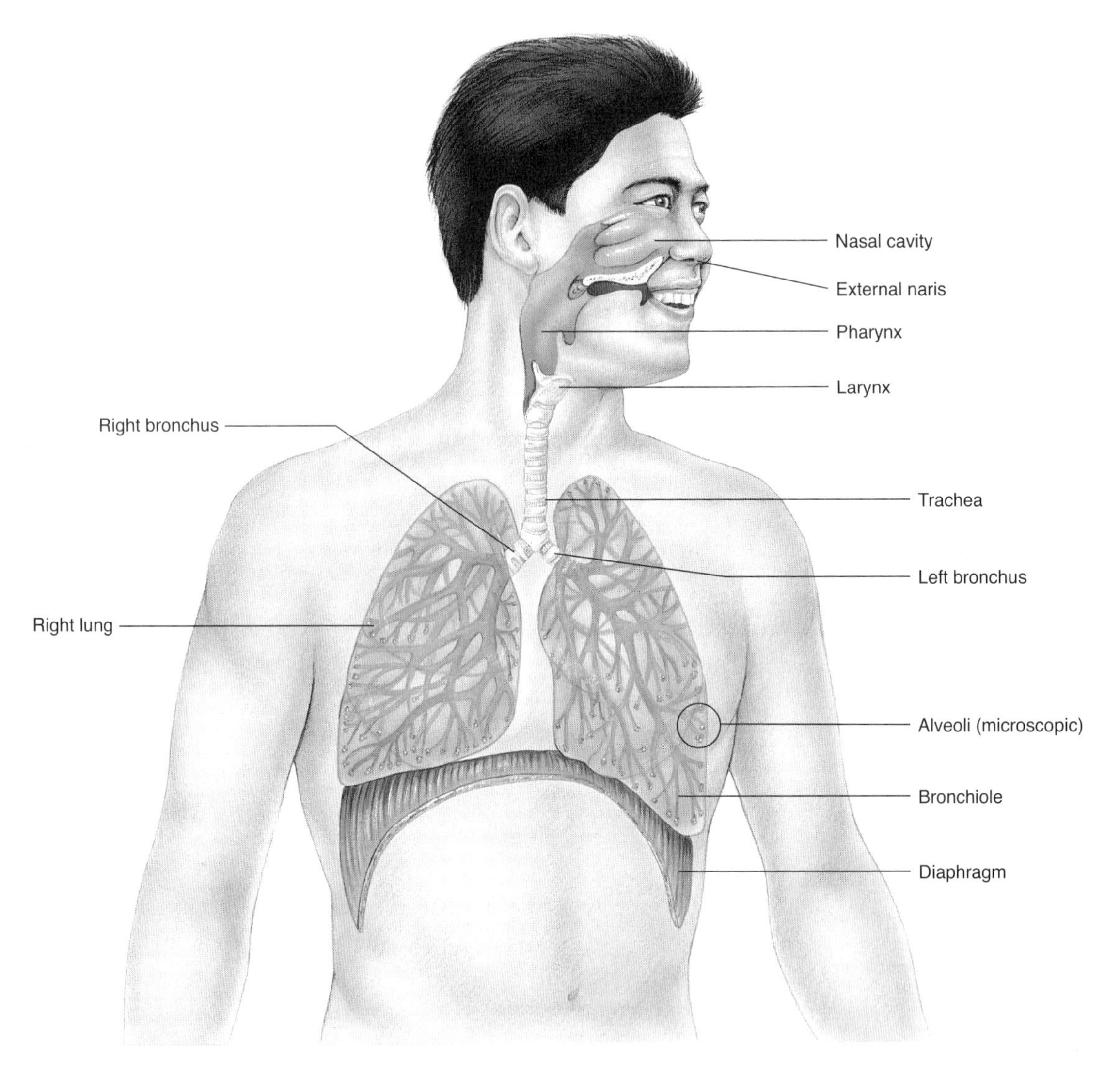

FIGURE 2-11 The organs of the respiratory system.

blood leaves the right ventricle, flows through the lungs where it becomes oxygenated, then returns to the left atrium of the heart.

Air is inhaled through the nose or mouth, travels down the throat, then passes down the trachea, through right and left bronchi, and finally into the alveoli (air sacs) of the lungs. The exchange of oxygen and carbon dioxide in the blood stream involves the respiration (inspiration and expiration) and the pulmonary blood circulation.

Some of the structures of the respiratory system are as follows:

The *nasal cavity* is the interior area of the nose. The area is lined with a sticky mucous membrane and has tiny hairs called cilia on the surface.

The *epiglottis* is a thin, leaf-shaped flap of cartilage located behind the tongue and prevents food from entering the larynx and the trachea (windpipe).

The *larynx* is the voice box and is located below and in front of the pharynx at the upper end of the trachea.

The *pharynx* is in the throat. It lies immediately below it and in front of esophagus. It is a cone-shaped cavity and lined with mucous membrane.

The *trachea* is the referred to as the windpipe. It is a fibro-cartilaginous tube lined with mucous membrane from the larynx to the bronchi.

The *esophagus* is the tube extending from the pharynx to the stomach. Food passes from the mouth into the stomach via the esophagus.

The *bronchi* are the air passages to the lungs. The lower end of the trachea separates into the right bronchus and the left bronchus. There is a difference between the two bronchi. The right bronchus is somewhat shorter, wider, and vertical in position.

The *pulmonary vessels* are the pulmonary arteries and veins. The pulmonary arteries take blood away from the right ventricle to the lungs for oxygen, and the pulmonary veins bring the oxygenated blood from the lungs to the left atrium.

The *pleural membrane* covers the lungs and is the lining to the chest cavity.

The *diaphragm* is the dome-shaped muscular partition between the thorax (chest) and the abdomen.

2.8 ANATOMY AND PHYSIOLOGY OF THE LUNGS

The lungs are surrounded by pulmonary vessels, bronchial vessels, and lymphatic vessels. The pulmonary artery extends about four to five centimeters beyond the apex of the right ventricle and divides into the right and left main branches, which supply blood to the respective lungs. These pulmonary arteries are more distensible than the pulmonary veins. A small amount of blood also flows into both lungs through several bronchial arteries and the particulate matter entering the alveoli is removed by the lymphatic vessels extending from all the supportive tissues of the lungs.

The lungs are a blood reservoir and, under different physiological and pathological conditions, can carry 50 to 200 percent of normal blood volume. The normal blood volume of the lungs is about 450 ml, which is approximately 9 percent of the total blood volume of the circulatory system. When a person exhales, high pressure is built up in the lungs and as much as 250 ml of blood is expelled from the pulmonary circulation into the systemic circulation. The volume of the systemic circulation is about seven times that of the pulmonary system, and any shift of blood from one system to the other affects the pulmonary system more than the systemic system.

The respiratory unit consists of respiratory bronchiole, alveolar ducts, atria, and alveoli and the walls of the unit are so thin that gaseous exchange takes place into and out of the blood flow. The oxygen from the alveoli diffuses into the red blood cells of the pulmonary circulation, then the carbon dioxide diffuses out of the red blood cells and is discharged into the air in the alveoli, to be excreted from the lungs.

2.9 DISEASES OF THE LUNGS

There are several major diseases of the lungs. Following is a list of the most common conditions:

Bronchitis is the inflammation or swelling of the airways of the respiratory system, particularly the airways of the lungs. There is an increase in the mucous production by the goblet cells. The normal amount of mucous in the airways catches and removes the dust and irritating particles when we breathe. However, the body produces the sticky, gel-like mucous more than normal when the airways are inflamed due to irritation and pollution. Bronchitis can be acute (sudden onset) or chronic (long term). The acute disease is usually due to viral infection; the chronic disease is due to constant irritation of the airways due to such things as smoking or air pollution.

Emphysema is chronic disease of the lungs when the alveoli and the elastic fibers break down or destruct. Alveoli are the air sacs that allow oxygen to enter the blood stream. When damaged, the body's ability to breathe is affected. The exchange of oxygen and carbon dioxide in the blood stream is impaired. With too much carbon dioxide in the blood, the person suffering from emphysema requires more oxygen, thus breathing becomes faster and more shallow. This shortness of breath is the primary symptom of this disease.

Chronic obstructive pulmonary disease (COPD) is the combination of chronic bronchitis and emphysema. The symptoms include constant coughing and shortness of breath. With the progress of the disease, the patient is unable to perform physical activities without experiencing shortness of breath.

2.10 ANATOMY AND PHYSIOLOGY OF THE NERVOUS SYSTEM

The central nervous system consists of the brain, spinal cord, and the network of nerves. Information flows from these nerves to the brain through the spinal cord and back again. The cranial nerves connect the brain to the head and the peripheral nerves branch out from the spinal cord to reach the organs and every other part of the body. **Figure 2-12a** and **Figure 2-12b** show the frontal and sagittal views of the nerves.

The nerves transmit information as electrical impulses to and from the brain, which allows us to hear, see, smell, taste, and touch. Some nerves carry information from the brain to the muscles for the body's movement.

Process of Communication Through Nerves

A nerve cell, also called a neuron, has a body (soma), spider-like dendrites, and a long, wire-like nerve fiber called an axon. The axon's branched ends then have button-shaped axon bulbs. These bulbs touch other nerve cells at junctions called synapses, as shown in **Figure 2-13a**. The impulses travel along the axon and jump across the synapses to other nerve cells at very high speeds. Sometimes, the impulses may be blocked from one neuron to the next or integrated with other impulses. They can even change from one impulse into repetitive impulses, as shown in **Figure 2-13b**.

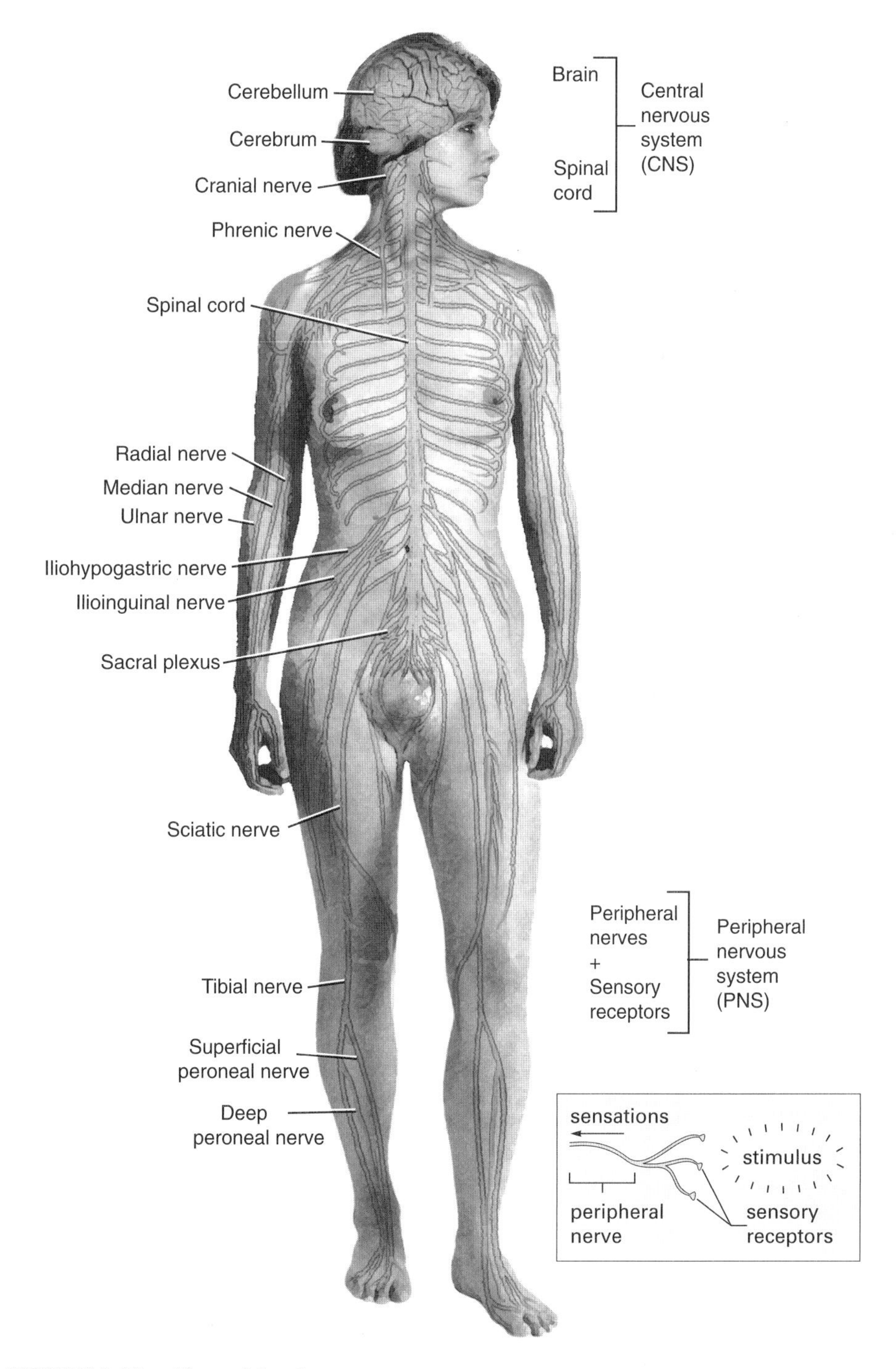

FIGURE 2-12a The peripheral nervous system.

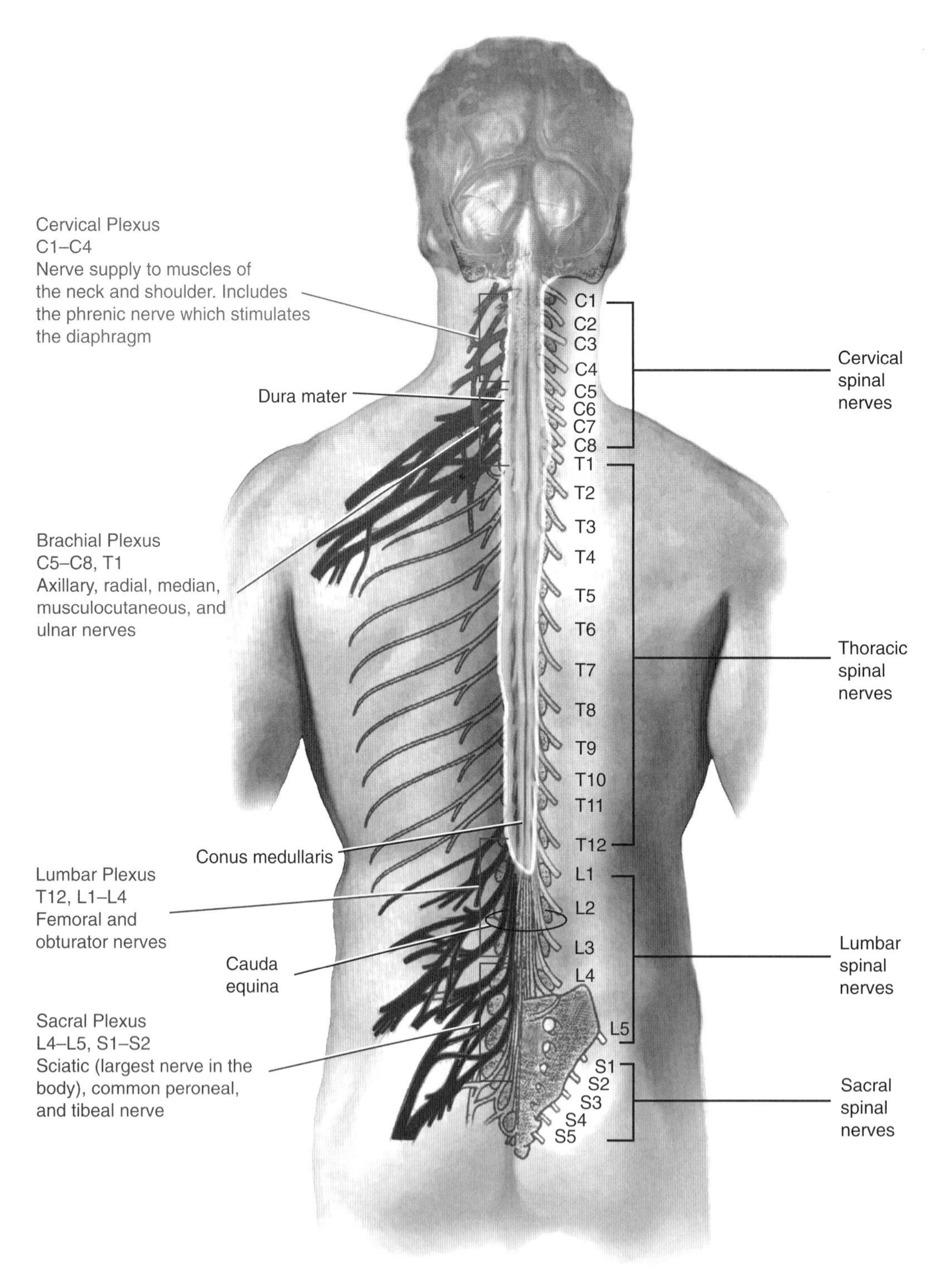

FIGURE 2-12b The spinal nerve plexus and important nerves.

FIGURE 2-13a A neuron, or nerve cell.

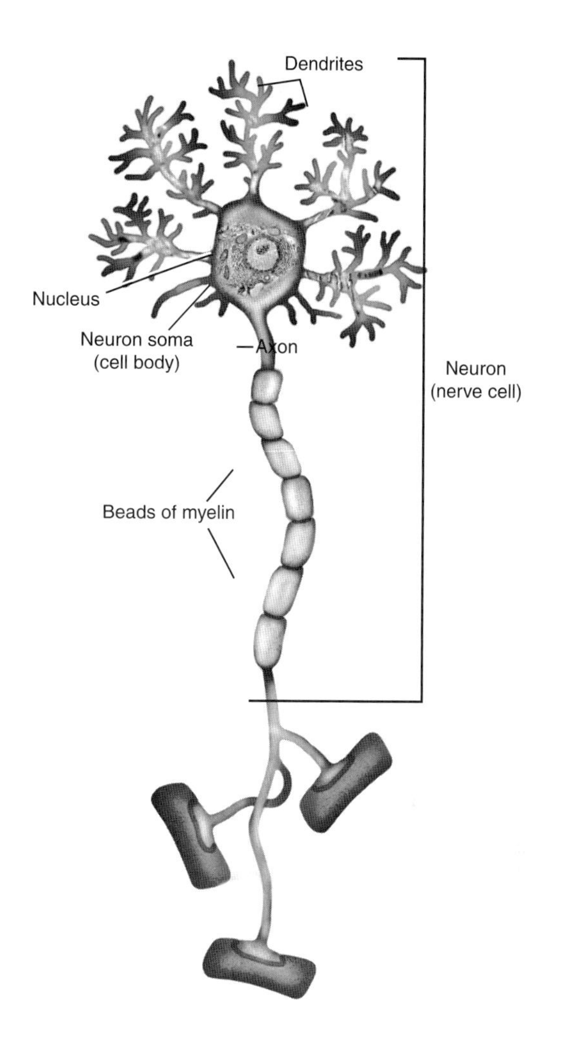

FIGURE 2-13b A simple "knee-jerk" reflex when the knee is tapped, resulting in the extension of the leg.

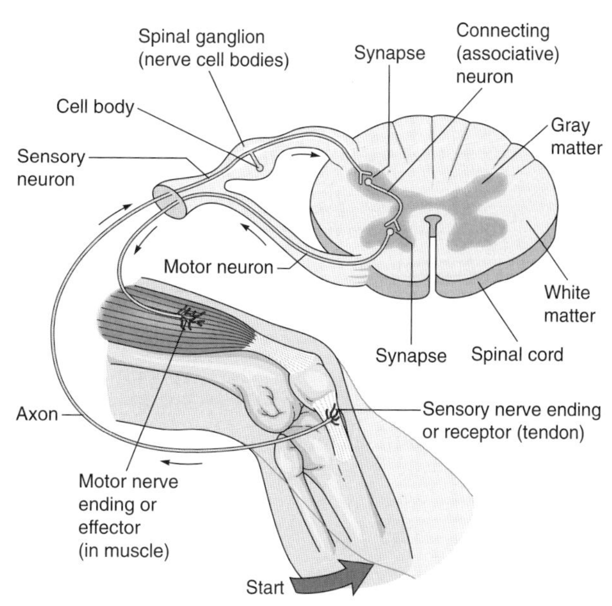

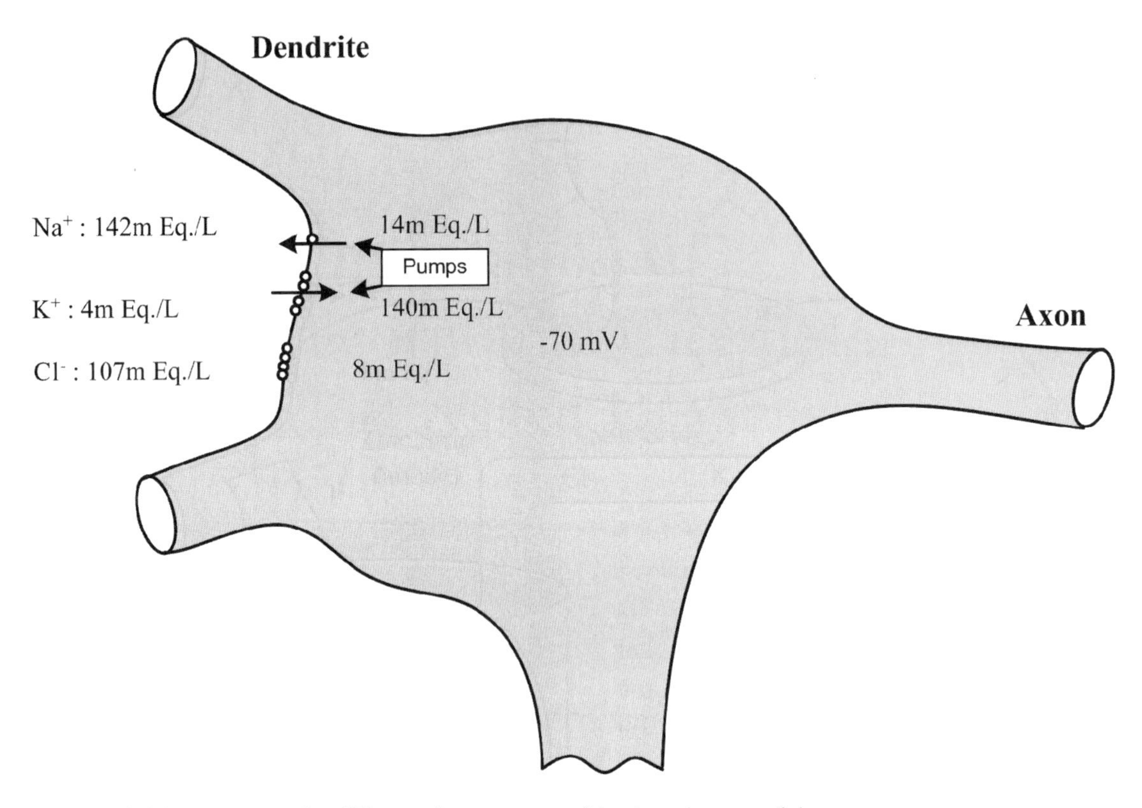

FIGURE 2-14a Concentration difference in a neuron resulting in action potential.

Figure 2-14a shows the process of a resting membrane potential of −70mV due to the distribution of sodium, potassium, and chloride ions across neuronal membrane. **Figure 2-14b** then shows the excited and inhibited neuron potentials.

2.11 ANATOMY AND PHYSIOLOGY OF THE BRAIN

The brain is the most complex organ in the human body. It produces our every thought, action, memory, feeling, and experience of the world. It is a jelly-like tissue and weighs approximately 3 pounds. There are nearly one hundred billion nerve cells, or neurons, in the human brain. The main parts of the brain are as follows:

The *cerebrum* surface is composed of gray and white matters, and the two hemispheres of the cerebrum are separated by a longitudinal fissure. Each hemisphere is then further divided into lobes. These lobes are the frontal lobe, parietal lobe, temporal lobe, and occipital lobe. Each lobe controls specific tasks through the neural paths. The tasks include muscular movements, sensory perception, and the evaluation and control of hearing, vision, smell, and thoughts.

The *brainstem* consists of the medulla oblongata, pons varolii, and the midbrain.

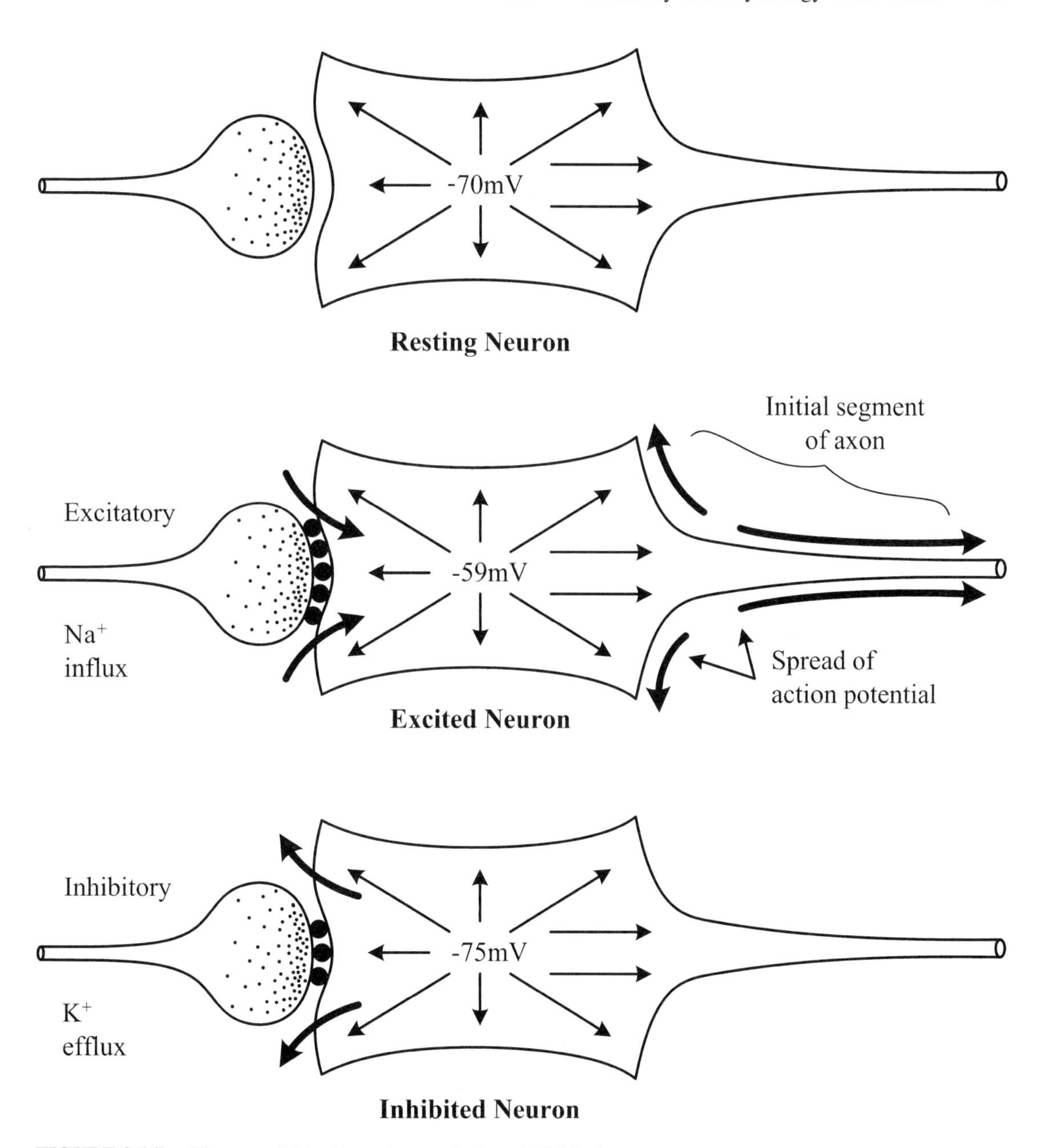

FIGURE 2-14b The potential in the resting, excited, and inhibited neurons.

The *cerebellum* controls muscular movements and the body's balance.

The *thalamus* is the relay station for the sensory impulses reaching the cerebral cortex from the spinal cord and other parts of the brain. The hypothalamus is a small structure that controls the autonomic nervous system. This is shown in **Figure 2-15**.

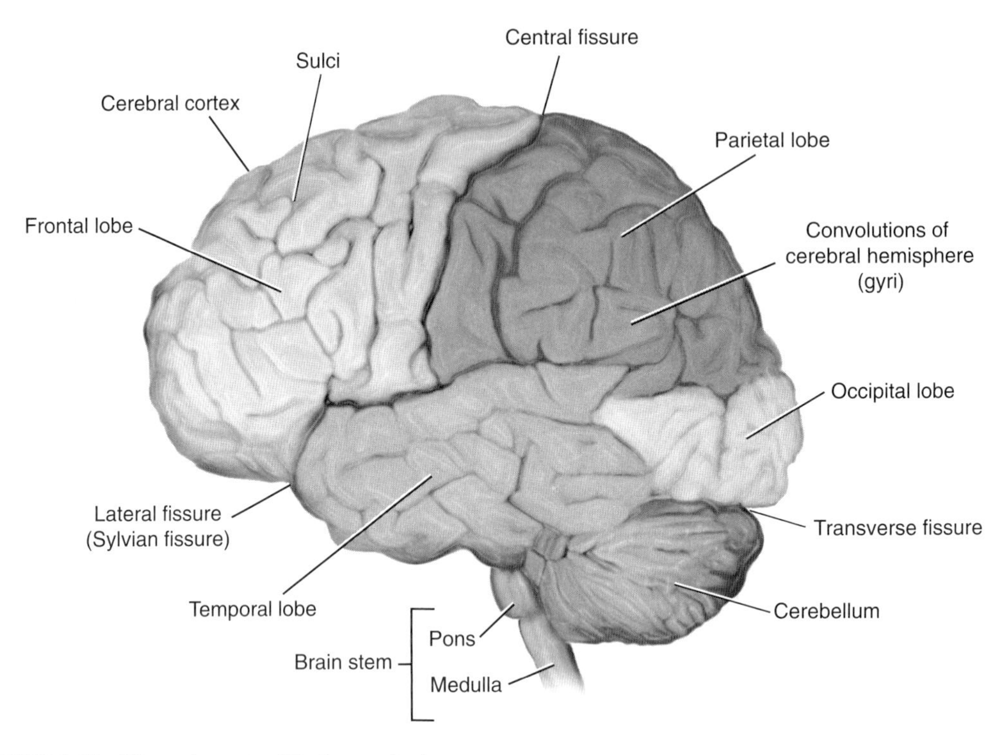

FIGURE 2-15 The main parts of the human brain.

We will turn our focus now to the characteristics of the brain. The action potential generated at the sensory organ neurons reaches the central nervous system through the spinal cord and then moves to the other neurons in the cerebral cortex. The integrative activities of these brain neurons then control the various functions of the human physiology. The cerebral cortex can be divided into the sensory cortex and the motor cortex for the functions of senses, perceptions, awareness, and types of motor controls.

2.12 DISEASES OF THE BRAIN

The brain is the control center of the body and it regulates the function of many organs. When the brain is healthy, it works quickly and automatically. However, when disease occurs, the results can be serious. Following is a list of common brain diseases:

Amyotrophic lateral sclerosis (ALS), also called Lou Gehrig's disease, is the progressive degeneration of motor cells in the brain and spinal cord.

Alzheimer's disease is a progressive and degenerative disease of the brain that results in impaired memory, thinking, and behavior and memory loss.

Meningitis is the inflammation of the meninges, the membranes that cover the brain.

Multiple sclerosis (MS) is a demyelinating disease marked by patches of hardened tissue in the brain or the spinal cord and associated especially with partial or complete paralysis and jerking muscle tremor. The patient is sometimes rendered unable to walk, speak, or write.

Muscular dystrophy (MD) is the progressive atrophy of muscle tissue, resulting in weakness and deformity.

Parkinson's disease (PD) is a chronic progressive disease marked especially by tremor of resting muscles, rigidity, slowness of movement, impaired balance, and a shuffling gait.

2.13 ANATOMY AND PHYSIOLOGY OF THE DIGESTIVE SYSTEM

There are at least three processes involved in the digestive system: the movement of food through the tract, the secretion of digestive juices, and the absorption of the food providing nutrients. **Figure 2-16** illustrates the alimentary tract that provides water, electrolytes, and nutrients to the body when food moves along the tract. Following is a list of the various parts of the digestive system and their different functions (see also **Figure 2-17**):

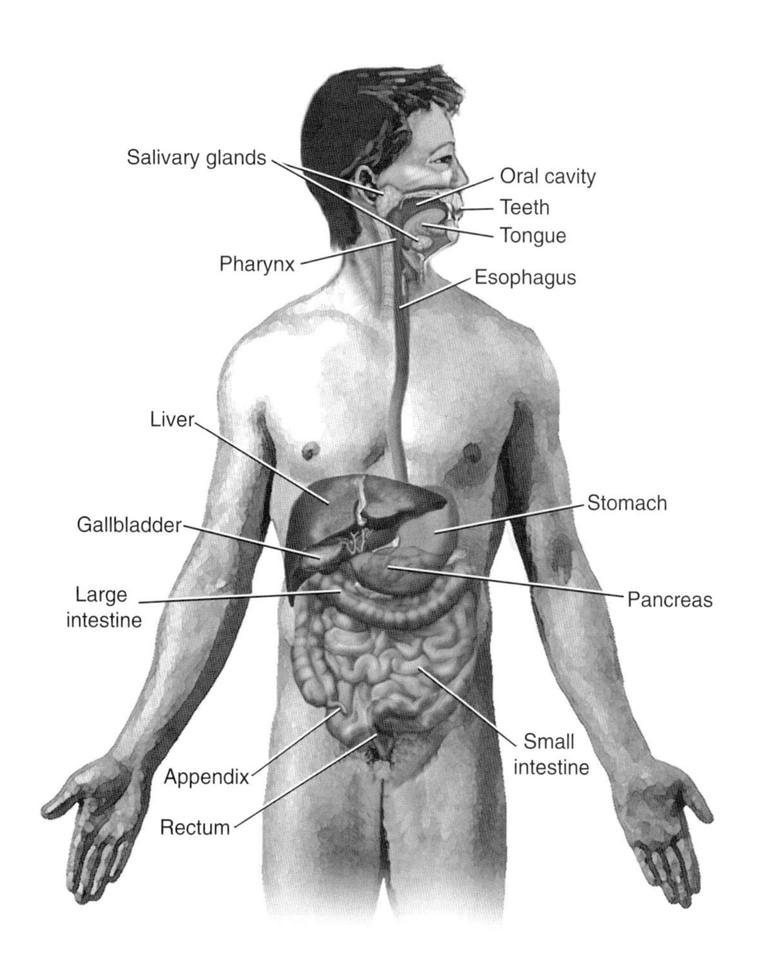

FIGURE 2-16 The structures of the digestive system.

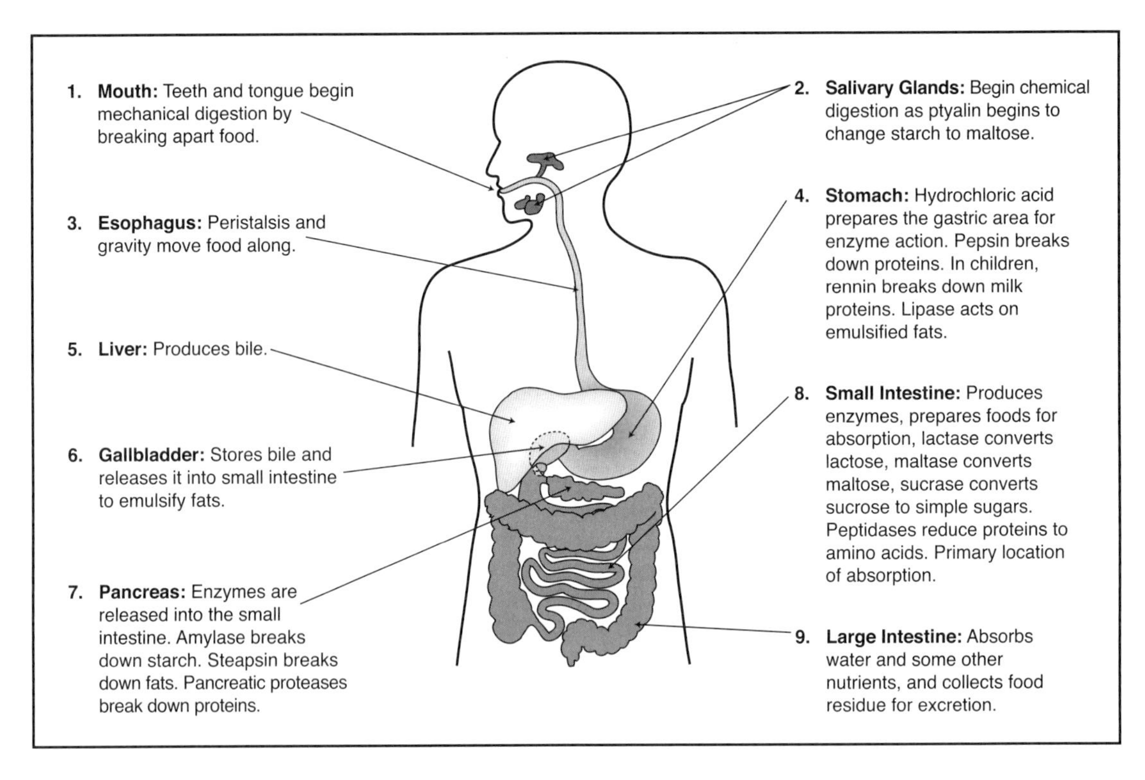

FIGURE 2-17 A simple overview of digestion.

The *mouth* is also called the oral cavity. It is lined with mucous membrane. The tongue, palate (soft and hard), cheek, and lips are part of this cavity. Its main functions include taste, the breakdown of food by mastication, and the chemical digestion of food by the salivary enzymes. Saliva also lubricates the food and controls bacteria.

The *salivary glands* consist of three pairs of glands: the parotid, the submandibular, and the sublingual. They each secret saliva into the oral cavity. The parotid glands are the largest salivary glands and are located on both sides of the face, in the front and below the ears. They secrete amylase into the mouth. The submandibular glands are located below the parotid glands near the lower jaw and they secrete mucin and ptyalin. Sublingual glands are the smallest and are located under the sides of the tongue. They secrete mucus without ptyalin.

The *esophagus* secretes mucus and transports food to the stomach. Smooth muscle contractions (peristalsis) push the food through the esophageal sphincter.

The *stomach* is the upper part of the abdominal cavity, located below the diaphragm. The stomach can be divided into an upper part, called the fundus, a middle part, called the body, and a lower part, called the pylorus. The opening from the esophagus to the stomach is through the cardiac sphincter, while the opening from the stomach to the duodenum is through the pyloric sphincter. Hydrochloric acid and gastric juices are released in the mucus layers of the stomach walls.

The *liver* is the largest organ of the body and is divided into left and right lobes. The liver is an essential organ that transforms poisons into less harmful substances. It stores excess carbohydrates as well as copper, iron, and several types of vitamins.

The *gallbladder* stores bile and releases it into the small intestine. The *pancreas* releases enzymes into small intestine. Bile emulsifies fats and enzymes break down fats, proteins, and carbohydrates.

The *intestinal tract* consists of the small intestine and the large intestine. The small intestine consists of duodenum, jejunum, and the ileum. Final absorption of food occurs in the small intestine. The ileum empties the semiliquid food into the large intestine. The large intestine consists of the ascending colon, the transverse colon, the descending colon, the sigmoid colon, the rectum, and the anal canal. The colons absorb water and nutrients and excrete food residue.

2.14 ANATOMY AND PHYSIOLOGY OF THE RENAL SYSTEM

The renal system consists of all the organs involved in formation and release of urine. It includes the kidneys, ureters, bladder, and urethra. The kidneys are bean-shaped organs, which help the body produce urine to get rid of unwanted waste substances. When urine is formed, tubes called ureters transport it to the urinary bladder, where it is stored and excreted via the urethra. They are also important in regulating our blood pressure and helping produce red blood cells. The renal system is shown in **Figure 2-18**. The kidneys perform two major functions:

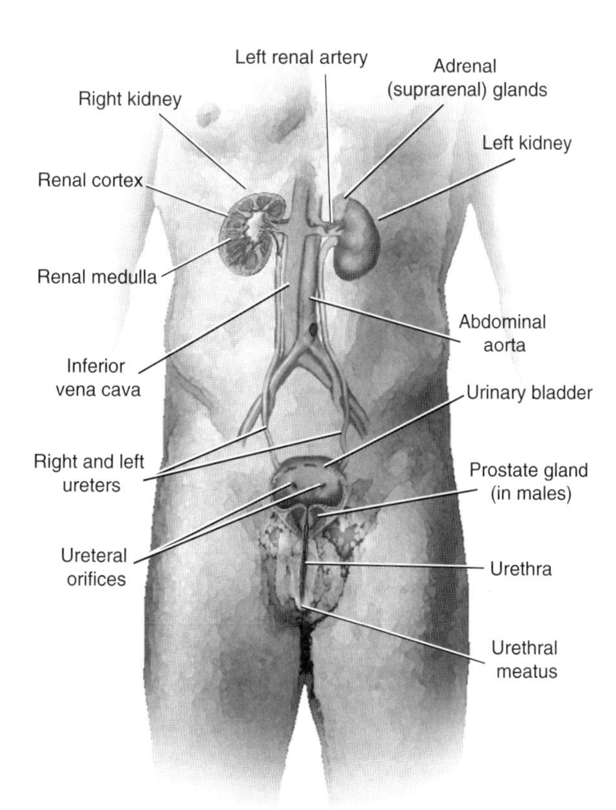

FIGURE 2-18 A simple structure of the urinary system.

1. They excrete the end-products of body metabolism.
2. They control the concentrations of body fluids.

The kidneys contain millions of nephrons. These nephrons form urine by three processes: filtration by the glomerulus, reabsorption within the renal tubules, and secretion by the tubular cells. **Figure 2-19** shows a functional diagram of a single nephron. The typical pressures in different parts of the nephron range from 100 mm Hg before the glomerulus to 0 mm Hg at the pelvis.

The blood flow through both kidneys is about 12 percent to 30 percent of the cardiac output in a resting person. If the cardiac output is 5,600 ml/minute, then the blood flow through both kidneys is about 1,200 ml/minute. The important parts of a nephron are the glomerulus, peritubular capillaries, vasa recta, loop of Henle, and the collecting duct.

The glomerulus filters water and dissolved substances from the plasma of the blood. There is an increased blood pressure in the glomerulus that allows the filtration process. Large

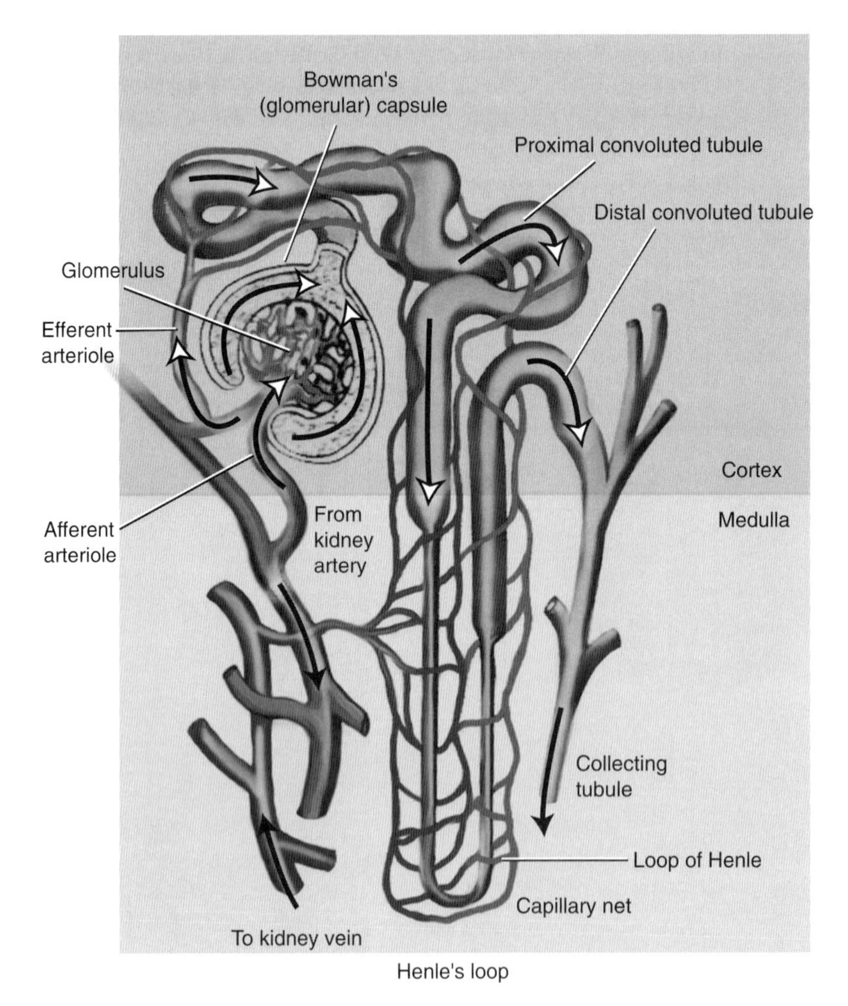

FIGURE 2-19 A simple structure of the nephrons.

proteins are not filtered. The filtrate is mostly water and the dissolved substances are sodium, potassium, calcium, magnesium, glucose, urea, uric acid, and other negatively charged ions.

The process of reabsorption of water and substances occurs throughout the renal tubule. The peritubular capillaries transport substances back into the blood. The descending loop of Henle reabsorbs water by osmosis, and the ascending loop reabsorbs sodium, potassium, and ions by the active transport.

Figure 2-20 shows a table of various organ characteristics.

~ Heart ~

Weight	7-15 ounces (200-425 grams)
Dimension	Measures about 120mm (4.75") in length, 90mm (3.5") in width at its broadest part, and 60mm (2.4") in thickness.
Circulation	The blood flow is controlled by four valves. Each opens to let the blood through when the chambers contract and then snaps shut to prevent it flowing back when they relax. The heartbeat sound comes from the opening and closing of these valves.
Muscles	Cardiac muscle. Muscular walls of the atriums and ventricles, known as the myocardium.
Unusual Fact	In a typical year, heart pumps approximately one million gallons (4.5 million litres).

~ Lungs ~

Weight	The right lung usually weighs about 625 gm and the left 567 gm., but much variation is met with according to the amount of blood or serous fluid. The lungs are heavier in the male than in the female
Dimension	Right lung proportion is approximately 55%, and left lung proportion is approximately 45%
Circulation	Pulmonary artery conveys the venous blood to the lungs; it divides into branches which accompany the bronchial tubes and end in a dense capillary net-work in the walls of the alveoli.
Unusual Fact	The total surface area of the alveoli (tiny air sacs in the lungs) is the size of a tennis court.

~ Liver ~

Weight	Largest and heaviest internal organ, weighing around 3.5 lb (1.6 kilos)
Dimension	Approximately the size of a football. Its greatest transverse measurement is from 20 to 22.5 cm. Vertically, near its lateral or right surface, it measures about 15 to 17.5 cm., while its greatest anterior-posterior diameter is on a level with the upper end of the right kidney, and is from 10 to 12.5 cm.
Circulation	Unlike any other organ, the liver has a double blood supply. Oxygenated blood from the heart to the liver, which needs about a quarter of the heart's total output - 1.75 pints (1 liter) a minute - comes via the hepatic artery. This subdivides into many branches within the liver to provide oxygen to all its cells. The portal vein also feeds the liver with blood. It carries nutrients from digested food which the liver either uses or stores.
Unusual Fact	It secretes up to two pints (1.14 liters) of bile daily to remove waste products

FIGURE 2-20 A table of characteristics of important organs: fact sheet. (*continued*)

~ Brain ~

Weight	1.4 kilos (three pounds)
Dimension	Average width = 140mm Average length =167mm Average height = 93 mm
Circulation	The cerebral arteries are derived from the internal carotid and vertebral, which at the base of the brain form a remarkable anastomosis known as the arterial circle of Willis.
Unusual Fact	Consists of 100 billion nerve cells, known as neurons

~ Kidneys ~

Weight	One kidney 140-170 grams (5-6 ounces).
Dimension	Each kidney is about 5 inches (13 centimeters) long and about 3 inches (8 centimeters) wide
Circulation	Blood flows into the kidneys through renal arteries, which come from the aorta. The renal arteries divide and sub-divide into ever smaller branches ending in coils known as glomeruli, which are capillaries that act as filters.
Unusual Fact	Approximately 400 gallons (1,800 liters) of blood are pumped through the kidneys every day

~ Pancreas ~

Weight	60 to 100 gm (2-4 ounces)
Dimension	6-10 inches (16-25 cm) long.
Circulation	Insulin, glucagon and other hormones are sent into the bloodstream to regulate blood sugar levels and other activities throughout the body.

FIGURE 2-20 (*concluded*)

SUMMARY

- This chapter included basic anatomy and physiology concepts for the reader including the six major systems of the human body: the cardiovascular system, circulatory system, respiratory system, nervous system, digestive system, and renal system.
- The main organs in the human body discussed in this chapter are the heart, lungs, brain, and kidneys.
- There are various diseases associated with the heart, including angina, arrhythmia, and cardiomyopathy.
- Diseases associated with the lungs include bronchitis, emphysema, and chronic obstructive pulmonary disease (COPD).
- Diseases associated with the brain include amyotrophic lateral sclerosis (ALS), Alzheimer's disease, and meningitis.

- The mechanics of engineering and human physiology are very similar. This chapter simplified the human systems in relation to the mechanics of engineering systems as follows:

Engineering term	Physiological system
Hydraulic	Cardiovascular
Pneumatic	Respiratory
Chemical	Biochemical
Computer	Central nervous
Communication and networking	Nervous
Mechanical	Biomechanical
Robotics	Hand-eye coordination
Fluid mechanics	Circulatory

MEDICAL TERMINOLOGY

The following is a list of medical terminology mentioned in this chapter.

Anterior: pertaining to the front of the body, or used to describe the forward part of an organ.

Diaphragm: a muscle that separates the thoracic from the abdominal cavity and is used in breathing.

Emphysema: a degenerative disease with no known cure that results in destruction of the walls of the alveoli; often attributed to smoking.

Endocardium: within the heart; lining of the heart.

Inflammation: a localized response to an injury or destruction of tissues characterized by heat, redness, swelling, and pain.

Lateral: toward the side of the body, away from the midline of the body.

Lymphatic vessels: vessels that resemble veins but have more valves.

Myocardium: the second layer of the heart that is involved in the contraction and relaxation causing a heartbeat.

Pericardium: the double-walled membranous sac that encloses the heart.

Posterior: pertaining to the back of the body, or used to describe the back part of an organ.

Prone: lying face down on the belly.

Pulmonary: a reference to or involving the lungs.

Pulmonary circulation: circulatory route that goes from the heart to the lungs and back to the heart.

Stenosis: narrowing; an abnormal narrowing of the opening of a heart valve.

QUIZ

1. To which structure(s) does the trachea lead?

a) Nasal cavity b) Liver c) Lungs d) Heart

2. True or False: The mechanical activity of the heart precedes the electrical activity.
   a) True b) False
3. If a plane divides the body into right and left parts, it is called a:
   a) Sagittal plane. b) Transverse plane. c) Frontal plane. d) None of the above.
4. The central nervous system consists of:
   a) The brain. b) The spinal cord. c) A network of nerves.
   d) All of the above.
5. Outer layers of the heart are called the:
   a) Endocardium. b) Myocardium. c) Pericardium. d) None of the above.
6. The natural pacemaker of the human body is the:
   a) AV node. b) SA node. c) Bundle of His. d) Right lung.
7. Urine is carried from the kidneys to the bladder by the:
   a) Nephron. b) Urethra. c) Glomeruli. d) None of the above.
8. Inflammation of the spinal cord is called:
   a) Myelitis. b) Encephalitis. c) Reye's syndrome. d) Meningitis.
9. Pulmonary edema is ______________________________.
10. Arteriosclerosis occurs when the arterial walls ____________________ because of the ____________________ elasticity.

PROBLEMS

1. Name the major blood vessels entering and exiting the heart, the chambers of the heart, and the valves of the heart.
2. Name the systemic and pulmonary blood circulation routes and the major diseases that can occur on these routes.
3. Describe the typical steps that occur in one cycle of the cardiac phase of contraction and relaxation.
4. Describe the sequence of processes involved in respiration.
5. Name the major parts of the brain and their functions.
6. Match the functions in the left column with appropriate parts of the body in the right column below.

   ____ moving muscles a) glomerulus
   ____ filtering water from blood plasma b) left atrium
   ____ storing vitamins c) gallbladder
   ____ storing bile d) brain
   ____ receiving oxygenated blood e) liver

7. Make an alphabetical list of the bones and their locations in the human skeletal system from an anterior view. Make a similar list from a posterior view.
8. Make a list of muscles and their locations in the human body from an anterior view. Make a similar list from a posterior view.

9. Make a list of nerves and their locations in the central nervous system. Also, make a list of nerves in the spinal nerve plexus.
10. Discuss the flow of the blood in a nephron starting at the afferent arteriole and ending at the collecting tubule.

CASE STUDIES

1. John is 57 years old. He indulges in eating doughnuts, cakes, and pies. He weighs 200 pounds and does not exercise. His recent annual medical exam showed that his blood glucose level after fasting was 165, his blood pressure was 160/95 mm Hg, and his LDL ("bad" cholesterol) level was 150. His doctor diagnosed him with diabetes and declared that his symptoms of high blood pressure and high cholesterol will probably develop into cardiovascular disease in the near future. However, he does not show any symptoms of diabetes at the present time.
   a) What is the physiology of diabetes and what organs are involved in controlling the blood sugar? Provide a detailed description.
   b) What are the symptoms of diabetes and why does John not show any symptoms?
   c) How does exercise help to control sugar levels, blood pressure, and cholesterol in the body?
2. Medical simulation using human models or mannequins is considered a learning tool for physiology education in many medical colleges. The ACCP (American College of Chest Physicians) Simulation Center in Illinois is a leader in simulation education using human patient simulators in providing hands-on learning opportunities for the practicing physicians. A case study may be done on the center and its simulation education with the emphasis on the clinical environment, cost, and the advantages of simulation.

RESEARCH TOPICS

1. Carbon monoxide poisoning kills many people each year. Analyze the problem and explain what physiological systems and organs are involved in this situation. What is poisoning? What other types of poisoning can occur to the human body?
2. There are differing reports regarding the effectiveness of the Atkins diet and its effect on people who choose this approach to weight loss. Collect data on this type of dieting and explain the physiological effects of the diet and what organs are affected in this process.
3. Cocaine baby syndrome seriously affects fetal development and newborn health. How do cocaine and other drugs affect the fetal anatomical and physiological processes? Collect data on this research topic.

CHAPTER 3

Biosignals and Noise

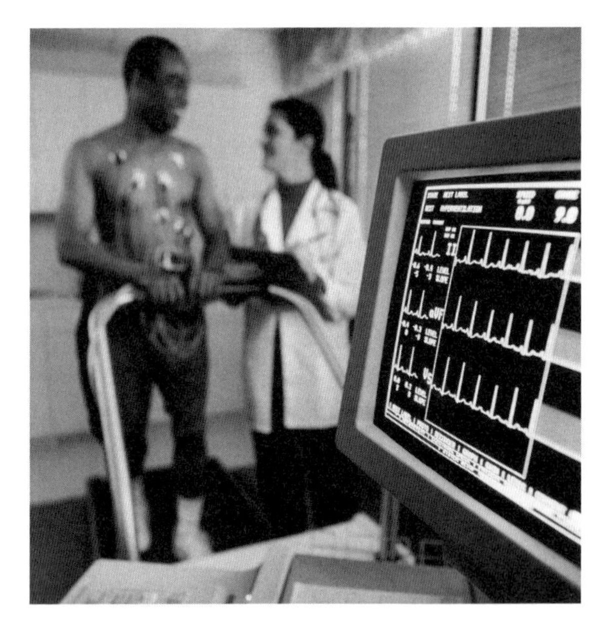

CHAPTER OUTLINE

OBJECTIVES

The objective of this chapter is to discuss the nature of biosignals and their presentations for display and recording. We will familiarize the reader with the conversion of a biosignal into a digital signal for the computer interface and we will explain the criterion of noise embedded onto a biosignal.

Upon completion of this chapter, the reader will be able to:

- Explain the phase shifts between two signals.
- Discuss the time-domain and frequency-domain concepts for biosignals.
- Describe types of biosignals.
- Compute signal-to-noise ratios.
- Compute noise figures.
- Compute a digital pattern for a biosignal.
- Compute Fourier series for a pulse train.

INTERNET WEB SITES

http://www.mathworks.com (The Mathworks™)
http://www.elsevier.com (Elsevier)
http://www.bsp.pdx.edu (Biomedical Signal Processing Laboratory of Portland State University)

INTRODUCTION

Biosignals are physiological events such as electrical, chemical, or mechanical activity that occur in the human body and that can be measured, displayed, and recorded. Electrical activity of the heart or brain, the beating of the heart, changes in glucose concentration in the blood, muscle contractions, and the blood flow in a stenotic (abnormally narrowing) vessel are all examples of biosignals. As there are various methods of acquiring these biosignals, there are various methods to present them in meaningful ways. The signals can be noisy. We must reduce the noise so that a meaningful signal can be evaluated.

This chapter discusses biosignals and non-biosignals and their properties. We will explain the fundamental concept of sinusoidal and rectangular pulse waves and discuss the presentation of the time-domain signal and the frequency-domain signal.

3.1 NATURE OF SIGNALS AND NOISE

Any practical signal consists of the sum of different sinusoids having different amplitudes, frequencies, and phases. A sinusoid is also called a sine wave function. Voice, music, video, and even biosignals all contain sinusoids. Whether voice or music sound waves, video optical waves, or biosignal electrical waves, they can all be displayed on an oscilloscope or on a monitor having the sum of several sinusoids. **Figure 3-1** shows a sinusoidal signal

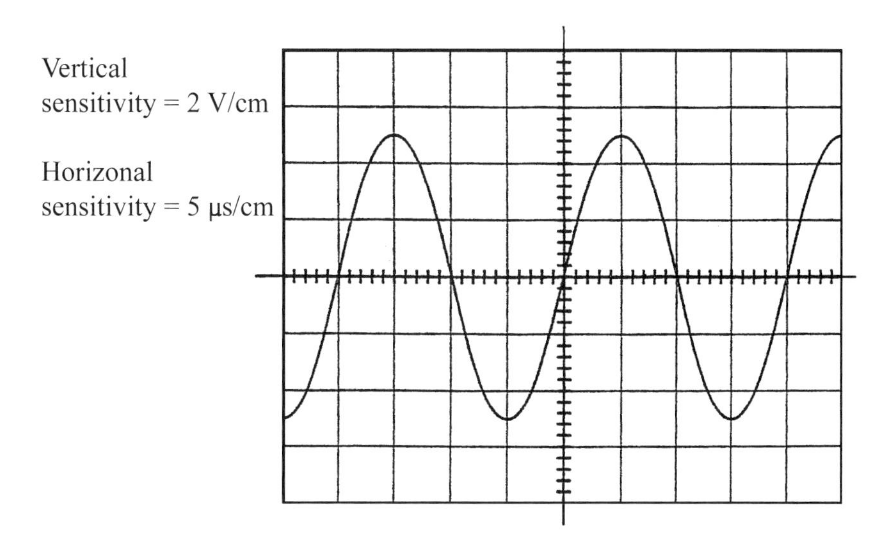

FIGURE 3-1 A sinusoidal signal shown on the scope.

on an oscilloscope. It is defined as having amplitude, frequency, and a phase. This signal is called an alternating current (AC) signal (compared to a constant and fixed direct current, or DC signal). You can compare it with another sinusoid in terms of amplitude, frequency, and phase.

On the oscilloscope, the amplitude of the sinusoid is displayed in volts (in the vertical axis), and its time is displayed in seconds (in the horizontal axis). The amplitude can be given as peak-to-peak amplitude or root-mean-square (RMS) amplitude. The RMS amplitude value is given as 0.707 of the peak amplitude of an AC signal. As the peaks of the signal are repeating, the frequency can be calculated as the inverse of the period or time between two peaks.

In **Figure 3-1,** the peak-to-peak amplitude is 10 V, and the time period for one complete cycle is 20 μsec (that is, the frequency of the signal is 50 kHz).

In the following sections, we will discuss the characteristics of sinusoidal signals. This information can then be applied to any biomedical signal, such as ECG or EEG.

1. **Sine wave**

The equation of an AC signal is given as:

$$V_S(t) = A \sin(\omega \times t) \qquad V_S(t) = A \sin(2\pi f t)$$

where $V_S(t)$ is the voltage AC signal with a peak amplitude of "A" volts and a frequency of "f" hertz. $\omega = 2\pi f$ is called the angular frequency (noted in radians).

2. **Add**

When we add two sinusoids of the same frequency, it results in a same-frequency signal but with the summation of their values in the real time. An example is shown in **Figure 3-2a.** Sine wave 1, $V_1(t)$, is added to another sine wave 2, $V_2(t)$, having the same frequency, and the result is shown as sine wave 3, $V_T(t)$.

When we add these two sinusoids with amplitudes of "A" and "B" but having the same frequencies, the equation can be written as:

$$V_T(t) = V_1(t) + V_2(t)$$
$$V_T(t) = A \sin(\omega \times t) + B \sin(\omega \times t)$$
$$V_T(t) = (A + B) \sin(\omega \times t)$$

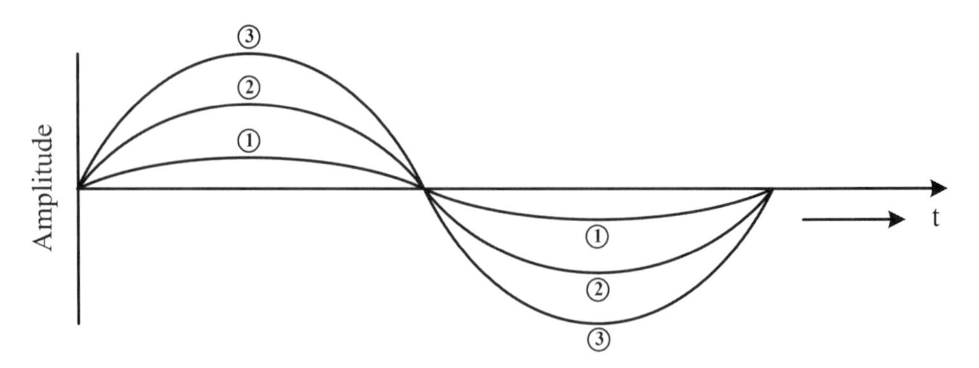

FIGURE 3-2a Summation of two sine waves of the same frequency but different amplitudes.

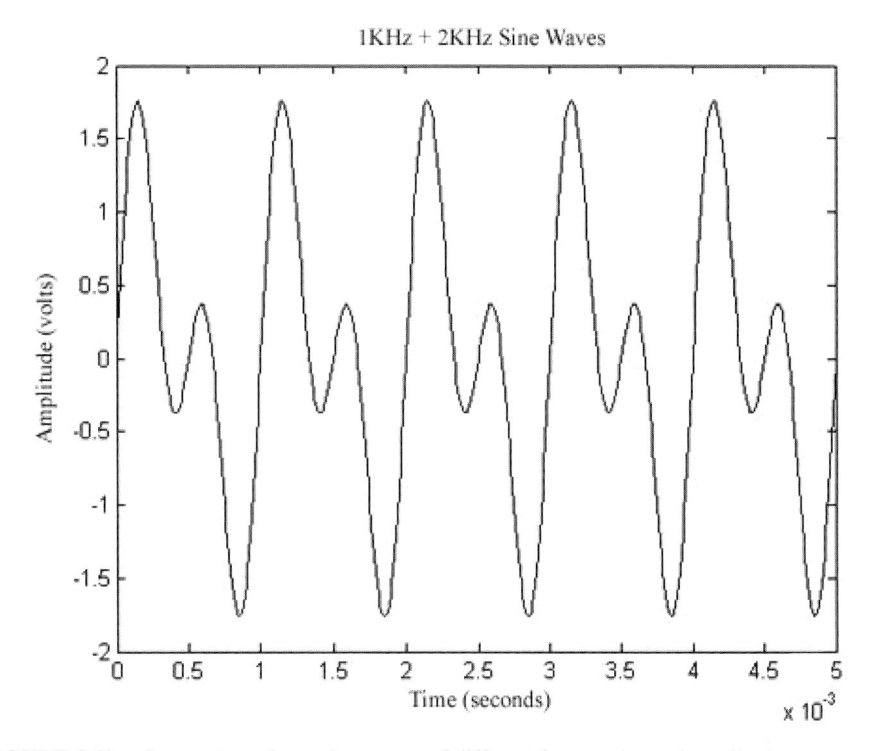

FIGURE 3-2b Summation of two sine waves of different frequencies and amplitudes.

We can also add two sine waves of different frequencies as shown in **Figure 3-2b.** The result of 1 kHz and 2 kHz sine waves looks periodic but does not add up to a 3 kHz sine wave.

3. **Add Phasor**

If two sinusoids have phase shifts, then adding them is equated as follows:

$$V_T\,(t) = A \sin(\omega \times t + \theta_1) + B \sin(\omega \times t + \theta_2)$$

where θ_1 and θ_2 are the phase angles of the two sinusoids in degrees. Furthermore, we can write:

$$V_T\,(t) = A \angle \theta_1 + B \angle \theta_2$$
$$V_T\,(t) = A \cos \theta_1 + jA \sin \theta_1 + B \cos \theta_2 + jB \sin \theta_2$$
$$V_T\,(t) = (A \cos \theta_1 + B \cos \theta_2) + j(A \sin \theta_1 + B \sin \theta_2)$$
$$V_T\,(t) = X + jY$$

where

$$X = A \cos \theta_1 + B \cos \theta_2$$

and

$$Y = A \sin \theta_1 + B \sin \theta_2$$

The peak amplitude M and phase angle θ can be determined as:

$$M = \sqrt{X^2 + Y^2}$$

$$\theta = \tan^{-1}\frac{Y}{X} \text{ degrees (in the proper quadrant)}$$

Finally, the V_T (t) can be written as:

$$V_T(t) = M \sin(\omega \times t + \theta)$$

4. **DC Offset**

An AC sine function can ride on a DC and the result is a DC offset sine wave shown in **Figure 3-3.** A sine wave is offset by a DC of +2 V. The DC offset can be a positive or a negative value. The equation can then be written as:

$$V_T(t) = DC + AC = A + B \sin(\omega \times t)$$

In the equation, the amplitude of the DC offset is **A** and the peak amplitude of the sine wave is **B**.

EXAMPLE Add two sinusoids given as:

$$3 \sin(\omega \times t + 30°) \text{ and } 2 \sin(\omega \times t - 60°)$$

$$V_T(t) = 3 \sin(\omega \times t + 30°) + 2 \sin(\omega \times t - 60°)$$
$$V_T(t) = 3 \angle 30° + 2 \angle -60°$$
$$V_T(t) = 3 \cos 30° + j3 \sin 30° + 2 \cos(-60°) + j2 \sin(-60°)$$
$$V_T(t) = [3 \cos(30°) + 2 \cos(-60°)] + j[3 \sin(30°) + 2 \sin(-60°)]$$
$$V_T(t) = [2.59 + 1] + j[1.5 - 1.73]$$
$$V_T(t) = 3.59 + j(-0.23)$$

Peak amplitude:

$$M = \sqrt{(3.59)^2 + (-0.23)^2}$$
$$M = 3.59$$

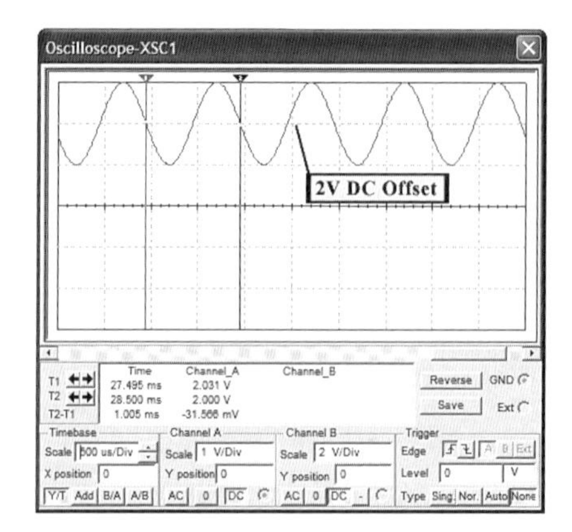

FIGURE 3-3 A sine wave with a DC offset.

Phase angle:

$$\theta = \tan^{-1}\frac{-0.23}{3.59}$$

$$\theta = -3.66°$$

Finally,

$$V_T\,(t) = 3.59\ \sin(\omega \times t - 3.66°)$$

■

5. Phase Lag and Lead

In comparing two sine waves, one wave may lead or lag with respect to the other in time. This can be represented as follows:

First Signal

$$V_1(t) = A\ \sin(\omega \times t)$$

As an example, if the second signal lags the first signal by 90 degrees, then the second signal can be written as

$$V_2(t) = B\ \sin(\omega \times t - 90°)$$

Thus, we can say $V_2(t)$ lags $V_1(t)$ by 90 degrees. Another way we may state this as $V_1(t)$ is leading $V_2(t)$ by 90 degrees. This is shown in **Figure 3-4.** Sine wave 1 is leading sine wave 2 by 90 degrees.

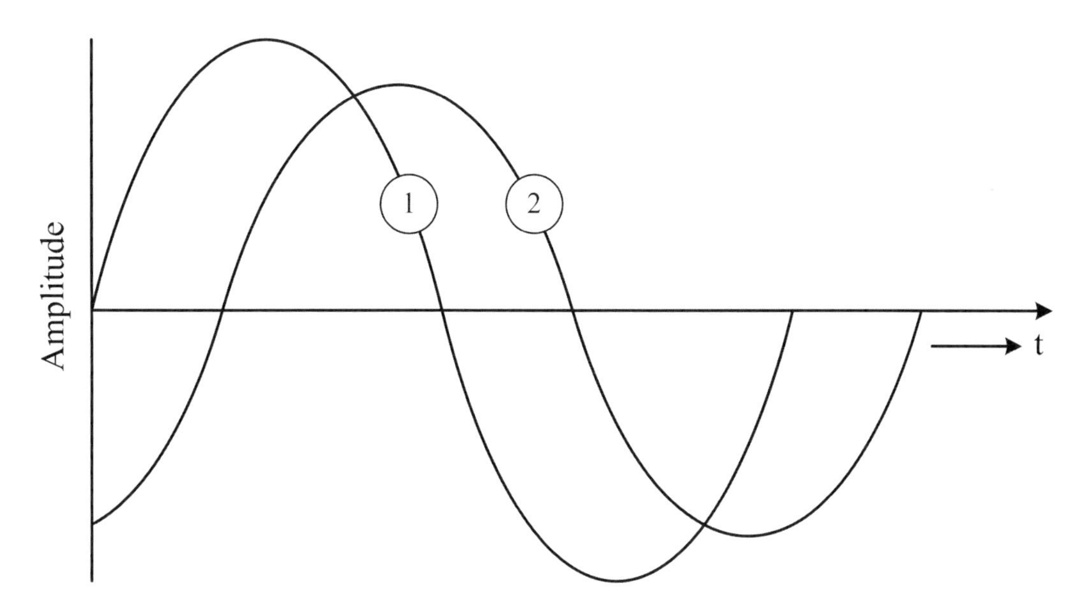

FIGURE 3-4 A phase shift between two sine waves.

3.2 TYPES OF SIGNALS

Figure 3-5 shows a voice signal, a music signal, and a biosignal. The music signal consists of many more frequencies than the voice signal or the biosignals. As the signal continues in real time, it is called an analog signal and is considered to have an infinite number of

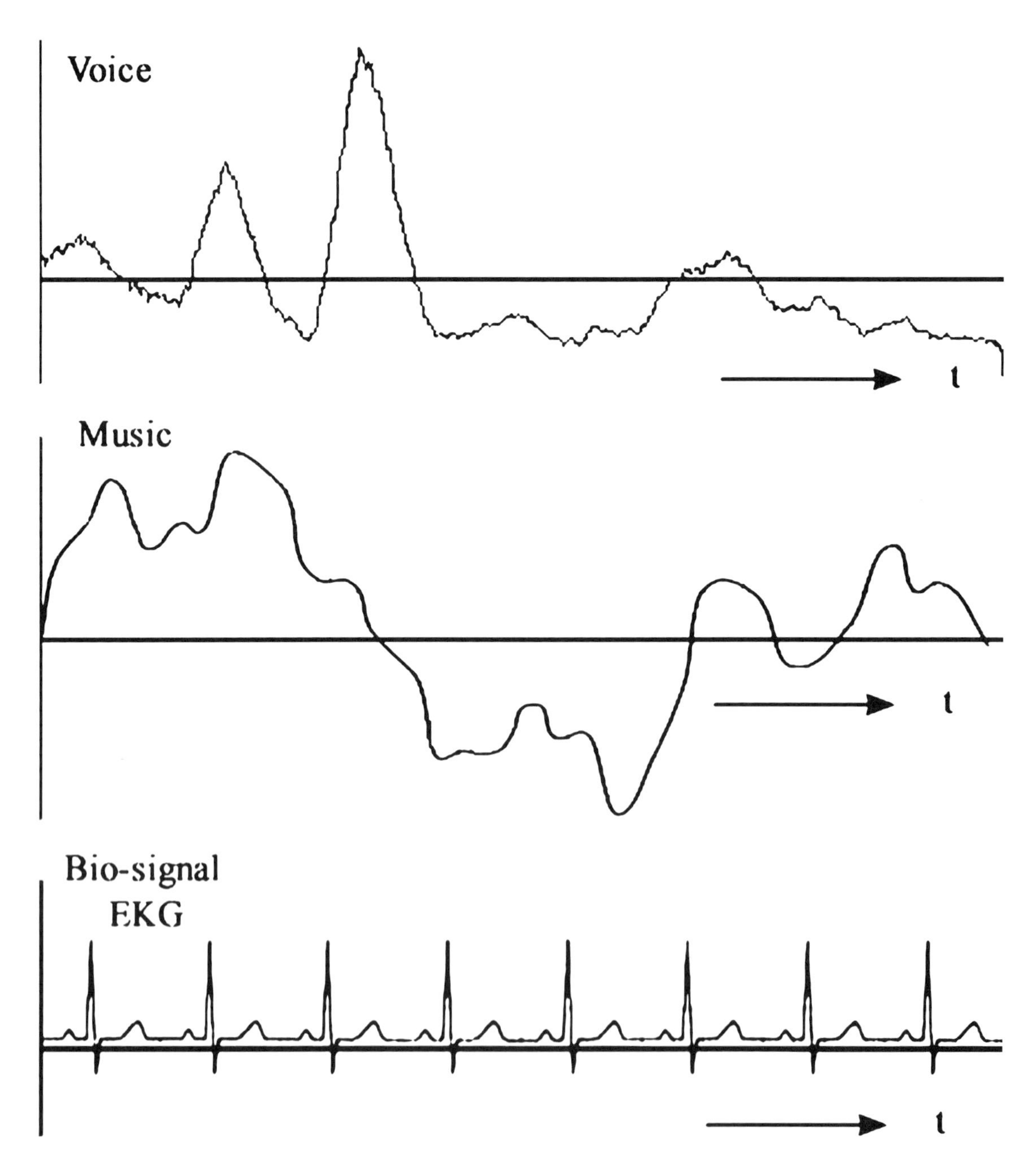

FIGURE 3-5 Various types of voltage signals shown in the time-domain.

samples. A sample is one value of the signal in the real time. A noncontinuous signal consists of a finite number of samples and is called a discrete signal. This signal can be converted into a digital signal.

Notice that the peaks of a biosignal are repeating and that we can call it a periodic signal. Voice and music are not periodic and their compositions have repeatable and nonrepeatable sine waves. However, some biosignals have the same set of sine waves repeating. This leads us to discuss the time-domain signal developing into a frequency-domain signal.

As each one of the aforementioned signals has several sine waves in its makeup, we can define bandwidth as the range of minimum to maximum frequencies in each signal. For example, a voice signal consists of any frequencies starting from DC to about 5 kHz, the bandwidth of the voice signal is then considered 5 kHz (Max = 5 kHz, Min = 0 kHz). Both voice and music signals are called audio signals. The range of audio signals is from DC to 20 kHz. Above 20 kHz, the signals are called ultrasound signals.

3.3 FREQUENCY-DOMAIN SIGNALS

The time-domain and frequency-domain of a signal are related by the Fourier series and Fourier transforms. The series provides the summation of sinusoidal signals with their amplitudes, frequencies, and phases to generate a periodic signal, whereas the Fourier transforms are for the nonperiodic signals. In **Figure 3-6a** and **Figure 3-6b,** time-domain and frequency-domain signals are shown when five sinusoids are added. The five sinusoids are 1 kHz, 2 kHz, 3 kHz, 4 kHz, and 5 kHz. The added signal is shown in time-domain and also in frequency-domain. The input to the spectrum analyzer is the signal shown in **Figure 3-6a** and the output of the spectrum analyzer is the signal's spectrum as shown in **Figure 3-6b.**

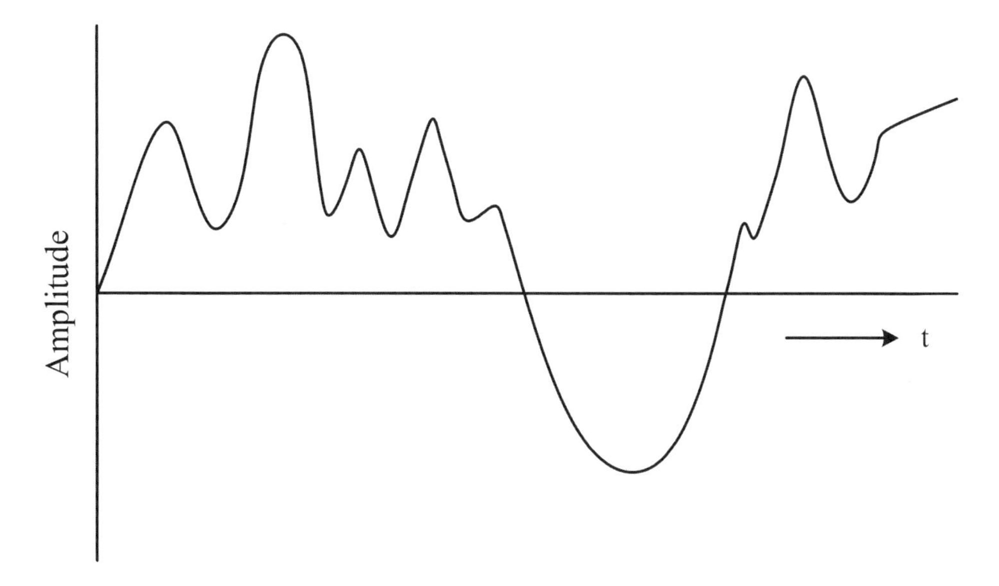

FIGURE 3-6a A representation of a voltage signal in the time-domain.

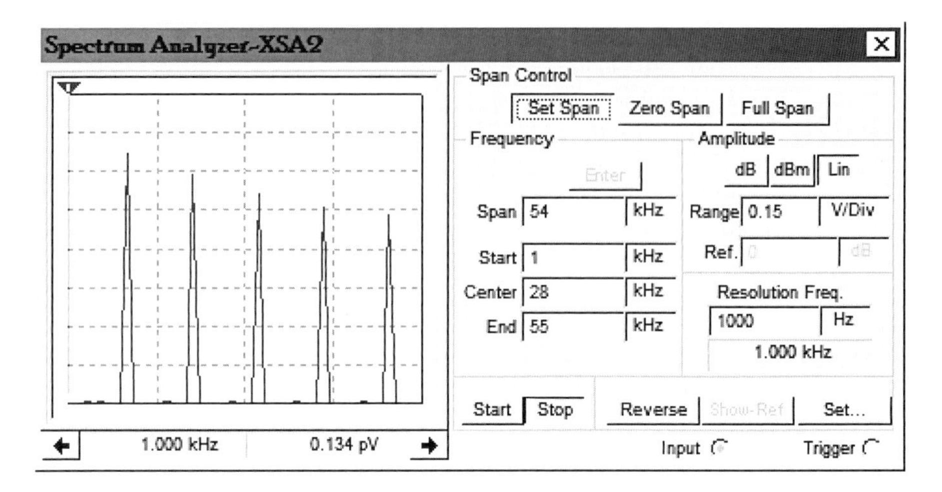

FIGURE 3-6b Spectral representation of the voltage signal shown in Figure 3-6a.

To understand how a signal is made up of sinusoids, we will look next into a simple example of a square wave. The square wave and its spectral are shown in **Figure 3-7.**

The square wave signal, x(t), has an amplitude of 5 V and a frequency of 1 kHz. It can be written as:

$$x(t) = a_0 + a_1 \cos(w_0 \times t) + a_2 \cos(2w_0 \times t) + a_3 \cos(3w_0 \times t) + a_4 \cos(4w_0 \times t) \ldots + \ldots + \ldots$$

where a_0 = the DC component of the square wave, calculated as:

$$a_0 = (\text{amplitude}) \times (\text{duty cycle})$$
$$a_0 = 5\text{V} \times 0.5$$
$$a_0 = 2.5\text{V}$$

$$\text{Duty cycle} = d = \frac{\text{Pulse width}}{\text{Time period}}, \text{ thus:}$$

$$d = \frac{\tau}{T}$$

$$d = \frac{0.5}{T}$$

$$d = 0.5$$

the fundamental frequency of x(t) is ω_0 (omega), thus:

$$\omega_o = 2\pi f$$
$$\omega_o = 2\pi(1 \text{ kHz})$$
$$\omega_o = 6.28 \times 10^3 \text{ radians}$$

Therefore, the second harmonic of x(t) can be written as:

$$2 \times \omega_o = 2 \times 2\pi(1 \text{ kHz})$$
$$2 \times \omega_o = 12.56 \times 10^3 \text{ radians}$$

Similarly, $3 \times \omega_0$ = the third harmonic of x(t).

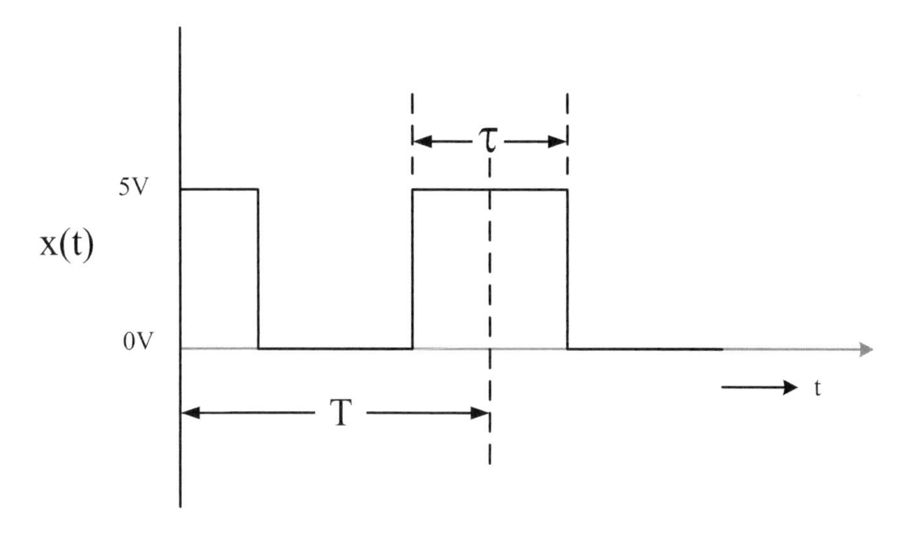

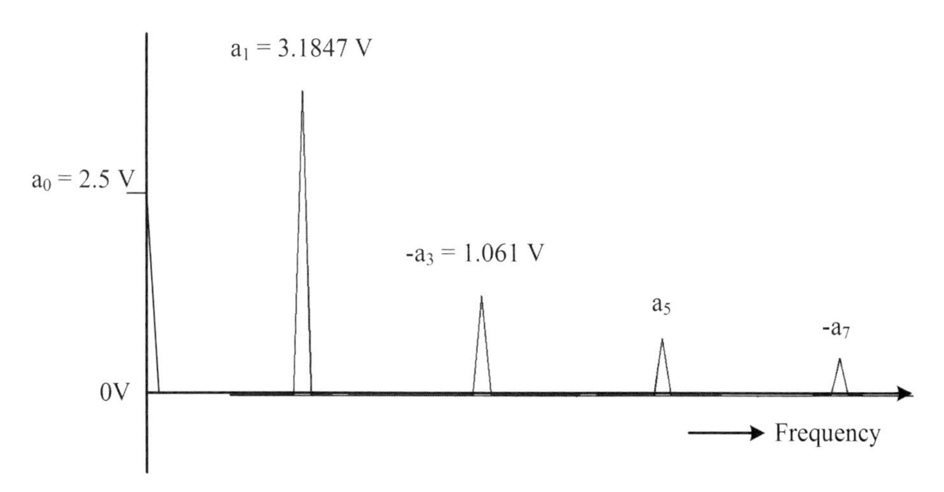

FIGURE 3-7 A square wave shown in time-domain and in the frequency-domain.

a_1 = the amplitude of the fundamental component of x(t), thus:

$$a_1 = 2 \times A \times d \times \frac{\sin(1 \times \pi \times 0.5)}{(1 \times \pi \times 0.5)}$$

$$a_1 = 2 \times 5 \times 0.5 \times \frac{\sin(1 \times \pi \times 0.5)}{(1 \times \pi \times 0.5)}$$

$$a_1 = 3.1847\text{V}$$

Similarly,

a_2 = the amplitude of the second harmonic, thus:

$$a_2 = 2 \times A \times d \times \frac{\sin(2 \times \pi \times 0.5)}{(2 \times \pi \times 0.5)}$$

$$a_2 = 2 \times 5 \times 0.5 \times \frac{\sin(2 \times \pi \times 0.5)}{(2 \times \pi \times 0.5)}$$

$$a_2 = 0$$

In general,

$$a_n = 2 \times A \times d \times \frac{\sin(n \times \pi \times d)}{(n \times \pi \times d)}$$

where n represents the harmonic for which you are seeking the amplitude ($n = 1, 2, 3 \ldots$).

As these frequency components make up x(t), we can determine the amplitude of x(t) at t = 0.1 second as a Fourier series.

EXAMPLE

$$x(t = 0.1 \text{ sec.}) = 2.5 + 3.1847 \times \cos(2 \times \pi \times 1000 \times 0.1) + 0.00 \times \cos(2 \times \pi \times 2000 \times 0.1) - 1.061 \times \cos(2 \times \pi \times 3000 \times 0.1) + \ldots$$

$$x(t = 0.1 \text{ sec.}) = 2.5 + (3.1847) \times (1.0) + (0.0) \times (1) - 1.061$$

$$x(t = 0.1 \text{ sec.}) = 2.5 + (3.1847) + 0 - 1.061$$

$$x(t = 0.1 \text{ sec.}) = 4.6237 \text{ V}$$

The result is close to the expected value of 5 V at t = 0.1 second. **Figure 3-7** shows the spectral of the symmetrical square wave. The even harmonics a_2, a_4, and so on are zeros and the spectrum analyzer inverts the negative terms such as a_3 and a_7.

■

3.4 BIOSIGNALS

The complex human body generates a variety of biosignals that can be acquired by biomedical transducers and electrodes. Following is a list with brief descriptions of some of these biosignals.

Biochemical signals can measure in real time the constant changes in the concentration of ions such as sodium, potassium, and calcium in the body. Several chemical processes can determine blood glucose levels, insulin levels, or pH and plot them in time.

Bioelectric signals are the action potentials due to changes in ion concentration. The action potential propagates through numerous muscle cells and various organs. The examples of ECG, EEG, and EMG are bioelectric signals that can be easily recorded.

Biomechanical signals can measure pressure in body functions such as blood pressure. The arterial and venous pressures are continuously changing and pressure sensors can detect these signals and monitor them on pressure monitors as real-time waveforms.

Biomagnetic signals are the magnetic fields that occur in the body such as in the brain, the heart, and the lungs. They are weak signals compared to ECG or EEG, but sophisticated magnetic detectors can detect them.

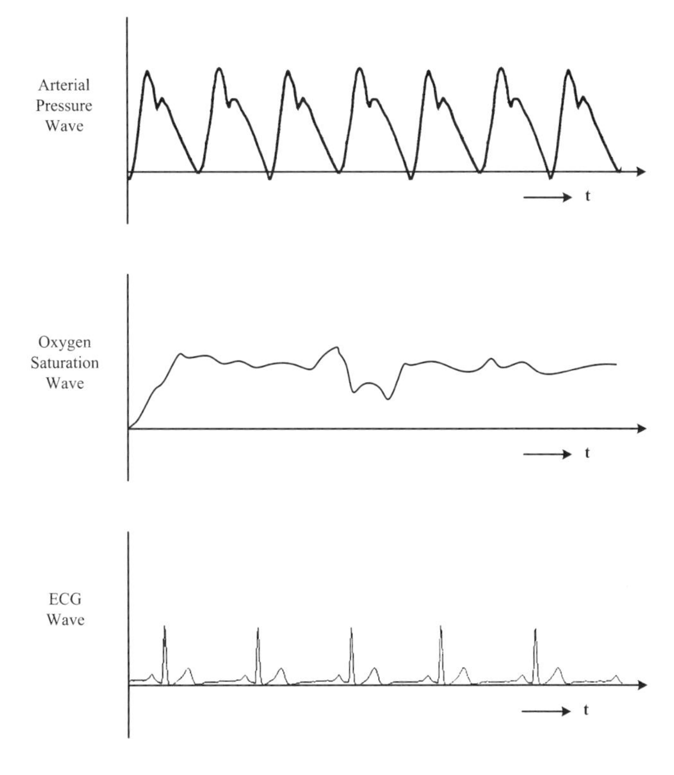

FIGURE 3-8 Various biosignals shown as voltage waveforms.

Bioacoustic signals measure distinctive sounds using microphones. The sound blood flow makes as it passes through heart valves opening and closing or the sound muscles and joints make against the skin are measured with bioacoustic signals.

Figure 3-8 shows various biosignals. The arterial blood pressure wave and the ECG wave are repetitive, whereas the oxygen saturation in the blood is not repetitive. These are acquired by specific electrodes and sensors and are very small-amplitude waves in the order of millivolts.

3.5 DIGITIZATION OF BIOSIGNALS

The aforementioned signals are all considered analog signals that cannot be sent to the computers or to the hospital networks without converting them into digital signals. These digital signals can be represented by binary and hexadecimal digits as ones and zeros. The following steps are taken to make an analog signal into a digital signal:

1. Sample the analog signal with the sampling rate at least two times the maximum frequency of the analog signal.
2. Convert the sampled signal into digits—typically eight digits (or bits) or more per sample.

The number of samples as well as the number of bits per sample is crucial in determining the resolution of the conversion from analog to digital.

An analog signal and a pulse signal are shown in **Figure 3-9a**. For sampling, these two signals are multiplied in time-domain and a series of samples of the analog signal results

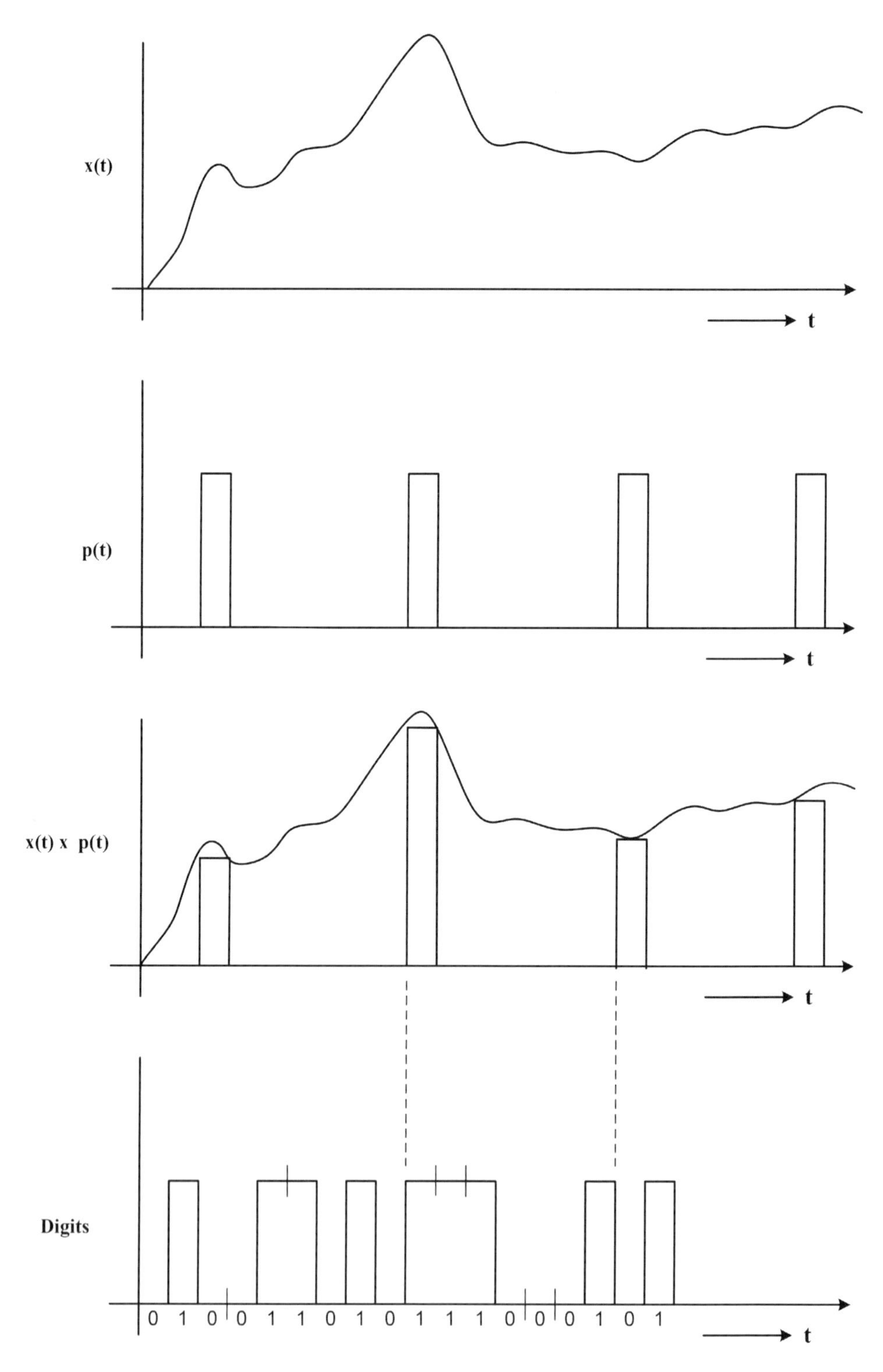

FIGURE 3-9a The digitization process of an analog signal x(t).

and is shown in **Figure 3-9a.** The digits are created based upon the height (or the amplitude) of these samples. Typically, the larger the amplitudes, the more binary ones will be in the digits. This is shown in **Figure 3-9b.** The digitization process is discussed next.

Digitization Process

Consider a three-bit analog-to-digital conversion process with the actual sample values of 1.6 V, 0.8 V, and 3.5 V. The three-bit conversion is based upon the eight quantized levels and the range of 0 V to 7 V. The result is the actual sample values rounded off to the quantized

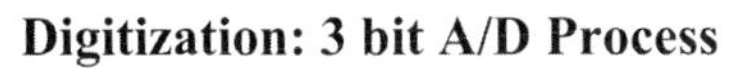

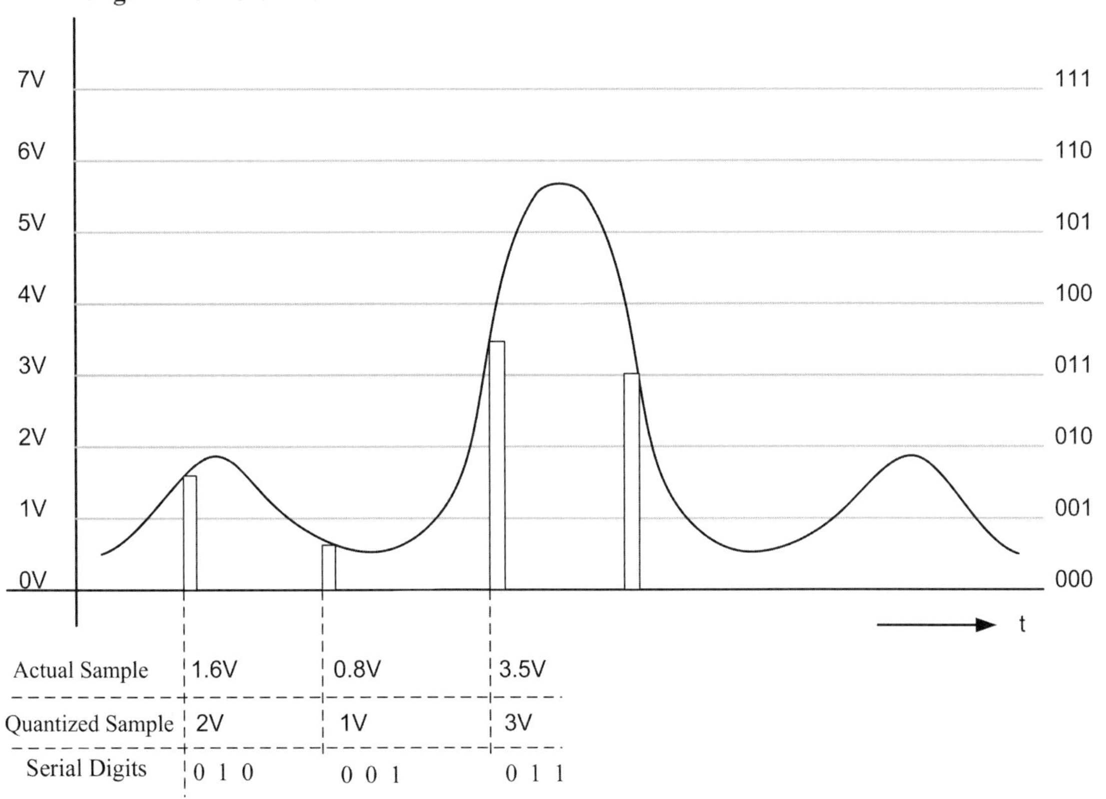

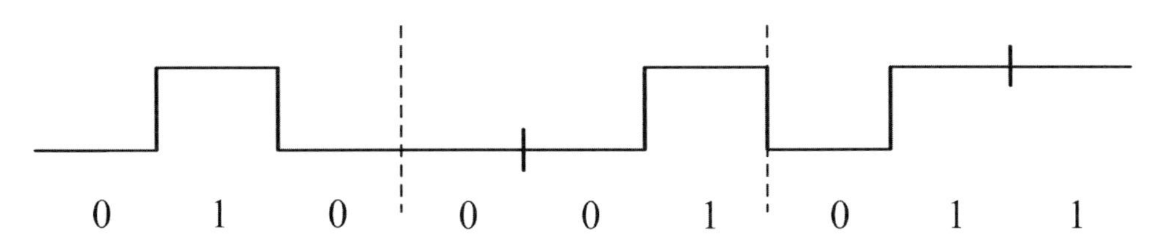

FIGURE 3-9b A three-bit digitization process.

level values equivalent to the specific digits. As shown in **Figure 3-9b,** the final digits are 010 001 011 for the corresponding sample values.

In general, we can digitize any analog signal by knowing the step size of the quantized levels and the amplitude range.

For a three-bit system (that is, the number of bits n = 3), and the range of 8 V, then the

$$\begin{aligned}\text{Step size} &= (2^{-n})\,(\text{Range})\\ &= (2^{-3})\,(8\ \text{V})\\ &= \left(\frac{1}{8}\right)\times 8\\ &= 1\ \text{V}\end{aligned}$$

We can describe the resolution as = 1 V/step = step size.

This digitization process can be improvised for a various number of digital systems and the given amplitude ranges.

3.6 TYPES OF NOISE

Figure 3-10 shows a noise voltage. It appears as random electrical fluctuations and is defined as any undesirable electrical energy. Most biosignals are low-frequency and low-amplitude signals; moreover, the random noise has all the frequencies (including the

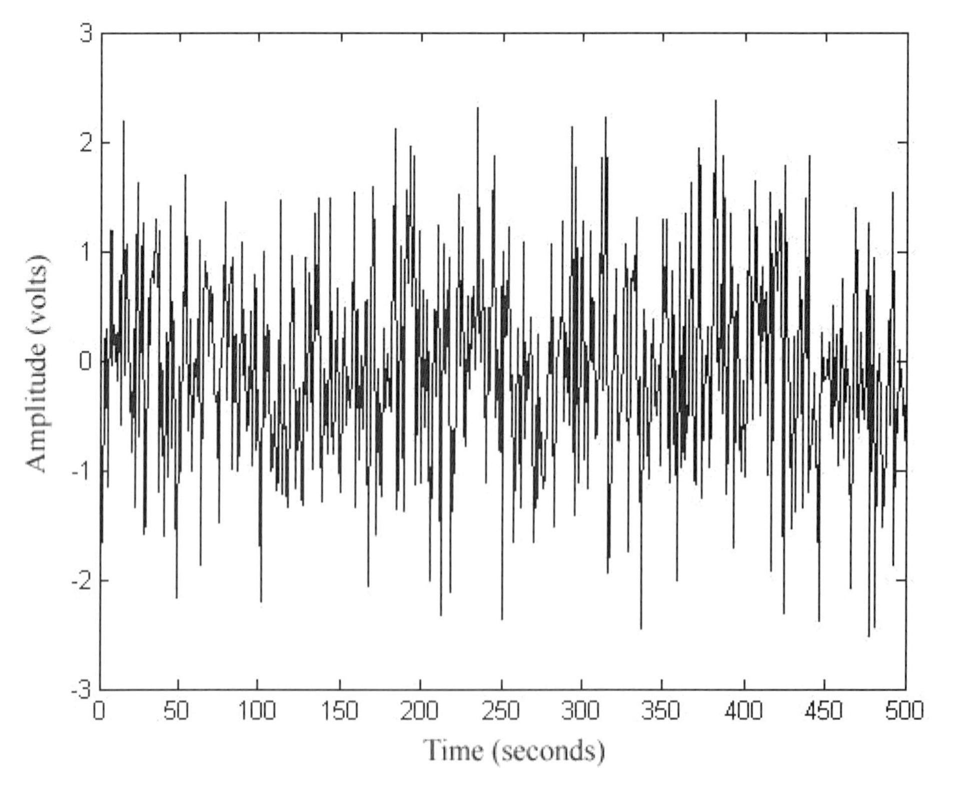

FIGURE 3-10 A white noise.

low-frequency range) and has low amplitudes. It is difficult to separate the actual signal from the noisy signal.

There are various noise sources in any electronic system that can corrupt the quality of the measured actual signal with unpredictable variations in measurements from moment to moment. From electric power fluctuations to interferences from RF radio transmissions, noise is also generated due to random thermal motion of molecules and the magnetic fields of the matter. Generally, the noise is not reproducible and it is not always the same—it can be unpredictable as we take measurements of the actual signals.

Some examples of noisy signals are given in the frequency-domain. **Figure 3-11a** shows a frequency plot of white noise and **Figure 3-11b** shows a frequency plot of pink noise. We can categorize a few important noise signals as follows:

White Noise

White noise has equal power spectral density at all frequencies. Its spectrum (shown in **Figure 3-11a**) is flat over a defined bandwidth.

The spectrum is flat out to about 20 kHz. The waveform contains frequency components of equal amplitude covering this 20 kHz range. Just as white light contains all visible color frequencies, white noise contains all of the audible sound frequencies.

White noise is also known as thermal noise. Free electrons within a conductor are in random motion as a result of receiving thermal energy. The average thermal noise power is proportional to the temperature of the conductor and the frequency bandwidth of the thermal noise. The relationship is given as:

$$P_n = K \times T \times B \text{ watts}$$

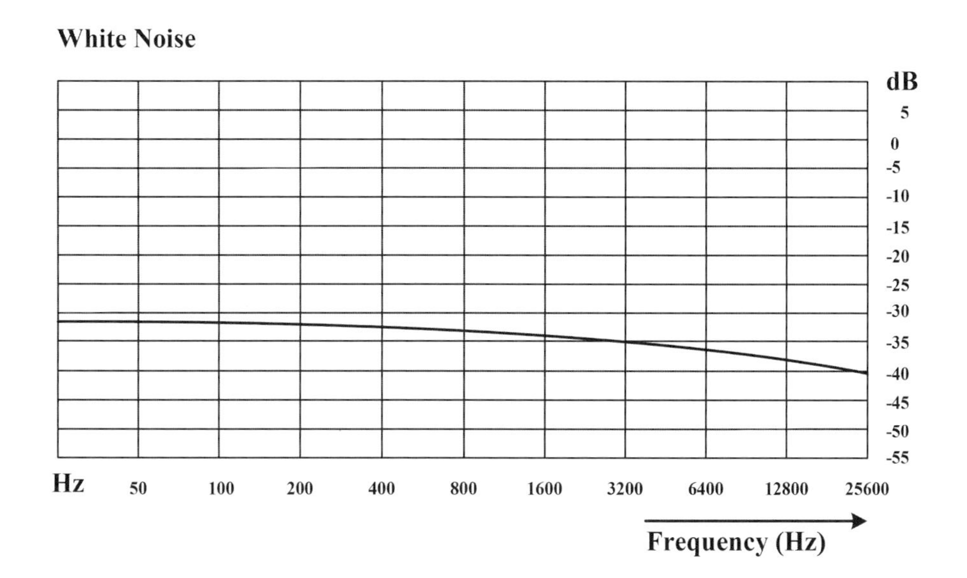

FIGURE 3-11a A frequency plot of white noise.

where,

P_n = Average thermal noise power in watts.
T = Temperature of the conductor in degrees kelvin
B = Bandwidth of the noise spectrum in hertz
K = Boltzmann's constant = 1.38×10^{-23} joules/kelvin

Shown below, the noise power generated in the conductor is interpreted by the hertz of the spectrum at room temperature (i.e., T = 290° K and 1 Hz of bandwidth).

$$\begin{aligned} P_n &= 1.38 \times 10^{-23} \times 290 \times 1 \\ &= 4 \times 10^{-21} \text{ watts} \end{aligned}$$

If the bandwidth changes, then for a bandwidth of 1 MHz,

$$\begin{aligned} P_n &= 1.38 \times 10^{-23} \times 290 \times 10^6 \\ &= 4 \times 10^{-15} \text{ watts} \end{aligned}$$

The noise power has increased with the larger bandwidth. Even though the noise power is small, the noise power in the biosignals seems also to be in the same order of magnitude.

The RMS signal power can be calculated for a source of 10 μV peak (as an example) with 50 Ω source resistance and 50 Ω load resistance.

$$P_S = \frac{[V_S \text{ peak}]^2}{2 \times (R_S + R_L)}$$

$$P_S = \frac{(10 \times 10^{-6})^2}{4 \times 50} \text{ watts}$$

$$= 5 \times 10^{-13} \text{ watts}$$

The signal-to-noise ratio for a 1 MHz bandwidth is then calculated as:

$$\frac{S}{N} = \frac{P_S}{P_n} = \frac{5 \times 10^{-13} \text{ watts}}{4 \times 10^{-15} \text{ watts}}$$

$$\frac{S}{N} = \frac{P_S}{P_n} = 1.25 \times 10^2$$

$$\frac{S}{N} = \frac{P_S}{P_n} = 125$$

Pink Noise

Pink noise is noise whose spectrum density (watts/hertz) varies as the inverse of the frequency considered. See **Figure 3-11b** for a frequency plot of pink noise. At certain frequency bands, pink noise has the same amount of energy, such as at 800 Hz to 1,600 Hz and 3,000 Hz to 6,000 Hz. However, the amount of energy in white noise is always equal, irrespective of bands.

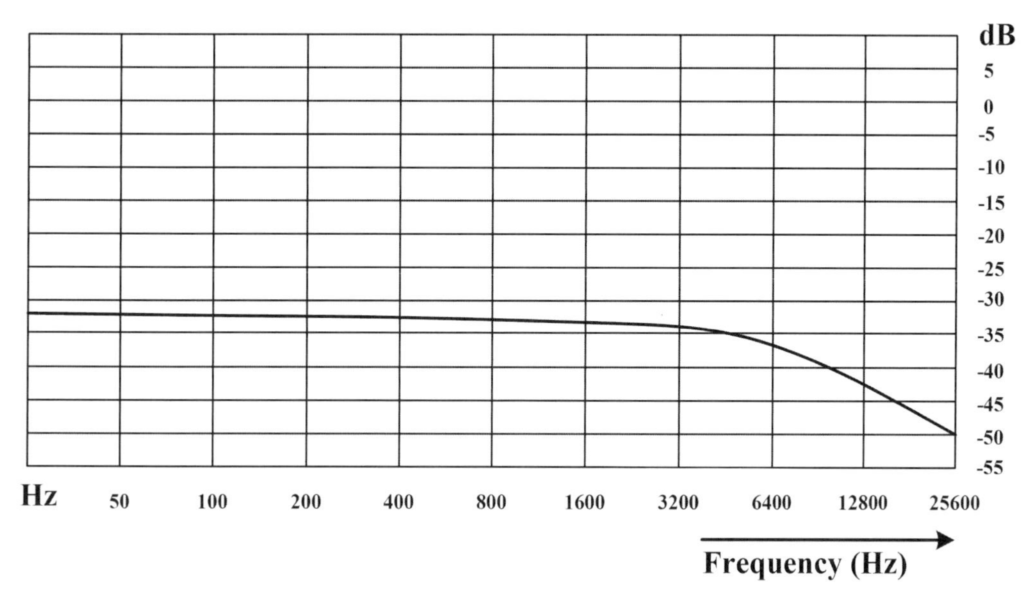

FIGURE 3-11b A frequency plot of pink noise.

3.7 PARAMETERS OF NOISE

Noise can be explained by parameters such as signal-to-noise ratio (SNR), noise figure, and noise temperature.

Signal-to-noise ratio (S/N ratio or SNR) is the ratio of the actual signal power to the noise power. This ratio indicates the magnitude of the noise power in comparison with the signal power and can be calculated at the input and output of the electronic devices.

Noise figure determines the degree of noisiness in an amplifier or any electronic device. An ideal amplifier should not add any internal noise to the actual signal that needs to be amplified. However, this is not possible; all amplifiers generate internal noise, which is amplified in addition to the actual signal. The degree of noise generation varies in different electronic amplifiers. Noise figure is the ratio of SNR at the input to the SNR at the output of the amplifier. Noise figure is also referred to as noise factor or noise ratio.

$$NF = (S/N)_i/(S/N)_o$$

Noise figure can also be defined in decibels:

$$NF(dB) = 10 \times \log(NF)$$

The larger the value, the higher the degree of noisiness in the electronic device such as an amplifier or a receiver.

Noise temperature is an equivalent temperature that will produce equivalent noise power. We can relate the noise figure to a noise temperature. This noise temperature is not the physical noise temperature of the device or amplifier at its input or output. As discussed earlier, the noise power is directly proportional to temperature in degrees kelvin and the noise power tends to zero out at zero degrees kelvin. In other words, if the electronic device adds no noise, then the signal-to-noise ratio is the same at the input and the output and the noise figure is 0 dB. The noise temperature of the device is then 0 degree kelvin and it is called a "cool" device. On the other hand, if the device adds to the incoming noise, the noise temperature will also increase and the device is no longer referred to as "cool." The noise temperature is given as T_e.

$$T_e = T(NF - 1)$$

where T = temperature of the environment and NF = noise figure as a ratio and not in decibels.

EXAMPLE A voltage amplifier is operating at a temperature of 20° C with a bandwidth of 20 KHz; determine the thermal noise power in watts. Also, determine the noise voltage when the internal resistance of the amplifier is 100 Ω and its load resistance is also 100 Ω.

The thermal noise power is given as:

$$N = K \times T \times B$$
$$N = (1.38 \times 10^{-23}) \times (20^\circ + 273^\circ) \times (2 \times 10^4)$$
$$N = 800.2 \times 10^{-19}$$
$$N = 8 \times 10^{-17}\ \text{W}$$

Also the noise voltage is given as:

$$V_N = \sqrt{4R_L KTB}$$
$$V_N = \sqrt{4 \times 100 \times 8 \times 10^{-17}}$$
$$V_N = 0.18\mu\text{V}$$

■

EXAMPLE The output signal voltage of an amplifier is 5 V and the output noise voltage is 0.005 V. Determine the signal-to-noise power ratio in decibels. Ignore the source resistance.

The formula of the signal-to-noise power ratio is given as:

$$\frac{S}{N} = \frac{P_{signal}}{P_{noise}} = \frac{P_s}{P_n}$$

This formula applies as:

$$\frac{S}{N}(\text{dB}) = 10 \log \times \left(\frac{\frac{V^2_{signal}}{R_L}}{\frac{V^2_{noise}}{R_L}} \right)$$

$$\frac{S}{N}(\text{dB}) = 10 \log \times \frac{V^2_{signal}}{V^2_{noise}} = 20 \log \times \frac{V_{signal}}{V_{noise}}$$

$$\frac{S}{N}(\text{dB}) = 20 \log \times \frac{5\ \text{V}}{0.005\ \text{V}}$$

$$\frac{S}{N}(\text{dB}) = 60\ \text{dB}$$

■

EXAMPLE A non-ideal amplifier has the following parameters:

Input signal power $= 5 \times 10^{-11}$ W

Input noise power $= 5 \times 10^{-20}$ W

Power gain of the amplifier $= 10^6$

Internal noise power (generated in the amplifier $= 5 \times 10^{-12}$ W

Determine the noise figure in decibels.

Since the input signal power and noise power are given, the input signal-to-noise power ratio is:

$$\frac{S}{N} = \frac{5 \times 10^{-11}\ \text{W}}{5 \times 10^{-20}\ \text{W}} = 10^9$$

$$\frac{S}{N}(\text{dB}) = 10 \log 10^9 = 90\ \text{dB}$$

At the output of the amplifier,

Output signal power

$$\text{output signal power} = (\text{power given}) \times (\text{input signal power})$$
$$\text{output signal power} = (10^6) \times (5 \times 10^{-11}\ \text{W}) = 5 \times 10^{-5}\ \text{W}$$

Output noise power

$$\text{output noise power} = (\text{gain}) \times (\text{input noise power}) + (\text{internal noise})$$
$$\text{output noise power} = (10^6) \times (5 \times 10^{-20}\ \text{W}) + (5 \times 10^{-12}\ \text{W})$$
$$\text{output noise power} = (5 \times 10^{-14}\ \text{W}) + (5 \times 10^{-12}\ \text{W})$$
$$= (0.05 \times 10^{-12}\ \text{W}) + (5 \times 10^{-12}\ \text{W})$$

$\frac{S}{N}$ and $\frac{S}{N}$dB

$$\frac{S}{N} = \frac{\text{output signal power}}{\text{output noise power}} = \frac{5 \times 10^{-5}\ \text{W}}{5 \times 10^{-12}\ \text{W}}$$

$$\frac{S}{N} = 0.99 \times 10^7$$

$$\frac{S}{N}(\text{dB}) = 10 \log \times (0.99 \times 10^7) \approx 70\ \text{dB}$$

Output noise power

$$\text{Noise Factor} = \text{NF} = \frac{\text{input}\ \frac{S}{N}}{\text{output}\ \frac{S}{N}}$$

$$\text{Noise Factor} = \frac{10^9}{10^7} = 100$$

Hence, the noise figure in decibels is calculated as:

$$\text{NF(dB)} = 10 \log 100 = 20\ \text{dB}$$

■

EXAMPLE Determine the noise temperature for a noise figure of 7 dB. The environmental temperature is 290 K.

$$\text{NF(dB)} = 10 \log \text{NF} = 7 \text{ dB}$$

$$\frac{7}{10} \text{ dB} = \log \text{NF}$$

$$\text{antilog}\left(\frac{7}{10}\right) = \text{NF}$$

$$\text{NF} = 5$$

Therefore, the noise temperature is:

$$\text{Te} = \text{T(NF} - 1)$$
$$\text{Te} = 290(5 - 1)$$
$$\text{Te} = 1{,}160 \text{ K}$$

or

$$\text{Te} = 1{,}160 - 273 = 887^\circ \text{ C}$$

■

3.8 EXAMPLES OF BIOMEDICAL NOISY SIGNALS

Figure 3-12a and **Figure 3-12b** show noisy ECG signals. In **Figure 3-12a,** the ECG signal is offset from the baseline due to DC noise generated due to an electrode not properly fixed on the skin surface. In **Figure 3-12b,** the ECG signal is corrupted with the 50 Hz and the

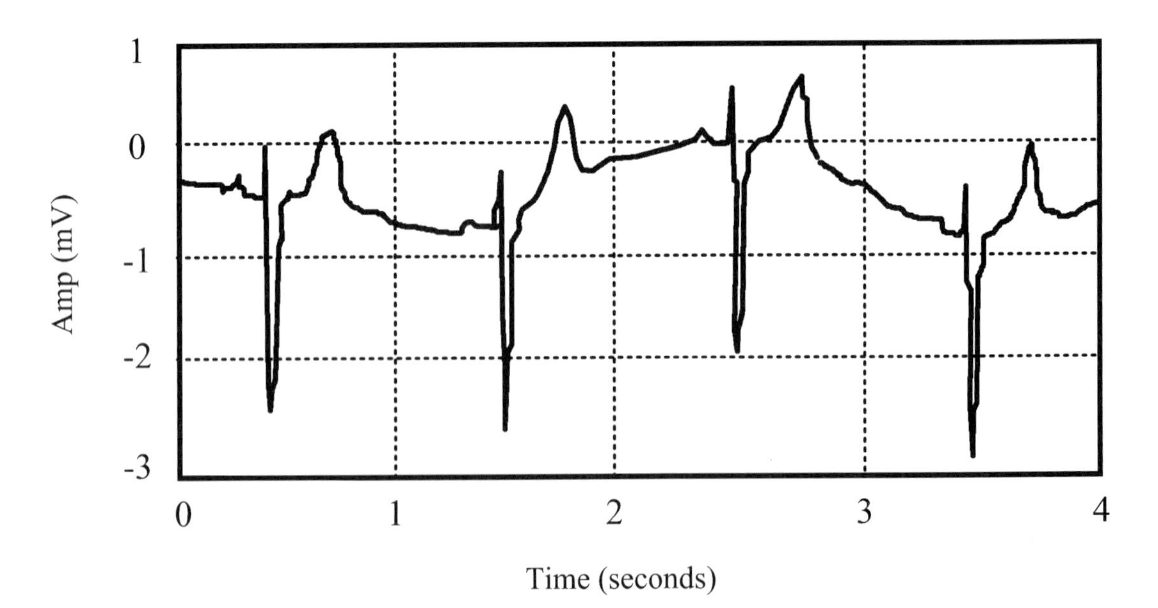

FIGURE 3-12a A wandering ECG signal.

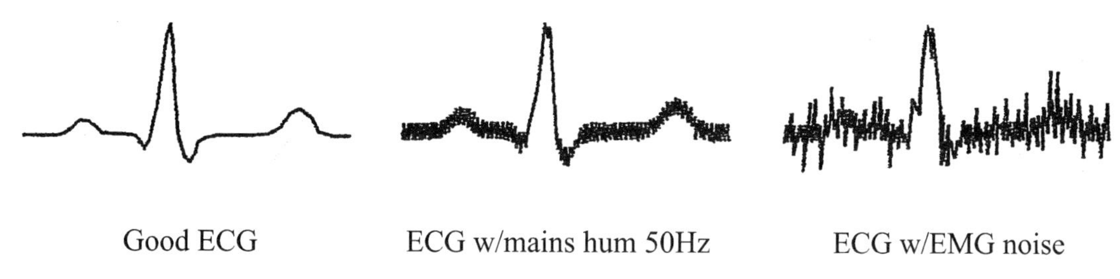

FIGURE 3-12b Noisy ECG signals.

EMG noises. In general, the acquired physiological signals are noisy signals and they are generated from different areas of the body. There is always a mixture of useful information and the unwanted noise in the measurement of the physiological signals. The use of electronic circuits and the computer software algorithms are always needed in acquiring the accurate information from this mixture of signals and the noise. In this chapter, we will only identify the noisy biosignals based upon the concepts discussed earlier.

SUMMARY

- Biosignals are physiological events such as electrical, chemical, or mechanical activity that occur in the human body and that can be measured, displayed, and recorded.
- Any practical signal consists of the sum of different sinusoids having different amplitudes, frequencies, and phases.
- The time-domain and frequency-domain of a signal are related by the Fourier series and Fourier transforms. The series provides the summation of sinusoidal signals with their amplitudes, frequencies, and phases to generate a periodic signal, whereas the Fourier transforms are for the nonperiodic signals.
- The most common type of bioelectric signal is ECG. Other signals such as biochemical, biomechanical, biomagnetic and the bioacoustic signals are used in biomedicine.
- Analog signals cannot be sent to computers or to hospital networks without converting them into digital signals. These digital signals can be represented by binary and hexadecimal digits as ones and zeros.
- Noise temperature is an equivalent temperature that will produce equivalent noise power. We can relate the noise figure to a noise temperature.

MEDICAL TERMINOLOGY

The following is a list of medical terminology mentioned in this chapter.

Audio signal: a waveform consisting of both high and low frequencies producing auditory sound. The signal can be converted to electrical signals by transducers with the ability to sense air pressure and vibrations.

Bandwidth: a range of frequencies, expressed in hertz (Hz), that can be carried on a transmission medium.

Biosignal: a biological function that is received through sensors and may be converted to electrical signals for analysis of the function.

Digital signal: a signal that is both discrete in time and quantized.

Digitized signal: a signal that has been converted from continuous time to a discrete time signal.

Discrete signal: a sampled continuous signal; the first process of the digital signal.

Frequency-domain: a signal strength that can be represented graphically as a function of frequency, instead of a function of time, pertaining to a method of analysis.

Harmonics: a frequency of the signal that is an integer multiple of the fundamental frequency (that is, if f is the frequency, then the harmonics are 2f, 3f, 4f, etc.).

Periodic signal: a signal that repeats its values after a defined time period.

Phase: the angular position of the signal within a cycle of the waveform.

Quantization: the conversion of a discrete signal (a sampled continuous signal) into one of finite steps or levels.

Resolution: a numerical value representing the quality of a signal to be reproduced back to its original waveform. It could also be considered the accuracy or dynamic range of a sensor's ability to detect minute biological changes.

Sampling: the process of converting a continuous time signal into a discrete signal by recording samples of the signal at set time intervals.

Sinusoidal signal: a smooth, continuously moving waveform that has positive and negative half-cycles that are generally symmetrical with respect to a reference. The waveform has a specified frequency in hertz (number of cycles per second) and specified amplitude.

Spectral: an efficient method to transform a time series into frequency.

Thermal noise: noise created by the movement and thus collision of electrons in a conductor. This disruption in the signal happens regardless of any applied voltage.

Time-domain: the analysis of mathematical functions, for real-life signals, with respect to time.

Video signal: a recoverable string of electrical impulses generated by the scanning of a two-dimensional image produced by optical conversion.

White noise: a random signal where the signal's power spectral density has equal power in any band, and at any center frequency, having a given bandwidth. This is similar to white light, which contains all frequencies.

QUIZ

1. Which biosignal is not periodic?

   a) Blood pressure. b) EEG. c) Mean blood pressure. d) Respiration.

2. A signal is represented by three parameters. What are they?

   a) ____________________

   b) ____________________

   c) ____________________

3. A sinusoidal voltage signal has a max height (amplitude) of 3 V and a frequency of 100 Hz. What is its value at t = 1 second?

   a) −2.99 V b) −1.52V c) −0.94V d) None of the above.

4. The number of levels in a seven-bit resolution is:
   a) 256 b) 128 c) 64 d) 32
5. The best sampling rate for a 10 Hz signal is:
   a) 20 Hz b) 40 Hz c) 60 Hz d) 80 Hz
6. An ECG signal, after amplification, has a range of −10 mV to +70 mV. What will be its range if noise offsets it by −20 mV?
7. What is the bandwidth of a normal ECG signal?
   a) 100 Hz. b) Less than 10 Hz. c) More that 10 Hz. d) None of the above.
8. How does pulse width (in the sampling process) relate to the number of harmonics?
9. A 40 Hz EEG signal is sampled by 100 Hz pulse, how many samples will be taken in one minute?
   a) 6,000 b) 4,000 c) 4,800 d) None of the above.
10. What is the resolution in a six-bit A/D conversion with a range of 10 V?

PROBLEMS

1. Write an equation of a signal that adds four sinusoidal signals and a DC offset: 1 kHz, 2 V(p-p); 6 kHz, 3 V(p); 10 kHz, 1.5 V(p); and 12 kHz, 5 V(p-p). The DC offset is −4 V. Also, determine the amplitude of the signal at time t = 0.1 second.
2. Determine the amplitude of a signal that adds three sinusoidal signals: $2\sin(\omega \times t + 45°)$, $-4\sin(\omega \times t - 78°)$, and $5\sin(\omega \times t - 22°)$. Given: frequency of the signal is 2 kHz and time t = 0.2 second.
3. For the given pulse signal shown in **Figure 3-13,** determine the frequencies and amplitudes of the third and eighth harmonic. Given: fundamental frequency = 2 kHz.

$$\text{Duty cycle} = \frac{\tau}{T} = 10\% = 0.1$$

$$\text{Amplitude} = 10\ \text{V}$$

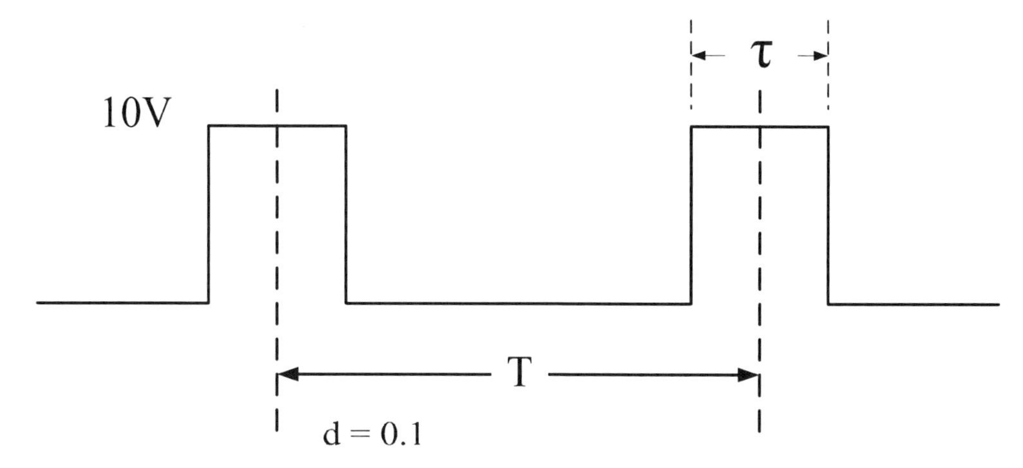

FIGURE 3-13 A rectangular wave.

4. For the given square wave shown in **Figure 3-14,** determine the amplitudes and frequencies of its first 10 harmonics. Now write the Fourier series for these harmonics. Given: fundamental frequency = 100 Hz

$$\text{Duty cycle} = \frac{\tau}{T} = 50\% = 0.5$$

$$\text{Amplitude} = 5\text{ V}$$

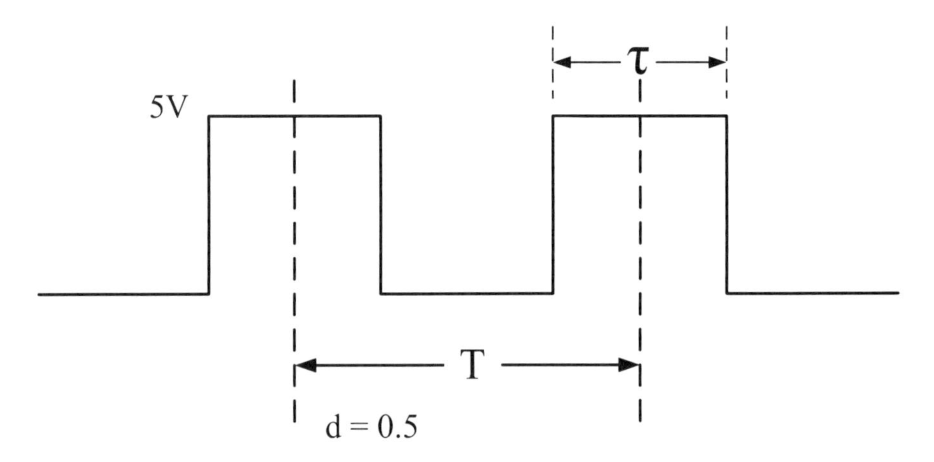

FIGURE 3-14 A square wave signal.

5. First, generate the square wave of Problem 4 with fundamental and its first five harmonics using MATLAB or any appropriate software. Next, generate the square wave with all harmonics as computed in Problem 4. Compare and contrast the two results.
6. For a six-bit A/D conversion, determine the digits for a 3.2 V analog sample when the full range is 0 V to 10 V.
7. For the binary 101101 digits, determine the analog voltage from the process given in Problem 6.
8. The sampling frequency of an EMG signal is 220 Hz. How many samples are taken in 1.2 minutes? What is the bandwidth of the EMG signal?
9. A biosignal has a minimum voltage of −20 mV and a maximum voltage of +85 mV. What is the resolution of an eight-bit A/D conversion process?
10. Thermal noise from a resistor is measured as 10×10^{-17} W for a given bandwidth and at a temperature of 30° C. Calculate noise power when the temperature is changed (a) to 40° C; (b) to 80° K.
11. Calculate the noise figure of an electronic system with a noise temperature of 100° C.
12. Make a table of equivalence between noise figure and the noise temperature starting with the noise figure of 1 dB and ending with the noise figure of 10 dB.

CASE STUDIES

1. Jack used a wireless Holter monitor for a month. His ECG signal was monitored through cell tower transmissions. The sensor was connected to the three chest leads and was sending signals to the wireless monitor placed in his pocket. This case raises several questions in regard to noise:

a) What types of noise can ruin a proper ECG signal in this wireless media?

b) There are two wireless links in this Holter system, one from the sensor to the monitor in his pocket, and the other from the monitor to the closest cell tower. Discuss the noise created due to Jack's movements and his daily chores that affect the ECG signal.

c) Compare the severity of various types of noise in this case.

2. Patients with different diseases have distinct voice signals and, in some cases, these voices are considered abnormal. Doctors can monitor these voice signals, particularly the laryngeal disease. These cases raise a few questions:

a) What are the abnormal voices in related diseases?

b) How do different voice signals look in time-domains and frequency-domains?

c) What are the various laryngeal diseases and what is the physiology of each? What is the pathology of each?

RESEARCH TOPICS

1. Differentiate Fourier series with Fourier transforms and develop equations for the Fourier transforms of the biosignals. Investigate advantages and disadvantages of the Fourier transforms in general, and then of the biosignal.

2. The physiological signals are a noisy mixture of several source signals arising from the body and there are a vast number of software products that can create more accurate medical profiles of the patient signals. Write a research paper that will include a medical software product for acquiring and processing the physiological signals and also the methodology/mathematical techniques used in the software.

3. Examples of voice waveforms and their frequency spectrum are useful information to understand the bandwidth and sampling requirements in signal processing. This research paper can be extended by collecting information on video waveforms and their spectrums.

4. Voice or speech recognition software and hardware from IBM and Dragon Systems helped the ability of a computer to interpret dictation. The speech patterns are stored in the digital database and compared with any new spoken word. The research paper should include the technology of A/D and D/A used in voice recognition by different companies.

CHAPTER 4

Biomedical Electronics: Analog

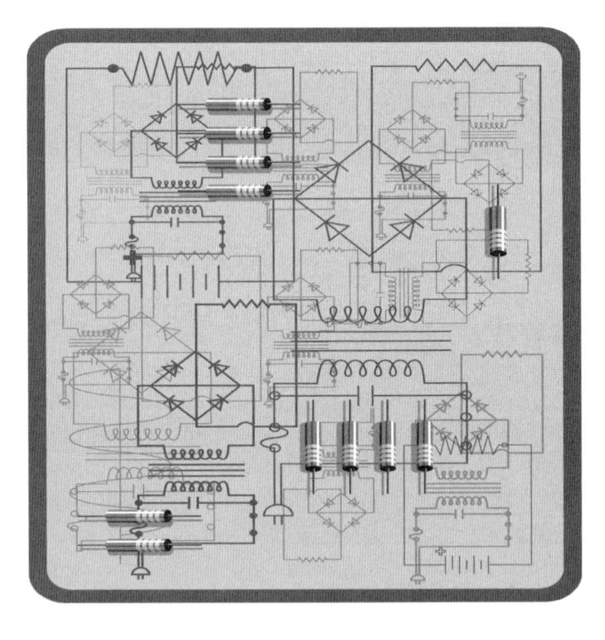

■ CHAPTER OUTLINE

■ OBJECTIVES

The objective of this chapter is to review the concepts of analog electronics and to gain an understanding of the electronic circuits and devices used in biomedical equipment and machines.

Upon completion of this chapter, the reader will be able to:

- Identify analog circuits.
- Identify reactances and impedances.
- Identify loading and max power problems in electronics.
- Identify DC and AC characteristics of operational amplifier ICs.
- Derive output for inventing or non-inventing amplifier.

INTERNET WEB SITES

http://www.ti.com (Texas Instruments)
http://www.national.com (National Semiconductor)
http://www.ni.com (National Instruments)

INTRODUCTION

This chapter is a review of the electronic principles as they apply to biomedical circuits and instrumentation. After reading this chapter, you should be familiar with the electronic workings of medical instruments. While medical instruments have circuit modules that can be replaced easily if they do not work properly, biomedical technicians and engineers need to know the concepts of the various circuits and their functions involving these modules. We begin this chapter discussing the basic circuit analysis with resistors, capacitors, and inductors. Next, we discuss semiconductor devices and their circuits. Finally, we discuss operational amplifiers and the use of op-amps in differentiators, integrators, waveshapers, Schmitt triggers, filters, and sensors.

Figure 4-1a shows the various types of analog electronic circuits used in medical equipment.

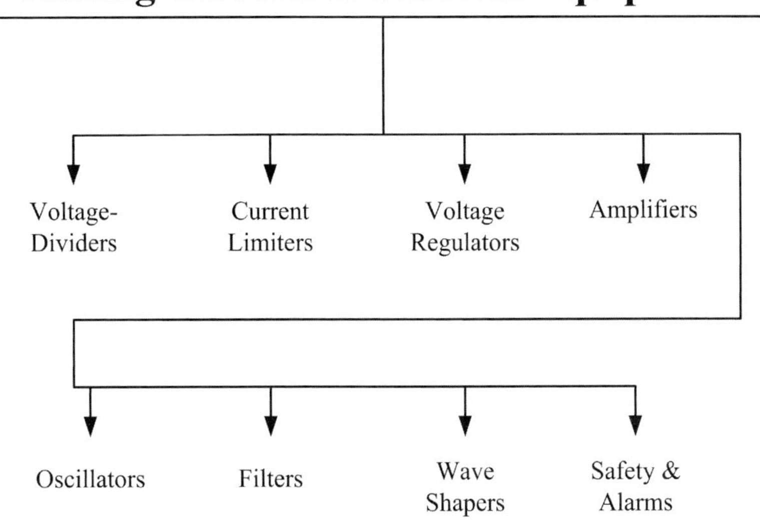

FIGURE 4-1a Analog circuits used in medical equipment.

Electronic circuits in biomedical applications with semiconductor devices, such as diodes, transistors, and operational amplifiers, can be divided into the following categories.

Amplifiers

Low-voltage medical signals can be amplified by semiconductor circuits so that they can be viewed on a scope or a monitor. An operational amplifier (op-amp) is an example of such a device. This type of device is referred to as an integrated device (also called an integrated chip, or IC) because it has several discrete transistors on its semiconductor wafer.

Waveshapers

Medical signals sometimes need waveshaping through comparators, rectifiers, and regulators such as op-amp comparators, diode rectifiers, Zener regulators, power supplies, and simple transformers.

Filters

There are various categories of op-amp filters used for filtering unwanted frequencies in medical signals. Most medical signals are low-frequency signals. Unwanted high frequencies need to be filtered out so that clean and accurate signals can be viewed for diagnostic purposes.

Safety and Alarms

Patient safety is a top priority. Many medical devices are equipped with features such as alarm circuits and isolation transformers.

Figure 4-1b shows some of the biomedical applications of various electronic circuits.

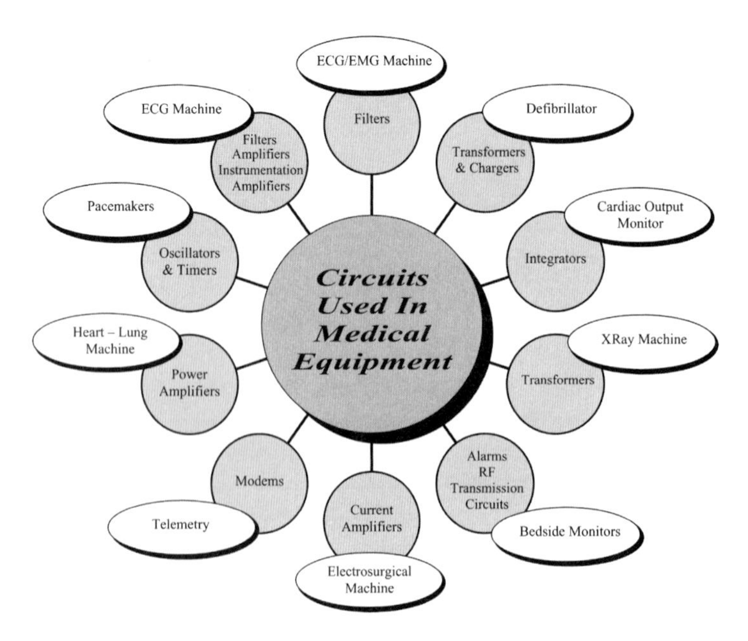

FIGURE 4-1b Various analog circuits used in medical equipment.

4.1 SERIES AND PARALLEL CIRCUITS

We use Ohm's law to relate voltage and current in a resistive circuit. This section explains the concepts of a series DC circuit and the concepts of a parallel DC circuit and we will learn how to calculate the total power delivered to the circuit and the power absorbed by a resistor in a series or a parallel circuit.

Ohm's law states the relationship among voltage, current, and resistance:

$$I = \frac{V}{R} \quad \text{or} \quad V = (I) \times (R) \quad \text{or} \quad R = \frac{V}{I}$$

where I is current, V is voltage, and R is the resistance in the circuit. The power is computed as

$$P = V \times I \quad \text{or} \quad \frac{V \times V}{R} \quad \text{or} \quad I \times R \times I$$

Series DC Circuit

The electronic components such as resistors, capacitors, and inductors all have properties that can restrict the amount of current flowing through them. All of these components exhibit the property of resistance to the flow of current. The property of resistance is measured in ohms. In capacitors and inductors, resistance is called reactance, as this property of resistance reacts to the applied signal frequency. The combination of resistance and reactance is called impedance. Impedance is measured also in ohms. Following is a discussion of the basic concepts of simple circuits.

A series circuit First, we will analyze a simple series resistive circuit with two resistors and a battery supplying a DC (direct current) voltage. This is shown in **Figure 4-2.**

Notice the ± polarities on the battery and the ground symbol.

V_S = Source voltage in volts (V)

I_S = Source current in amperes (A)

R_1, R_2 = Resistors in ohms (Ω)

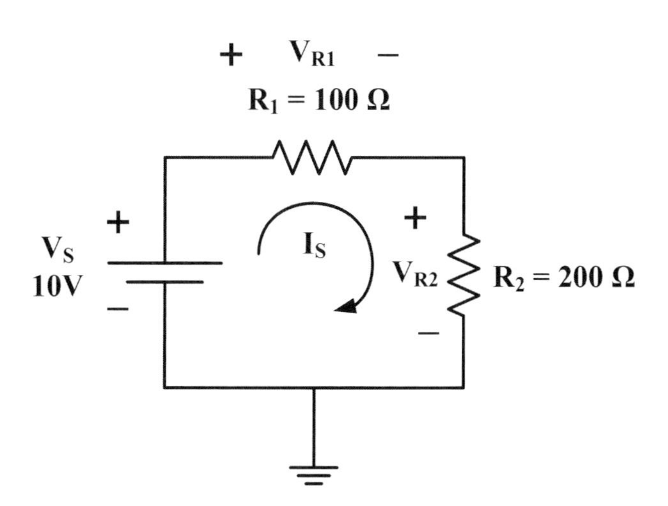

FIGURE 4-2 A simple series circuit.

Using Ohm's law:

$$I_S = \frac{\text{Applied Source Voltage}}{\text{Total Resistance in the circuit}} = \frac{V_S}{R_T} \text{ amperes or mA}$$

$$V_{R1} = \text{Voltage drop across } R_1 = R_1 \times I_S$$

$$V_{R2} = \text{Voltage drop across } R_2 = R_2 \times I_S$$

$$P_T = \text{Total power delivered to the circuit} = I_S \times V_S \text{ in watts or Joules/second}$$

$$P_{R1} = \text{Power absorbed by the resistor } R_1 = V_{R1} \times I_S \text{ in watts}$$

Voltage divider rule The other way to find the voltage drop across any resistor is to use the voltage divider rule.

Voltage drop across a resistor = (applied voltage to the circuit) × (resistance of the resistor) / (total resistance in the circuit).

$$V_{Rx} = V_S \times \frac{R_X}{R_T}$$

As an example, we will compute the current and the voltage drop across each resistor for the circuit in **Figure 4-2** with the given source voltage and values of resistances.

$$\text{Current} = I_S = \frac{10\text{ V}}{100\ \Omega + 200\ \Omega} = \frac{10\text{ V}}{300\ \Omega} = \frac{1}{30}\text{ Amps}$$

Voltage drop across 100 ohm resistor

$$\frac{1}{30}\text{ Amps} \times 100\ \Omega = 3.33\text{ V}$$

Voltage drop across 100 ohm resistor using the voltage divider rule

$$10\text{ V} \times \frac{100\ \Omega}{300\ \Omega} = 3.33\text{ V}$$

Notice the same voltage is determined by using the voltage divider rule.

Similarly, we can find the voltage drop across the 200 ohm resistor

$$10\text{ V} \times \frac{200\ \Omega}{300\ \Omega} = 6.67\text{ V}$$

If there are three resistors in series, we can find individual drops and their sum will be equal to the source voltage.

EXAMPLE See **Figure 4-3**, where the source voltage equals the sum of voltage drops across each resistor.

$$V_S = V_{R1} + V_{R2} + V_{R3}$$

$$V_S = \frac{100\ \Omega}{600\ \Omega} \times 10\text{ V} + \frac{200\ \Omega}{600\ \Omega} \times 10\text{ V} + \frac{300\ \Omega}{600\ \Omega} \times 10\text{ V}$$

$$V_S = \frac{1}{6} \times 10\text{ V} + \frac{1}{3} \times 10\text{ V} + \frac{1}{2} \times 10\text{ V}$$

$$V_S = 1.67\text{ V} + 3.33\text{ V} + 5\text{ V}$$

$$V_S = 10\text{ V}$$

Note: the larger the resistor value, the greater the voltage drop.

The rule of the summation of drops to the applied voltage is called Kirchhoff's voltage law.

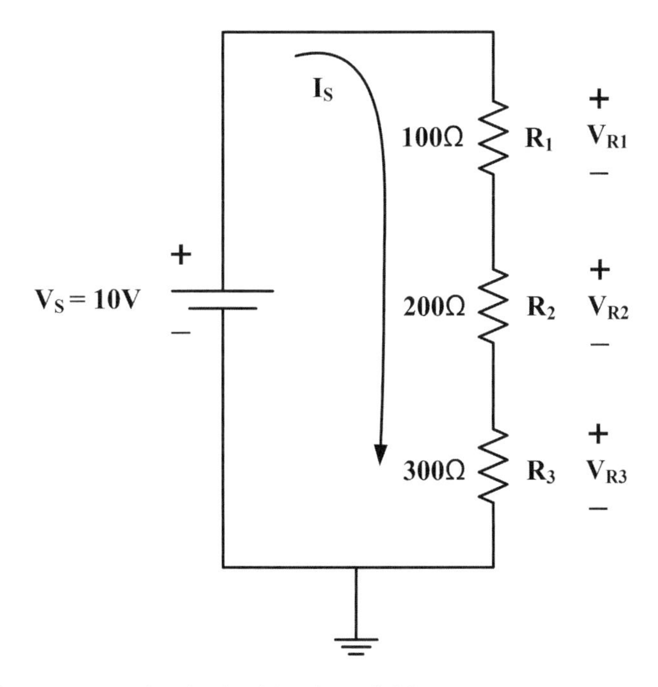

FIGURE 4-3 A simple series circuit with voltage divisions.

A parallel DC circuit **Figure 4-4** shows two resistors in a parallel. The voltage drop across each resistor will be the same as the applied voltage; the current will be different. The total current in the circuit will be the summation of these two currents.

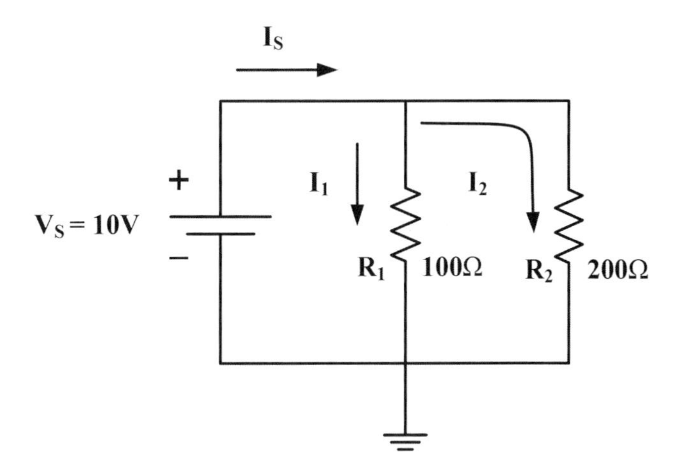

FIGURE 4-4 A simple parallel circuit with current divisions.

Current through the 100 Ω resistor = (applied voltage) / resistance

$$\frac{10\ \text{V}}{100\ \Omega} = 0.1\ \text{A}$$

Current through 200 ohm resistor

$$\frac{10\ \text{V}}{200\ \Omega} = 0.05\ \text{A}$$

Total current in the circuit

$$0.1\ \text{A} + 0.05\ \text{A} = 0.15\ \text{A}$$

Also, the total current I_S can be determined by first finding the total resistance in the circuit.

$$R_T = \text{total resistance in the parallel circuit} = \left(\frac{1}{R_1} + \frac{1}{R_2}\right)^{-1} = 66.7\ \Omega$$

$$I_S = \frac{V_S}{R_T} = \frac{10\ \text{V}}{R_T} = \frac{10\ \text{V}}{66.7\ \Omega} = 0.15\ \text{A}$$

Current divider rule If applied current to the circuit is given instead of applied voltage, we can determine the individual current through each resistor by the current divider rule.

Current through a resistor in a parallel circuit with two resistors = (applied current to the circuit) × (parallel opposite resistance) / (total resistance in the circuit).

Therefore, the current through the 100 Ω resistor in **Figure 4-4** is

$$0.15\ \text{A} \times \frac{200\ \Omega}{300\ \Omega} = 0.1\ \text{A}$$

If there are more than two resistors in a parallel circuit, then we have to either combine them before the current divider rule is applied or we can use the following formula:

$$I_X = \frac{R_T}{R_X} \times I_S$$

where R_T is the total resistance of the parallel circuit.

EXAMPLE Determine the current (I) and the voltage (V) drop across the 10 Ω resistor for the circuit of **Figure 4-5a.**

We can redraw the circuit as shown in **Figure 4-5b.**

$$\text{Total resistance } R_T = 5\ \Omega + 10\ \Omega + 5\ \Omega = 20\ \Omega$$

Total voltage (source) in the circuit

$$V_T = 20\ \text{V} - 10\ \text{V} = 10\ \text{V}$$

Total current in the circuit

$$I_T = \frac{V_T}{R_T} = \frac{10\ \text{V}}{20\ \Omega} = 0.5\ \text{A}$$

Voltage drop across the 10 Ω resistor is

$$V_{10\Omega} = (I_T) \times (10\ \Omega)$$
$$V_{10\Omega} = (0.5\ A) \times (10\ \Omega)$$
$$V_{10\Omega} = 5\ V$$

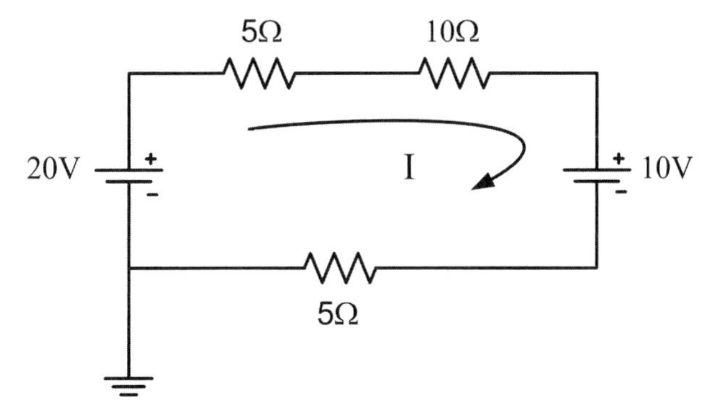

FIGURE 4-5a More than one power supply in a series circuit.

■

EXAMPLE Determine the voltage drop across the 10 Ω resistor using the voltage divider rule for the circuit in **Figure 4-5b.**

$$V_{10\Omega} = \frac{10\ \Omega}{R_T} \times V_T = \frac{10\ \Omega}{20\ \Omega} \times 10\ V = 5\ V$$

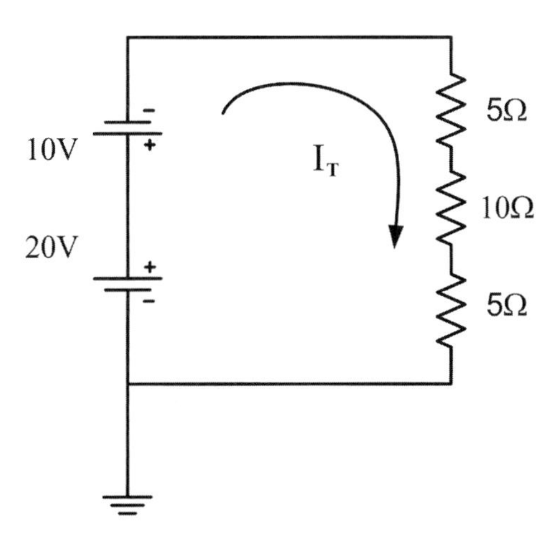

FIGURE 4-5b Rearranging power supplies of the circuit in Figure 4-5a.

■

EXAMPLE Find the total resistance and the current through the 10 Ω resistor for the circuit in **Figure 4-6a.**

Total resistance in the circuit is,

$$R_T = 5\ \Omega + \text{sum of parallel resistance}$$

$$R_T = 5\ \Omega + \left(\frac{1}{5\ \Omega} + \frac{1}{5\ \Omega} + \frac{1}{10\ \Omega}\right)^{-1}$$

$$R_T = 5\ \Omega + (0.2 + 0.2 + 0.1)^{-1}\ \Omega$$
$$R_T = 5\ \Omega + (0.5)^{-1}\ \Omega$$
$$R_T = 5\ \Omega + 2\ \Omega$$

$$R_T = 7\ \Omega \qquad I_T = \frac{10\ \text{V}}{7\ \Omega} = 1.43\ \text{A}$$

Now, we will use the current divider rule to find current through the 10 Ω resistor as shown in **Figure 4-6b.**

The current divider rule is used between the two resistors so we can combine the 5 Ω resistors as 2.5 Ω as shown in **Figure 4-6b.**

This leads us to the current divider rule:

$$I_{10\Omega} = \frac{\text{opposite resistance}}{\text{sum of resistances}} \times (1.43\ \text{A})$$

$$I_{10\Omega} = \frac{2.5\ \Omega}{2.5\ \Omega + 10\ \Omega} \times (1.43\ \text{A})$$

$$I_{10\Omega} = \frac{2.5\ \Omega}{12.5\ \Omega} \times (1.43\ \text{A})$$

$$I_{10\Omega} = 0.286\ \text{A}$$

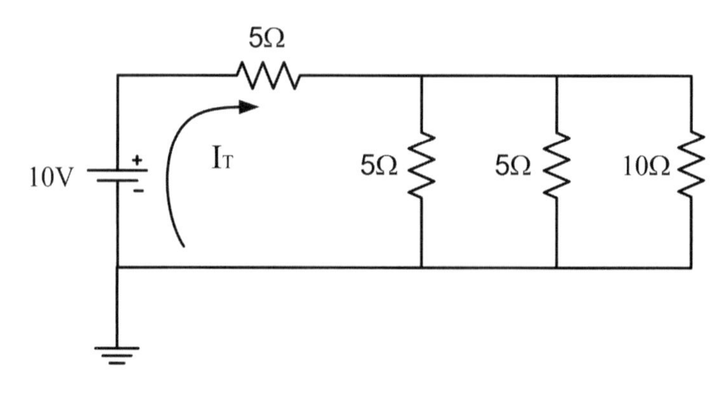

FIGURE 4-6a A simple series-parallel circuit.

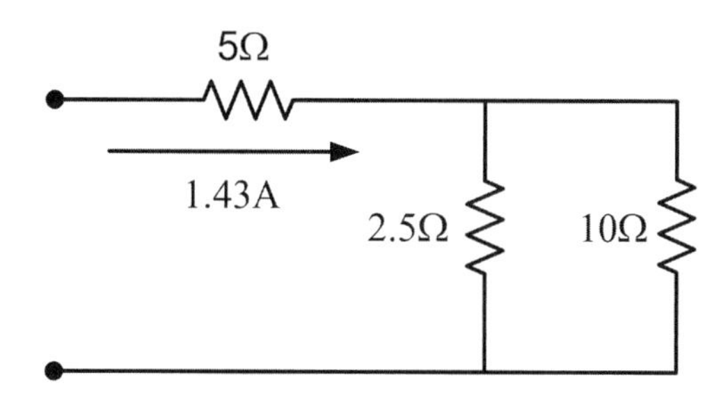

FIGURE 4-6b Simplifying the circuit of Figure 4-6a.

4.2 SERIES DC CAPACITIVE AND INDUCTIVE CIRCUITS

Capacitors and inductors are used in medical circuits for slow build up of voltage or current as delay components. They are used also in suppressing certain frequencies of a signal.

As we apply a DC voltage to a capacitor, the charge slowly builds up across the capacitor in approximately five time constants. The time constant in a capacitive circuit is a multiplied quantity of capacitance, and the total resistance of the circuit and its unit is in seconds. **Figure 4-7** shows a series capacitive circuit and the voltage and current.

A Series Capacitive Circuit

R = Series resistance in ohms (Ω)

C = Capacitance in microfarads (μF)

V_S = Source voltage

I_S = Source current

τ = Time constant = R × C in seconds

5 Time constants = 5 R × C

FIGURE 4-7 A simple RC series circuit.

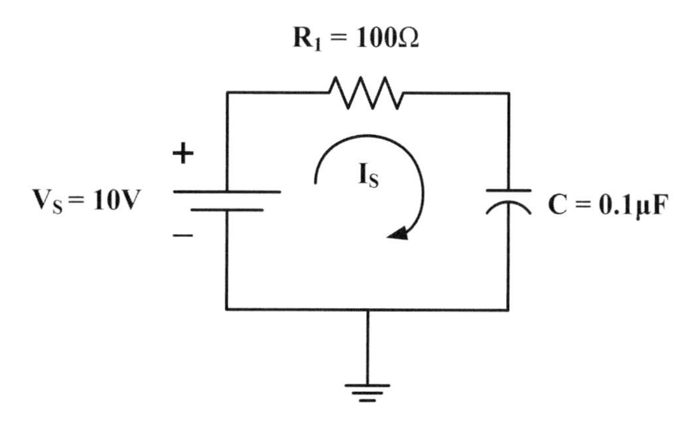

In the circuit of Figure 4-7,

Time constant $(\tau) = R \times C$

$$(\tau) = 100\ \Omega \times 0.1\ \mu F$$
$$(\tau) = 100 \times 0.1 \times 10^{-6}\ sec$$
$$(\tau) = 10\ \mu s$$

A Series Inductive Circuit

Similarly, we can find the current build up in an inductor shown in **Figure 4-8.**

L = Inductance in henries (mH)

R = Resistance in ohms (Ω)

V_S = Source voltage

I_S = Source current

τ = Time constant $= \frac{L}{R}$ sec

A universal time constant curve is shown in **Figure 4-9.** It can be used to compute the voltage or current build up in either capacitive or inductive circuits. The voltage or current is shown at each time constant before the maximum build up.

4.3 SUMMARY TABLE OF DC CONCEPTS

Device/Measurement	Action	Result
Series resistors	Simply add them together	R_T is larger than any single resistor value
Parallel resistors	Add them after inverting each value of the resistor, then invert the result	R_T is less than any single resistor value
Voltage drop in a series resistive circuit	The sum of drops equals the total source voltage	As the resistor value goes up, the value of the voltage drop also increases making them directly proportional
Currents in parallel circuits	Sum of branch currents equals the total current	As the resistor value goes up, the current value goes down making them inversely proportional
Capacitor	Voltage charges in a capacitor	Time constant $= R \times C$
Inductor	Current builds up in an inductor	Time constant $= \frac{L}{R}$

4.4 REACTANCES AND IMPEDANCES

The capacitors and inductors are frequency-dependent electronic components, but the resistors are frequency-independent components. The reactance of a capacitor is inversely proportional to the applied signal frequency. That is, the capacitor is a short at very high

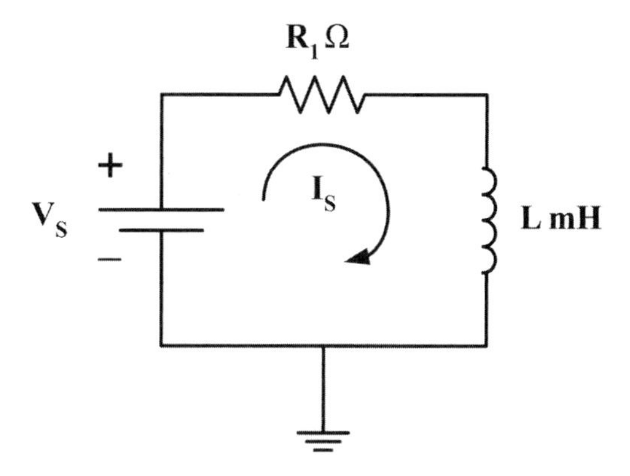

FIGURE 4-8 A simple RL series circuit.

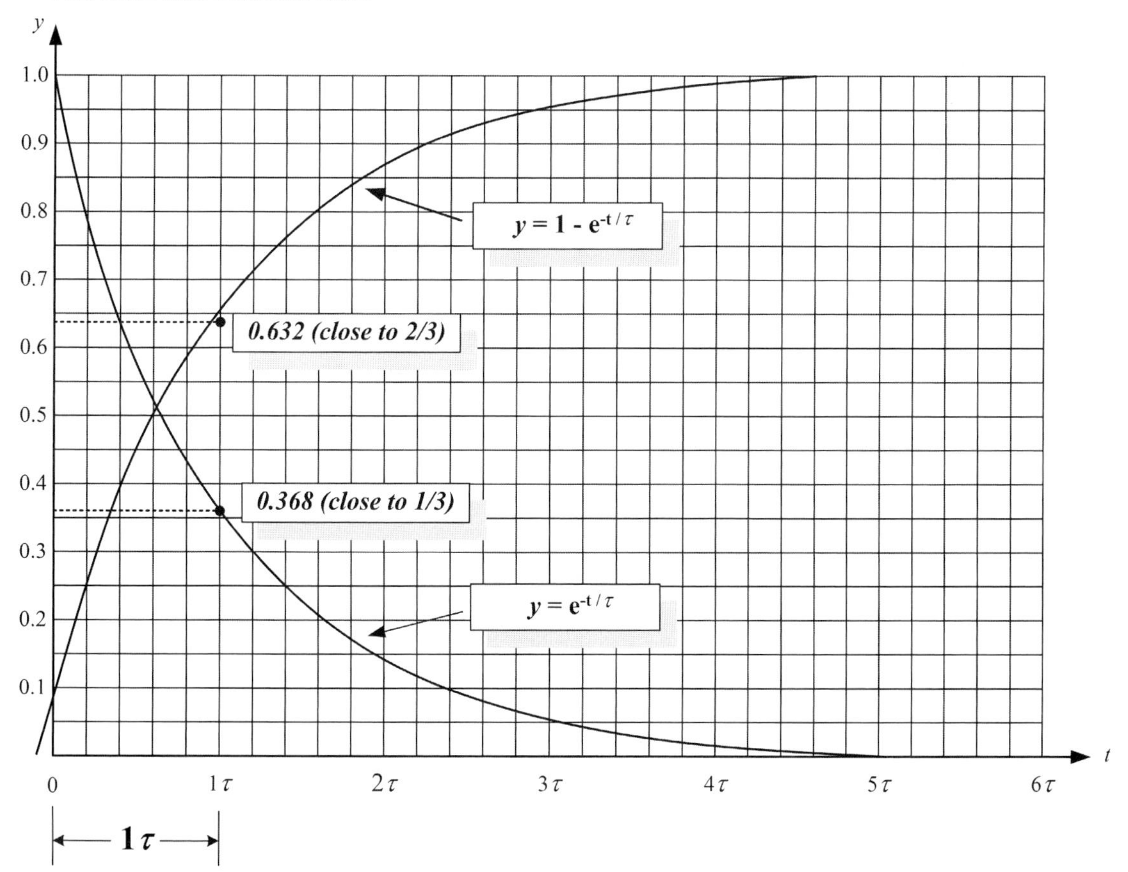

FIGURE 4-9 A universal time-constant chart.

frequencies. The reverse is true for the inductors—the inductor acts as a short at low frequencies. An ideal short exhibits a zero-ohm resistance.

When we apply an AC signal to a capacitor or an inductor, their AC resistances are called reactances and are given as follows:

$$X_C = \frac{1}{2 \times \pi \times f \times C}$$

$$X_L = 2 \times \pi \times f \times L$$

f = Frequency of the applied sig

X_C and X_L are capacitive reactance and inductive reactance, respectively, and are measured in ohms (Ω).

Capacitors and inductors are different from resistors and exhibit AC current and voltage relationships differently. In purely resistive circuits, AC current and voltage are in sync (meaning that they start and end at the same time; but this does not happen in capacitive or inductive circuits). These are called phasor relationships between current and voltage for the resistive, capacitive, and inductive circuits and are shown in **Figure 4-10a, Figure 4-10b,** and **Figure 4-10c.** The current in a capacitor leads the voltage across it by 90°. But the reverse is true in an inductor. The voltage across an inductor leads the current by 90°

Next, we discuss a series RC circuit with an AC signal applied. In the series AC circuit, resistance and reactance add up, the sum of these being noted as impedance. **Figure 4-11** shows the circuit and the calculations that follow.

$$X_C = \frac{1}{2 \times \pi \times f \times C}$$

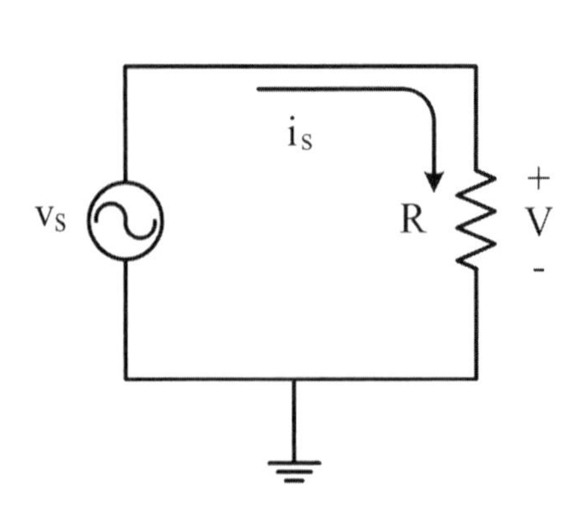

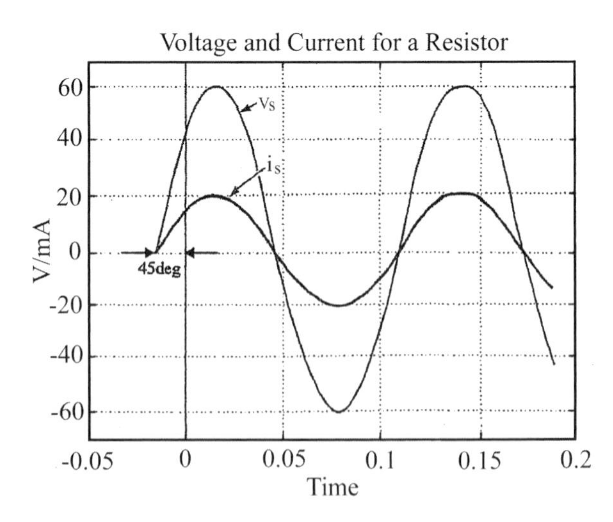

FIGURE 4-10a Voltage and current waveforms in a resistive circuit.

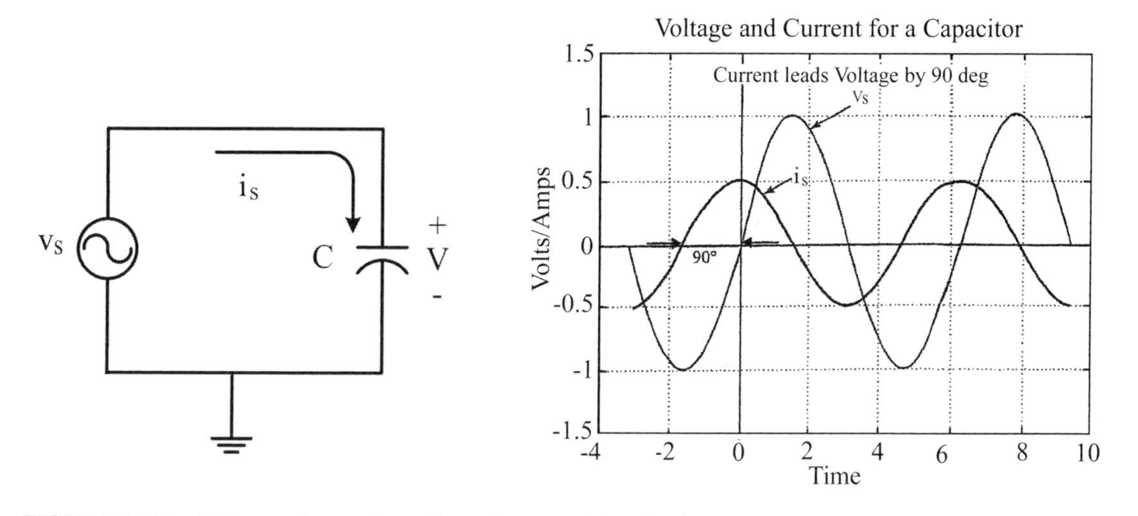

FIGURE 4-10b Voltage and current waveforms in a capacitive circuit.

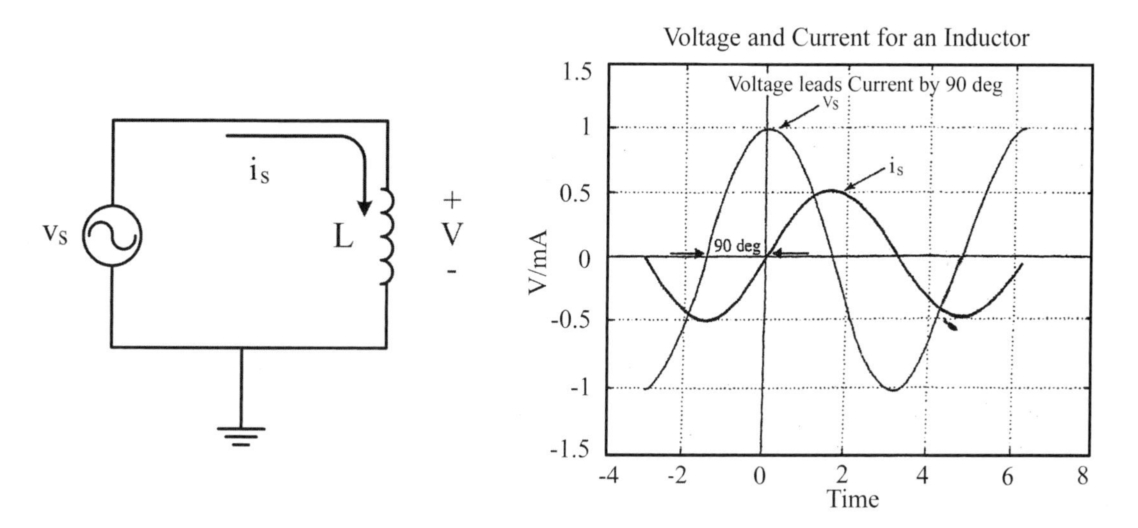

FIGURE 4-10c Voltage and current waveforms in an inductive circuit.

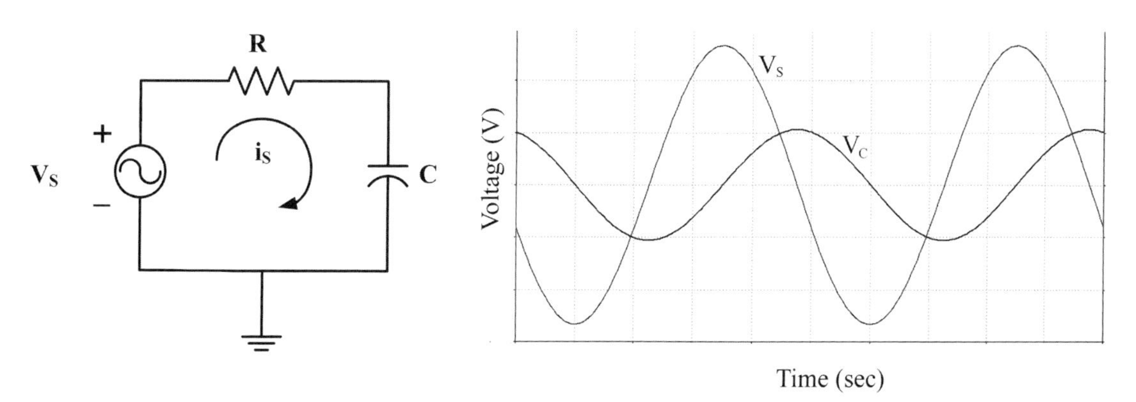

FIGURE 4-11 Voltage and current waveforms in an RC series circuit.

Total impedance (Z_T) in the circuit:

$$Z_T = R\angle 0° + X_C\angle - 90°$$
$$Z_T = R[\cos 0° + j\sin 0°] + X_C[\cos(-90°) + j\sin(-90°)]$$
$$Z_T = R[1] + X_C[-j]$$
$$Z_T = (R - jX_C)\Omega$$

$$I_S = \frac{V_S\angle 0°}{Z_T} \text{ Amps}$$

$$V_R = (R \times I_S) \text{ Volts}$$

$$V_C = [(-jX_C) \times (I_S)] \text{ Volts}$$
$$V_C = [X_C\angle - 90°] \times I_S \text{ Volts}$$

EXAMPLE Refer to **Figure 4-12a.** With R = 4.7 KΩ and C = 6.47 μF, calculate voltage drops across the resistor and the capacitor.

$$X_C = \frac{1}{2\pi \times f \times C} = \frac{1}{2\pi\,(3\text{ kHz}) \times (6.47\ \mu\text{F})} = 8.2\ \text{K}\Omega$$

$$Z_T = R - jX_C = (4.7\ \text{K}\Omega\angle 0°) - (j8.2\ \text{K}\Omega\angle - 90°) = 9.45\ \text{K}\Omega\angle - 60.18°$$

$$I_S = \frac{V_S\angle 0°}{Z_T} = \frac{6\angle 0°\ \text{V}}{9.45\ \text{K}\Omega\angle - 60.18°} = 634.92\ \mu\text{A}\angle 60.18°$$

$$V_R = R \times I_S = (4.7\text{K}\Omega\angle 0°) \times (634.92\mu\text{A}\angle 60.18°) = 2.98\angle 60.18°\ \text{V}$$

$$V_C = (-jX_C) \times I_S = [X_C\angle - 90°] \times I_S = (8.2\text{K}\Omega\angle - 90°) \times (634.92\mu\text{A}\angle 60.18°)$$
$$V_C = 5.21\text{V}\angle - 29.82°$$

The result is shown in vector form and in time in **Figure 4-12b** and **Figure 4-12c.**

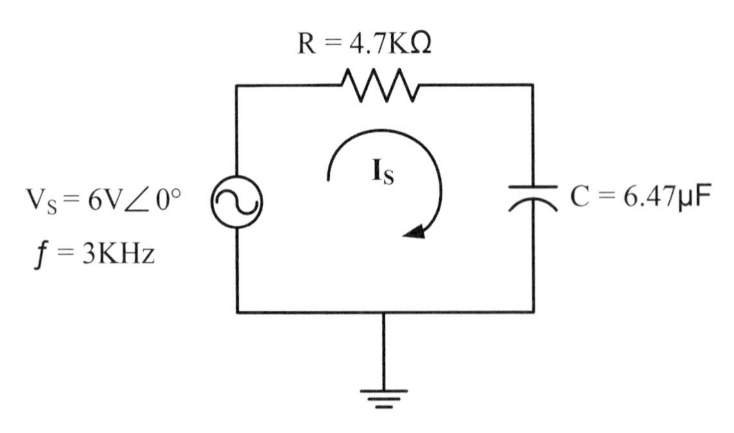

FIGURE 4-12a RC series circuit with AC power supply.

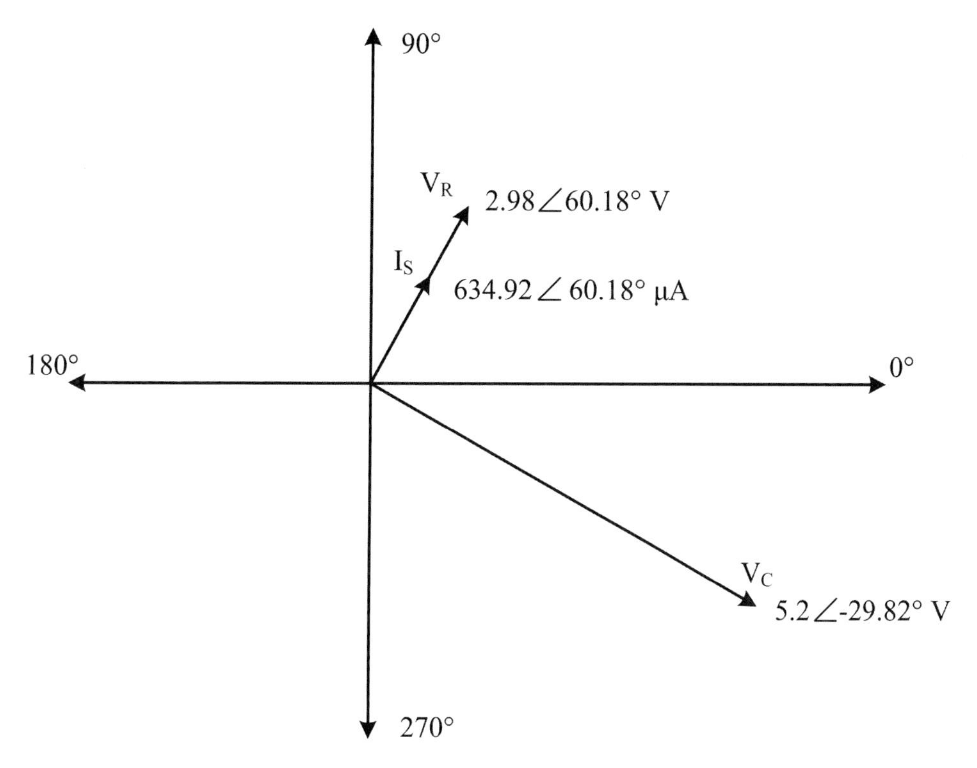

FIGURE 4-12b Vector diagram for the circuit in Figure 4-12a.

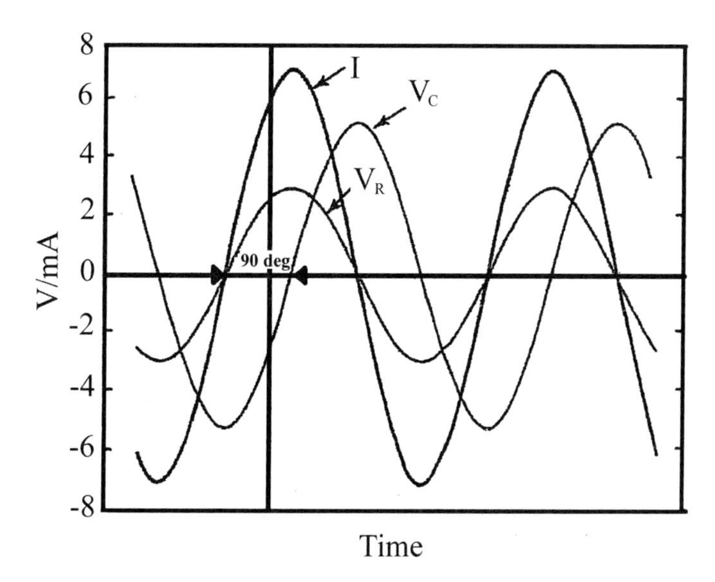

FIGURE 4-12c Voltage and current waveforms for the circuit in Figure 412a.

■

EXAMPLE Determine current and voltage drops for the circuit in **Figure 4-13a.** First, we will find the inductive reactance.

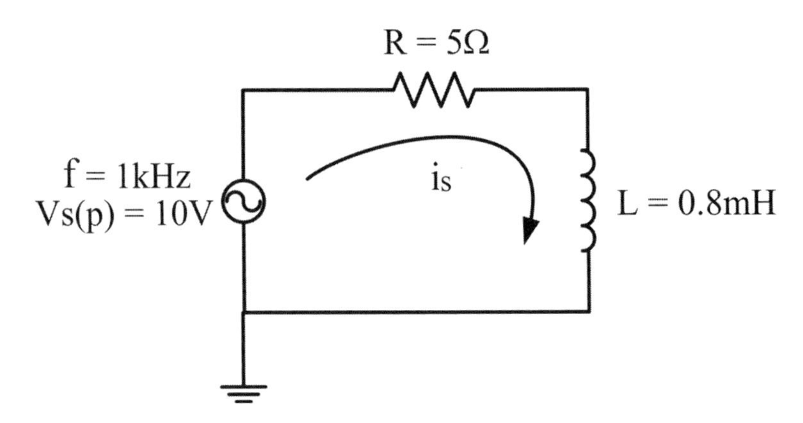

FIGURE 4-13a A series RL circuit with an AC power supply.

$$X_L = 2 \times \pi \times f \times L$$
$$X_L = 2 \times \pi \times 1\text{ kHz} \times 0.8\text{ mH}$$
$$X_L = 6.28 \times 1 \times 10^3 \times 0.8 \times 10^3$$
$$X_L = 5\ \Omega$$

$$Z_T = R + jX_L = (5\ \Omega \angle 0°) + (5\ \Omega \angle 90°)$$
$$Z_T = 7.07\ \Omega \angle 45°$$

$$I_S = \frac{V_S(p)\angle 0°}{Z_T}$$
$$I_S = \frac{10\text{ V}\angle 0°}{7.07\ \Omega \angle 45°}$$
$$I_S = 1.414\text{ A} \angle -45°$$

$$V_R = R \times I_S$$
$$V_R = (5\ \Omega \angle 0°) \times (1.414\ \Omega \angle -45°)$$
$$V_R = 7.07\text{ V} \angle -45°$$

$$V_L = (j \times X_L) \times (I_S)$$
$$V_L = (X_L \angle 90°) \times (1.414\text{ A} \angle -45°)$$
$$V_L = 7.07\text{ V} \angle 45°$$

If we add these voltage drops, the result will be the source voltage of 10 V∠ 0°. See **Figure 4-13b.**

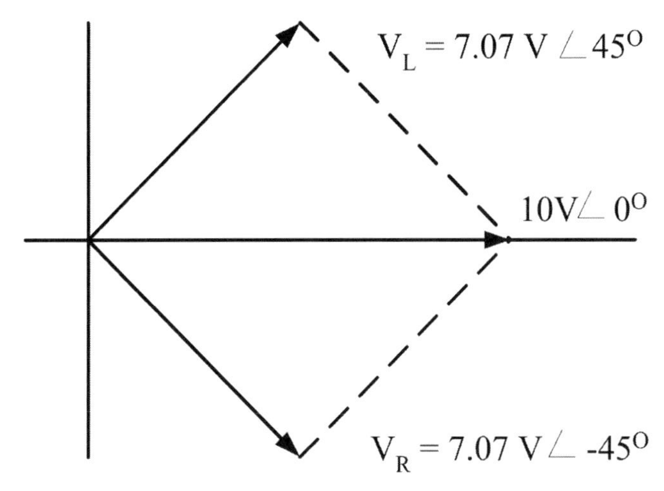

FIGURE 4-13b Vector diagram for the circuit in Figure 4-13a.

■

4.5 SUMMARY TABLE OF AC CONCEPTS

Device/Measurement	Action	Result
Inductor	Inductive voltage leads the current by 90°	The inductor is open at high frequency
Capacitor	Capacitive current leads the voltage by 90°	The capacitor acts as a short at high frequency
Resistor	$R\ \Omega\angle 0°$	Real number
Capacitive reactance	$X_C\Omega\angle -90°$	$-J\ X_C\Omega$
Inductive reactance	$X_L\Omega\angle 90°$	$+J\ X_L\Omega$
Capacitive circuit	$R - J\ X_C$	$R\angle 0° + X_C\angle -90°$
Inductive circuit	$R + J\ X_L$	$R\angle 0° + X_L\angle 90°$

4.6 BRIDGE CIRCUIT

A bridge circuit, as shown in **Figure 4-14a,** has various applications in electronics and medical instruments. It is used in DC and AC applications to detect small changes in a balanced network where voltages and currents are equal in adjacent branches. It is widely used in medical transducers, rectifiers, and regulators. The circuit is explained in the following section.

In the balanced condition of $V_O = 0V$:

Equation (1). $I_3 \times R_3 = I_4 \times R_4$

Because there is no current in the midsection, $I_3 = I_1$ and $I_4 = I_2$

also, $V_S = V_1 + V_3 = V_2 + V_4$

because $V_3 = V_4$ and $V_1 = V_2$

Equation (2). $I_1 \times R_1 = I_2 \times R_2$

Equation (3). $I_3 \times R_1 = I_4 \times R_2$ because $I_1 = I_3$ and $I_2 = I_4$

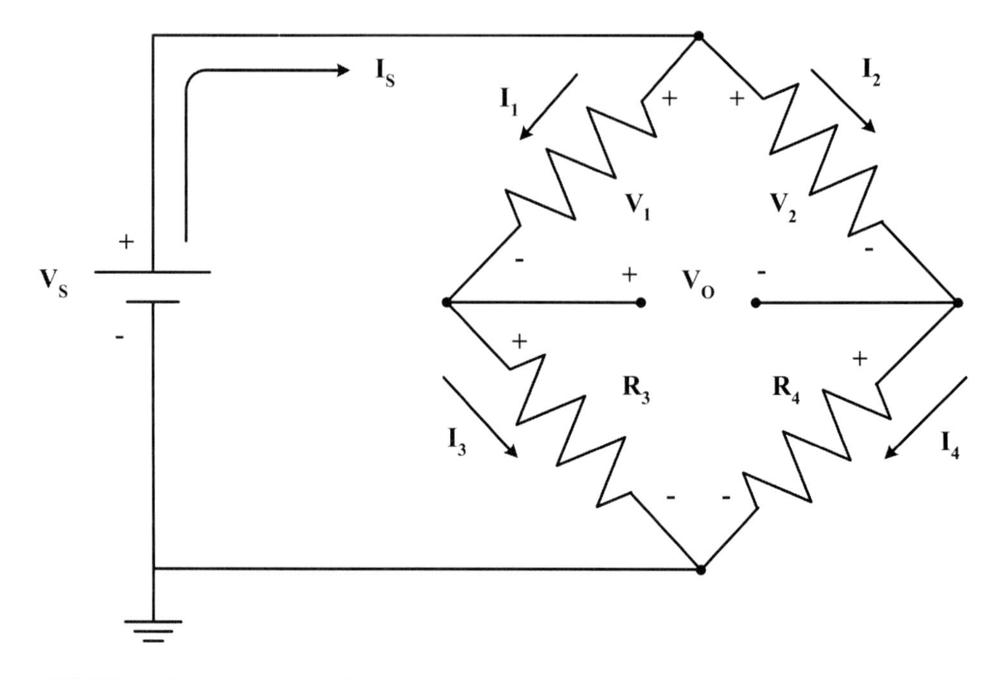

FIGURE 4-14a A bridge circuit.

Combining Equation 1 and Equation 3:

$$I_3 = \frac{I_4 \times R_4}{R_3} \text{ and } I_3 = \frac{I_4 \times R_2}{R_1}$$

That is,

$$\frac{I_4 \times R_4}{R_3} = \frac{I_4 \times R_2}{R_1}$$

Thus,

$$\frac{R_4}{R_3} = \frac{R_2}{R_1} \text{ or } \frac{R_1}{R_2} = \frac{R_3}{R_4} \text{ or } \frac{R_1}{R_3} = \frac{R_2}{R_4}$$

The result states that if the ratios are equal, then the bridge will be balanced and the output will be zero volts.

As an application, one of the resistors is replaced by a transducer resistance in a normal condition. When the condition is abnormal, the resistance of the transducer will change, and the output voltage will not remain zero. The output therefore detects the abnormality.

The following **Figure 4-14b** is an example of a temperature transducer in a bridge circuit. Assume the temperature is 70° F and the corresponding transducing resistor is 100 KΩ.

At an unbalanced condition

$V_0 = V_3 - V_4$ = negative voltage when R_1 = 110 KΩ (Temperature @ 72° F)
$V_0 = V_3 - V_4$ = positive voltage when R_1 = 90 KΩ (Temperature @ 68° F)

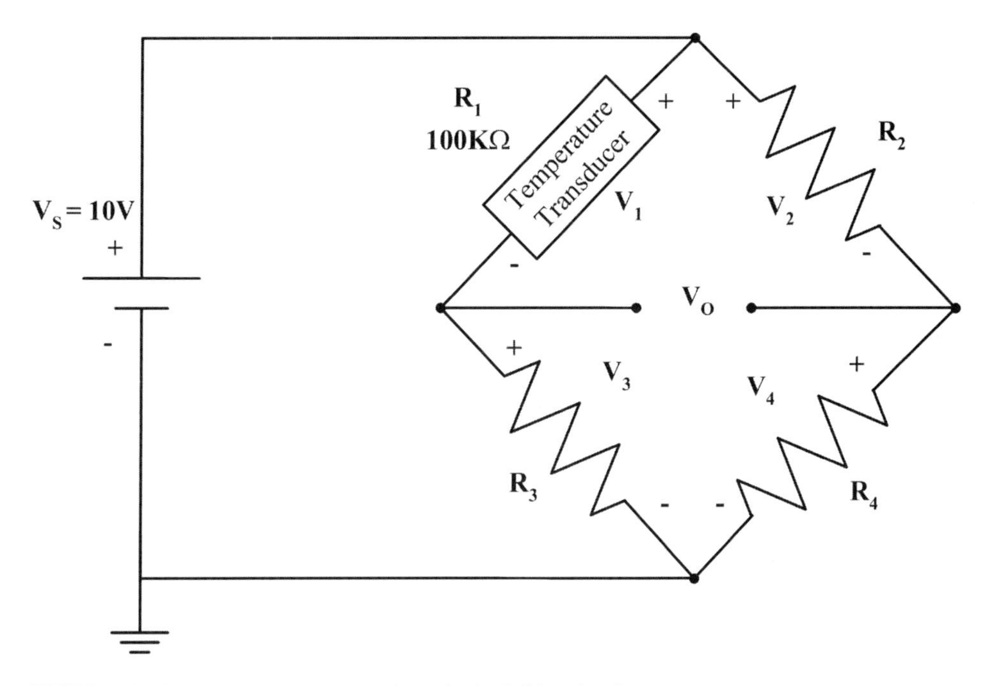

FIGURE 4-14b A temperature transducer in the bridge circuit.

4.7 LOADING PROBLEM IN ELECTRONICS

We can now explain the loading problem in electronic circuits. The concept is that the internal source resistance should be minimal compared to the load impedance in an electronic circuit. If the source resistance is not minimal, then there will be a voltage drop across the source resistance and the actual voltage of the source will be small across the load.

Figure 4-15a shows a no-load condition.

FIGURE 4-15a A series circuit without a loading problem.

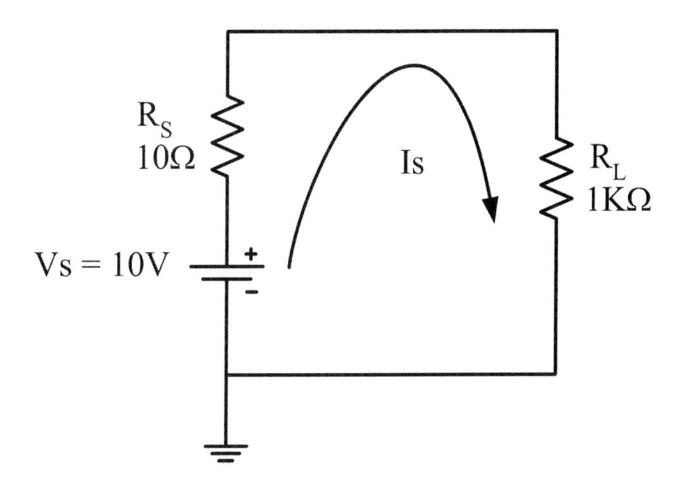

Notice $R_L >> R_S$ and the source voltage of 10 V is almost all delivered to the load (R_L). There is a negligible voltage that drops across R_S.

$$V_{R_L} = \frac{R_L}{R_L + R_S} \times V_S = \frac{1{,}000\ \Omega}{1{,}010\ \Omega} \times 10\ V = 9.9\ V$$

and the current in the system is

$$I_S = \frac{V_S}{R_L + R_S} = \frac{10\ V}{1{,}010\ \Omega} = 0.0099\ A$$

What this means is that the source is not loaded by the circuit, and the intended source voltage remains across the load. The current in the circuit is negligible.

Figure 4-15b shows a loading condition. If we change the load resistance to 10 Ω in the circuit, then the intended supply voltage to the circuit will drop to 5 V instead of 10 V. The current in the circuit will increase to 0.5 A from 0.0099 A in the no-loading circuit.

This is unacceptable in electronic applications and is called a loading problem.

In general, the loading problem needs to be reduced, not increased. To avoid the loading problem, the load resistance should be very large compared to the internal resistance of the source.

4.8 MAX POWER TRANSFER PROBLEM IN ELECTRONICS

There is another concept of the max power transfer to the load or to the circuit. In this case, the source resistance and the load resistance should be equal.

Maximum power transfer in electronics is needed when maximum power is intended to be delivered to the load by the source. This is achieved by ensuring that the load resistance is equal to the internal resistance of the source. We can prove this by the following example.

For **Figure 4-16a,** we will compute power across the load.

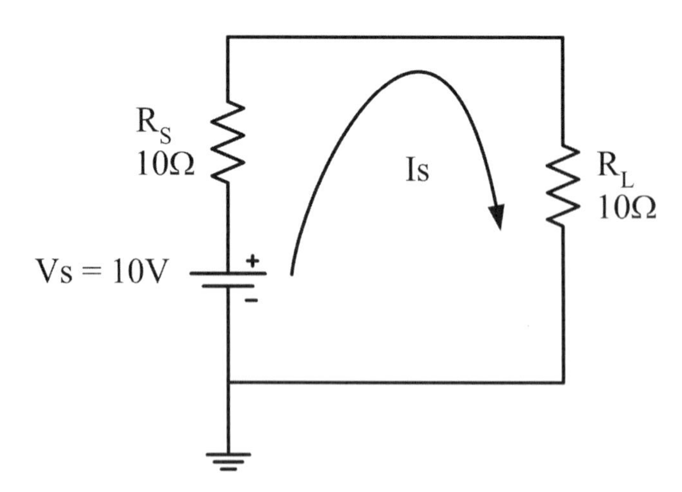

FIGURE 4-15b A series circuit with a loading problem.

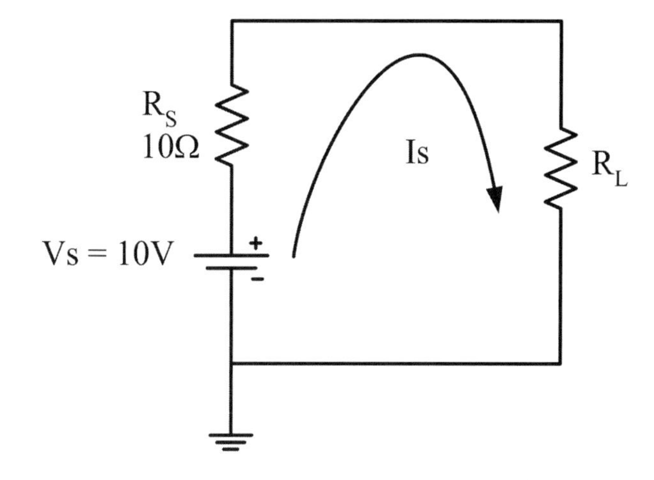

FIGURE 4-16a A series circuit to compute max power across the load resistance.

The following chart shows the effect of load on a circuit. As R_L becomes larger, current decreases and voltage increases. We could simply state that current is inversely proportional to R_L and voltage is directly proportional to R_L.

R_S Fixed 10 Ω	**R_L**	$I_S = \frac{V_S}{R_S + R_L}$	V_{R_L}	$P_{R_L} = (V_{R_L}) \times (I_S)$
10 Ω	1 Ω	$\frac{10\text{ V}}{11\ \Omega} = 0.91$ A	0.91 V	0.83 W
10 Ω	2 Ω	$\frac{10\text{ V}}{12\ \Omega} = 0.83$ A	1.66 V	1.38 W
10 Ω	3 Ω	$\frac{10\text{ V}}{13\ \Omega} = 0.77$ A	2.31 V	1.77 W
10 Ω	4 Ω	$\frac{10\text{ V}}{14\ \Omega} = 0.71$ A	2.84 V	2.01 W
10 Ω	5 Ω	$\frac{10\text{ V}}{15\ \Omega} = 0.67$ A	3.35 V	2.24 W
10 Ω	10 Ω	$\frac{10\text{ V}}{20\ \Omega} = 0.5$ A	5 V	2.5 W
10 Ω	50 Ω	$\frac{10\text{ V}}{60\ \Omega} = 0.167$ A	8.35 V	1.39 W
10 Ω	100 Ω	$\frac{10\text{ V}}{100\ \Omega} = 0.09$ A	9.9 V	0.89 W

Notice that in the example above the max power is delivered only when $R_L = R_S =$ 10 Ω. Power to the load decreases when $R_L > 10\ \Omega$ and when $R_L < 10\ \Omega$.

In general, a maximum power graph can be plotted as shown in **Figure 4-16b.**

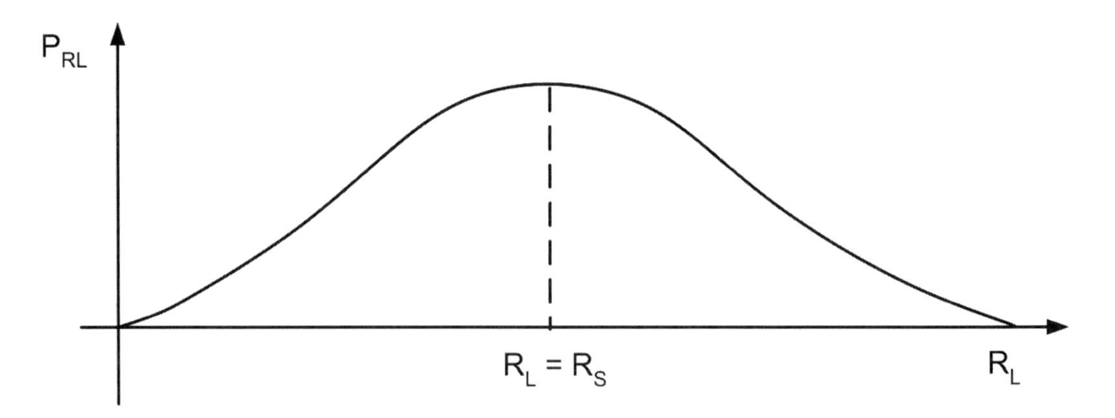

FIGURE 4-16b A power graph with a changing load resistance.

Next, let's move the discussion to semiconductor diodes and their applications in rectification and power regulation. We will start with a diode rectifier.

4.9 SEMICONDUCTOR DIODE RECTIFIER

A regular diode can rectify a signal in the sense that the positive or a negative part of the signal can be attenuated. A diode is a semiconductor device made up of silicon wafer doped with impurities such as antimony or indium. Its characteristics are as follows.

A diode has positive and negative polarities and is ON when its positive polarity is connected to the positive terminal of a power supply. This state is known as forward-biased and the current can flow in the circuit as shown in **Figure 4-17a**. There is drop of approximately 0.7 volts across the silicon diode.

The diode can also be in the OFF condition. This is when the diodes negative polarity is connected to the positive terminal of the supply voltage. This configuration inhibits current from flowing in the circuit, as shown in **Figure 4-17b.**

When the current cuts off in the circuit, the diode is in the reverse-bias mode.

FIGURE 4-17a A forward-biased diode circuit.

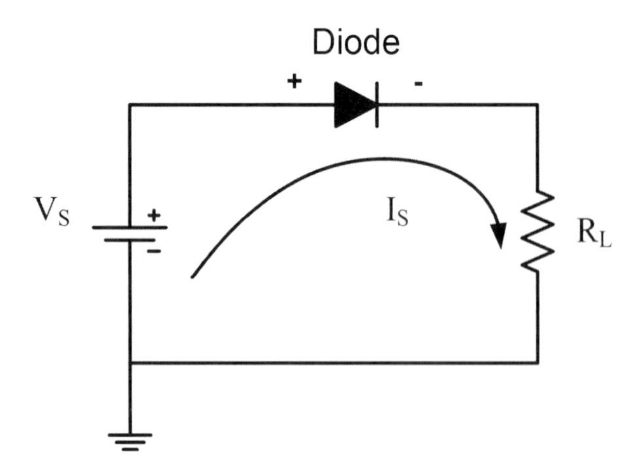

FIGURE 4-17b A reverse-biased diode circuit.

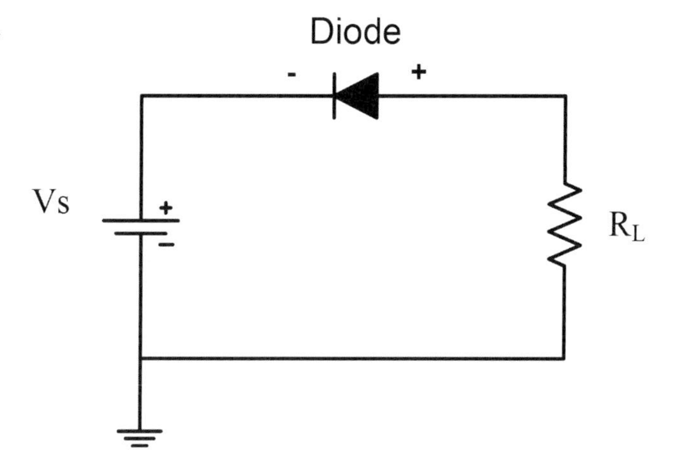

For an example, a square wave is applied to a diode circuit, and the output across R_L is shown in **Figure 4-17c.**

We can see that during the positive cycle of the input square wave, the diode is forward-biased and the current flows in the circuit to develop the output voltage. However, the current is cut off during the negative half of the input square-wave cycle.

4.10 ZENER DIODE REGULATOR

Another type of semiconductor diode is called a Zener diode and can also be made in the forward- or reversed-bias. Mainly, the Zener diode is used in the reverse-bias mode where a large current can flow through it. Note that even though the regular diode could be used in reverse-bias mode, it could not handle large current flow without damage to itself. A Zener diode circuit is shown in **Figure 4-18a.**

The types of reverse mode Zener diodes are 1.5 V, 3 V, 5 V, and many more. Once the current becomes large enough, a breakdown occurs, known as breakdown current. The Zener, once in this state, maintains the reverse voltage and a large reverse current. The following example explains the Zener process.

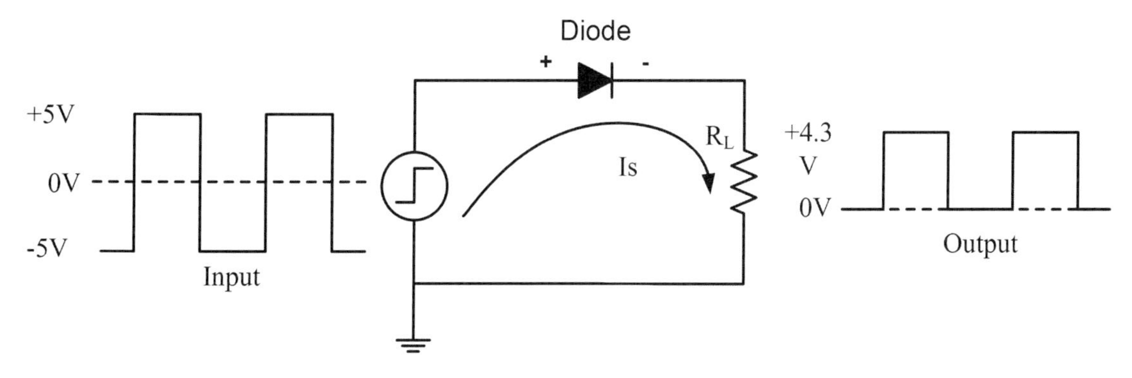

FIGURE 4-17c A bipolar square wave applied to a forward-biased diode circuit.

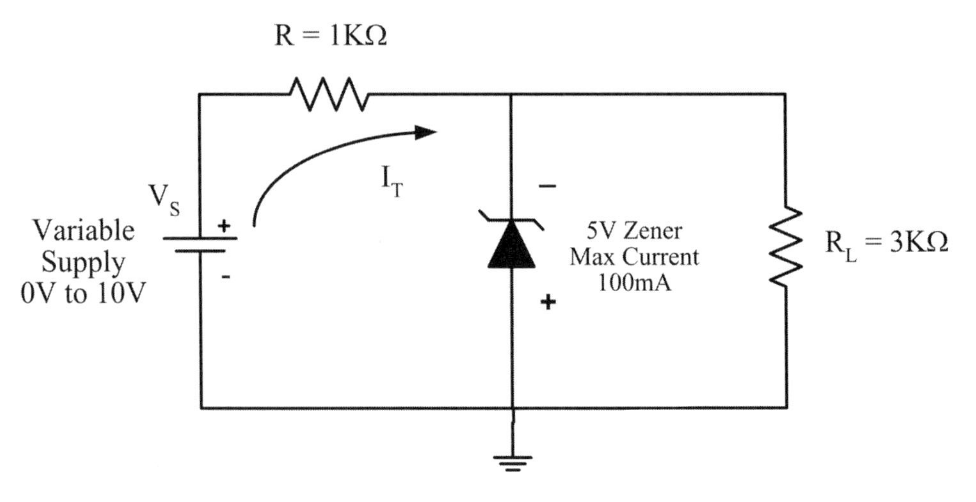

FIGURE 4-18a A Zener diode circuit.

When $V_S < 5$ V, there is no current through the Zener diode, as shown in **Figure 4-18b.** The Zener acts like an open circuit and the voltage drops across the resistors are:

$$V_{1K\Omega} = \frac{1\ K\Omega}{1\ K\Omega + 3\ K\Omega} \times 4\ V = 1\ V$$

$$V_{3K\Omega} = \frac{3\ K\Omega}{3\ K\Omega + 1\ K\Omega} \times 4\ V = 3\ V$$

and

$$I_T = \frac{4\ V}{4\ K\Omega} = 1\ mA$$

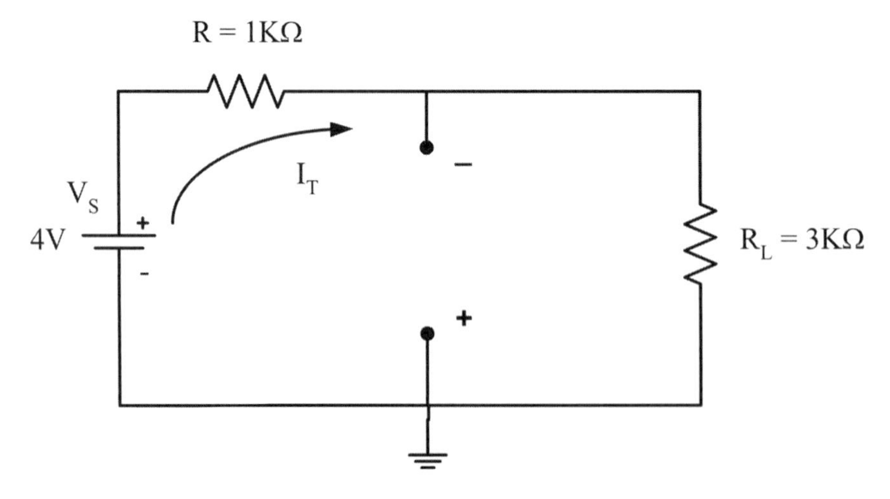

FIGURE 4-18b Forward-bias to the Zener circuit of Figure 4-18a.

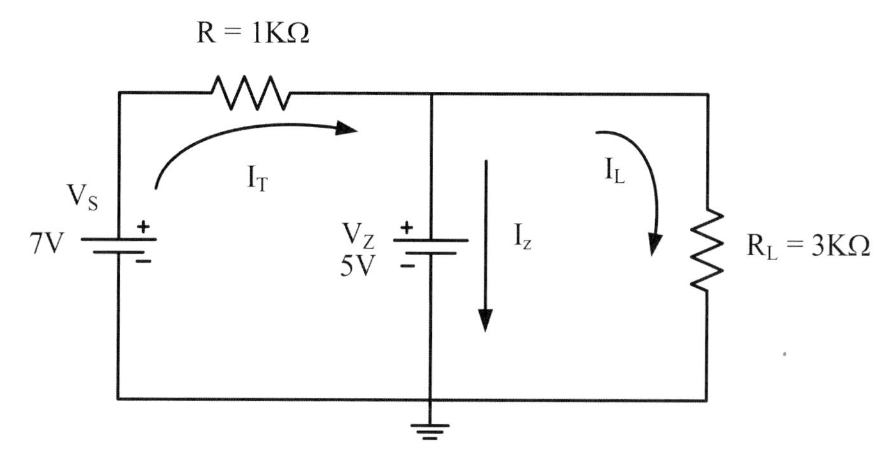

FIGURE 4-18c Reverse-bias to the Zener circuit of Figure 4-18a.

But as $V_S > 5$ V, the situation changes and the voltage drops are as shown in **Figure 4-18c.**

The Zener now acts as a DC regulator of 5 V and the load R_L maintains a current of 5 V/3 KΩ (that is, 1.67 mA).

$$V_{1K\Omega} = 7\text{ V} - 5\text{ V} = 2\text{ V}$$

$$I_T = I_Z + I_L = \frac{2\text{ V}}{1\text{ K}\Omega} = 2\text{ mA}$$

$$I_L = \frac{5\text{ V}}{3\text{ K}\Omega} = 1.67\text{ mA}$$

$$I_Z = I_T - I_L = 2\text{ mA} - 1.67\text{ mA} = 0.33\text{ mA}$$

Depending on the load resistance, the input DC power supply V_S needs to be adjusted until the Zener diode breaks down in its reverse bias. In the above example, even V_S of 6 V will not break the Zener diode because I_T is not yet 1.67 mA. For proper operation, the total current should be more than the load current. With the breakdown, the Zener current operates within its minimum and maximum values given by the manufacturer.

4.11 TRANSFORMER AND THE REGULATED POWER SUPPLY

A regulated power supply converts conventional 110 V AC line voltage to a DC level. This DC level can range from 1.5 V to 12 V or higher and the level is regulated by the use of proper Zener diodes. To start, the circuit consists of a transformer, a rectifier, and a filter. The circuit of **Figure 4-19a** represents a full-wave rectifier.

At point A the voltage is:

$$V_A = V_2 - 1.4\text{ V}$$

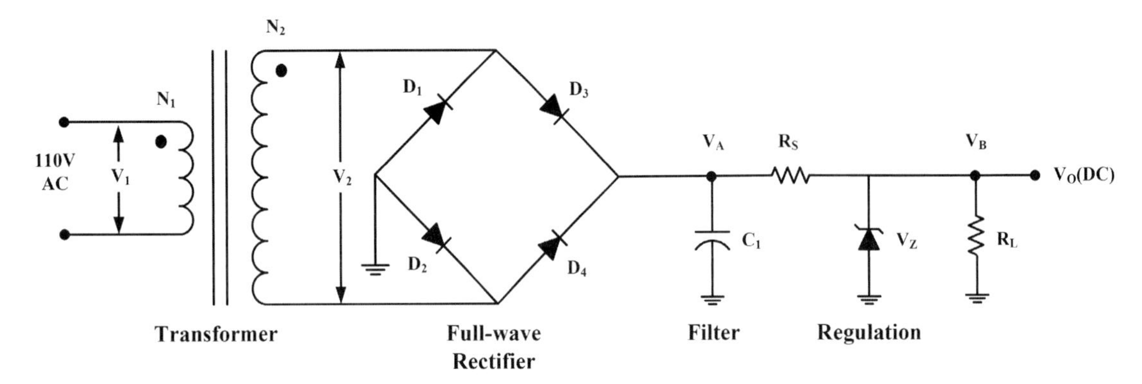

FIGURE 4-19a A DC voltage regulator circuit.

The drop of 1.4 V is due to the voltage drops across the two Zener diodes: both D_2 and D_3 in the positive AC cycle or D_1 and D_4 in the negative AC cycle.

At point B:

$$V_B = \text{the Zener voltage} = V_Z = V_O(\text{DC})$$

The transformer is a step-down device and V_2 is related to V_1 with respect to the turns-ratio N_1 and N_2.

That is,

$$\frac{V_2}{V_1} = \frac{N_2}{N_1}$$

V_1 and V_2 are both sine-wave waveforms. A set of timing diagrams is shown at different parts of the circuit in **Figure 4-19b.**

V_1 is the input voltage at the primary, whereas V_2 is the step-down voltage at the secondary.

As an example,

$$\frac{N_2}{N_1} = \frac{1}{10} \text{ and } V_Z = 3 \text{ V}$$

end after voltage drops across two diodes, V_A and V_B are given as:

$$V_A = 14.1 \text{ V (p)}$$
$$V_B = 3 \text{ V d.c.}$$

4.12 BIPOLAR JUNCTION TRANSISTOR (BJT) AND FIELD-EFFECT TRANSISTOR (FET) CIRCUITS

The bipolar-junction transistor (BJT) is an extension of the diode from a PN junction semiconductor into an NPN or PNP junction device. It has three leads: emitter, base, and collector pins. The device amplifies a small signal with the input at the base and the amplified output at the collector. In **Figure 4-20a,** a BJT amplifier circuit is shown. The input V_i is provided at the base (junction of a capacitor and two resistors). The output is amplified and out of phase with respect to input at the collector (junction of C_3 and R_3). The emitter is grounded through R_4. The DC power is provided through $+V_{CC}$.

FIGURE 4-19b Timing-diagram of the voltages in the circuit of Figure 4-19a.

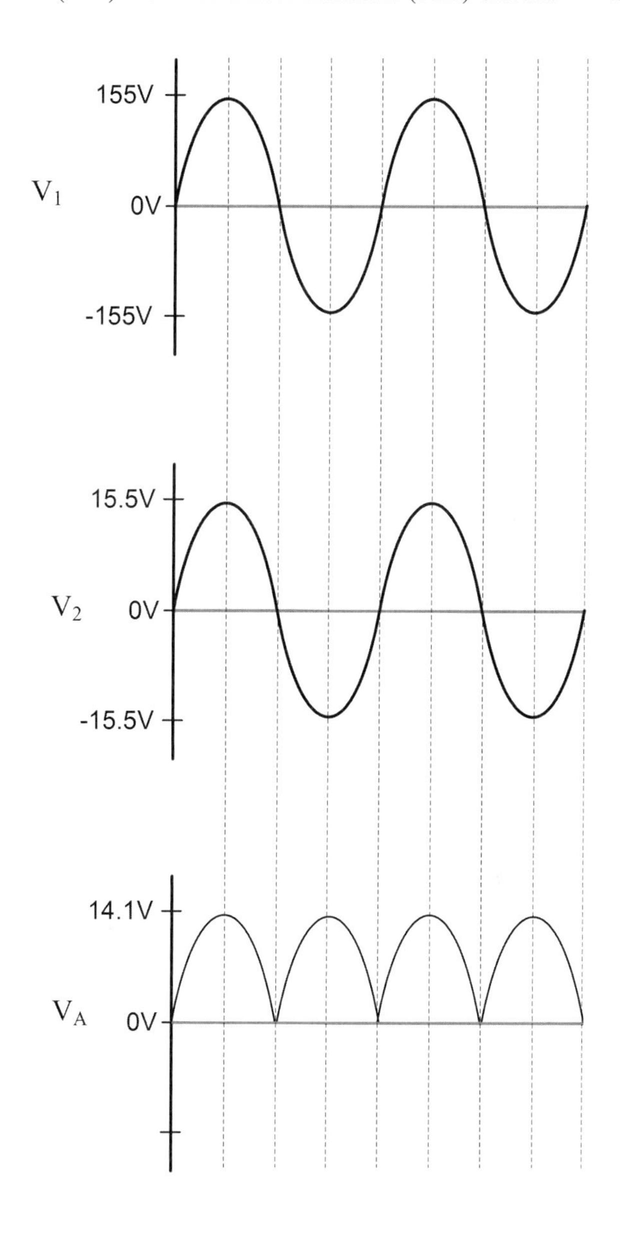

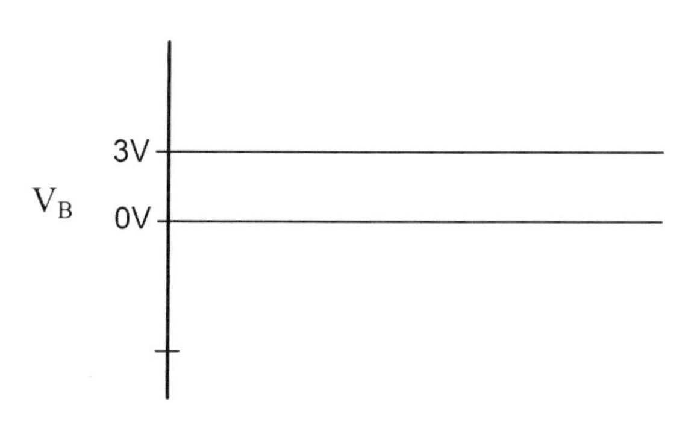

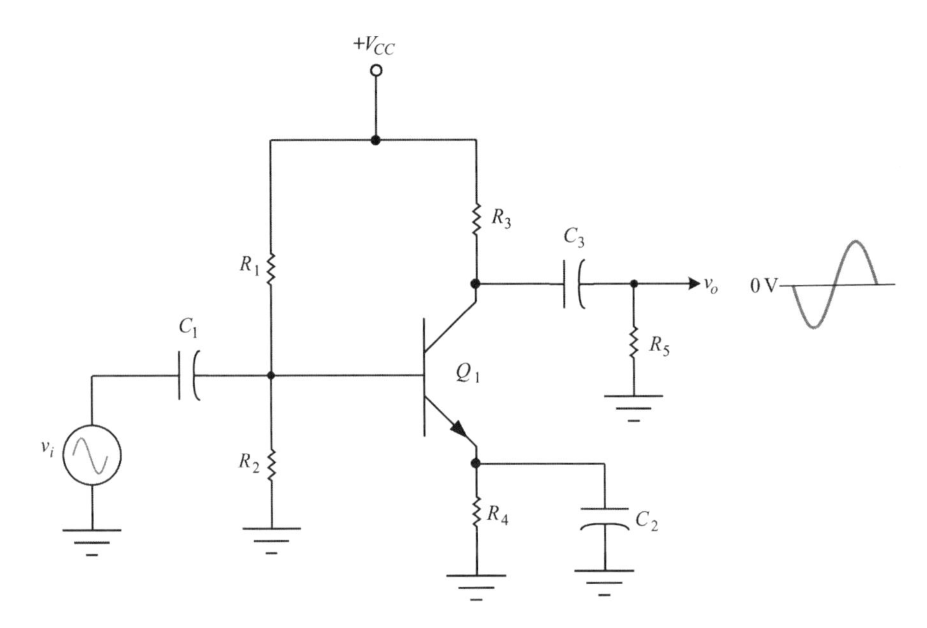

FIGURE 4-20a A bipolar-junction transistor (BJT) amplifier circuit.

The values of resistors around the transistor Q_1 are based upon the operational currents; they are the base current and collector current. The BJT is a current-controlled device and it provides a current gain of the order of 100. That means for the base current of 10 μA at the base, the output collector current is 1,000 μA. Around this DC operation of the BJT circuit, a signal can now be imposed for the purpose of the amplification.

The voltage gain of a BJT amplifier is given as:

$$A_V = -\beta \times \frac{R_5 \| R_3}{h_{ie}}$$

where $A_V = \dfrac{V_o}{V_i}$

β = current gain of the transistor

h_{ie} = input resistance between base and the emitter

R_5 = load resistance

R_3 = collector resistance

When capacitor C_2 is not connected across the emitter resistor R_4, the voltage gain drops tremendously and the voltage gain is given as:

$$A_V = -\beta \times \frac{(R_5 \| R_3)}{(h_{ie} + \beta \times R_4)}$$

The other circuit is shown in **Figure 4-20b.** This is the FET circuit with resistors around the three-lead FET. The input is at the gate G, output at drain D, and the control at the source S. This is similar to a BJT amplifier but it provides a larger input impedance

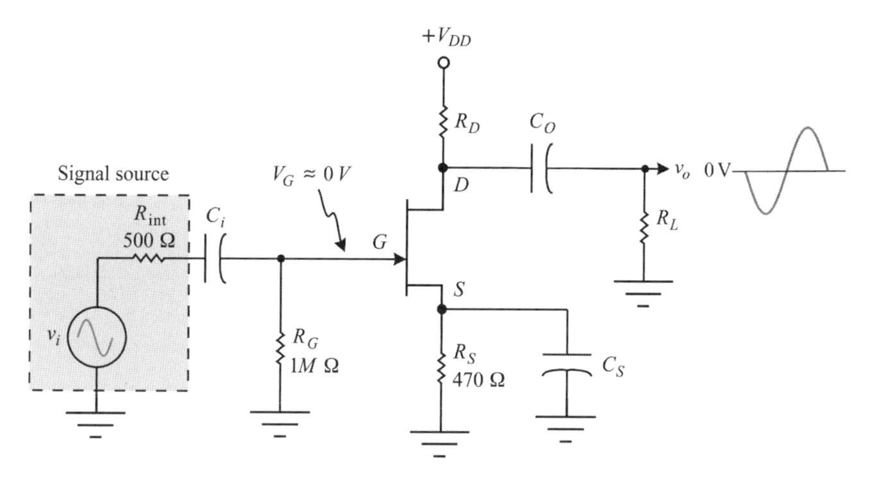

FIGURE 4-20b A field-effect transistor (FET) amplifier circuit.

(to the input signal) and faster switching (ON/OFF) operations. Field-effect transistors are voltage-controlled devices (for example, any change of voltage at gate G will provide a large change of the output voltage at drain D).

$$A_V = -g_m \times R_L || R_D$$

Where A_V = voltage gain of the amplifier $= \dfrac{V_o}{V_i}$

g_m = transconductance gain of the JFET in amp/volt

R_L = load resistance

R_D = drain resistance

The voltage gain drops when the source-capacitor C_S is removed from the circuit and the formula is then given as:

$$A_V = -g_m \times (R_D || R_L) / (1 + g_m \times R_S)$$

where R_S is the source resistance.

4.13 OPERATIONAL AMPLIFIER AND VARIOUS CONFIGURATIONS

Figure 4-21 shows the op-amp as two inputs and one output device with +V and −V DC power supplies. It is eight-pin integrated general purpose LM741 IC with the output voltage V_{out} as a linear output between −V and +V voltage saturations. The general characteristics of an op-amp can be given as:

1. Inverting input is labeled with a minus sign, and the non-inverting input is labeled with a + sign.
2. The difference between the inverting and non-inverting inputs is approximately a zero volt. In addition, there is no current flow between them, i.e., no current enters at inverting and non-inverting inputs.

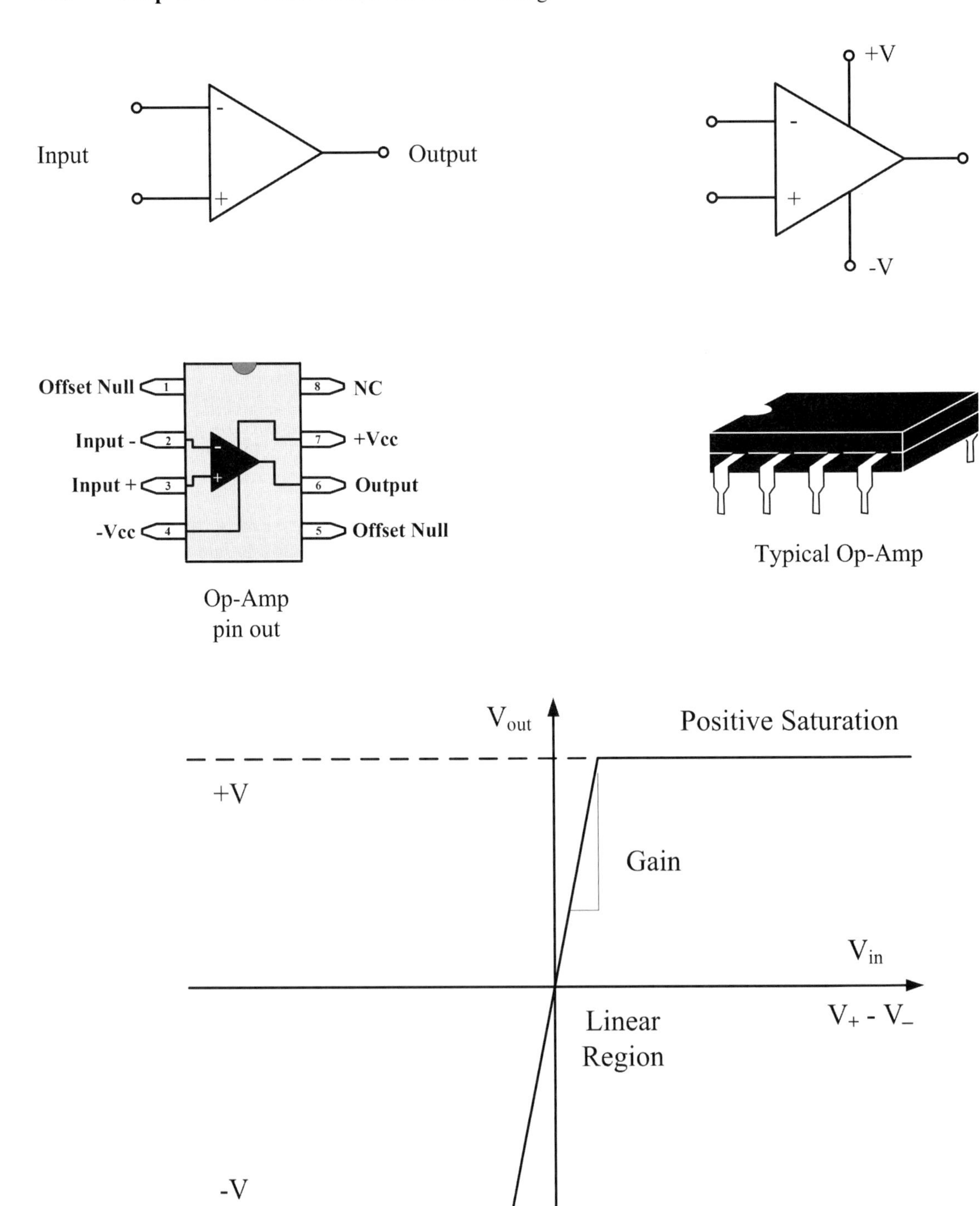

FIGURE 4-21 Pin out of a typical op-amp chip.

3. The LM741 op-amp has become the industry's standard and its open-loop voltage gain is about 2×10^5, and the bandwidth is 1 MHz. The ideal voltage gain and the bandwidth of an op-amp should be infinite.
4. The ideal input resistance must be infinite ohms, whereas the output resistance must be zero ohms. In LM741 op-amp, though, the input resistance is 2 MΩ and the output resistance is approximately 75 Ω.

The following discusses how op-amp will be used in circuits such as comparators, inverting and non-inverting amplifiers and filters. The derivations will be provided for the reader to understand the input-output relationships in op-amp circuits. We will start with a comparator circuit.

1. **VOLTAGE COMPARATOR**

As there is no feedback from the output terminal to the input terminals, this circuit is called an open-loop circuit. The voltage comparator is meant to compare two inputs, one at the inverting terminal and the other at the non-inverting terminal. The output of the op-amp will reach +V volts when the voltage at the non-inverting input is slightly larger than the voltage at the inverting input. Conversely, the output will be –V volts when inverting input is slightly more than the non-inverting input. The circuit is shown in **Figure 4-22.**

That is,

$$V_1 > V_2 \text{ then } V_{OUT} = +V$$
$$V_2 > V_1 \text{ then } V_{OUT} = -V$$

When comparator uses positive feedback, it is referred to as a Schmitt trigger. It has much more skeeter noise immunity than simple gen-loop op-amp voltage comparators.

FIGURE 4-22 An op-amp voltage comparator.

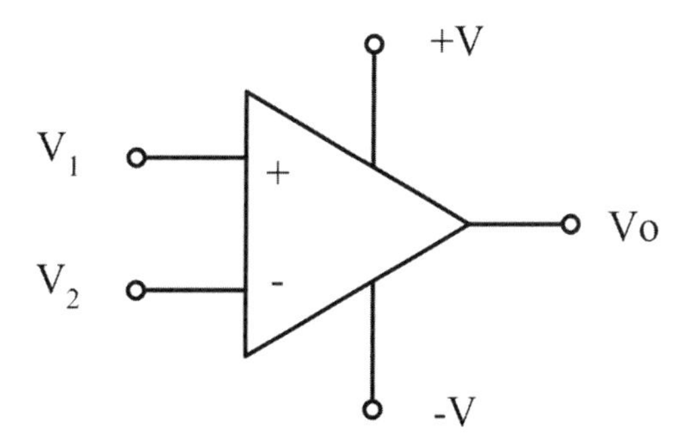

2. **INVERTING AMPLIFIER**

The output is an amplified signal by some gain of the inverting input. Also, the phase of the output is 180 degrees out of phase of the inverting input. The gain depends upon the ratio of the feedback resistance to the input resistance. The larger the ratio, the more gain, but the output can never be more than +V or less than –V voltage. As physiological signals are small-amplitude voltages, they are amplified before they can be displayed on the monitors (in **Figure 4-23a**).

With the inverting input at virtual ground:

$$I_1 = \frac{V_{in} - 0}{R_1}$$

$$I_2 = \frac{0 - Vo}{R_2}$$

$I_2 = I_1$ (no current enters at the inverting input)

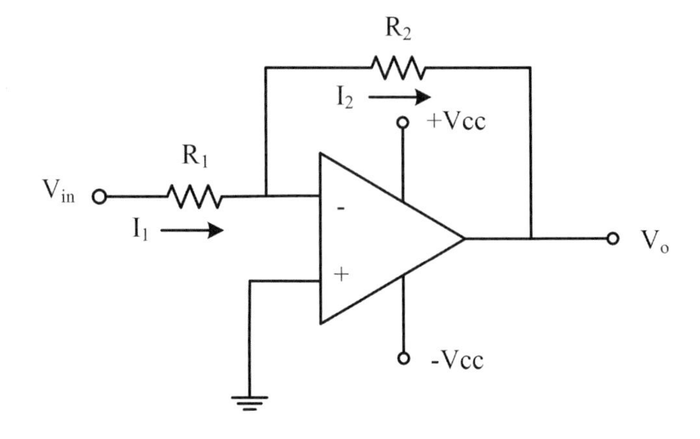

FIGURE 4-23a An op-amp inverting amplifier.

Using these three equations,

$$\frac{V_{in}}{R_1} = \frac{-Vo}{R_2} \quad \text{so} \quad Vo = \frac{-R_2}{R_1} \times V_{in}$$

Simplifying,

$$\text{Output Voltage} = -\ (\text{Input Voltage}) \times \text{Gain}$$

where

$$A_V = \text{Voltage Gain} = -\frac{R_2}{R_1}$$

3. **NON-INVERTING AMPLIFIER**

In **Figure 4-23b,** a non-inverting amplifier is shown. This is another type of op-amp configuration where the output and input are in phase, but the gain still depends upon the ratio of feedback and input resistances. The inverting and non-inverting configurations both are used in differential and instrumentation amplifiers. One of the main reasons

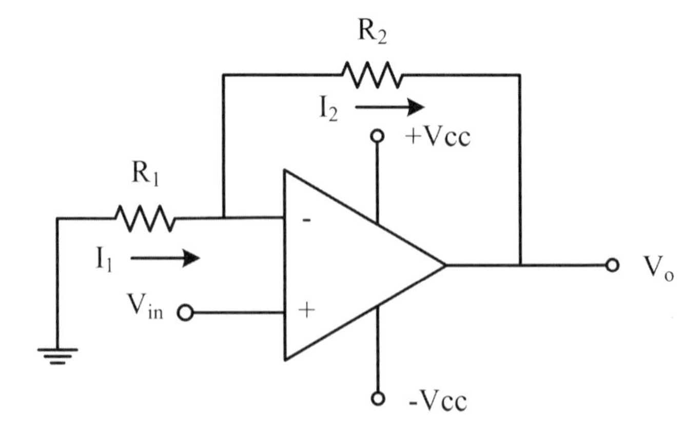

FIGURE 4-23b An op-amp non-inverting amplifier.

this circuit is widely used is that it provides a very large input resistance to the source compared to the inverting amplifier.

The calculations for a non-inverting amplifier are as follows:

With the inverting input the same as the non-inverting input, V_{in}

$$I_1 = \frac{0 - V_{in}}{R_1} \qquad \text{hence, } I_2 = I_1$$
$$I_2 = \frac{V_{in} - Vo}{R_2}$$

Simplifying,

$$\frac{-V_{in}}{R_1} = \frac{V_{in} - Vo}{R_2} = \frac{V_{in}}{R_2} - \frac{Vo}{R_2}$$
$$\frac{-V_{in}}{R_1} - \frac{V_{in}}{R_2} = \frac{-Vo}{R_2}$$

Or

$$\frac{V_{in}}{R_1} + \frac{V_{in}}{R_2} = \frac{Vo}{R_2}$$
$$V_{in}\left(\frac{R_2 + R_1}{R_1 \times R_2}\right) = \frac{V_O}{R_2}$$

Finally,

$$V_{in}\left(1 + \frac{R_2}{R_1}\right) = V_O$$

Therefore,

$$\text{output voltage} = (1 + \text{gain}) \times \text{input voltage}$$
$$A_V = 1 + \left(\frac{R_2}{R_1}\right)$$

4. SUMMING AMPLIFIER

Several signals can be added or subtracted together in the summing amplifier configuration. The output is the sum of all the inputs, and this can be done when inputs are at an inverting or a non-inverting terminal.

See **Figure 4-24** for a summing amplifier.

The non-inverting input is zero volts, as it is connected to ground; thus the inverting input is also at virtual ground.

$$I_1 = \frac{V_1 - 0}{R_1} = \frac{V_1}{R_1} \qquad I_2 = \frac{V_2 - 0}{R_2} = \frac{V_2}{R_2}$$
$$I_3 = \frac{V_3 - 0}{R_3} = \frac{V_3}{R_3} \qquad I_4 = \frac{0 - Vo}{R_4} = \frac{-Vo}{R_4}$$

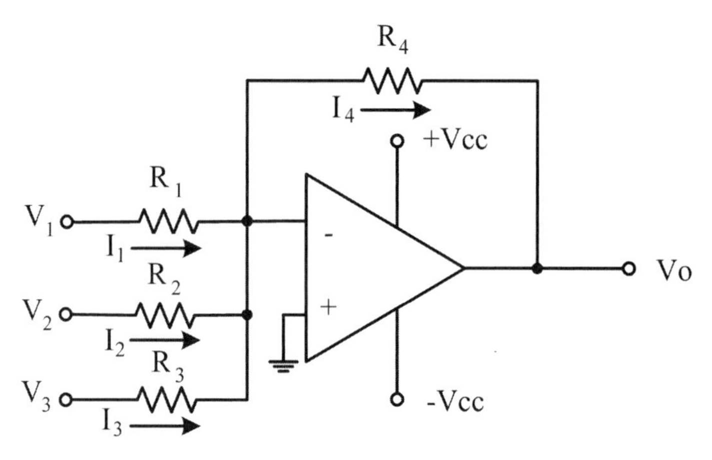

FIGURE 4-24 A summing amplifier.

Also,

$$I_4 = I_1 + I_2 + I_3$$

or

$$I_4 = \frac{V_1}{R_1} + \frac{V_2}{R_2} + \frac{V_3}{R_3} = \frac{-Vo}{R_4}$$

Finally,

$$Vo = -\left(\frac{R_4}{R_1} \times V_1 + \frac{R_4}{R_2} \times V_2 + \frac{R_4}{R_3} \times V_3\right)$$

5. **DIFFERENTIAL AMPLIFIER**

In this circuit, the difference of two inputs, one at the inverting terminal and the other at the non-inverting terminal, can be provided at the output. The word "differential" has nothing to do with the derivative of the inputs as in differential calculus. A circuit of a differential amplifier is shown in **Figure 4-25a** and the calculations are performed as follows:

The non-inverting input can be calculated as:

$$V_{R2} = \frac{R_2}{R_1 + R_2} \times V_2 \text{ (using the voltage divider rule)}$$

As before, the inverting input is the same as the non-inverting input, thus:

$$I_1 = \frac{V_1 - V_{R2}}{R_1}$$

$$I_2 = \frac{V_{R2} - V_O}{R_2}$$

$$I_1 = I_2$$

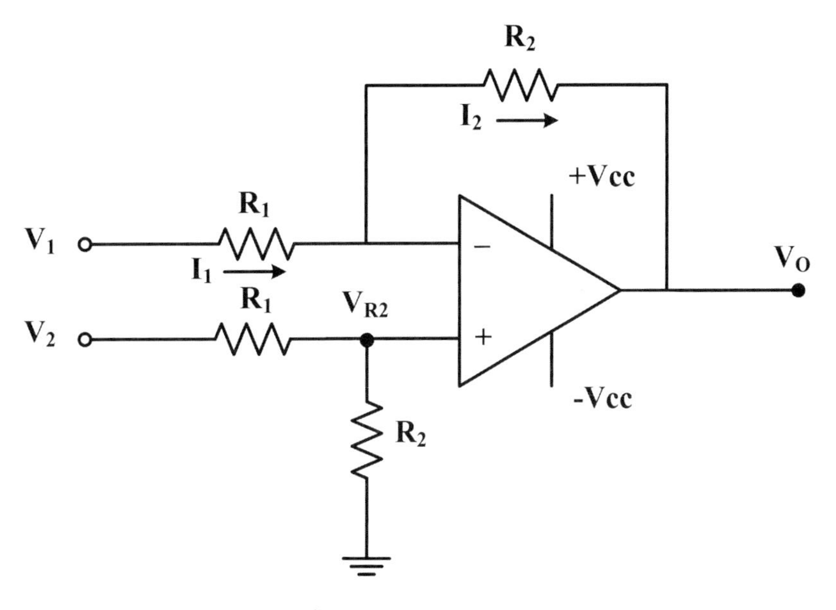

FIGURE 4-25a A differential amplifier.

Using these three equations we find,

$$\frac{V_1 - V_{R2}}{R_1} = \frac{V_{R2} - Vo}{R_2}$$

$$\frac{-Vo}{R_2} = \frac{V_1}{R_1} - \frac{V_{R2}}{R_1} - \frac{V_{R2}}{R_2}$$

$$\frac{-Vo}{R_2} = \frac{V_1}{R_1} - V_{R2}\left(\frac{1}{R_1} + \frac{1}{R_2}\right)$$

$$\frac{-Vo}{R_2} = \frac{V_1}{R_1} - V_{R2}\left(\frac{R_1 + R_2}{R_1 \times R_2}\right)$$

$$\frac{-Vo}{R_2} = \frac{V_1}{R_1} - \frac{R_2 \times V_2}{R_1 + R_2} \times \left(\frac{R_1 + R_2}{R_1 \times R_2}\right)$$

$$\frac{-Vo}{R_2} = \frac{V_1}{R_1} - \frac{V_2}{R_1}$$

$$Vo = R_2 \times \frac{(V_2 - V_1)}{R_1}$$

Finally,

$$Vo = (V_2 - V_1) \times \frac{R_2}{R_1}$$

In other words, the difference of inputs $\times$ gain $=$ output voltage.

6. INSTRUMENTATION AMPLIFIER

This circuit is very stable in its operation and uses the inverting, non-inverting, and differential configurations all in the same circuit. The circuit is shown in **Figure 4-25b** and the calculations are as follows:

Using the superposition principle:

$$V_{OUT1} = \left(1 + \frac{R_2}{R_1}\right) \times V_1 - \frac{R_2}{R_1} \times V_2$$

$$V_{OUT2} = \left(1 + \frac{R_3}{R_1}\right) \times V_2 - \frac{R_3}{R_1} \times V_1$$

If

$$R_5 = R_7 \text{ and } R_4 = R_6$$

then

$$Vo = (V_{OUT2} - V_{OUT1}) \times \frac{R_5}{R_4}$$

We can further simplify these equations if R2 = R3, then,

$$V_{OUT1} - V_{OUT2} = \left[\left(1 + \frac{R_2}{R_1} + \frac{R_3}{R_1}\right) \times V_1\right] - \left[\left(1 + \frac{R_2}{R_1} + \frac{R_3}{R_1}\right) \times V_2\right]$$

$$V_{OUT1} - V_{OUT2} = \left[\left(1 + \frac{2 \times R_2}{R_1}\right) \times V_1\right] - \left[\left(1 + \frac{2 \times R_2}{R_1}\right) \times V_2\right]$$

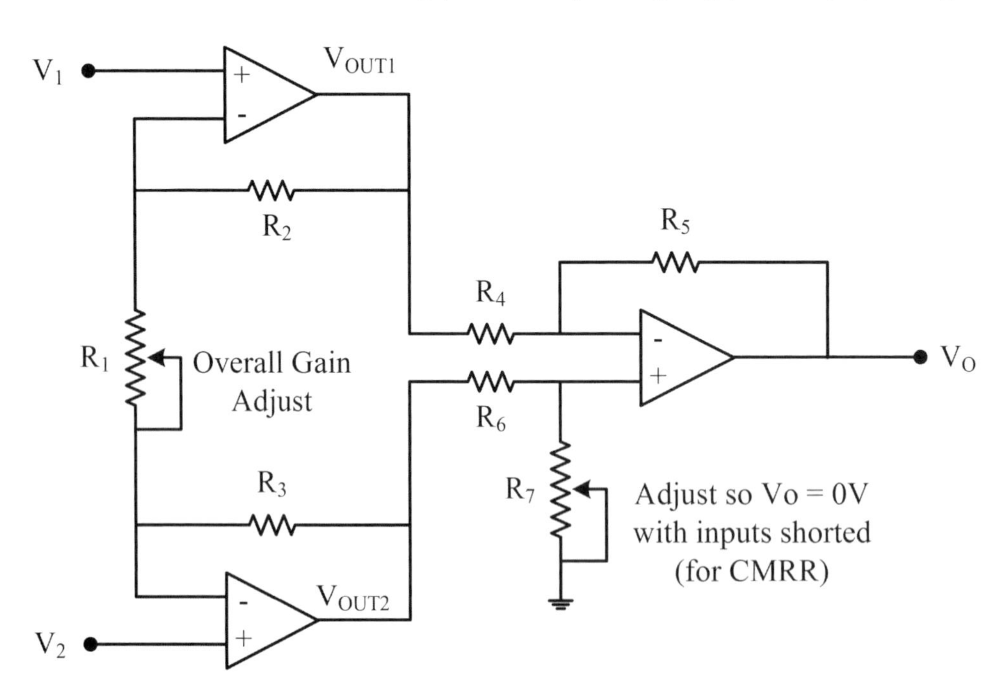

FIGURE 4-25b An instrumentation amplifier.

So,

$$V_{OUT1} - V_{OUT2} = (V_2 - V_1) \times \left(1 + \frac{2 \times R_2}{R_1}\right)$$

Finally,

$$V_O = (V_2 - V_1) \times \left(1 + \frac{2 \times R_2}{R_1}\right) \times \frac{R_5}{R_4}$$

7. POWER AMPLIFIER

The previous circuits amplify voltages from input to the output, but they do not amplify appreciably the power of the signals. The following power amplifier circuit can increase the power from input to the output in the range of several watts. The power amplifier can drive electronic circuits such as medical infusion pumps or medical monitors.

A circuit and its calculations are shown in **Figure 4-26.**

$$V_{OUT} = \left(1 + \frac{R_2}{R_1}\right) \times V_{IN}$$

AC output power:

$$P_{OUT}(RMS) = \frac{[V_{OUT}(peak)]^2}{2 \times R_L}$$

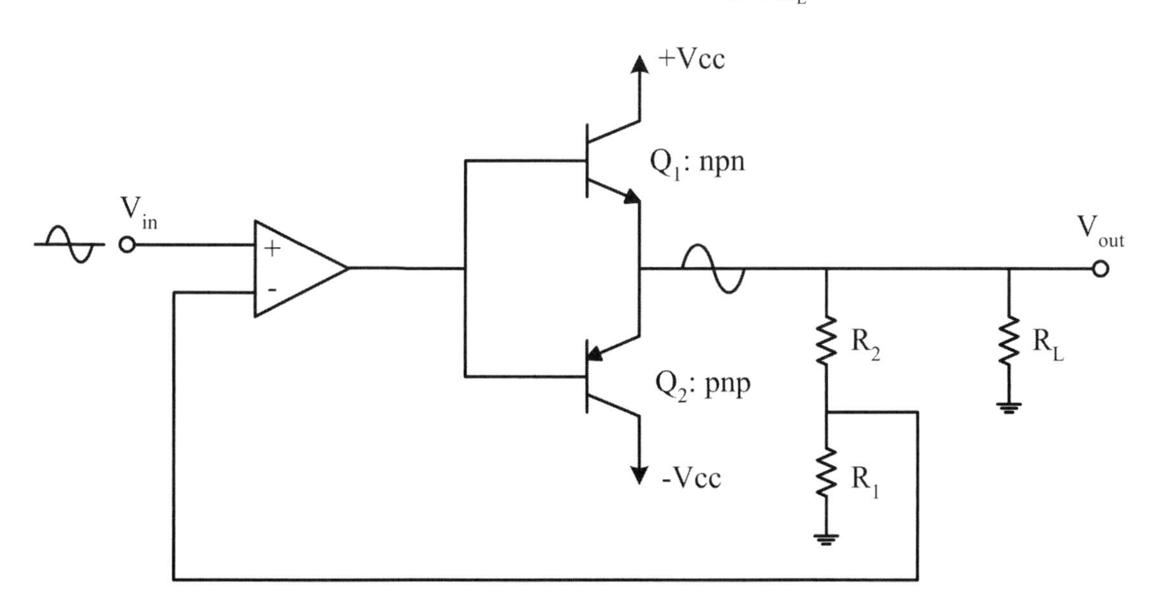

FIGURE 4-26 A push-pull power amplifier.

8. ISOLATION AMPLIFIER

In an isolation amplifier configuration, the AC power line is isolated from the amplifier circuit in the medical equipment for electrical safety reasons and also to eliminate any

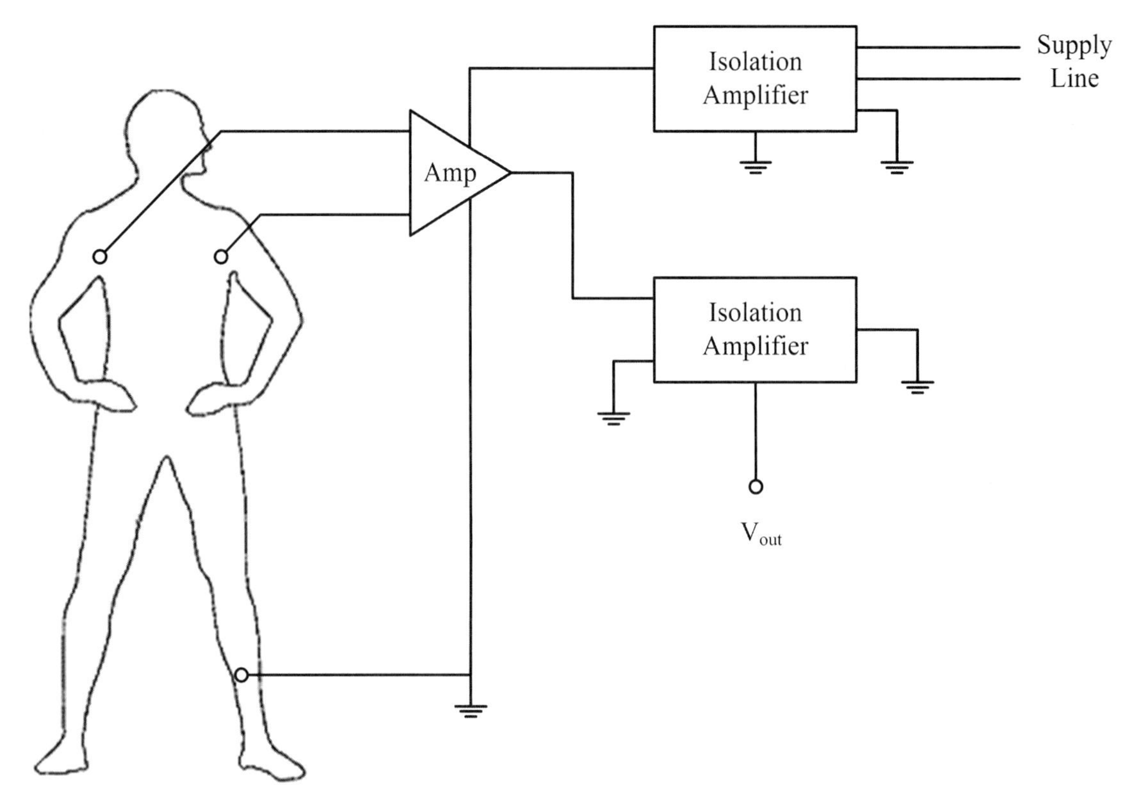

FIGURE 4-27 An isolation amplifier.

60 Hz interference noise in the biopotential recordings. The isolation provides very high impedance at the line frequency.

Figure 4-27 provides an isolation amplifier configuration where the AC line supply is isolated from the DC supply to the bioamplifier of the ECG signal. Also, the output of the amplifier is isolated from the recorder of the ECG signal. The isolation can be achieved by opto-coupling or transformer-coupling or even the capacitive-type coupling.

4.14 DC AND AC CHARACTERISTICS OF OPERATIONAL AMPLIFIER ICs

It is important to know which op-amp chip is better suited for various applications, not only in terms of input and output resistances or open-loop gains, but also in terms of its DC and AC characteristics. Regarding DC, we will discuss the offset voltage, offset current, and the supply voltage rejection ratio. Regarding AC, we will discuss common-mode rejection ratio, slew rate, and gain-bandwidth product.

V_{IO}

Input offset voltage (or DC offset voltage) is the voltage difference between the two input terminals of the op-amp. Ideally, voltage of the non-inverting terminal should be equal to the voltage of the inverting terminal. However, in practical op-amps, these voltages are not equal. DC offset voltage is typically ≈ 2 mV (in most op-amps). Erratic DC offset voltage can change the medical signal amplification in a differential amplifier circuit.

I_{IO}

The input offset current is the difference between the two input currents at the terminals. Ideally, the difference should be equal to zero. The value of this offset current in a general all-purpose op-amp is typically ≈ 10 to 20 nA.

Power Supply Voltage Rejection Ratio

Power supply voltage rejection ratio (PSRR) measures how well the op-amp rejects noise, hum, or ripple coming from the DC power supply. It is computed as follows:

$$PSRR = \frac{V_{CC1} - V_{CC2}}{V_{IO1} - V_{IO2}}$$

and

$$PSRR(dB) = 20 \log(PSRR)$$

V_{CC1} and V_{CC2} are the two values of the DC power supply provided to the op-amp, and V_{IO1} and V_{IO2} are the corresponding DC offset voltages. The larger the ratio of PSRR, the more desirable the op-amp is for medical application. That is to say, the larger the ratio, the greater the rejection of undesirable effects of the power supply.

The value of PSRR in a general use op-amp is typically ≈ 95 dB.

Common-mode Rejection Ratio

Common-mode rejection ratio (CMMR) is an important parameter of any op-amp. It is the measure of how well the op-amp rejects the common signal (such as noise) superimposed on two separate inputs in a differential amplifier circuit.

In a differential amplifier: $V_O = (V_1 - V_2) \times$ gain.

If the same noise is added (or superimposed) to both V_1 and V_2, the output should still be the same.

$$V_O = [(V_1 + \text{Noise}) - (V_2 + \text{Noise})] \times \text{Gain}$$
$$V_O = (V_1 - V_2) \times \text{Gain}$$

In practice, common noise may not be rejected by an op-amp. The calculation of CMRR suggests that the larger the figure, the better the degree of noise rejection.

$$CMRR = \frac{\text{differential gain}}{\text{common mode gain}}$$

$$CMRR = (\text{differential gain}) \times \frac{\text{input voltage in common mode}}{\text{output voltage in common mode}}$$

and

$$CMRR(dB) = 20 \log (CMRR)$$

A common-mode noise input is shown in **Figure 4-28a.**

In a 741 op-amp, CMRR is about 90 dB.

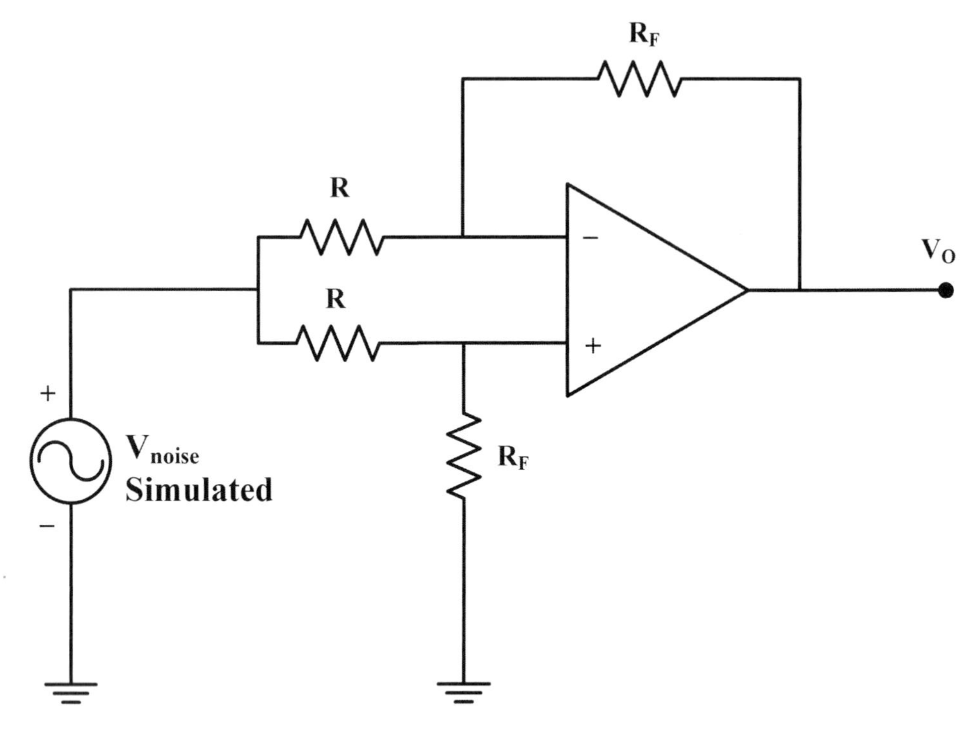

FIGURE 4-28a Common-mode rejection ratio (CMRR) circuit.

Slew Rate

Slew rate suggests the maximum state of change of the output voltage in time. For the 741 op-amp, the output cannot change faster than 0.5 V/μsec. For superior slew rate in some op-amps, this rate can go as high as 50 V/μsec. For superior slew rate, the output immediately follows the input.

Gain-bandwidth

A gain-bandwidth product is also called the bandwidth of the op-amp. This is the measure of frequency response pertaining to any op-amp, from low to high frequency inputs.

Refer to **Figure 4-28b.** Notice that the larger the bandwidth, the better the response of the op-amp.

Here, $BW_2 > BW_1$ and G = gain, hence,

$$GWB_2 = (G) \times (BW_2) \text{ and } GWB_1 = (G) \times (BW_1)$$

For a 741 op-amp GWB = 1 MHz with unity gain, whereas the 351 op-amp has a GWB = 4 MHz.

4.15 ACTIVE FILTERS, DIFFERENTIATORS, INTEGRATORS, AND ALARM CIRCUITS

Op-amps can be used for low-pass, high-pass, band-pass, and notch filters and are called active filters. The frequency-dependent components such as inductors and capacitors are used in these circuits. After amplification of the physiological signals, filtering of low

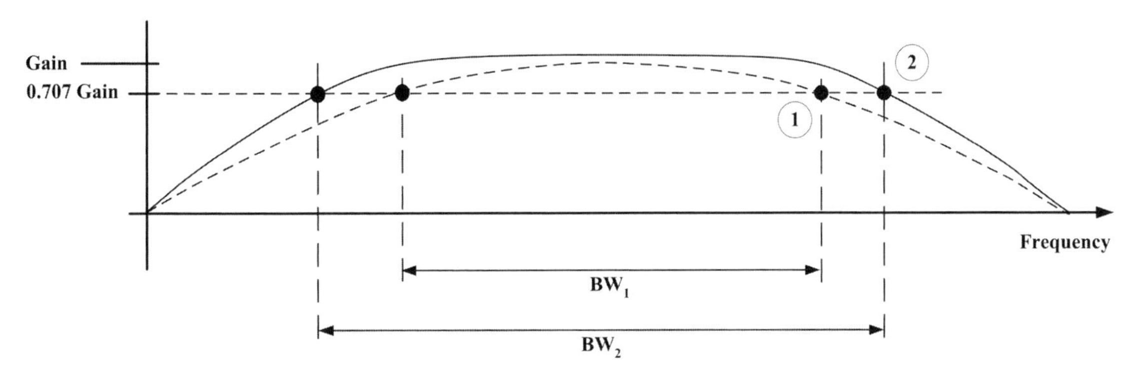

FIGURE 4-28b Gain-bandwidth diagram.

frequencies or high frequencies is needed in various applications. Examples of first-order and second-order low-pass filters are explained next.

First-order, Low-pass Filter

In **Figure 4-29a,** a first-order filter is shown. In this circuit, the first RC section is the low-pass filter. Here the R_1R_2 section is the non-inverting amplifier gain. This gain is:

$$A_V = (1 + R_1 / R_2)$$

For the filter section, using the voltage-divider rule:

$$\frac{V'_{IN}}{V_{IN}} = \frac{-jX_C}{R - jX_C} = \frac{1}{1 - \dfrac{R}{jX_C}} = \frac{1}{1 + \dfrac{jR}{X_C}} = \frac{1}{1 + j2\pi f \times RC}$$

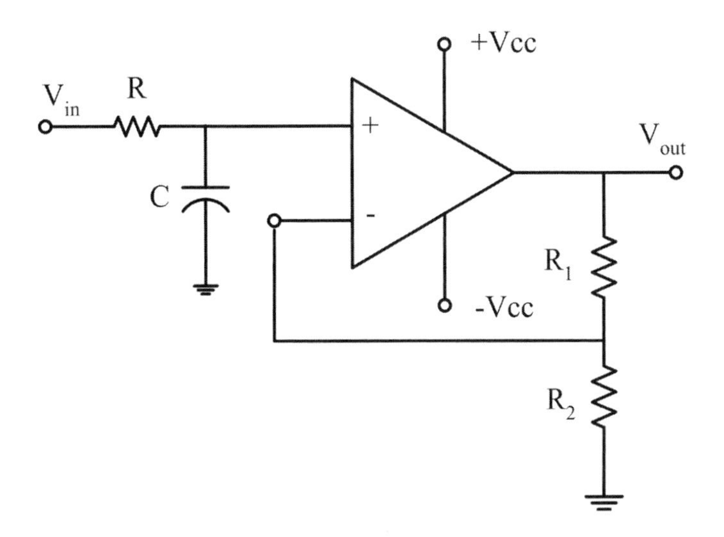

FIGURE 4-29a First-order active filter.

where

$$X_C = \frac{1}{2\pi fC} \text{ or } \frac{1}{\omega C}$$

Combining the filter section with the gain provider, the final output V_{OUT} is as follows:

$$\frac{V_{OUT}}{V_{IN}} = \frac{V'_{IN}}{V_{IN}} \times \frac{V_{OUT}}{V'_{IN}} = \frac{1}{1 + j2\pi f \times RC} \times A = \frac{A}{1 + j\omega RC}$$

Finally,

$$V_{OUT} = \frac{A \times V_{IN}}{1 + j\omega RC}$$

As the frequency (f) increases, V_{OUT} decreases; that is, the lower frequencies can pass through, but the higher frequencies cannot.

Second-order, Low-pass Filter

Figure 4-29b shows the second-order filter and that there are two filter sections, R_1C_1 and R_2C_2. Here R_3R_4 are the non-inverting gain circuit.

For this second-order circuit:

$$V_{OUT} = \frac{A \times V_{IN}}{(1 - \omega^2) + j\alpha\omega}$$

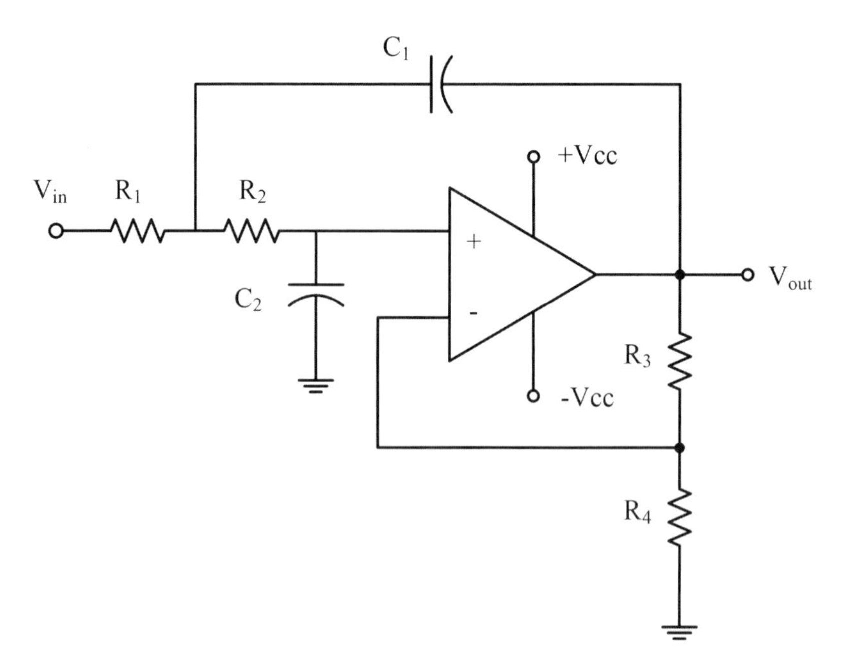

FIGURE 4-29b Second-order active filter.

where

$$A = 1 + \frac{R_3}{R_4}$$

$$\omega = 2\pi f$$

$$\alpha = \frac{R_2C_2 + R_1C_2 + R_1C_1(1 - A)}{\sqrt{R_1R_2C_1C_2}}$$

Notice that the term ω^2 in the denominator suggests that V_{OUT} will decrease easier as frequency increases in comparison to the first-order LPF.

Differentiator

A differentiator circuit provides output as the derivative of the input. In differential calculus, the derivative process is to determine the slope or the positive or negative change of the signal with respect to time. In an ECG machine, the slope of the QRS complex can be determined by a differentiator circuit. Differentiator circuit is shown in **Figure 4-30a.**

The current through a capacitor is given as:

$$i_C = C \times \frac{dV_C}{dt} = C \times \frac{d(V_{IN} - V'_{IN})}{dt}$$

where

$$V'_{IN} = 0 \text{ thus ic} = C \times \frac{dV_{IN}}{dt}$$

The current through a resistor is given as:

$$i_R = \frac{V'_{IN} - V_{OUT}}{R} = \frac{0 - V_{OUT}}{R} = \frac{-V_{OUT}}{R}$$

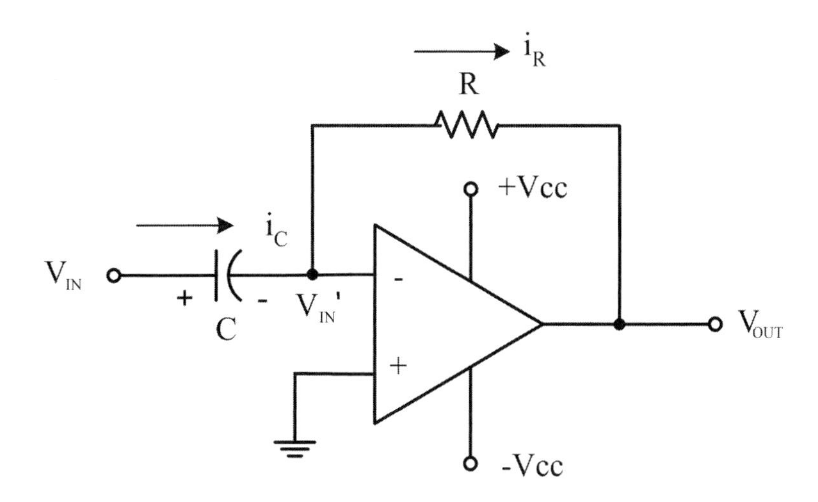

FIGURE 4-30a A differentiator circuit.

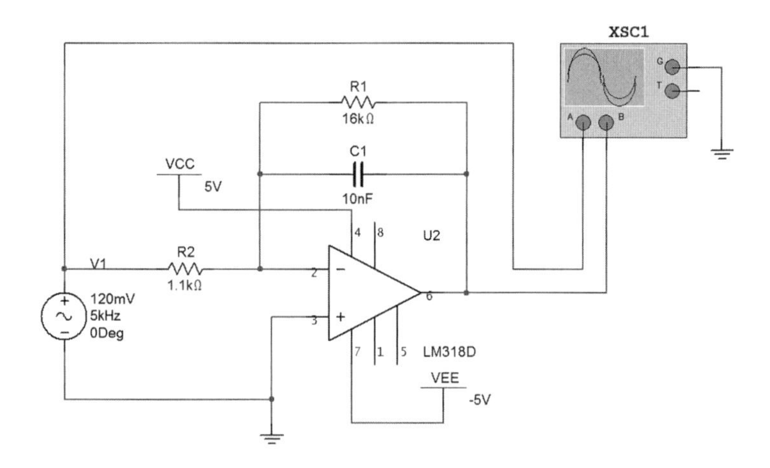

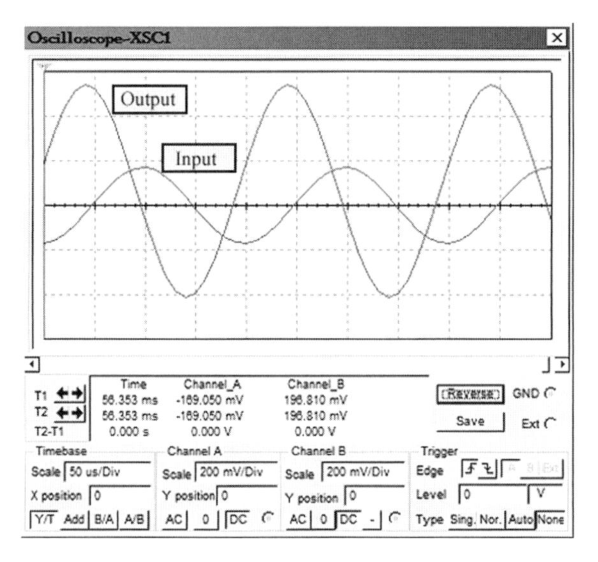

FIGURE 4-30b A sine-wave input to a differentiator circuit in MULTISIM.

Given these two equations of i_R and i_C, we know they are equal, so

$$\frac{-V_{OUT}}{R} = C \times \frac{dV_{IN}}{dt}$$

thus

$$V_{OUT} = -RC \times \frac{dV_{IN}}{dt}$$

MULTISIM software simulation of a differentiator circuit shows the differentiation of a sine-wave and a square-wave input in **Figure 4-30b** and **Figure 4-30c.** In Figure 4-30b, the derivative of the input sine wave is the output cosine wave. Similarly, in Figure 4-30c, the derivative of the square wave is the positive and negatives impulses.

Integrator

Integration is the process of finding "area under the curve," and it may represent a single integrated value of a signal starting from time $t = t_1$ to time $t = t_2$, where $t_1$and t_2 are the starting and the ending times of the integration process. In a cardiac output machine, the

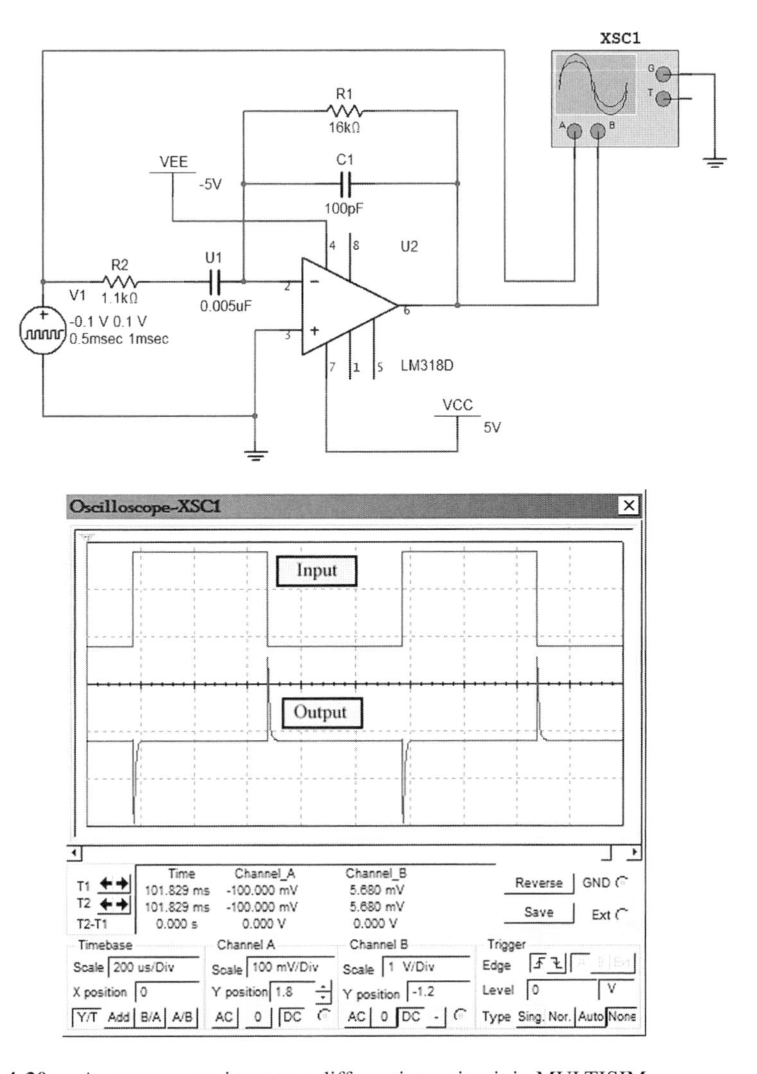

FIGURE 4-30c A square-wave input to a differentiator circuit in MULTISIM.

cardiac output signal is integrated between two points to determine whether its integrated value is in the normal range. See **Figure 4-31a.**

Given that $V'_{IN} = 0$ as the non-inverting terminal is at ground potential,

$$i_R = \frac{V_{IN} - V'_{IN}}{R} = \frac{V_{IN} - 0}{R} = \frac{V_{IN}}{R}$$

$$i_C = C \times \frac{dV_C}{dt} = C \times \frac{d(V'_{IN} - V_{OUT})}{dt}$$

or

$$i_C = C \times \frac{d(-V_{OUT})}{dt} = -C \times \frac{dV_{OUT}}{dt}$$

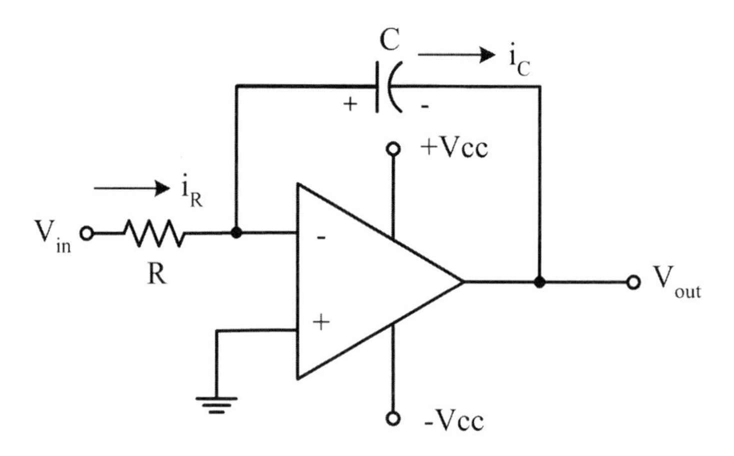

FIGURE 4-31a An integrator circuit.

Thus,

$$i_C = i_R$$

and

$$-C \times \frac{dV_{OUT}}{dt} = \frac{V_{IN}}{R}$$

Integrating both sides will result in:

$$-C \times V_{OUT} = \frac{1}{R}\int V_{IN} \times dt$$

$$\text{i.e., } V_{OUT} = -\frac{1}{RC}\int V_{IN} \times dt$$

MULTISIM simulation of an integrator circuit with sine- and square-wave inputs is shown in **Figure 4-31b** and **Figure 4-31c**. The integration of a sine wave is an inverted cosine wave, as shown in Figure 4-31b. Also, the integration of a square wave is a triangular wave, as shown in Figure 4-31c.

Oscillator

There are several op-amp oscillator circuits that generate sine-wave or square-wave oscillations or signals. These circuits use the principle of positive feedback to generate oscillations at specific resonant frequencies. See **Figure 4-32.**

Frequencies of Oscillation (f_O)

$$f_O = \frac{0.065}{RC}$$

and

$$\text{Gain} = \frac{R_2}{R_1} = 29$$

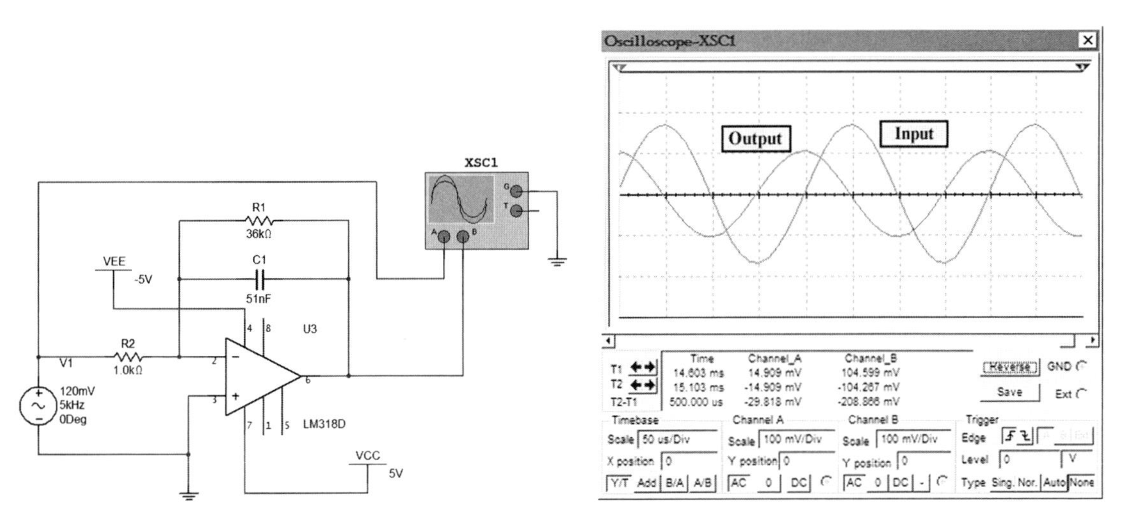

FIGURE 4-31b A sine-wave input to an integrator circuit in MULTISIM.

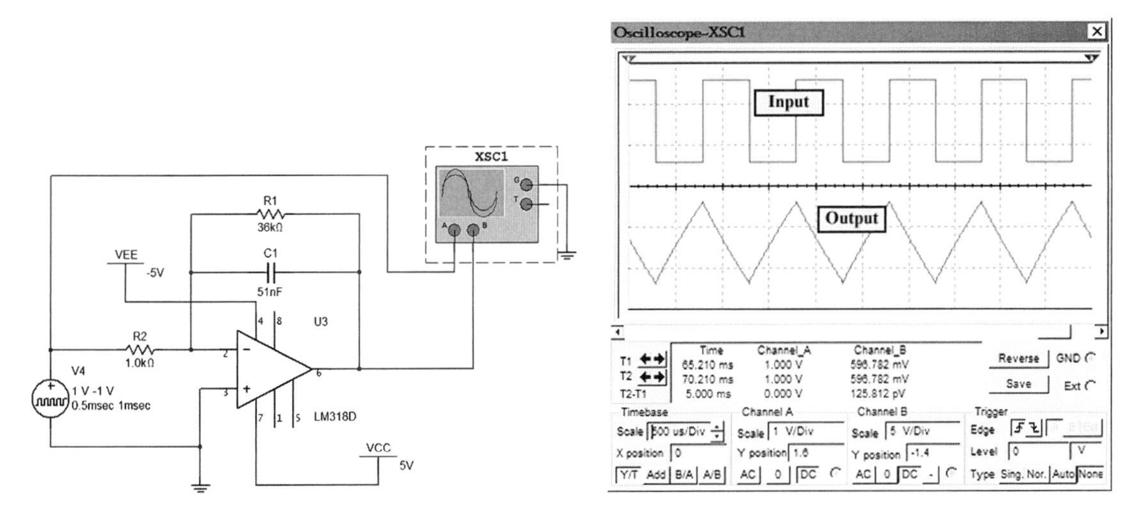

FIGURE 4-31c A square-wave input to an integrator circuit in MULTISIM.

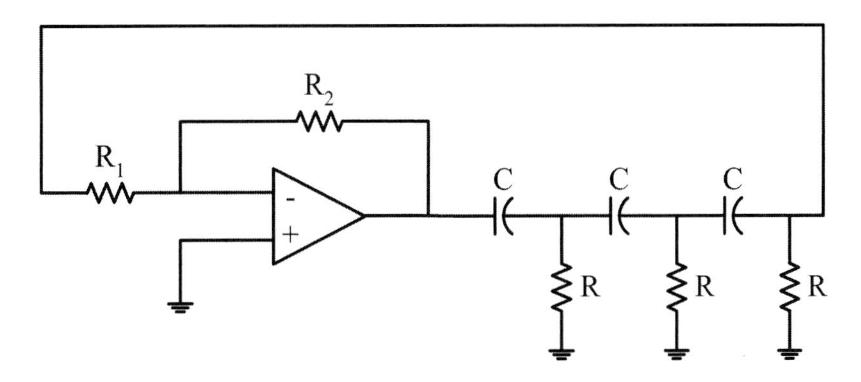

FIGURE 4-32 An RC phase-shift oscillator.

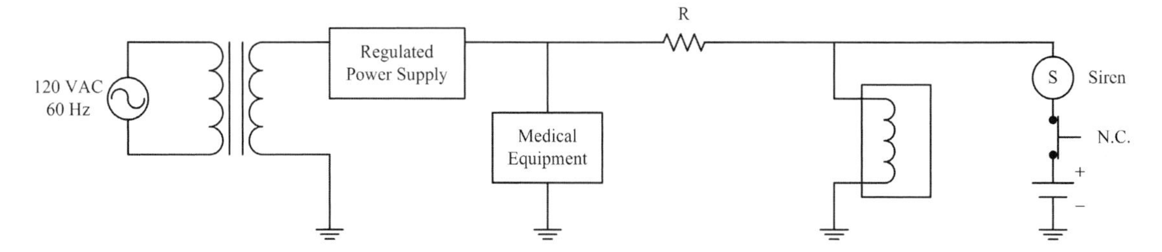

FIGURE 4-33 An alarm circuit.

Electronic Alarm Circuits

Various types of electronic alarm circuits are employed in medical equipment when the AC power is lost to the machine. The alarm may typically be a relay circuit with contacts to produce an audible, visual, or even a physical signal that warns the patient or nurse that AC power has failed. Such an alarm circuit is shown in **Figure 4-33.** Apart from warning, the alarm circuit turns on an uninterruptible backup DC power supply producing hours of power to the machine in emergency.

SUMMARY

- There are many types of analog circuits used in medical equipment. Some of the most commonly used are voltage dividers, current limiters, amplifiers, oscillators, filters, and waveshapers.
- The electronic components such as resistors, capacitors, and inductors all have properties that can restrict the amount of current flowing through them. All of these components exhibit the property of resistance to the flow of current. The property of resistance is measured in ohms.
- Maximum power transfer in electronics is needed when maximum power is intended to be delivered to the load by the source. This is achieved by ensuring that the load resistance is equal to the internal resistance of the source.
- One type of semiconductor diode is called a Zener diode. It is usually made in the reverse-bias mode where a large current can flow through it.
- Low-voltage medical signals can be amplified by semiconductor circuits such as operational amplifiers (op-amps) so that they can be viewed on a scope or a monitor.
- Op-amps are used in differentiators, integrators, waveshapers, Schmitt triggers, filters, and sensors.

TECHNICAL TERMINOLOGY

The following is a list of technical terminology mentioned in this chapter.

Amplitude: a nonnegative scalar measurement of a wave's magnitude of oscillation (i.e., measurement of the waveform magnitude starting at zero).

Analog signal: a variable signal continuous in both time and amplitude.

Digital: a conversion of analog signal into a discrete signal in time, defined as either a 1 or a 0, indicating on or off. These 1s and 0s can be stored and recalled to be converted back into usable information.

Filter: a device intended to remove unwanted signal components and/or enhance wanted ones. Electronic or audio filters can be: passive or active, analog or digital, discrete-time (sampled) or continuous-time, linear or non-linear, infinite impulse response (IIR type) or finite impulse response (FIR type).

Oscillator: an electronic device capable of generating a recurring waveform, or a digital process used by a synthesizer to generate the same.

Rectifier: an electrical device, comprising one or more semiconductor devices (such as diodes) converting alternating current to direct current.

Regulator: a device used to regulate the output of a device, such as voltage or current. This device is designed to automatically maintain a constant voltage level or a constant current level. It may be used to regulate one or more AC or DC voltages.

Transformer: an electrical device that transfers energy from one circuit to another by magnetic coupling with no moving parts. These devices are used to convert between high and low voltages (and currents), to change impedance, and to provide electrical isolation between circuits.

QUIZ

1. Which following circuit is used in amplifying a weak ECG signal?

a) Transformer circuit. b) Differential amplifier circuit.
c) Non-inverting amplifier circuit. d) None of the above.

2. True or False: The voltage drop across a large resistance is always more.

a) True. b) False.

3. True or False: The current through a larger resistance is always more.

a) True. b) False.

4. The total resistance of a 10 KΩ and 20 KΩ in parallel is ________________.

a) 15 KΩ b) 30 KΩ c) 6.67 KΩ d) 12 KΩ

5. True or False: A signal loads down (that is, gets smaller) when load resistance is larger than the source resistance.

a) True. b) False.

6. The voltage gain in a differential amplifier is ________________.

a) $R_F = R_I$ b) R_F/R_I c) R_F/R_F d) None of the above

Note: R_F and R_I are the feedback and input resistances, respectively.

7. The integration of sin(wt) in an integrator is ________________.

a) $-\cos(wt)$ b) $\cos(wt)$ c) $\sin^2(wt)$ d) $-\sin(wt)$

8. When the input to a differentiator is sin (wt), the output is ________________.

a) $-\cos(wt)$ b) $\cos(wt)$ c) $\cos^2(wt)$ d) $-\cos^2(wt)$

9. A capacitor fully charges in ________________.

a) One time constant. b) Three time constants. c) Four time constants.
d) Five time constants.

10. A power source having a source resistance of 50 Ω delivers maximum power to a load having a resistance of ________________.

a) 50 Ω b) 100 Ω c) 120 Ω d) 150 Ω

PROBLEMS

1. For the RC circuit of **Figure 4-11,** resistance R = 10 KΩ, capacitance C = 2 nF, and the source voltage V_S = 5 V (peak) from DC to 100 kHz. Determine the cut-off frequency of the circuit and plot the voltage gain (Bode plot) curve on semi-log paper using at least 10 frequency values between 100 Hz and 20 kHz.
2. For the RL circuit of **Figure 4-13a,** determine the cut-off frequency and plot the voltage gain (Bode plot) curve on semi-log paper using at least 10 frequency points starting at 100 Hz and ending at 10 kHz. Given source voltage V_S(p) remains constant at 10 V(p) between 100 Hz and 10 kHz.
3. For the bridge circuit shown in **Figure 4-14a,** determine the output voltage (V_O) when $R_1 = R_2 = R_3$ = 150 KΩ, R_4 = 50 KΩ, and the applied voltage V_S = 20 V.
4. For the Zener diode circuit in **Figure 4-18a,** determine the total current when R = 2 KΩ, R_L = 5 KΩ, and V_S = 4 V.
5. Determine the output voltage for the circuit given in **Figure 4-20a.** Given: R_3 = 2 KΩ, R_5 = 5 KΩ, input resistance of the transistor h_{IE} = 1.2 KΩ, current gain of the transistor β = 100, and the input voltage V_I = 100 mV (peak). Also, determine the output voltage when load resistance R_5 and the emitter capacitor C_2 are removed from the circuit.
6. For the circuit of **Figure 4-20b,** determine the output voltage V_O when drain resistance R_D = 1.5 KΩ, load resistance R_L = 10 KΩ, transconductance gain of the JFET g_m = 0.1 amp/volt, and the input voltage is 0.15 V (peak).
7. Determine CMRR in decibels for the circuit in **Figure 4-25a.** In the differential mode, V_1 = 2 V, V_2 = −3.1 V, and V_O = −11.1 V. Also, in the common-mode, V_1 = 1 V, V_2 = 1 V, and V_O = 0.00014 V. Given R_1 = 2 KΩ and R_2 = 20 KΩ.
8. For the **Figure 4-29a,** determine V_O when R = 2 KΩ, C = 0.1μF, R_1 = 4 KΩ, and R_2 = 2.2 KΩ. The input voltage is 5 V (peak) at 3.9 kHz.
9. For the second-order filter shown in **Figure 4-29b,** determine the output voltage when the components are: R_1 = 1 KΩ, C_1 = 0.1 μF, R_2 = 2 KΩ, C_2 = 0.15 μF, R_3 = 10 KΩ, and R_4 = 2 KΩ. The input voltage is 2 V and the frequency is 1 kHz.
10. Determine the time constant in the circuit in **Figure 4-34.** Also, find the voltage across the capacitor at one time constant.

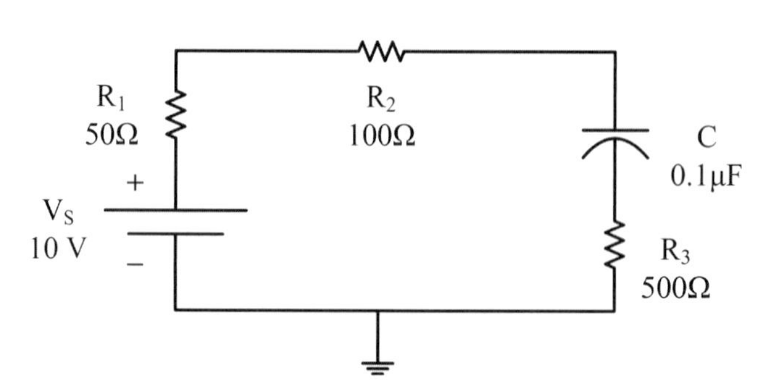

FIGURE 4-34 An RC circuit with a DC power supply.

11. Determine the current in the circuit given in **Figure 4-35.**

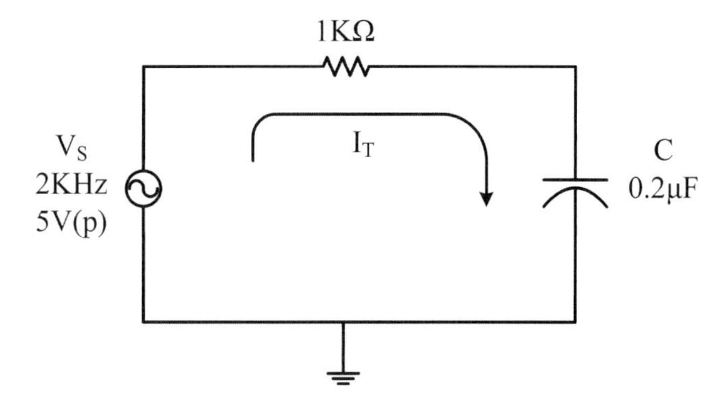

FIGURE 4-35 An RC circuit with an AC power supply.

12. Determine the output voltage of the following circuits as shown in **Figures 4-36a, 4-36b, 4-36c,** and **4-36d.**

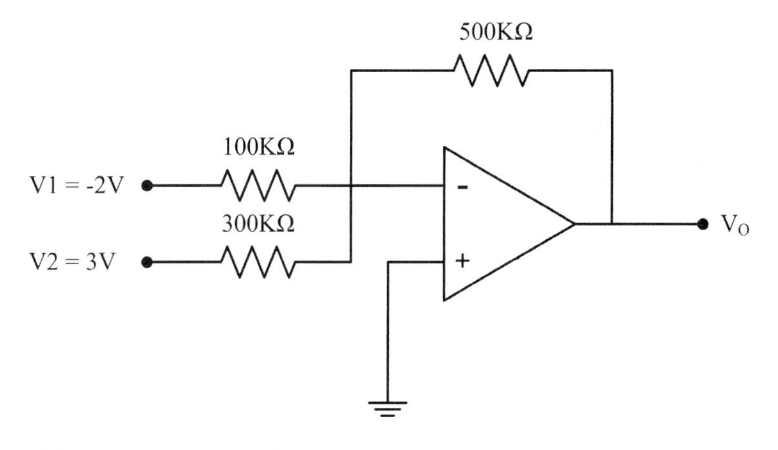

FIGURE 4-36a A summing amplifier.

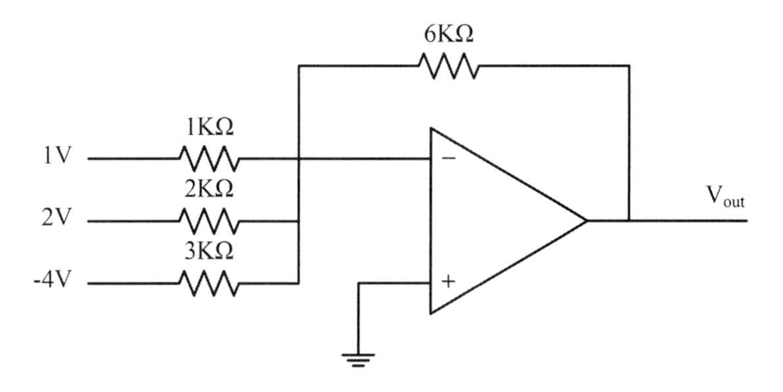

FIGURE 4-36b A summing amplifier.

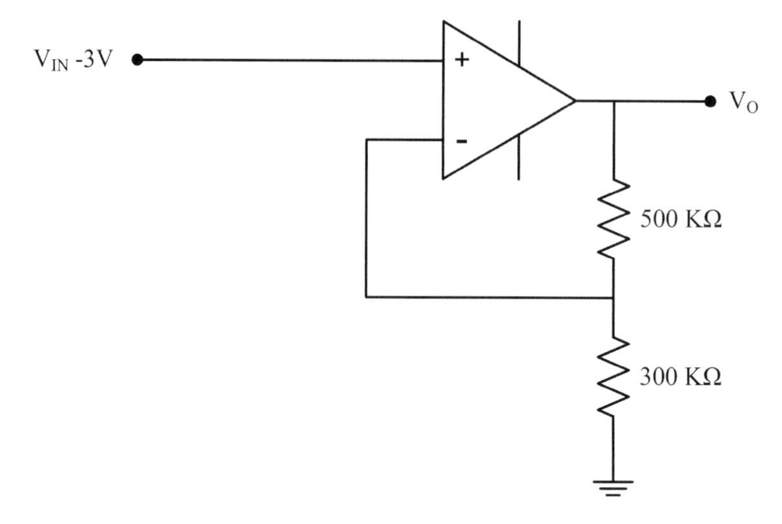

FIGURE 4-36c A non-inverting amplifier.

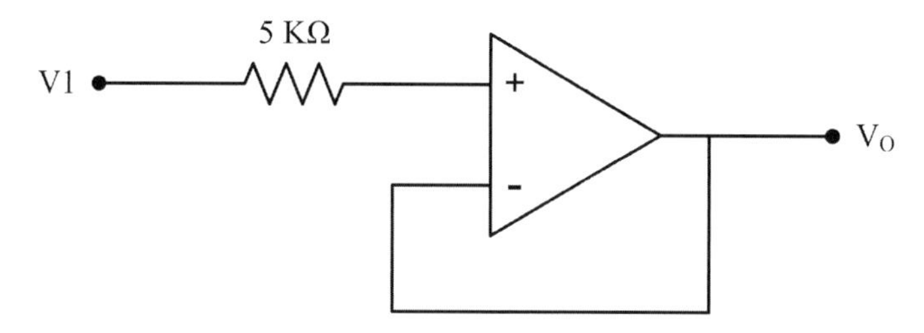

FIGURE 4-36d A buffer circuit.

13. Determine the voltage at points 1, 2, and 3 for the circuit shown in **Figure 4-37.**

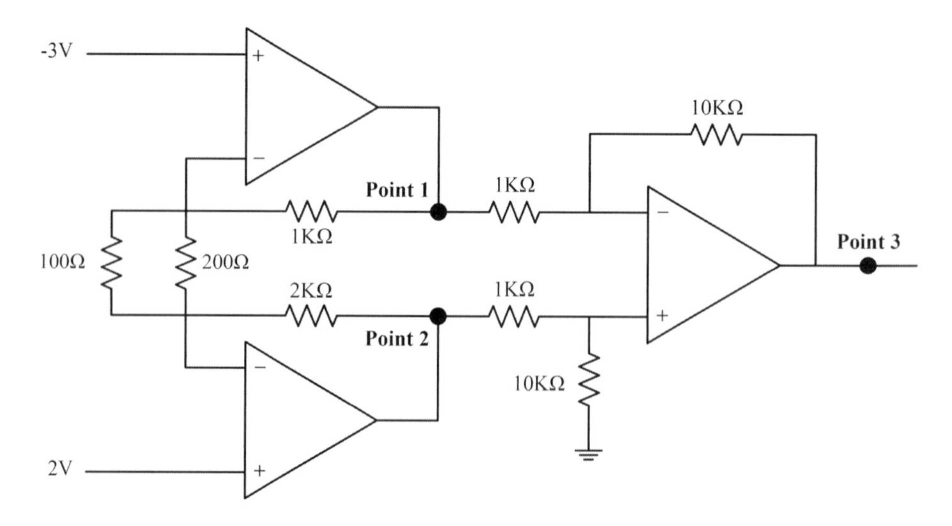

FIGURE 4-37 An instrumentation amplifier.

14. Sketch the output waveform for the given input as shown in **Figure 4-38a.**

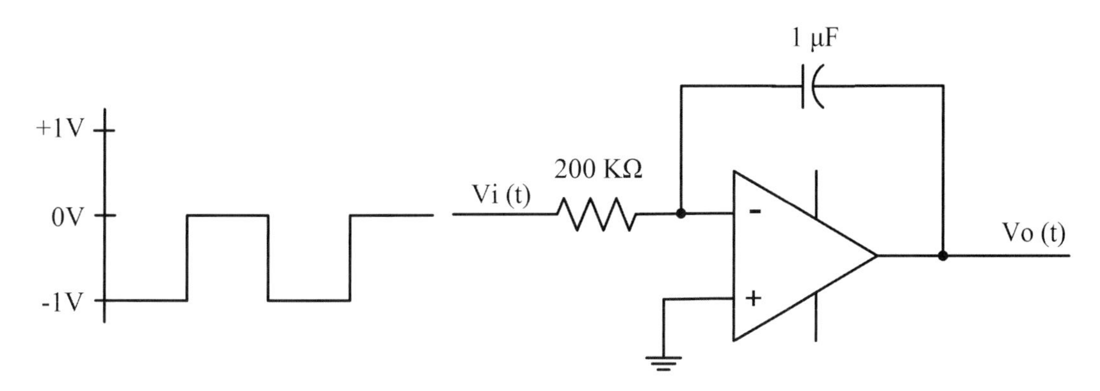

FIGURE 4-38a Input to an integrator circuit.

15. Find the total output voltage for the integrator shown in **Figure 4-38b.** Integrate between t = 0 and t = 5 seconds.

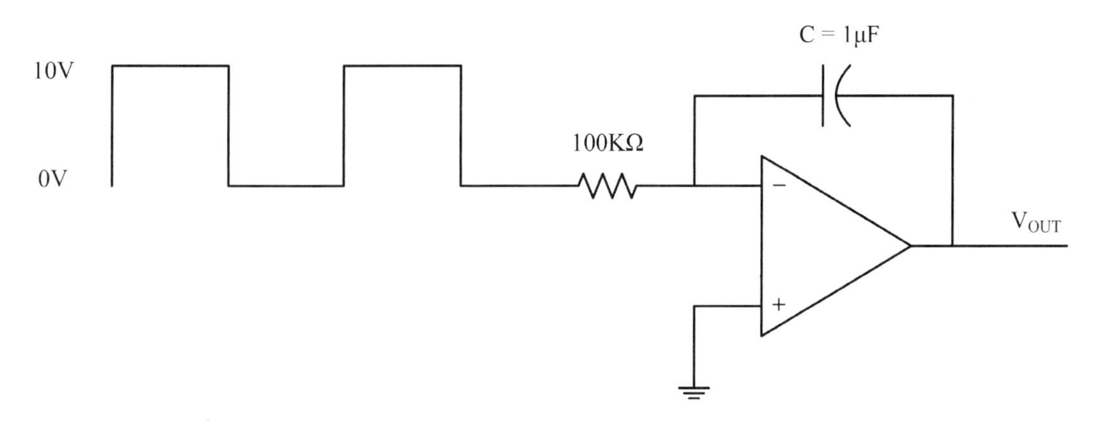

FIGURE 4-38b Input to an integrator circuit.

16. Rough sketch the output of an integrator, given the input signal sketch in **Figure 4-38c.**

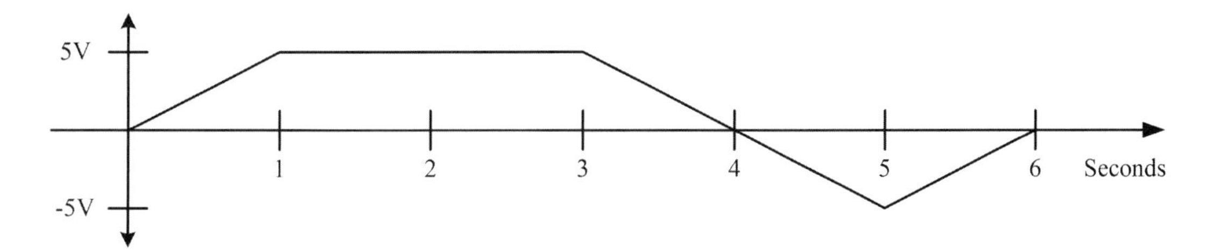

FIGURE 4-38c Input a waveshape to an integrator.

17. Rough sketch the output of a differentiator with the input signal as shown in **Figure 4-38c.**

18. Determine the output of the differentiator shown in **Figure 4-39.**

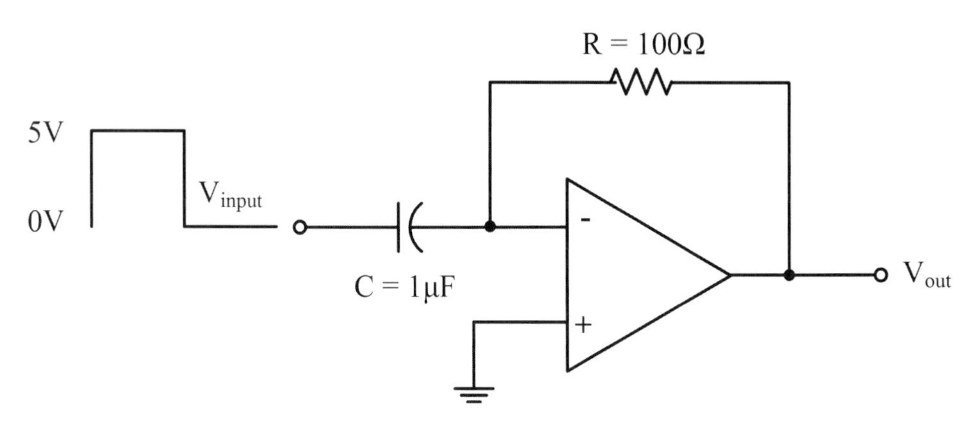

FIGURE 4-39 A differentiator circuit.

19. Design a non-inverting amplifier with a gain of 12 when the input signal has an internal resistance of 100 Ω.

20. Determine the total resistance of the circuit shown in **Figure 4-40.** Also, determine the RMS current in the 1 KΩ resistor when the input voltage is 10 V (peak).

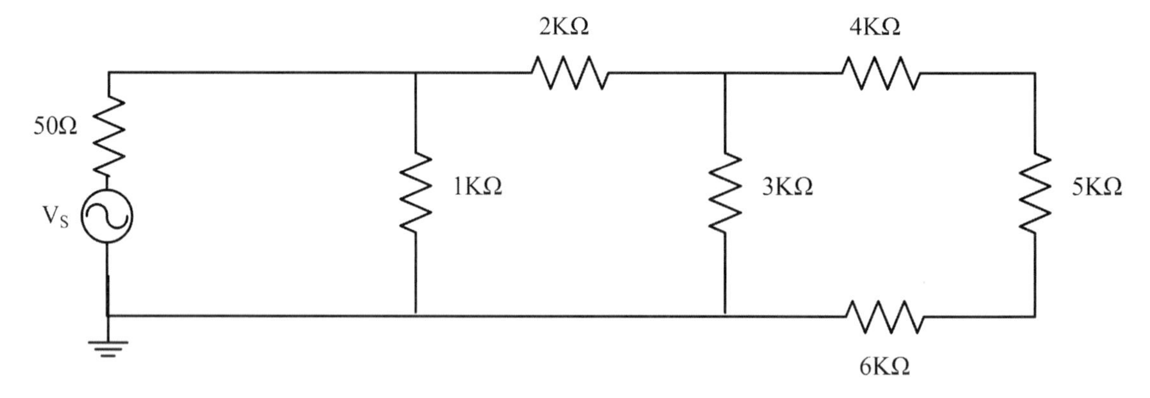

FIGURE 4-40 A series/parallel circuit.

CASE STUDY

An elderly man who suffers from high blood pressure and diabetes has a medical emergency locket on him at all times. The patient also has a stent inserted into the right side of his heart by catheterization. Recently, he felt pain in his chest and considered that he was having a heart attack. He pushed the medical emergency button; however, no emergency assistance arrived. Fortunately, this was a false alarm. There are several possibilities for the malfunctions with the emergency medical device he is using. Name a few of them and explain possible remedies. (Hint: Possible problems may be a weak battery or the wireless circuits may not be working properly.)

RESEARCH TOPICS

1. Develop a performance criterion in using operational amplifier chips from at least two or three vendors in the evaluation of amplifying a small AC or DC voltage. The op-amp chip can be connected in an inverting or non-inverting amplifier mode. The performance criterion must be detailed and should compare with the chips from the various vendors.
2. Develop the same as in the previous research topic, but explore the use of differential amplifier or instrumentation amplifier mode. In this project, two inputs will be used.
3. Design a notch filter using op-amps, resistors, and capacitors. Also, determine the quality factor of the notch filter and discuss how to change the quality factor for a specific application.
4. Implement the MATLAB or LABVIEW simulation of a second-order band-pass filter and show its time-domain and the frequency-domain analysis.

CHAPTER 5

Biomedical Electronics: Digital

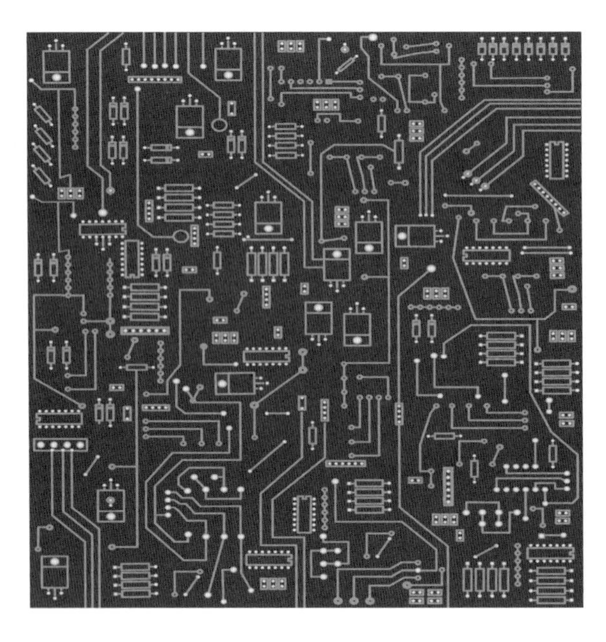

CHAPTER OUTLINE

OBJECTIVES

The objective of this chapter is to provide the reader with a review of digital circuits and microprocessors commonly used in medical instruments. This chapter includes computer hardware and software concepts for medical data processing.

Upon completion of this chapter, the reader will be able to:

- Determine the output of a D/A converter.
- Determine the output of an A/D converter.
- Discuss the tables of various logic gates.

- Differentiate the output of various flip-flops.
- Discuss the architecture of a microprocessor.
- Discuss the components of a computer.

INTERNET WEB SITES

http://www.computer.org (Institute of Electrical and Electronics Engineers [IEEE] Computer Society)
http://www.acm.org (Association of Computing Machinery)
http://www.aitp.org (Association of Information Technology Professionals)
http://www.pcworld.com (PC World Magazine [online version])
http://www.microsoft.com (Microsoft)
http://www.pcmag.com (PC Magazine)
http://www.intel.com (Intel Corporation)

INTRODUCTION

Most biomedical instruments consist of both analog and digital circuits and a conversion between the two is often necessary. The process of digitization is based on the sampling of an analog signal, with the signal's resolution dependent on how many samples are taken in one second. This means that the higher the number of samples, the better the resolution. This chapter discusses analog-to-digital converters, digital-to-analog converters, digital gates and flip-flops, registers, microprocessors, computer hardware, and computer software.

5.1 DIGITAL ELECTRONICS IN BIOINSTRUMENTATION

Digital circuits and analog circuits have distinct differences. Digital circuits are based on discrete voltage levels, whereas analog circuits depend on continuously varying voltages. There are at least two ways to understand the use of digital electronics in biomedical instruments: the first is to understand digital and microprocessor circuits as individual units; the second is to understand computers and computer interfaces. **Figure 5-1** shows an example of analog-to-digital conversion and the computer interface for the automatic external defibrillator (AED) biomedical device. This figure shows also the digitization of the ECG signal and the computer control of the defibrillation signal. The instrumentation/operational amplifiers receive the analog ECG signal from the electrodes and pass it to the analog-to-digital converter (ADC) chip for conversion into serial digits. The digits are then sent to the computer through a universal serial bus (USB) interface. Computer software determines when and what kind of shock pulse should be given to the patient based upon the ECG signal. Notice the high-voltage transformer circuit and the current controller. This example illustrates the importance of digital electronics in medical instrumentation.

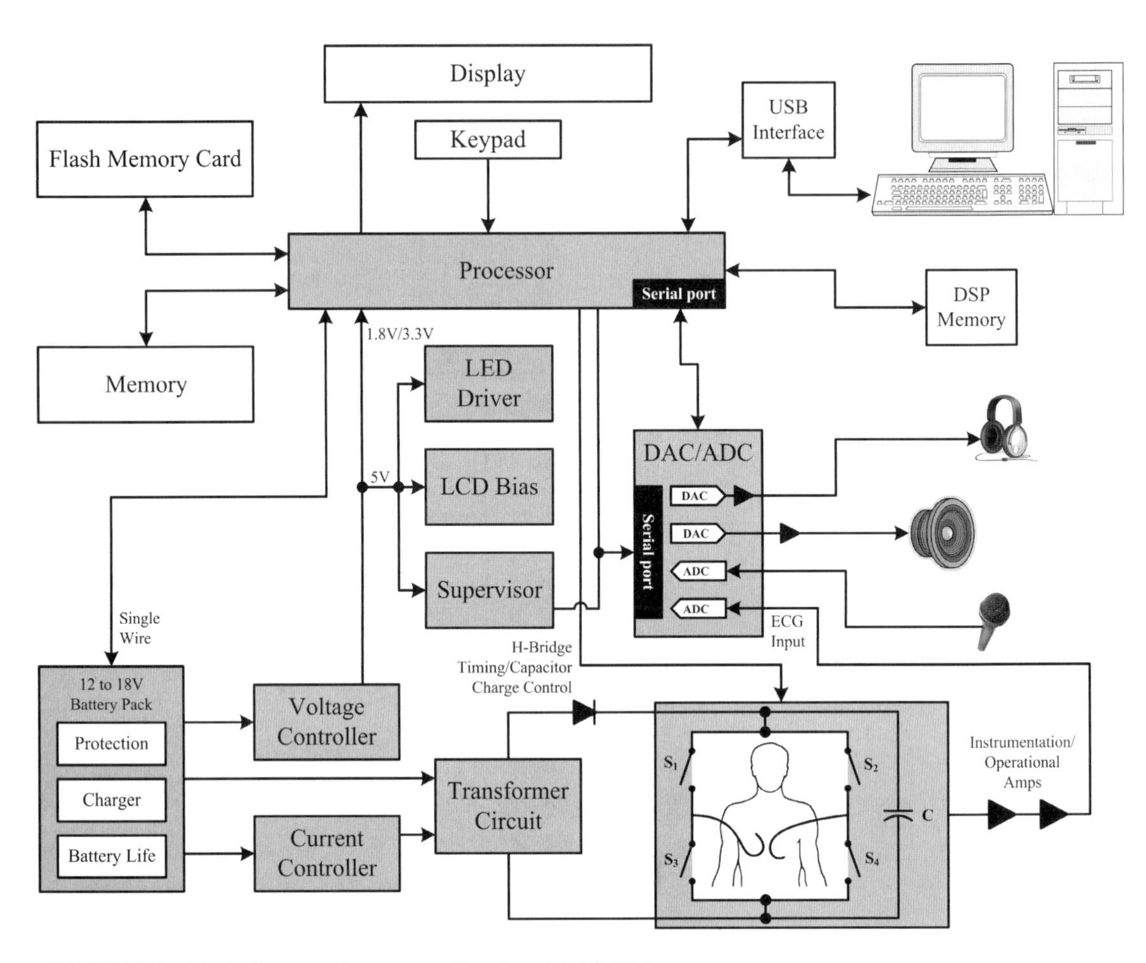

FIGURE 5-1 Block diagram of an automatic external defibrillator.

5.2 ADVANTAGES OF DIGITAL CIRCUITS

Digital circuits (also called digital systems or logic circuits) have numerous advantages over analog circuits in electronics.

1. Digital circuits are less noisy than analog circuits. They are affected less by noise because the noise level in most applications is below the discrete level of binary one (1). That is, the noise is considered as binary zero (0).
2. Digital circuits are programmable and can be interfaced easily with microprocessors and computers. Software loaded on computers or microprocessors can drive or program any digital circuit, which is not possible with analog circuits.
3. Digital circuits have large-scale integration (LSI). It is possible to build large digital circuits on small-size integrated circuits (ICs).
4. Digital circuits are regenerative. Because of the nature of digital signal, the discrete levels can be regenerated or repeated easily in digital circuits.

5. Digital circuits provide better storage than analog circuits. Digital memory devices have superior quality and are immune to noise so information can be stored and retrieved without degradation.

However, there are disadvantages in using digital circuits. To preserve the resolution of an analog signal, digital circuits depend on the proper sampling rate and the number of bits used in each sample. It is also more expensive to manufacture digital circuits if the quantity is small. Additionally, digital circuits may use more energy in some applications compared to analog circuits.

5.3 DIGITAL-TO-ANALOG CONVERTERS

Digital-to-analog converters (DAC) incorporate a ladder network of resistors. The parallel digits are interfaced to this ladder network and its analog output can then be amplified by an op-amp circuit. As analog-to-digital converters use DAC circuits for the digitized result, we will first explain an R/2R resistor ladder network as a DAC circuit. We will then discuss the ADC circuit. An example of a four-bit D/A circuit is given in **Figure 5-2a.**

Assume

$$R = 10\ K\Omega,\ \text{then}\ 2R = 20\ K\Omega$$

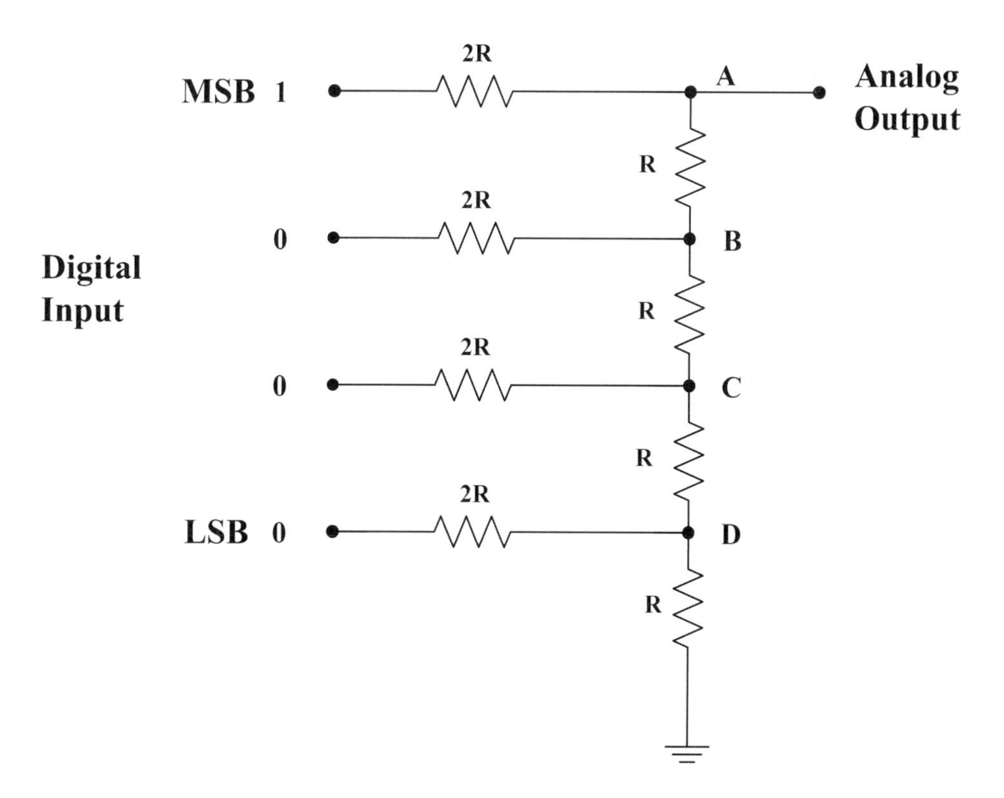

FIGURE 5-2a R/2R ladder network with an input of 1000 bits.

The most significant bit (MSB) is a binary 1, which is 5 V. The least significant bit (LSB) is binary 0, or 0 V (ground).

At point D in the circuit, 2R and the 2R resistors are in parallel, thus resulting in the value of R.

At point C, the lower section adds up to 2R (i.e., R + R in series). Sequentially, as we reach point A, the equivalent circuit becomes more simplified, as shown in **Figure 5-2b.**

The resulting analog output is then 2.5 V in the voltage divider network. Thereby, a digital pattern of 1000 results in an analog voltage of 2.5 V. Similarly, for the digital pattern of 0100, the result is 1.25 V. This is shown in the circuit analysis in **Figure 5-2c.**

At point B, the equivalent circuit is as shown in **Figure 5-2d.**

The circuit can also be redrawn, as shown in **Figure 5-2e, Figure 5-2f,** and **Figure 5-2g.**

With the above discussion in mind, a four-bit table can be shown as:

1	1	1	1	=	4.6875 V
1	1	1	0	=	4.375 V
1	1	0	1	=	4.0625 V
1	1	0	0	=	3.75 V
1	0	1	1	=	3.4375 V
1	0	1	0	=	3.125 V
1	0	0	1	=	2.8125 V
1	0	0	0	=	2.5 V
0	1	1	1	=	2.1875 V
0	1	1	0	=	1.875 V
0	1	0	1	=	1.5625 V
0	1	0	0	=	1.25 V
0	0	1	1	=	0.9375 V
0	0	1	0	=	0.625 V
0	0	0	1	=	0.3125 V
0	0	0	0	=	0 V

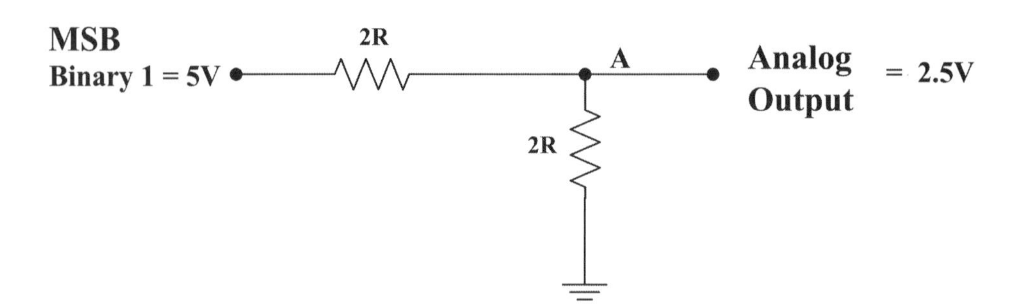

FIGURE 5-2b Simplified R/2R ladder network for Figure 5-2a circuit.

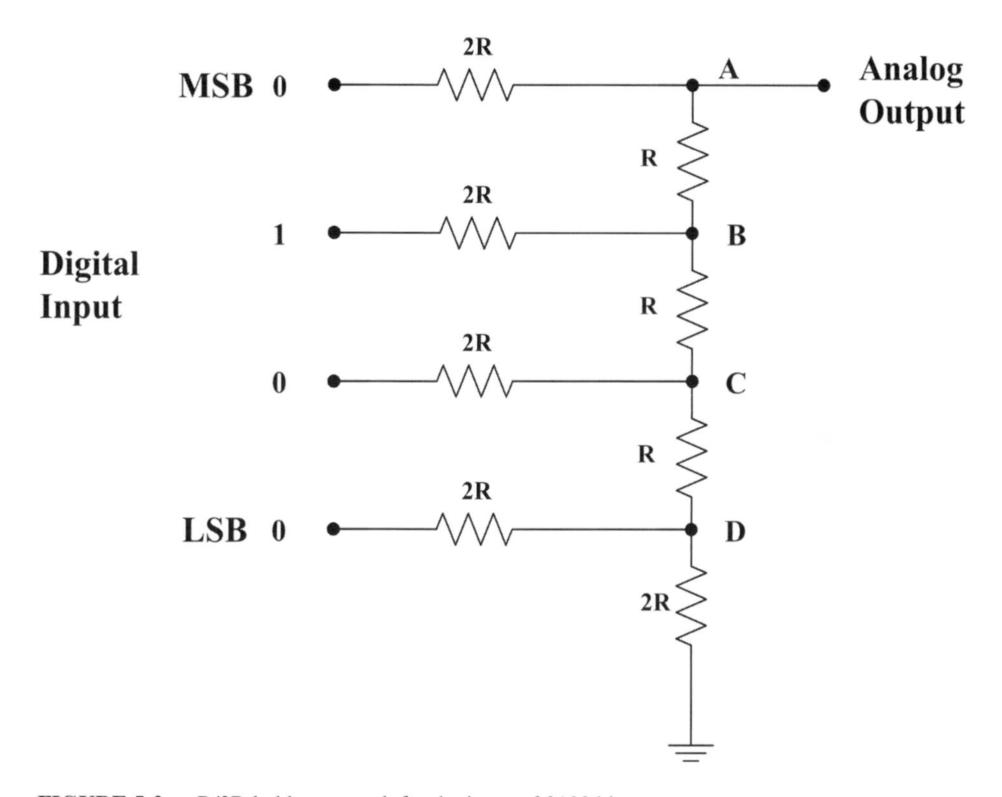

FIGURE 5-2c R/2R ladder network for the input of 0100 bits.

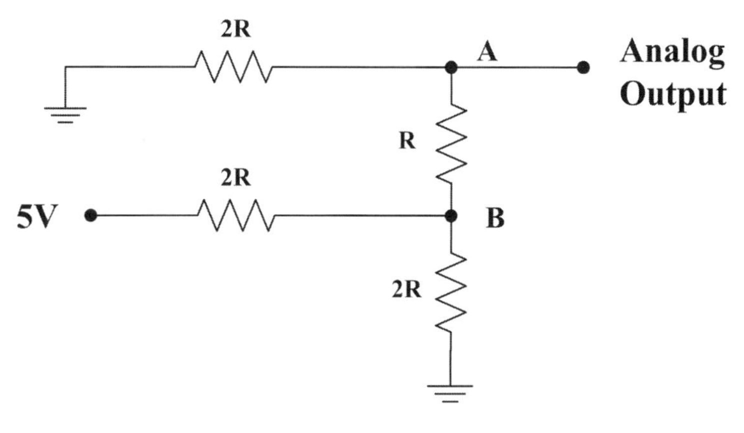

FIGURE 5-2d Simplified network of Figure 5-2c.

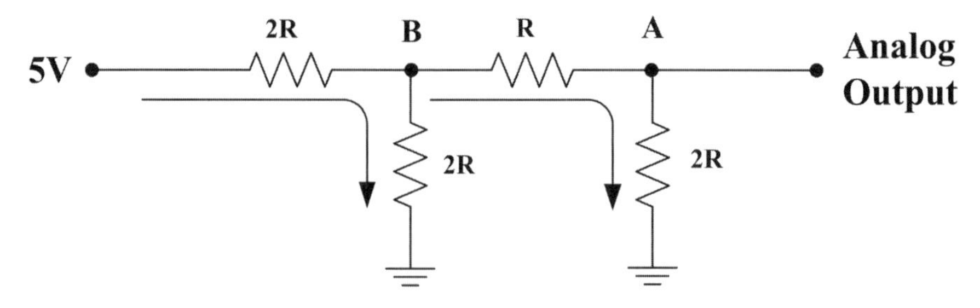

FIGURE 5-2e Simplified network of Figure 5-2d.

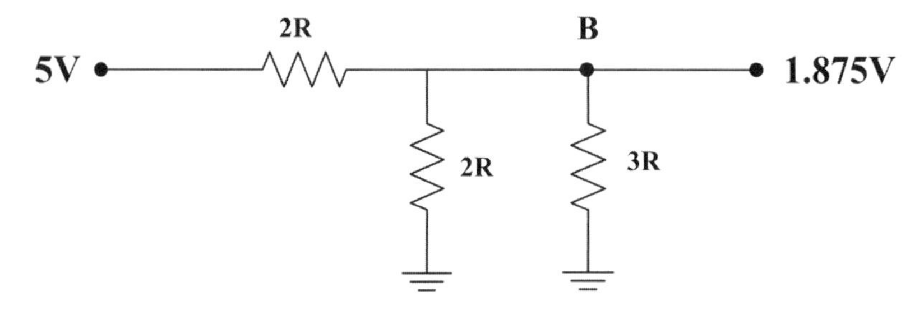

FIGURE 5-2f Simplified network of Figure 5-2e.

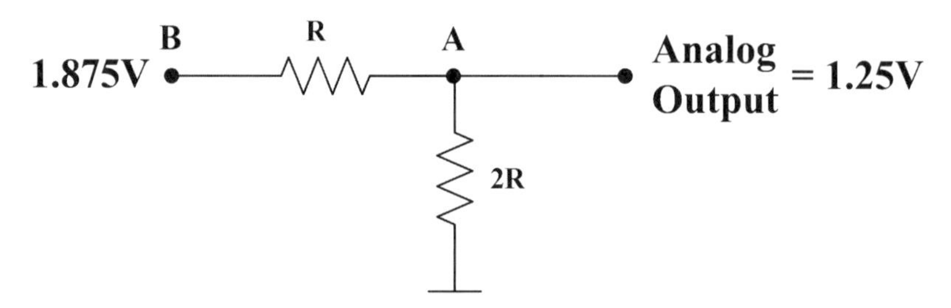

FIGURE 5-2g Simplified network of Figure 5-2f.

The step size is given as $(2^{-n}) \times$ voltage range, where n = number of bits. When n = 4, the step size is $(2^{-4}) \times 5$ V = 0.3125 V. The digits of 0001 result in the first step size of 0.3125 V.

The example of a 4-bit DAC can be extended to more popular 8-bit, 12-bit, or 16-bit DACs. The resolution is better with the larger number of bits because the step size gets smaller and the digital pattern is closer to the actual sample analog value.

5.4 ANALOG-TO-DIGITAL CONVERTERS

The successive approximation type of analog-to-digital converters (ADC) may take more time in converting analog signals into digits, but the resolution is superior to flash ADCs or slope ADCs. An example of a successive approximation circuit is provided in this section. **Figure 5-3** shows a block diagram circuit of a four-bit successive approximation ADC.

The analog signal is X and the process of successive approximation generates a digital signal. Four 1-bit shift registers are triggered with the clock input. The shift registers latch to the successive approximation register (SAR) and the SAR latches to the DAC.

Each bit shifts from left to right. After four shifts, the tri-state buffer output displays the final DAC input bits as a digital output. The comparator output sets or resets the bits of the SAR after each comparison of the X and Y bits (Y is the DAC output). For the four-bit ADC, there will be four comparisons between X and Y.

Assume that the input is a 3-V analog sample. Determine the digits in a four-bit A/D converter.

Comparison	X	Y	DAC Input	Comment
1	3 V	2.5 V	1000 MSB↑	Clock starts X > Y MSB is not reset
2	3 V	3.75 V	1100 MSB↑	X < Y Bit is reset
3	3 V	3.25 V	1010 MSB↑	X < Y Bit is reset
4	3 V	2.8125 V	1001 MSB↑	X > Y Last bit is not reset

The final digital output = 1001

We can improvise this process for an eight- or higher-bit A/D converter.

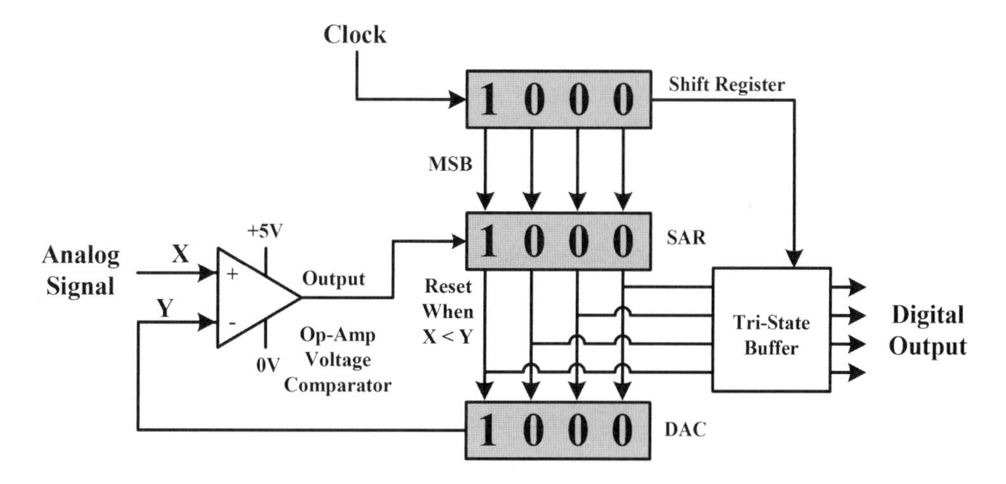

FIGURE 5-3 A block diagram of a successive approximation ADC.

5.5 DIGITAL SIGNAL PROCESSING (DSP) CHIPS

Digital signal processing (DSP) chips are the special types of microprocessor chips (a set of digital circuits on a single semiconductor chip) to handle digital audio and video data in real-time applications. In computers, these chips perform operations such as removing noise and creating compact files or video files and releases the CPU to perform other tasks. DSP chips can be programmed and are used today in cell phones, medical devices, MP3 players, packet-switched networks, and digital cameras. They are manufactured by such companies as Texas Instruments, Motorola, Analog Devices, and Lucent Technologies.

5.6 DIGITAL LOGIC CIRCUITS

The signals in digital electronics have two discrete values called binary values. Ideally, binary 0 means a value of 0 V and binary 1 means a value of 5 V. Binary logic in digital systems is the manipulation and processing of binary information resembling mathematical operations of addition and multiplication. Boolean algebra in digital operations is shown in **Figure 5-4** in truth tables and in the form of symbols of digital circuits. "A" and "B" are the inputs and "Q" is the output in all of these operations. Each one of these variables can assume a binary value of 0 or 1.

Buffer:

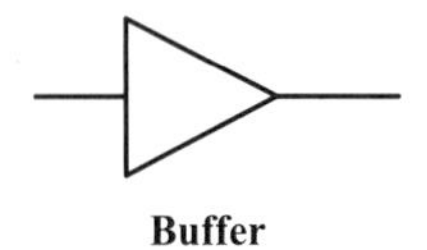

Buffer

A buffer is used to produce a binary value equal to the binary value of the input. It is used for power amplification of the input signal.

Buffer	
Input A	Output Q
0	0
1	1

Inverter:

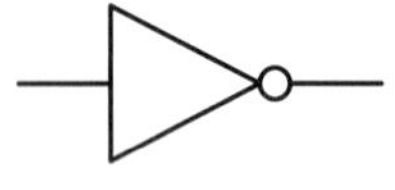

Inverter or NOT gate

The inverter circuit inverts the logic binary 0 into binary 1 or vice versa. It is represented by a small circle or "bubble" at the output of simple function gates and produces the NOT or complementary function of such gates.

Inverter	
Input A	Output Q
0	1
1	0

AND gate:

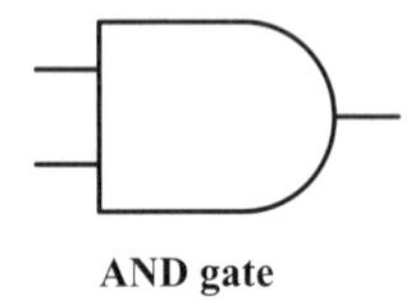

AND gate

The AND gate is a product generator. The output is binary 1, when all inputs are 1. Any other combination of 1s and 0s will output logic 0. Consider multiplying the AND gate inputs. The product of this multiplication is the output.

AND Gate		
Input A	Input B	Output Q
0	0	0
0	1	0
1	0	0
1	1	1

FIGURE 5-4 Logic gates and their truth tables. (*continued*)

NAND gate:

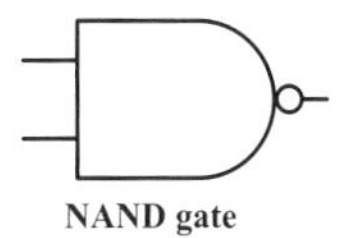

The NAND gate is the complement of the AND function. It is also called NOT-AND.

NAND Gate		
Input A	Input B	Output Q
0	0	1
0	1	1
1	0	1
1	1	0

OR gate:

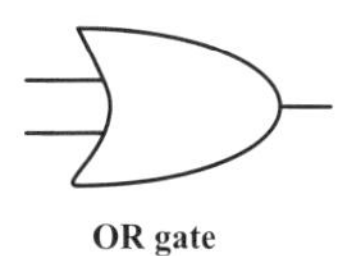

The OR gate operates similarly to addition or mathematical sum. The output is always binary 1 when one of the inputs is binary 1.

OR Gate		
Input A	Input B	Output Q
0	0	0
0	1	1
1	0	1
1	1	1

NOR gate:

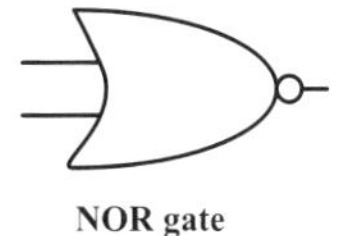

The NOR gate is the complement of the OR function. It is also called NOT-OR.

NOR Gate		
Input A	Input B	Output Q
0	0	1
0	1	0
1	0	0
1	1	0

Exclusive OR gate (XOR):

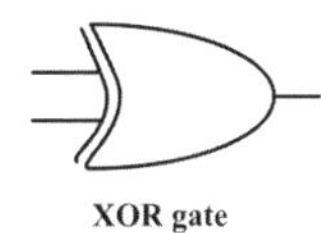

The XOR gate is similar to the OR gate; however, it excludes the combination of both inputs being equal to 1. This circuit is called anti-equivalence. That is, when two binary inputs are equal, the output is always 0.

XOR Gate		
Input A	Input B	Output Q
0	0	0
0	1	1
1	0	1
1	1	0

Exclusive NOR gate (XNOR):

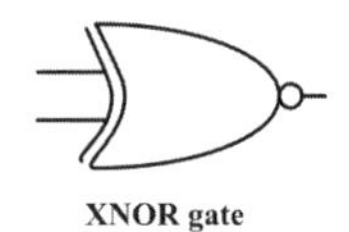

The XNOR gate is the complement of the XOR function.

XNOR Gate		
Input A	Input B	Output Q
0	0	1
0	1	0
1	0	0
1	1	1

FIGURE 5-4 *(continued)*

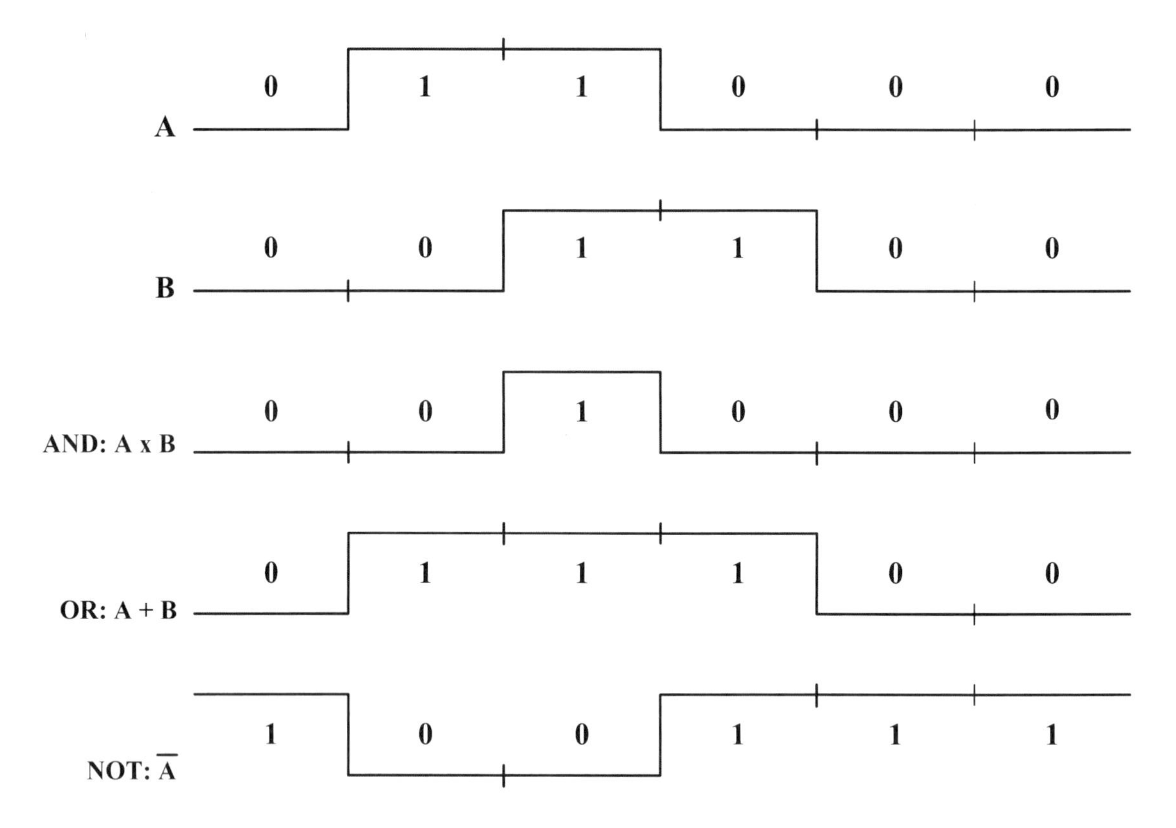

FIGURE 5-5 Timing diagrams of AND, OR, and INVERTER circuits.

An example of the input and output operations in these logic circuits can be explained as time-domain signals in **Figure 5-5.**

A and B are input digits to AND, OR, and inverter logic gates in time. For each one of these gates, the output is shown that follows the truth table of the gate.

5.7 REGISTERS AND FLIP-FLOPS

In digital electronics, the memory elements are devices that store the binary information. A register is such a group of binary storage cells. A group of flip-flops constitutes a single register, and each flip-flop can store one bit of information—either a binary 0 or a binary 1. A flip-flop can maintain its binary state indefinitely until an input signal directs it to switch its state.

Two basic flip-flop circuits are shown in **Figure 5-6a** and **Figure 5-6b.** One is with two NOR gates and the other is with two NAND gates. A feedback path is created when the output of one gate is coupled to the input of the other gate. Each flip-flop has two outputs, Q and $\overline{Q}$, and two inputs, R (reset) and S (set). These circuits are also called RS flip-flops or SR latches. There are varieties of flip-flops. The major differences among

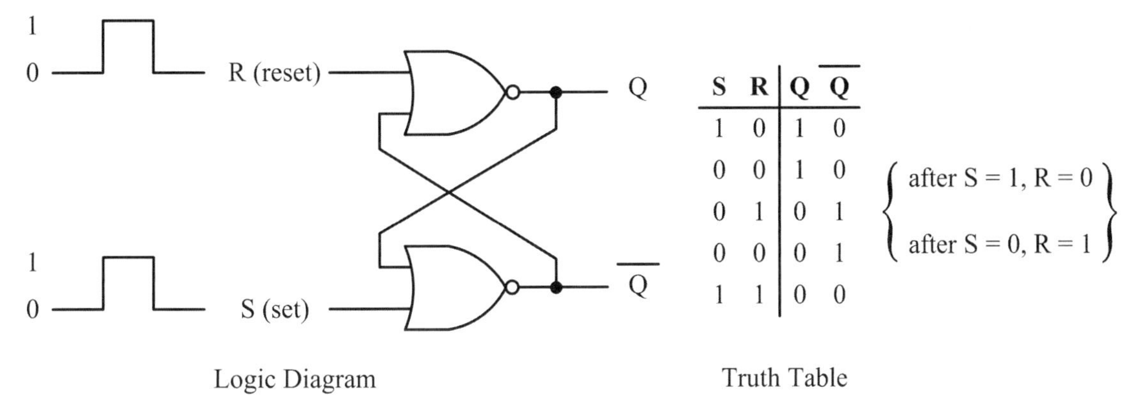

FIGURE 5-6a Flip-flop circuit using two NOR gates.

the varieties are due to the number of inputs and the manner in which the output state changes.

In normal operation of the NOR gate flip-flop, set and reset inputs should not be binary 1 simultaneously. Similarly, the inputs of the NAND gate flip-flop should not be binary 0 and the condition should be avoided. In analyzing a NOR gate flip-flop, for example, assume S = 1 and R = 0; then gate 2 output $\overline{Q}$ must be 0 (following the logic of a NOR gate: if any input is 1, the output is 0). $\overline{Q}$ is cross coupled to gate 1 input and that makes Q of gate 1 to be binary 1 (following the logic of a NOR gate: if inputs are all 0s, output is binary 1). Now, when set input returns to a 0, $\overline{Q}$ is still 0, both inputs of gate 1 are still 0 and so Q remains a binary 1.

The above example illustrates the concept of a changing state in digital electronics. The truth tables are provided in NOR and NAND gate flip-flops. Other popular flip-flops are D flip-flops and JK flip-flops and they can be clocked also by external clock

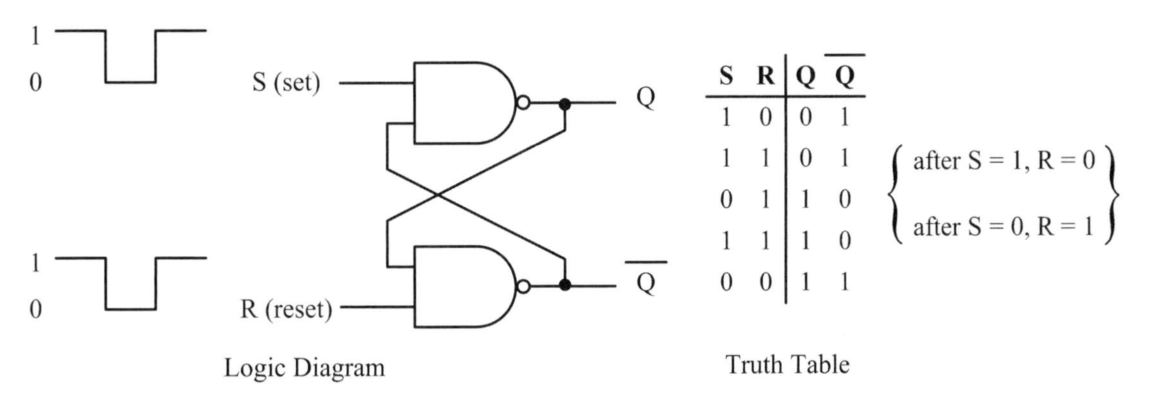

FIGURE 5-6b Flip-flop circuit using two NAND gates.

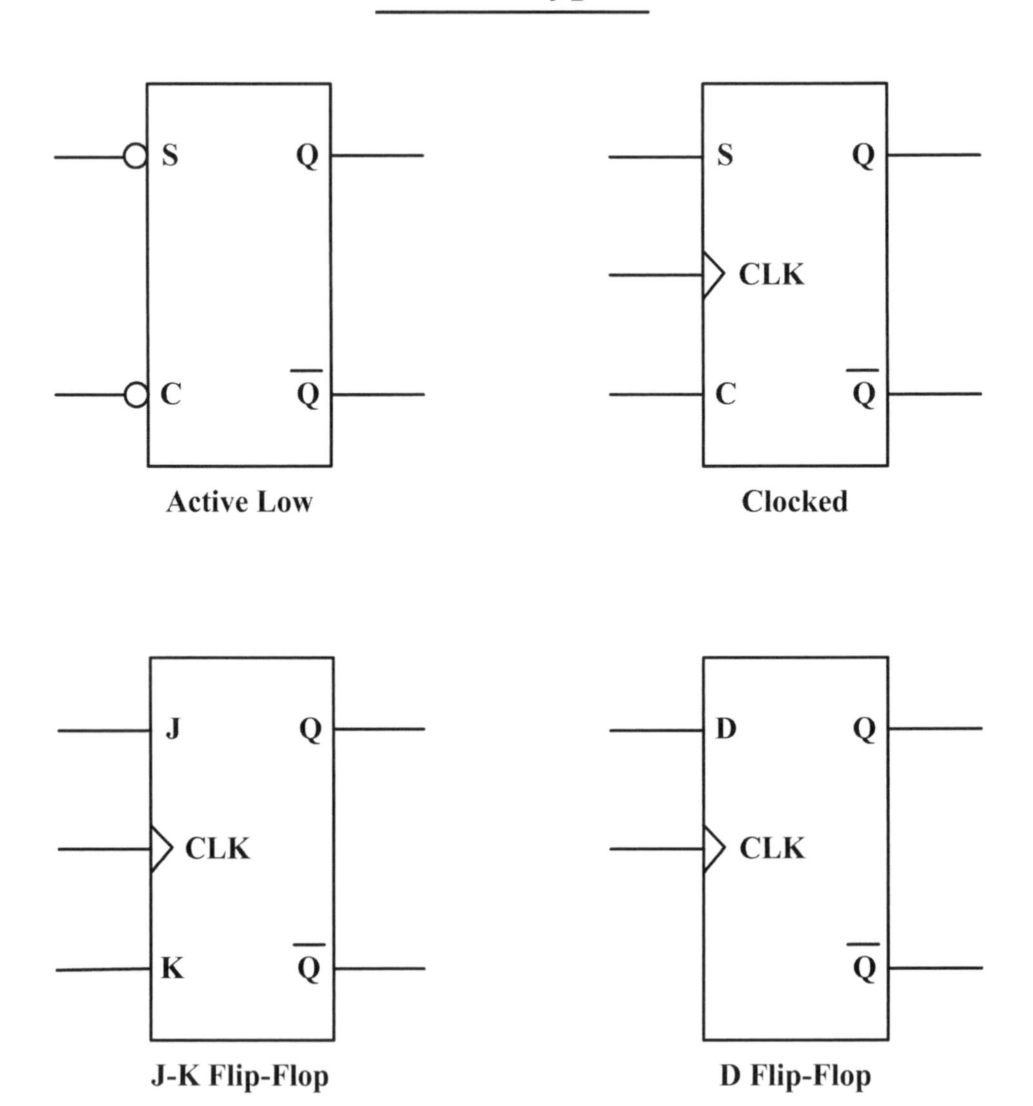

FIGURE 5-6c Latch types.

pulses as inputs to the set and reset terminals. Different latch types are shown in **Figure 5-6c.**

Next, we discuss the operation of a clocked JK flip-flop, which is more easily understood with a truth table and timing diagrams, as shown in **Figure 5-7.**

1. Inputs J, K, and the external clock are 0 initially. Assume output Q = 1.
2. As the clock pulse edges to binary 1, and J = 0 and K = 1 at point "a," the JK flip-flop output is reset to 0.

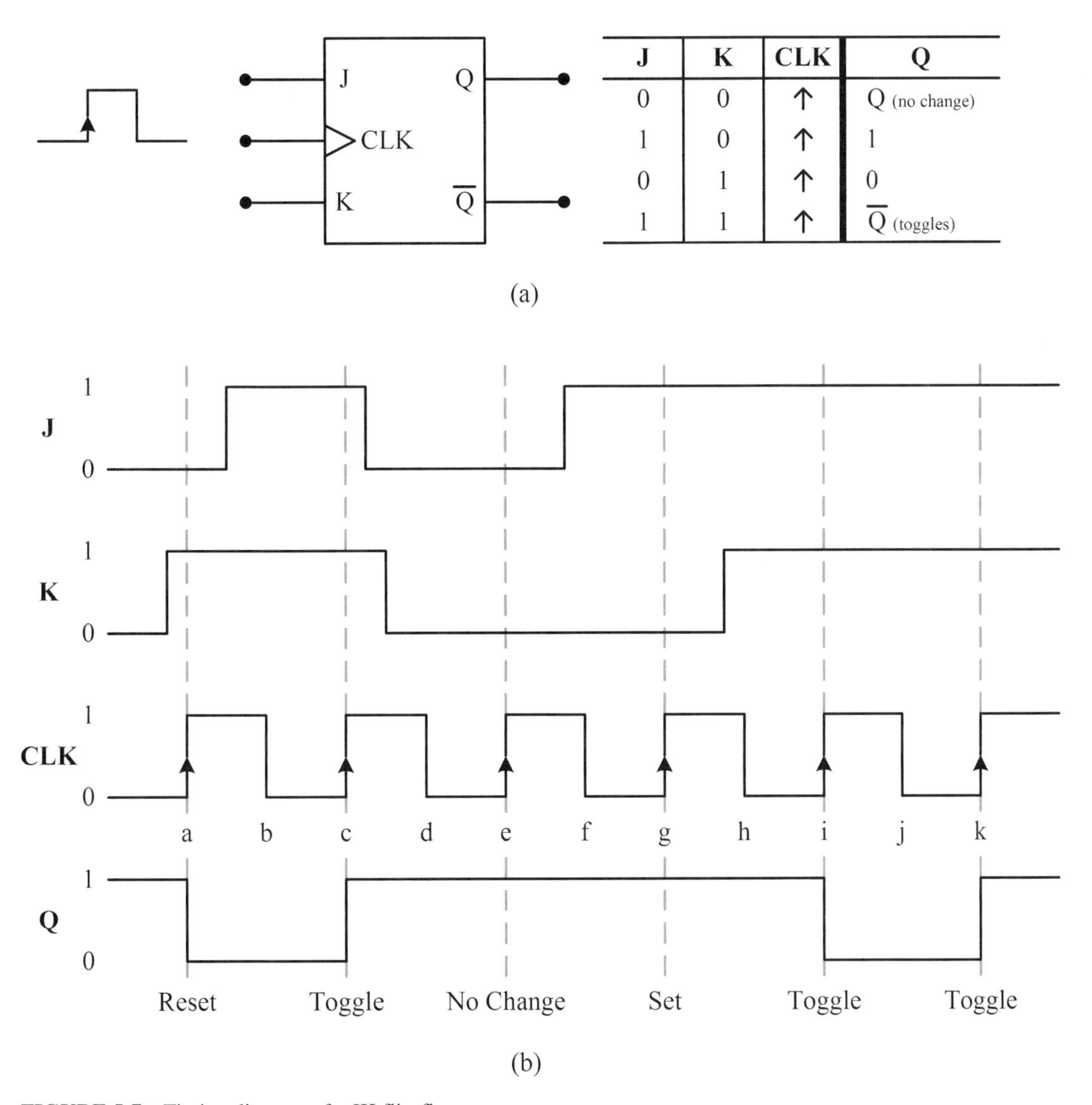

J	K	CLK	Q
0	0	↑	Q (no change)
1	0	↑	1
0	1	↑	0
1	1	↑	$\overline{Q}$ (toggles)

FIGURE 5-7 Timing diagram of a JK flip-flop.

3. At the second clock pulse at point "c," the flip-flop toggles to the opposite state and Q becomes 1. (The new value is the inverse of the previous condition and is called a toggle operation.)
4. At the third clock pulse, at point "e," J = 0 and K = 0; no change occurs at the flip-flop output.
5. At point "g," J = 1 and K = 0. The output Q is still set to be 1 and continues to be binary 1.
6. At the fifth clock pulse (point i), J and K both are 1, flip-flop toggles to the opposite condition and changes to binary 0.

Next, we combine several flip-flops to make a register that stores binary values and holds digital information as data.

The example of a four-bit shift register is now provided with four clocked flip-flops connected in series. Data of binary 1 is shifted from the leftmost JK flip-flop to the rightmost flip-flop due to the clocked shift pulses. This is shown in **Figure 5-8.** Note that

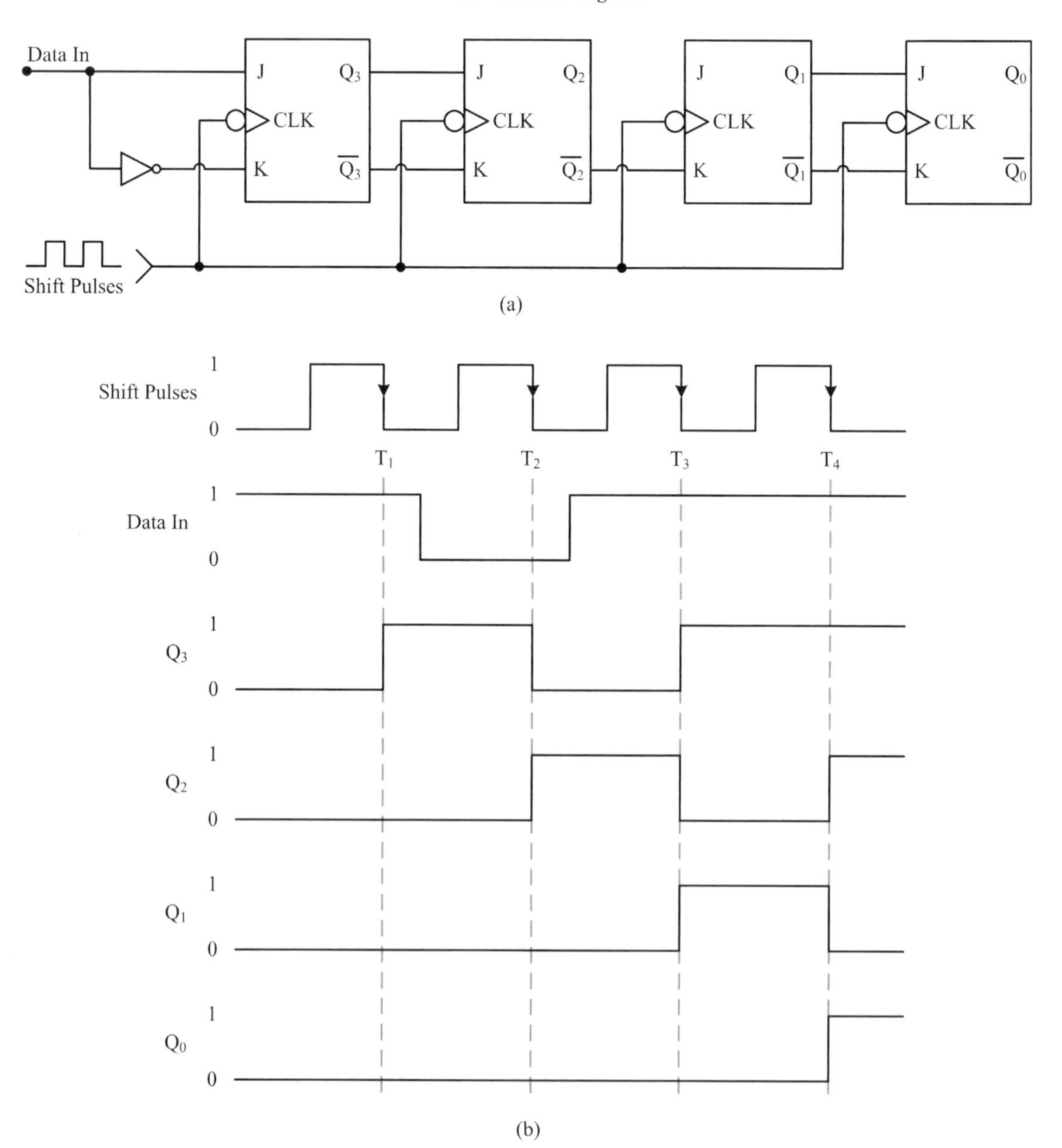

FIGURE 5-8 Timing diagram of a four-bit shift register.

the output of Q_3 transfers to Q_2, Q_2 transfers to Q_1, and so on. Each output follows the conditions present on its J and K inputs when the clock goes from positive to negative transition.

5.8 MEMORY AND STORAGE

There are mainly two types of memory used in microcomputers: read-only memory (ROM) and random-access memory (RAM). Read-only memory is used to store data and programs. Once stored, the data cannot be changed. However, RAM stores data that can be changed frequently. Random-access memory is further divided into static RAM and dynamic RAM. Static RAM needs constant power supply, while dynamic RAM needs only periodic power supply.

Every memory location can hold one byte (eight bits of data). A 64K RAM memory means that $64 \times 1{,}024 = 65{,}536$ bytes are then available for data storage. A memory area may be partitioned into RAM and ROM areas requiring several RAM and ROM chips. The following section provides descriptions of some of these chips.

5.9 MULTIPLEXING AND DISPLAY

Seven-segment display is a common readout method found in medical instruments. It can illuminate up to seven addressable bars. The arrangement is two rectangles having vertical and horizontal segments with the seventh segment in the middle, as shown in **Figure 5-9.** The display is referred to also as letters A to G with a decimal point shown in **Figure 5-10.** These are generally arrays of illuminating light-emitting diodes (LEDs) or liquid crystal displays (LCDs).

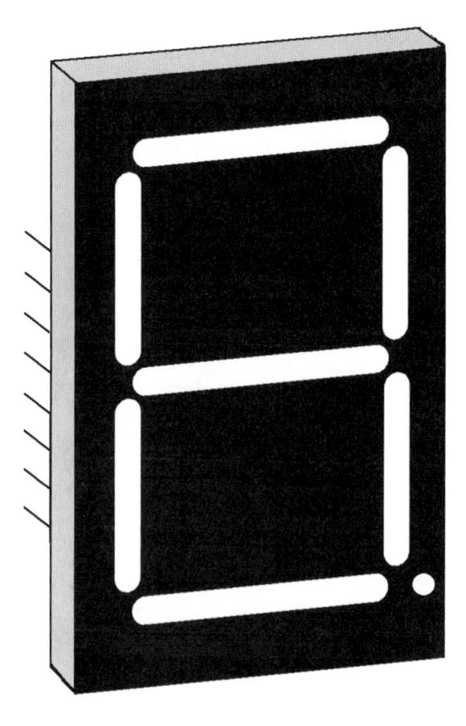

FIGURE 5-9 A seven-segment display component, with decimal point.

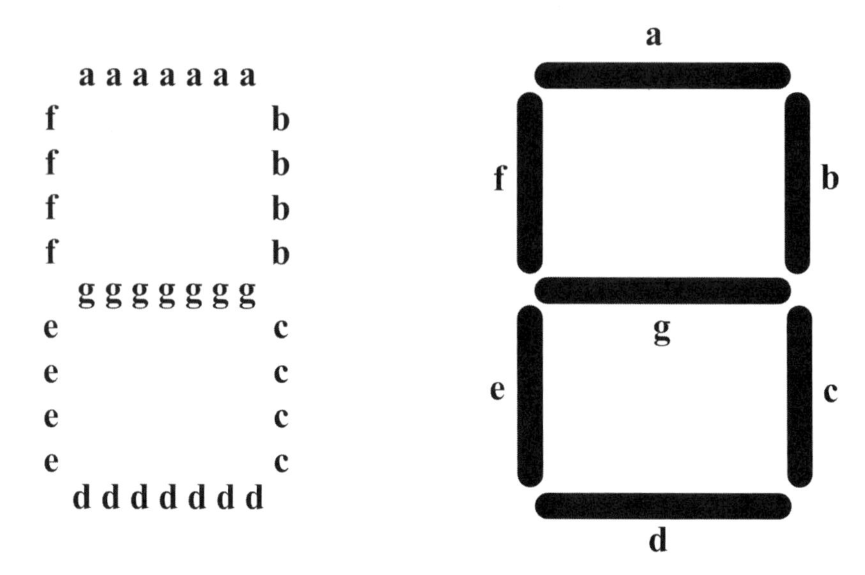

FIGURE 5-10 Segments of the seven-segment display.

In **Figure 5-11a,** all the cathodes of the LEDs are connected together as a common lead. The other end of each LED is interfaced to a power supply and a digital circuit. This is a common-cathode seven-segment unit. However, as shown in **Figure 5-11b,** a common-anode unit is also possible. Certain logic circuits and configurations are compatible with either common-cathode or common-anode LEDs.

5.10 MICROPROCESSORS

A microprocessor (sometimes abbreviated as µP) is a set of digital logic circuits built on a single semiconductor chip or integrated circuit (IC). One or more of these microprocessors build the central processing unit (CPU) in computers and in embedded systems such as in cars, traffic lights, ECG machines, cell phones, and so on. Before the 1970s, electronic CPUs were bulky switching devices with few transistors. However, with the advent of microprocessors, the number of transistors in CPUs grew to thousands—even millions!

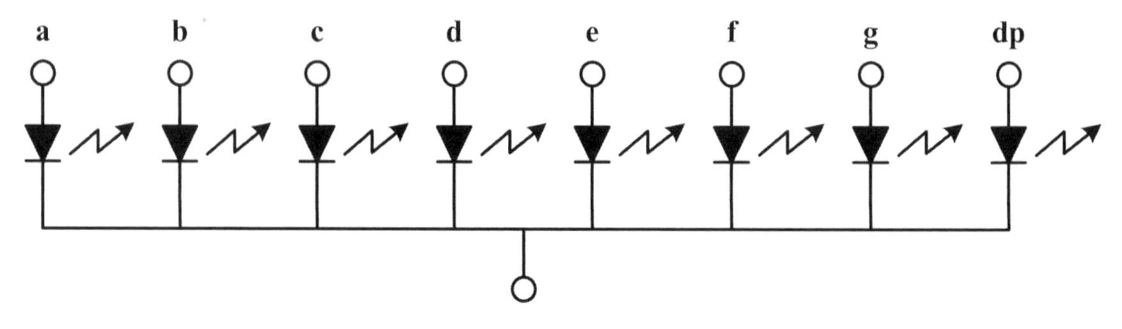

FIGURE 5-11a Common-cathode LED array.

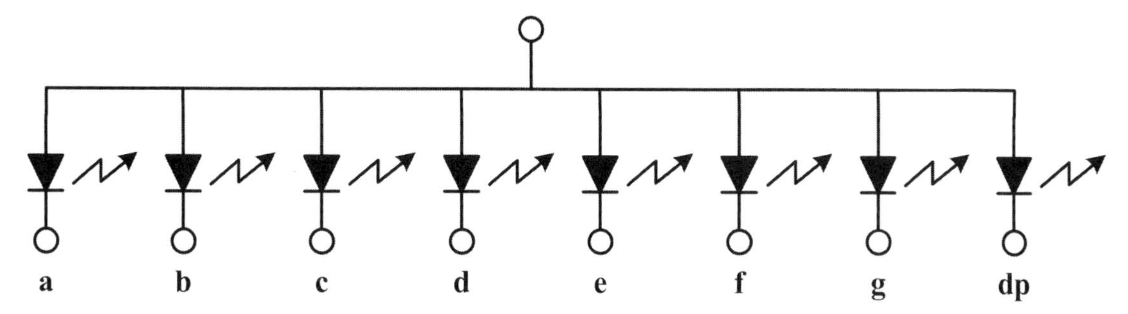

FIGURE 5-11b Common-anode LED array.

Figure 5-12 to **Figure 5-15** show a general microprocessor internal structure and then a specific microcontroller chip. A general-purpose microprocessor requires external support chips, whereas a microcontroller chip can store its program and data on the chip itself. As shown in **Figure 5-12,** the internal structure of a microprocessor consists of data, address, and control buses, and a vast array of registers—all involved in its decision making. A microcontroller chip implements all of the components of a computer—input and output, control, and memory—all in one chip. **Figure 5-13** shows the pin diagram of the PIC18F242 microcontroller. This chip uses its assembly language and the conversion to the C language for the

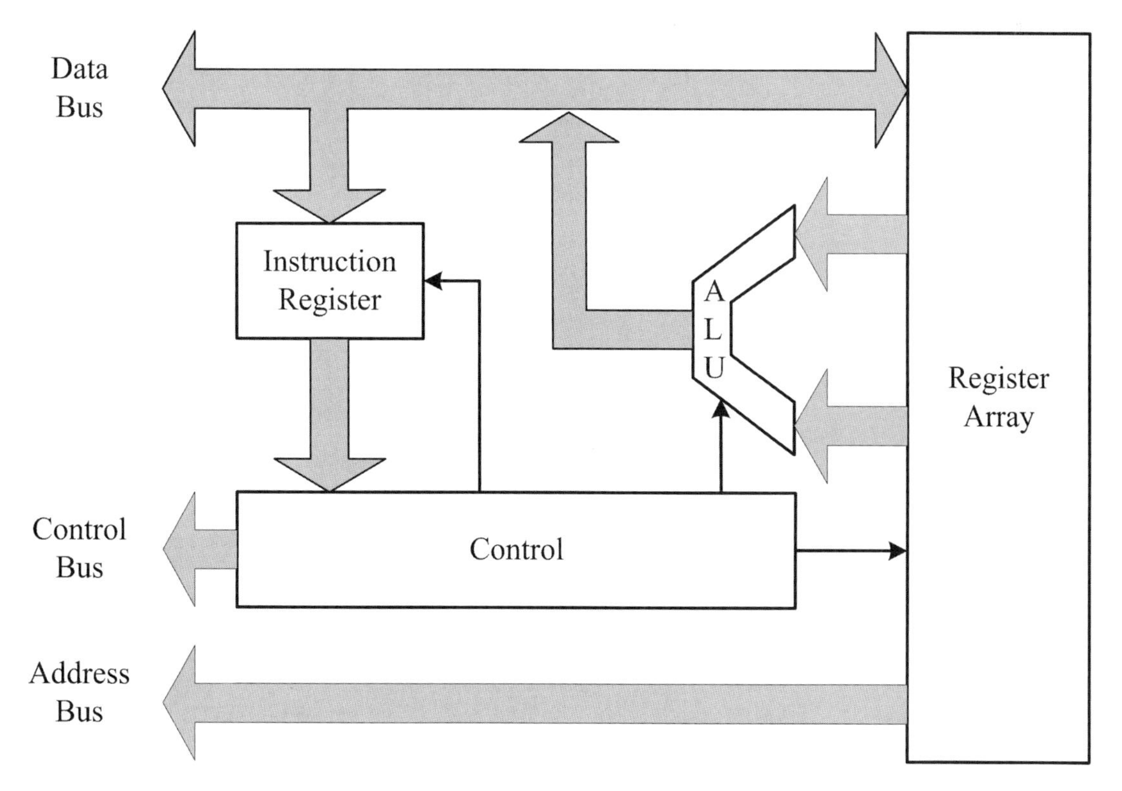

FIGURE 5-12 Internal structure of a microprocessor.

FIGURE 5-13 PIC18F242 pin diagram.

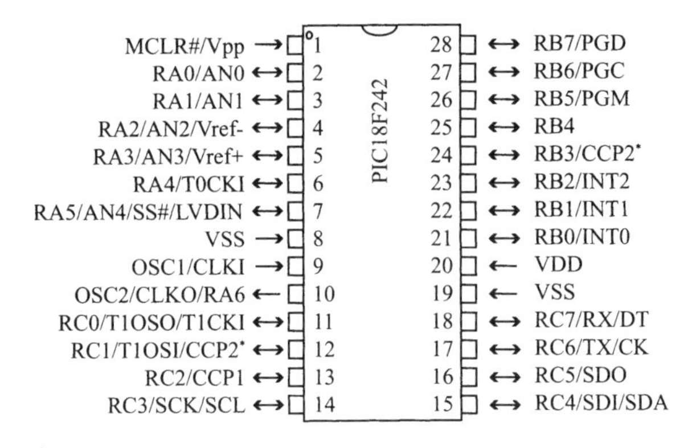

*RB3 is the alternate pin for the CCP2 pin multiplexing

Figure redrawn by author from PIC18Fxx2 datasheet (DS39564B), Microchip Technology Inc.

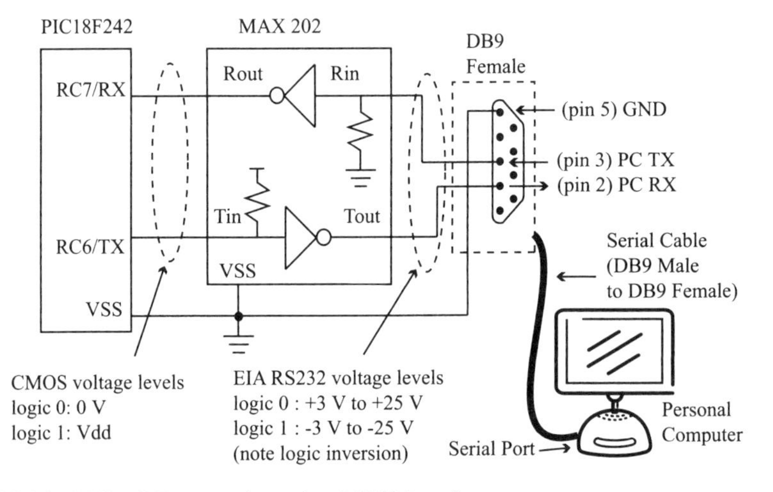

FIGURE 5-14 PIC to PC connection using RS232 interface.

FIGURE 5-15 Internal structure of the PIC18F242.

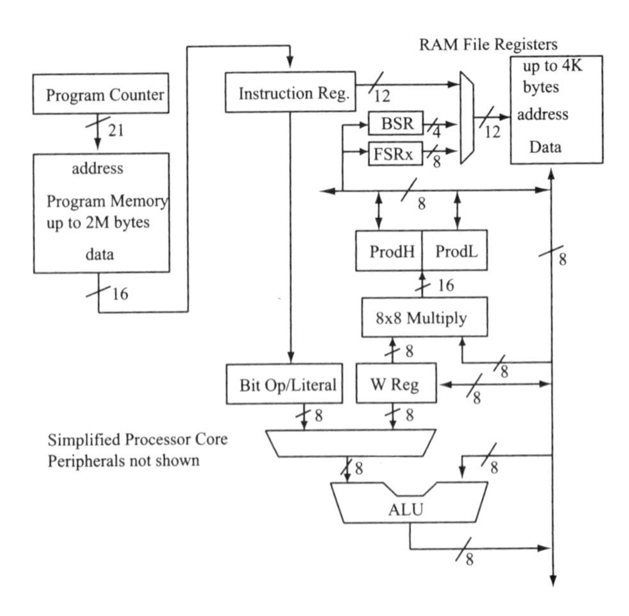

interface operations. OSC pins are the main clock source for the device; the RAn, RBn, and RCn pins are parallel port IO bidirectional pins; AN pins are the analog inputs for the A/D converters; and the MCLR resets the device when low. In **Figure 5-14,** an RS232 communication link is established from the PIC to a PC. MAX202 converts RS232 logic levels to the CMOS logic levels. **Figure 5-15** shows the simplified architectural diagram of the PIC18F242. The size of internal data paths is eight bits; therefore, this PIC is referred to as an eight-bit microcontroller chip. The instruction set defines 75 instructions, of which the majority require 16-bit operations. ALU is the arithmetic logic unit and the BSR is the bank select register.

5.11 COMPUTERS

In computers, the data is manipulated by a series of instructions called a program or software. Digital logic circuits perform the manipulation; memory and input and output peripheral devices are stored in ROM and RAM (as previously mentioned). The microcomputer, based on a microprocessor chip, is the most common type of computer. It is commonly called a personal computer (PC). However, there are other types of computers. Mainframe and minicomputers are used for large-scale data manipulations and parallel processing such as for telephone switching, airline reservations, banking, and for the military.

Figure 5-16 and **Figure 5-17** show various computer types and general computer architecture. Today, laptops are widely used and palm-held computers called personal

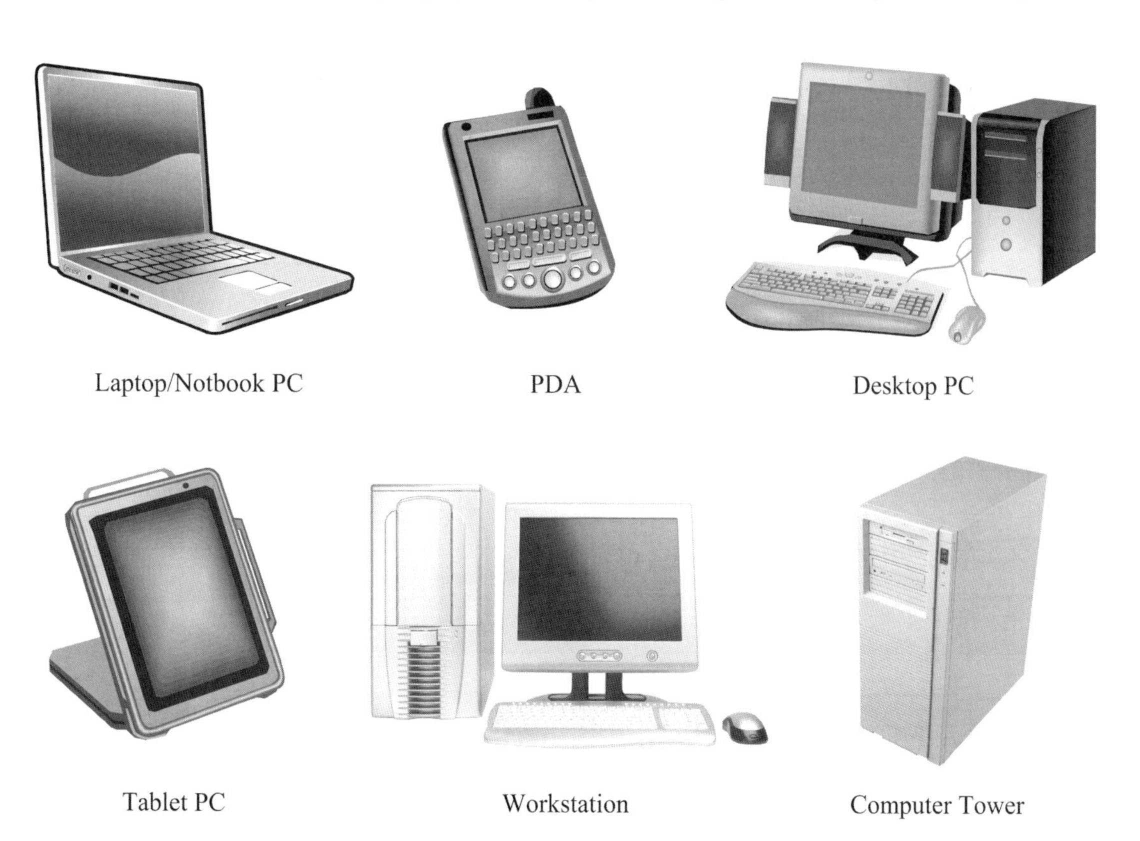

FIGURE 5-16 Computing devices.

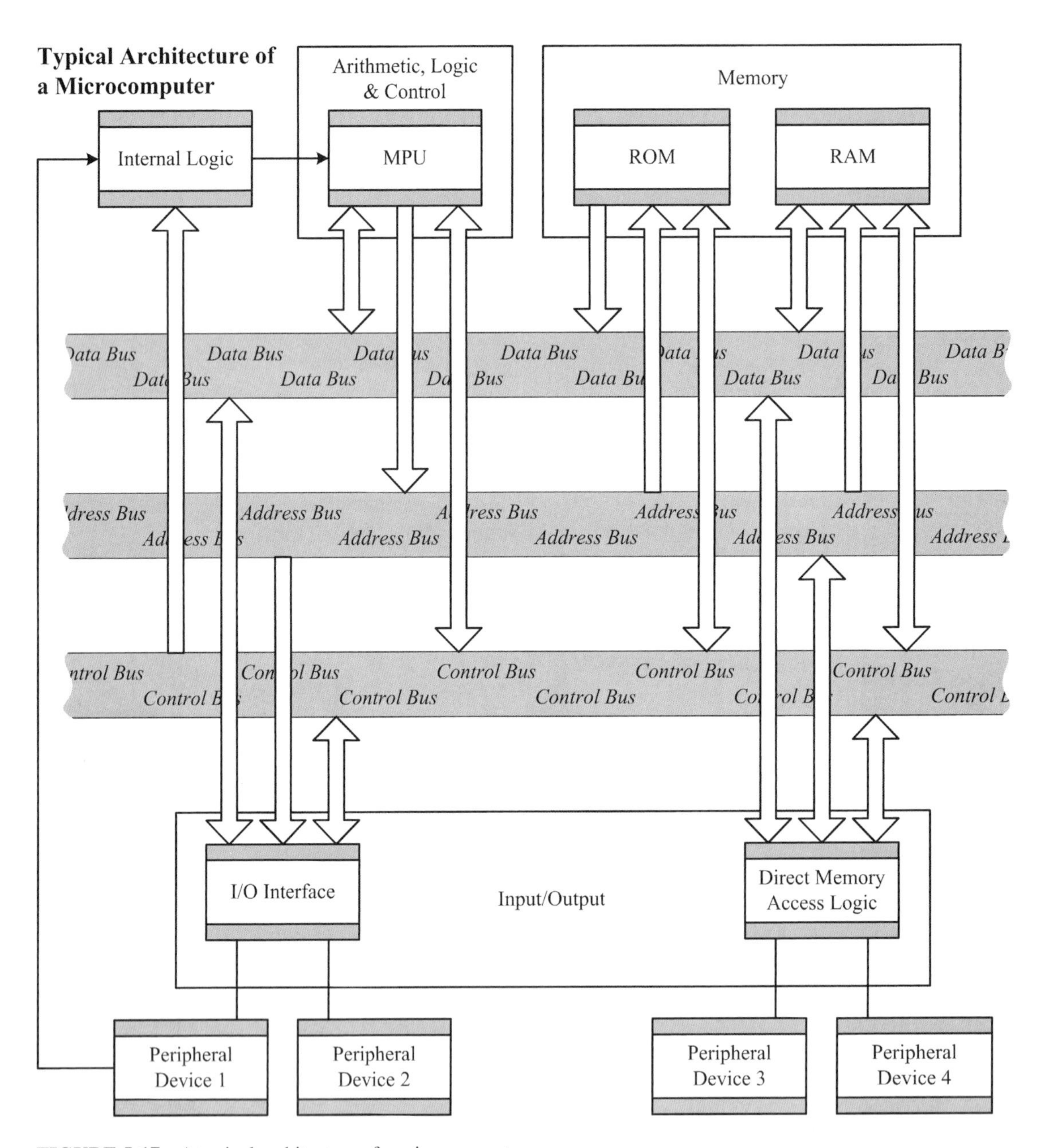

FIGURE 5-17 A typical architecture of a microcomputer.

digital assistants (PDAs) are convenient ways to search databases and to access the Internet. While the microprocessor is the heart of a computer, there can be more than one microprocessor in a computer. Peripheral devices such as printers and keyboards can interface with a computer. A printer is considered an output device, while a keyboard is considered an input device. The memory units RAM and ROM connect to the data, address, and the control buses.

5.12 COMPUTER HARDWARE

The physical components of a computer are called its hardware. This hardware includes the computer's digital circuitry. Software installed onto the computer then instructs the data manipulation within its digital circuitry. A typical personal computer has the following physical parts:

The **motherboard,** also called the system board, includes the CPU, RAM, BIOS, PCI, and USB buses. This hardware is placed on slots.

Input devices are user-interface devices such as the keyboard, the mouse, a joystick, a game pad, an image scanner, or a webcam.

Output devices are devices such as a printer, a monitor, a speaker, or a headset. Data is provided to these types of devices as text, display, or audio output to the user.

The **power supply** is the box with a transformer, a fan, and the regulator circuit.

Internal storage is where data is kept on the hard disk and disk controller.

Controllers are accessible in the computer, such as a video display controller, drive controller, and bus controller. The video display controller generates the horizontal and vertical synchronization timing signal for the video RAM, whereas the drive controller allows the CPU to communicate with the hard disk and other drives in the computer. The bus controller monitors the system board's temperature and voltage.

Drives such as CD-ROM drive, DVD, floppy disk drive, Zip drive, flash drive, and tape drive are available on the computer.

A **computer network** allows several computers to be connected to each other through copper or fiber cables, Network Interface Cards (NICs) and the modems. The computers can send or receive files, e-mails, texts, or videos on the network.

A **sound card** allows the computer to create and record high-quality sound.

5.13 FLOWCHART AND COMPUTER SOFTWARE

Figure 5-18 shows a simple programming flowchart and is an example of how a program (or software code) is written. The flowchart shows the given problem and the several steps involved in solving the problem. In this example, if the worker's pay is more than $500, then a check must be written; if less than $500, cash is provided. Based upon the steps, codes in a specific language are then written.

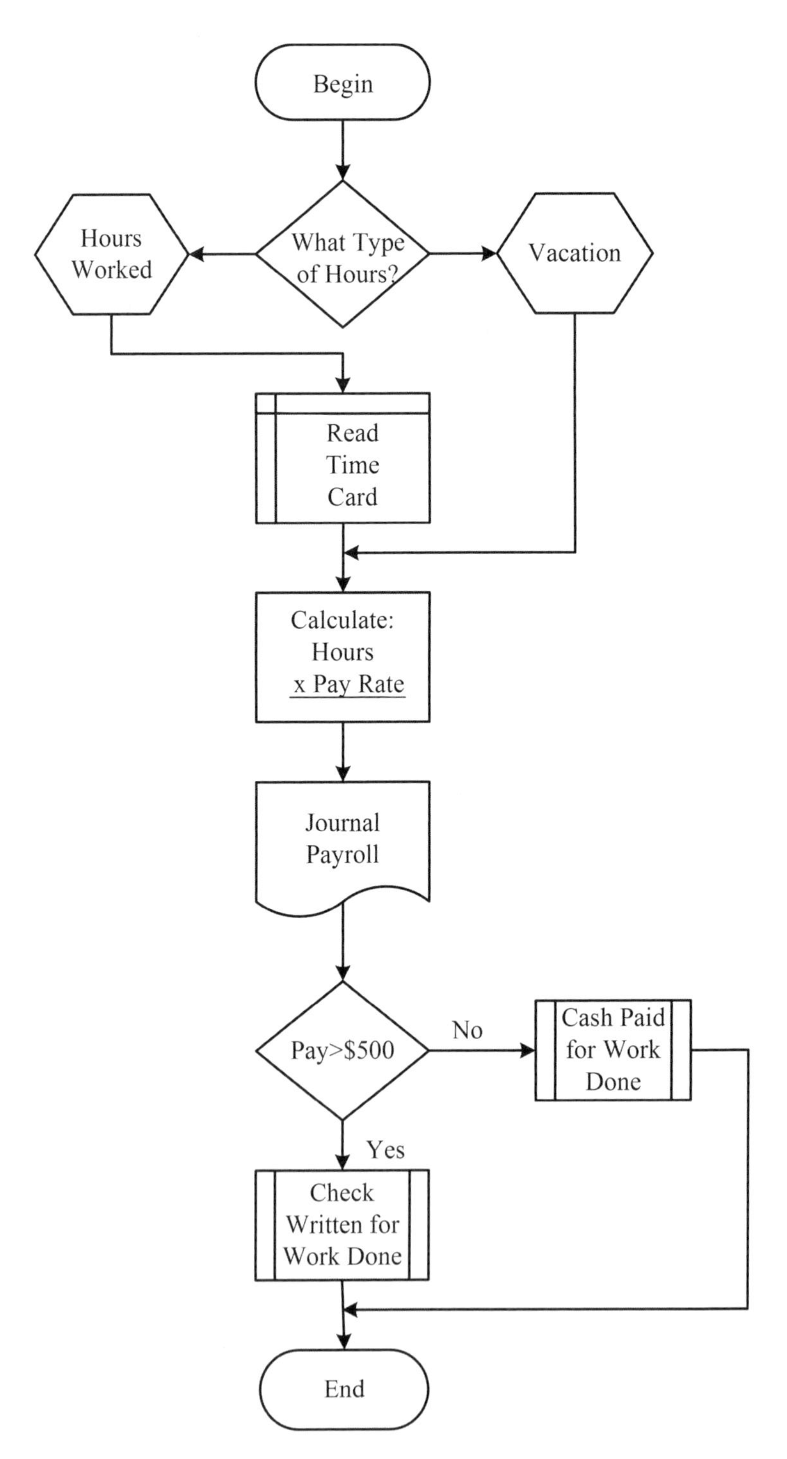

FIGURE 5-18 A programming flowchart.

SUMMARY

- Digitization of any biomedical analog signal is compatible with acquiring it for computer or microprocessor interface.
- An R/2R ladder network converts parallel digits into an analog signal. The size of the ladder depends on the number of parallel bits used in the process. The successive-approximation register bit is set or reset based on the comparison of the input analog sample with the DAC output.
- Logic gates include OR, exclusive-OR, AND, NAND, and inverter circuits. Flip-flops are made of these gates. The J-K flip-flop is a refinement of the RS flip-flop in that the indeterminate state of the RS type is defined in the JK type.
- A microcontroller chip is more versatile than a microprocessor chip because the RAM, ROM, ADC, and DAC can all reside on a single micro-controller chip.
- The computer hardware includes RAM, ROM, hard drives, display monitor, keyboard, and the mouse. The software codes are stored and retrieved from the memory storage devices.

TECHNICAL TERMINOLOGY

Bandwidth: a measure of the capacity of a communications channel. The greater a channel's bandwidth, the more information it can carry in a given amount of time. Bandwidth can also relate to resolution. Bandwidth is usually stated in bits per second (bps), kilobits per second (Kbps), or megabits per second (Mbps).

Compatible: ability of the software or the hardware to connect with each other; also called software or hardware compatibility.

Computer programming: the method of writing algorithms in the form of a set of commands that can later be compiled and interpreted in order to run a task. Programming requires logic, but has elements of science, mathematics, and engineering. Also referred to as coding.

Display: a display device or an information display device for visual presentation of images (including text) acquired, stored, or transmitted in various forms. The three types of displays are analog electronic displays, digital electronic displays, and 3D displays.

Flowchart: a schematic representation of a process. Flowcharts are commonly used to visualize the content better or to find flaws in a process.

Medical monitor: hardware that is an automated medical device that senses a patient's vital signs and displays the results. In critical care units of hospitals, it allows continuous supervision of a patient without continuous attendance, thus improving patient care.

Memory: an electronic holding place for instructions and data that a computer's microprocessor can reach quickly. Random-access memory (RAM) holds memory as long as power is supplied to the device (volatile). Read-only memory (ROM) stores the data permanently even when power is disconnected (nonvolatile).

Network: a system of interconnected electronic components, circuits, software, and devices enabling communication among them for the transfer of data.

Resolution: the level at which detail can be captured or presented such as in sound, optics, signals, displays, or in the function of medical devices.

Speed: a communication speed at which data can be transferred from one device to another using media such as CAT5 cable, Bluetooth wireless, T1 line, or a 10Base-T Ethernet connection.

Storage: a device that holds user data that has been saved or that will be saved for later use. Storage is slower than memory.

Thermal noise: noise created by the movement and collision of electrons in a conductor. This noise can change the characteristics of an actual signal.

QUIZ

1. The samples of a medical signal are:

a) A series of pulses with a frequency the same as the frequency of the medical signal.

b) A series of pulses that is proportional to the amplitude of the medical signal.

c) A series of digits proportional to the frequency of the medical signal.

d) All of the above.

2. Resolution is:

a) The number of bits per sample. b) The number of samples per second.

c) Both a and b. d) None of the above.

3. In a four-bit ADC, if 0001 is 0.3125 V, then 1110 is:

a) 5 V. b) 4.375 V. c) 4.6875 V. d) None of the above.

4. For a six-bit D/A converter, 100000 represents:

a) 5 V b) 2.9 V c) 2.5 V d) 0 V

5. The quantized levels in the A/D SAR process are 1 V and 2 V. If the analog sample is 1.5 V, it would be approximated to:

a) 2 V b) 0 V c) 1 V d) 5 V

6. The input to an R/2R ladder network in a D/A converter is:

a) Serial digits. b) Parallel digits. c) Both a and b. d) None of the above.

7. A tri-state buffer in digital means:

a) The output is 0 or 1. b) The output is 1 or 0.

c) The output is 1, high-Z, or 0. d) None of the above.

8. A two-input NAND will have a low output only when:

a) Both inputs are high. b) Both inputs are low.

c) Both inputs are different. d) Both a and c.

9. The output of the logic circuit shown in **Figure 5-19** is:

a) (A + B) + C. b) $(\overline{AB})$ C. c) $\overline{AB}$ + C. d) None of the above.

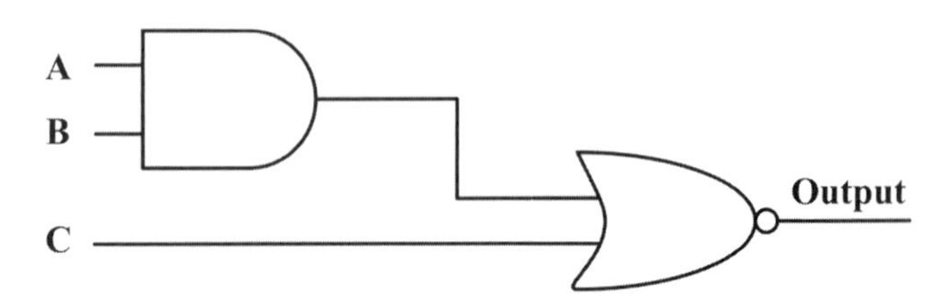

FIGURE 5-19 A logic circuit.

10. RAM and ROM in a computer are:

a) The same

b) Both erasable.

c) Different: RAM is erasable, ROM is not erasable.

d) None of the above.

PROBLEMS

1. Determine the step size for a 12-bit A/D converter having a range of 10 V. Also, convert an analog sample of 4.3 V into the 12-bit digits.
2. For an eight-bit D/A converter having a range of 5 V, convert 10110101 into an analog sample value.
3. How many quantized levels are possible in a 16-bit A/D converter? What is the normalized value of the quantized step size in mV? Show the block diagram of the successive approximation 16-bit A/D converter.
4. Draw the block diagram of a successive approximation six-bit A/D converter having a range of 0 V to 6 V, and determine the approximation steps for an analog sample of 2.9 V.
5. An analog signal consists of a 1 kHz and a 3.2 kHz spectral. Determine the Nyquist (minimum sampling) rate of sampling and the approximate number of samples for the duration of two minutes of the signal. Also, provide an example of the aliasing problem for the signal.
6. For a six-bit D/A converter, draw an R/2R ladder network and determine the output voltage for 010000 input using the circuit analysis method.
7. Simplify the logic circuit shown in **Figure 5-20.**

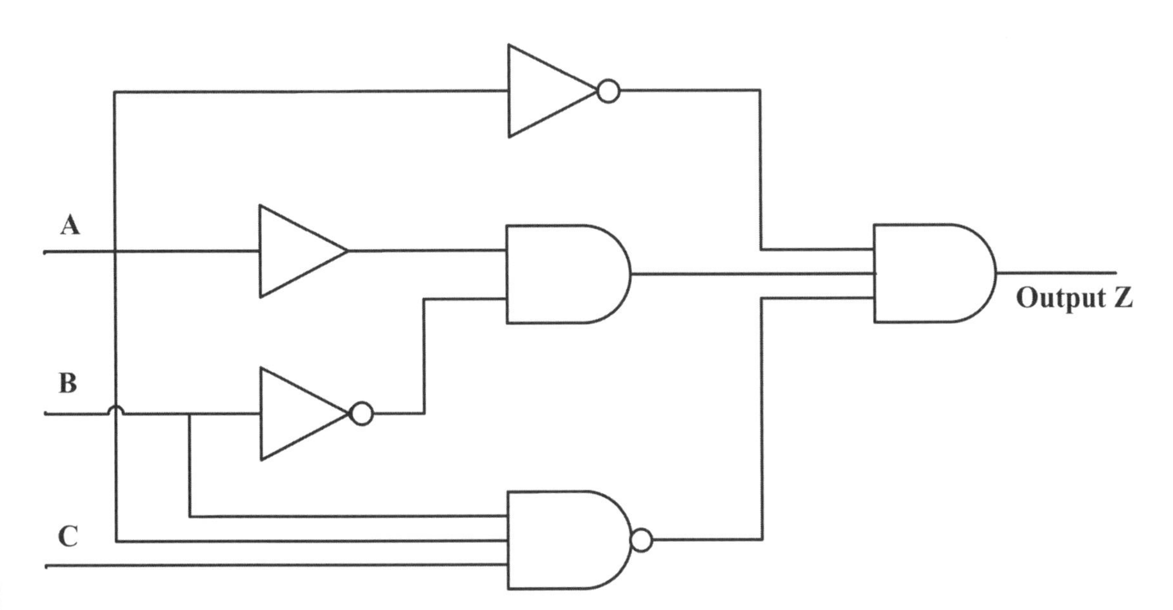

FIGURE 5-20 A logic circuit.

8. Determine the output Q and complete the truth table for the circuit shown in **Figure 5-21.**

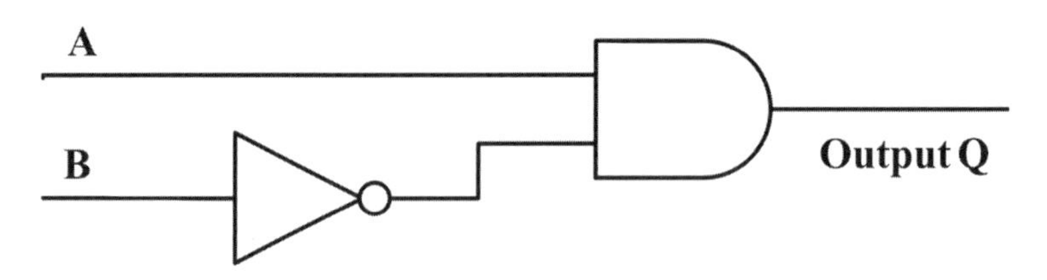

FIGURE 5-21 A logic circuit.

9. Design a logic circuit whose output is HIGH only when a majority of its inputs are HIGH. Assume the circuit has three inputs.
10. Design a logic circuit whose output is HIGH when a majority of inputs X, Y, and C are LOW.
11. Show the timing diagram of the output for the inputs given in **Figure 5-22.**

FIGURE 5-22 Timing diagrams of a three-input AND gate.

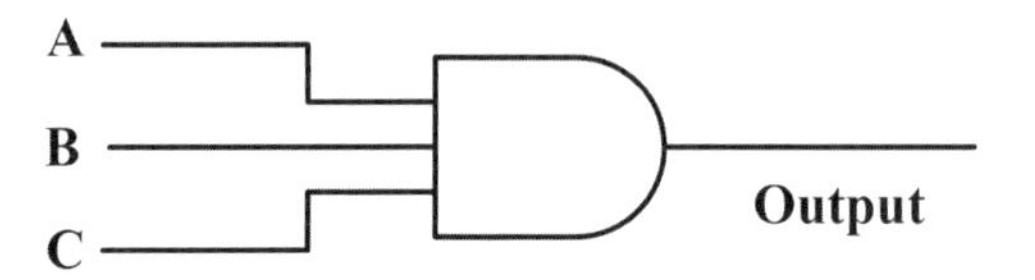

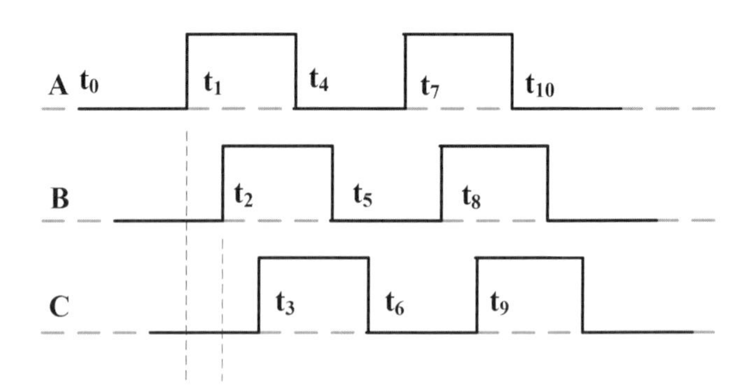

12. Show the timing diagram of the output of an exclusive-OR gate for the inputs A, B, and C given in **Figure 5-22.**
13. Show the logic circuit of a clocked RS flip-flop with four NAND gates. Also, determine the truth table.
14. Draw the logic network for the function F = (A&B) | C and show the truth table. The symbol | is for the OR logic operation.

15. Compare and contrast at least two microcontroller chips in terms of resolution, memory, number of ADC channels, serial and parallel ports, and any additional information about the chips. Use the Internet and the vendor Web sites for this assignment.

CASE STUDIES

1. A patient is complaining about his pacemaker that is programmed from his doctor's office. His complaint is that he has to call the doctor frequently for setting adjustments. The settings include the timing and the intensity of the pacemaker pulses. The following questions can be explored in the case study:
   a) How is digital circuitry involved in the pacemaker setting?
   b) Is the setting done through a telephone or through a wireless medium?
   c) What could be the reasons for any frequent changes needed on the pacemaker?
2. A radiologist cannot read a patient's x-ray images that are interfaced, processed, and displayed on the computer and holds the biomedical technician responsible for the unacceptable reading. What did the biomedical technician do wrong? The case study should answer the following questions:
   a) What are the characteristics of an x-ray image compared with a biomedical signal?
   b) How is an image interfaced to a computer?
   c) What does the technician do to the image so that the image is acceptable to the radiologist?

RESEARCH TOPICS

1. Sampling rates and the resolution in terms of number of bits per sample can destroy or bring back an analog signal with compatible or incompatible DACs. Develop a protocol for the following experiments or simulations: 8-bit ADC and 8-bit DAC; 16-bit ADC and 16-bit DAC; 16-bit ADC and 16-bit DAC. Analog input is a sine wave of 3 kHz and the sampling rate is fixed with a rate of 8 kHz. The research report should include the impact on the resolution for various frequency signals and the criterion of Nyquist (minimum sampling) rates.
2. Develop a list of biomedical devices or instruments that use embedded microprocessors or microcontroller chips and a list that does not include these types of chips.

CHAPTER 6

Biomedical Electrodes, Sensors, and Transducers

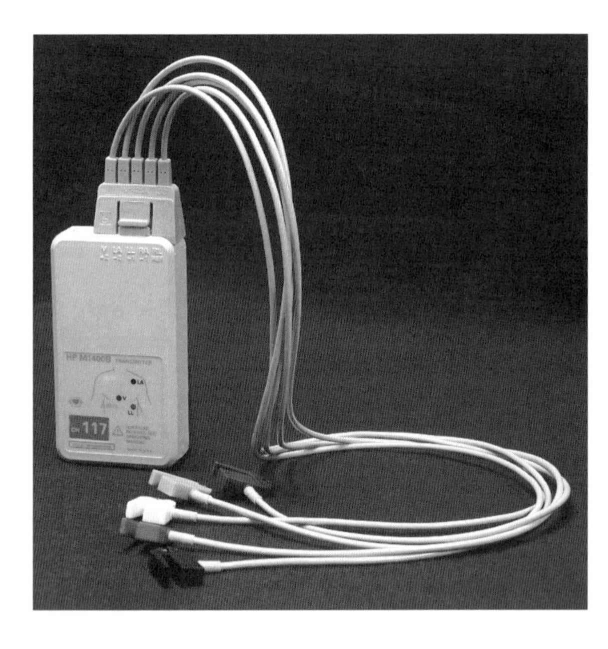

CHAPTER OUTLINE

OBJECTIVES

The objective of this chapter is to introduce the reader to the theory and types of medical electrodes, sensors, and transducers used in health care.

Upon completion of this chapter, the reader will be able to:

- Define and compare sensors, transducers, and electrodes.
- Explain the types of biomedical electrodes.
- Draw a model of an electrode.
- Explain oxidation and reduction reactions.

- Discuss the types of pressure transducers.
- Explain the various types of temperature transducers.

INTERNET WEB SITES

http://www.medicaldesign.com (MD Medical Design Magazine)
http://www.medcompare.com (Medcompare)

INTRODUCTION

Biomedical instruments that measure signals from the human body use devices called electrodes, sensors, and transducers. Biomedical electrodes are used in ECG, EEG, EMG, defibrillators, and external pacemakers. Sensors, such as thermistor devices, detect and respond to physical stimulus such as temperature, pressure, or motion, while the transducer uses these sensors in its electrical or electronic circuit to generally produce a corresponding electrical signal. This chapter discusses the various electrodes, sensors, and transducers used by medical devices and compares resolution and the manufacturing technology of these devices.

6.1 DEFINITION OF BIOMEDICAL ELECTRODES, SENSORS, AND TRANSDUCERS

Figure 6-1 provides examples of a nonbiomedical electrode, sensor, and transducer and **Figure 6-2** shows a biomedical electrode, sensor, and transducer. An electrode is a solid electric conductor through which an electric current enters or leaves an electrolytic cell or other similar medium. Electrodes can be used to detect electrical activity such as brain waves.

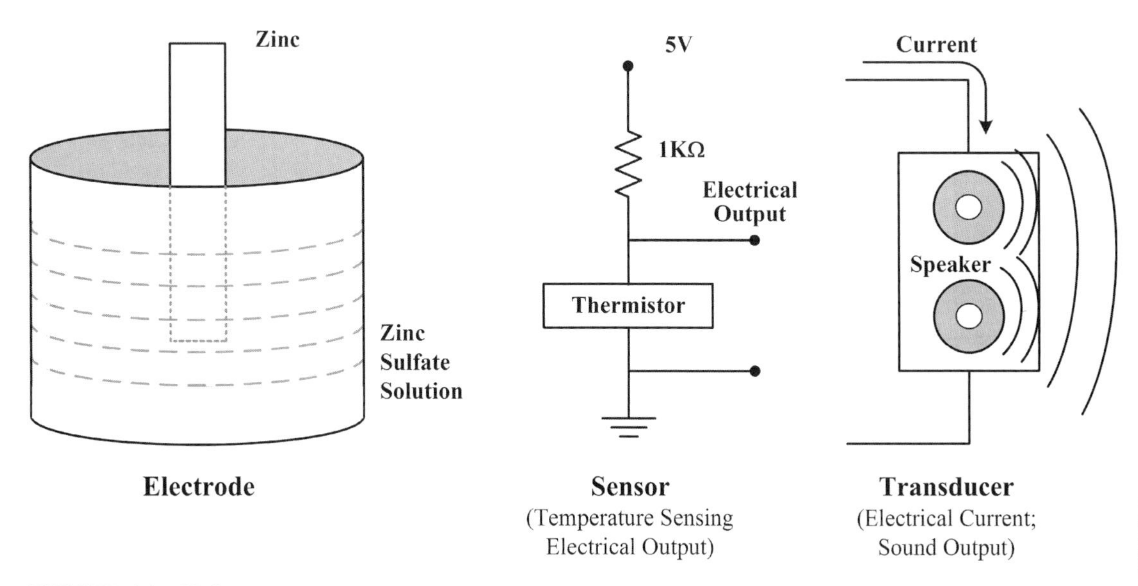

FIGURE 6-1 Various sensors.

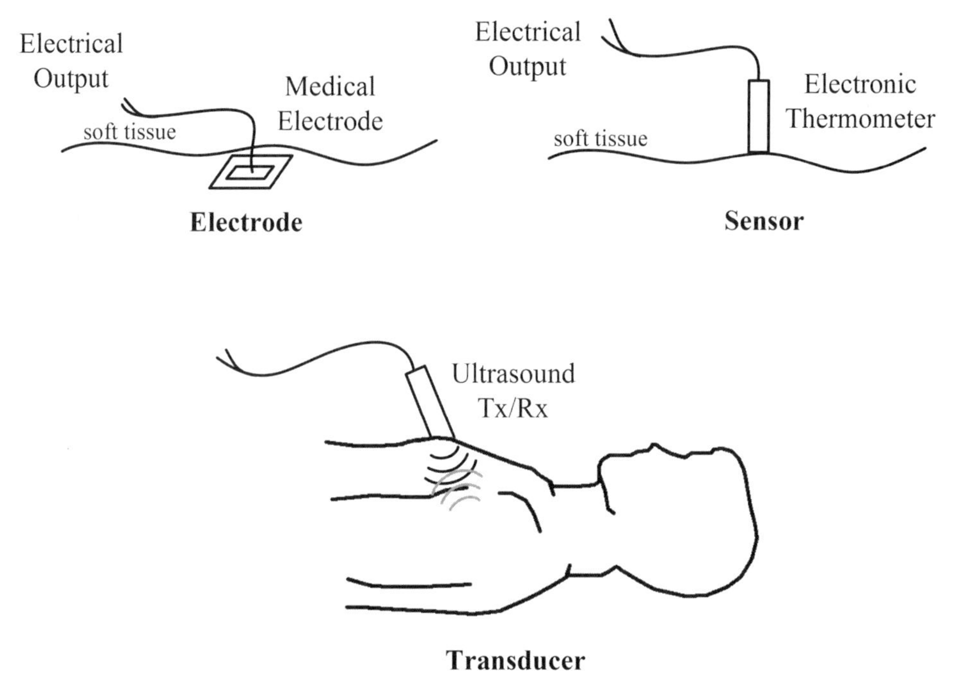

FIGURE 6-2 Sensors in medical devices.

A transducer converts one type of energy to another type of energy. The word "sensor" is derived from "to perceive," whereas transducer means "to lead across." A sensor is a device that detects a change in a physical stimulus and turns it into a signal for measurement. A transducer is a device that transfers power or energy from one system to another in similar or in different form. In some cases, a sensor can be a type of a transducer. For our purposes in this textbook, a sensible distinction is made to use "sensor" for the sensing element itself and "transducer" for the sensing element plus the associated circuitry. For clarity in defining biomedical sensors and transducers, we can determine that the final output of a transducer is an electrical signal and a sensor is part of a transducer unit. The sensor senses, or detects, and responds to a physical stimulus such as temperature, pressure, or motion; the transducer uses this sensor in its electrical or electronic circuit to produce a corresponding electrical signal.

For example, a temperature sensor such as a thermistor device senses the temperature around it by changing its electrical resistance, but then the transducer puts this sensor in its voltage divider network to generate the proportional voltage. Thus, the voltage across the thermistor is proportional to the temperature. In some cases, this voltage-temperature relationship can be inverted (that is, as the temperature increases, the voltage across it decreases).

Figure 6-3 shows a sensor, input and output transducers, and a modifier. The type of energy is sensed and the input transducer changes the signal into an electrical signal. A modifier then amplifies it and the output transducer presents the signal in a proper format to a recorder or a monitor. Often these three components are housed as one and the combined unit is called simply a transducer.

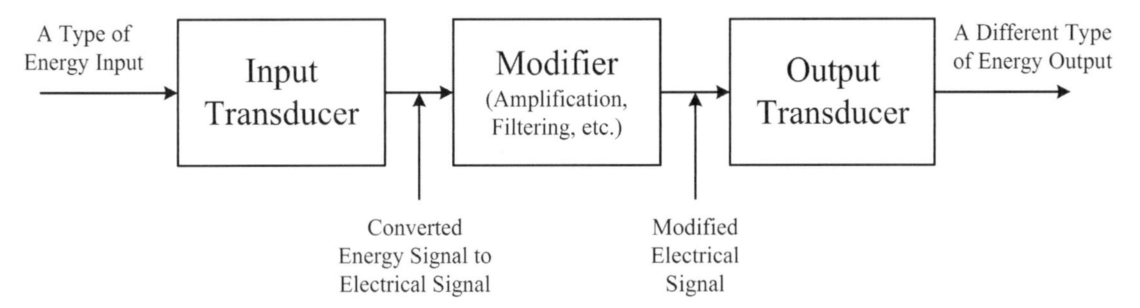

FIGURE 6-3 A block diagram of human-machine interface.

An electrode, however, is a conductor that makes a contact with a nonmetallic electrolyte for the flow of electrical current in the circuit. The input and output of an electrode are electrical. However, the same cannot be said for transducers and sensors.

6.2 BIOMEDICAL ELECTRODES

An electrode is a conductor that makes a contact with a nonmetal, such as an electrolyte or a semiconductor or even a vacuum. In an electrochemical cell, an electrode is either an anode or a cathode. When the electrode is an anode, the oxidation process occurs on the electrode. When the electrode is a cathode, the reduction process occurs on the electrode (the same electrode may act as an anode or a cathode depending on whether oxidation or the reduction process is occurring). **Figure 6-4** explains the charge density at the interface of the skin and the metal electrode. This process is similar to the oxidation and reduction

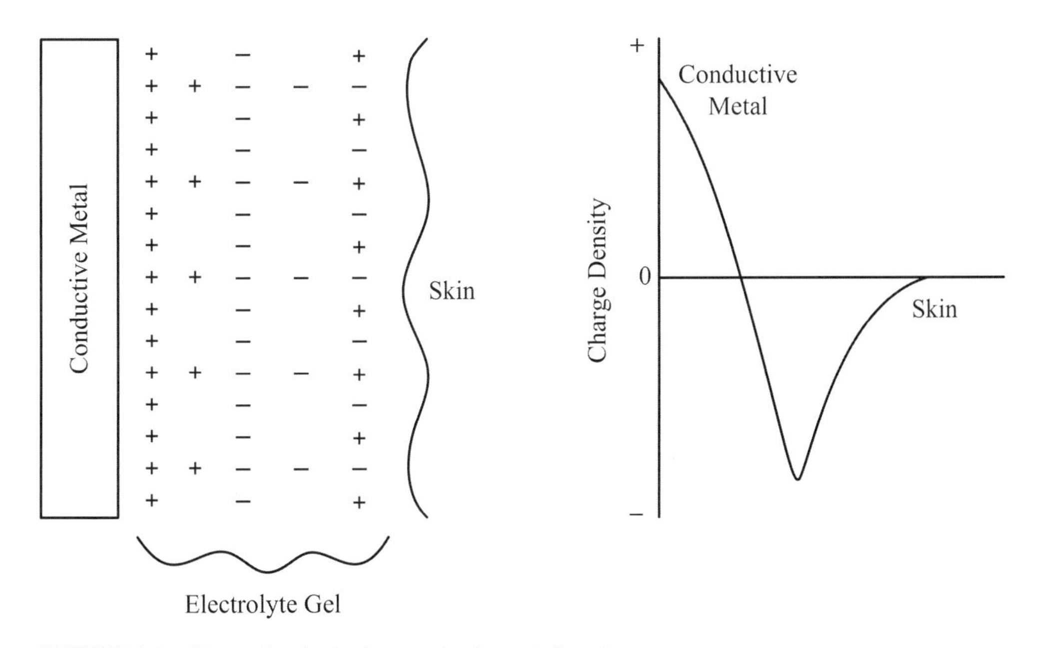

FIGURE 6-4 Charge density in the muscle-electrode interface.

in an electrochemical cell, in semiconductor diodes, or in vacuum tubes where the anode is the positive polarity and the cathode is the negative polarity.

Biomedical electrodes are used in ECG, EEG, EMG, defibrillators, external pacemakers, and many more. These electrodes are conductors that make contact with soft tissues and muscles.

6.3 THEORY OF ELECTRODES

A biomedical electrode such as an ECG electrode placed on the surface of the skin or a muscle is an electrochemical cell where a chemical reaction occurs between the electrode and an electrolyte. The electrolyte is a solution that reacts with the electrode to form ions, through which current can pass more easily.

See **Figure 6-5a**, showing an electrode immersed in an electrolyte. The electrode is silver and the electrolyte is a solution of silver chloride. Due to chemical reaction, a half-cell potential of E_{hc1} is established with respect to a reference electrode. For comparison, see **Figure 6-5b**, showing an ECG electrode placed on human skin. Here, the human skin, soft tissues, and muscles exhibit the characteristics of electrolytes.

The electrochemical cell is divided into the voltaic cell and the electrolytic cell. In the voltaic cell, the chemical reaction generates an electric current, but in the electrolytic cell, the chemical reaction uses the electric current. Most biomedical electrodes on the skin surface are like voltaic cells, such as ECG and EEG electrodes placed on the chest or scalp. However, the electrodes for electric stimulation of body muscles behave as electrolytic cells because the muscle uses the external electric source.

FIGURE 6-5a Electrodes in an electrolyte.

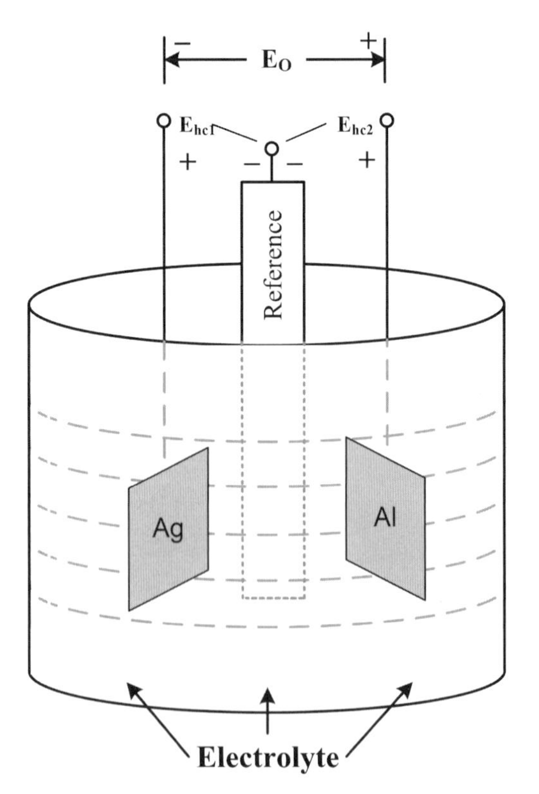

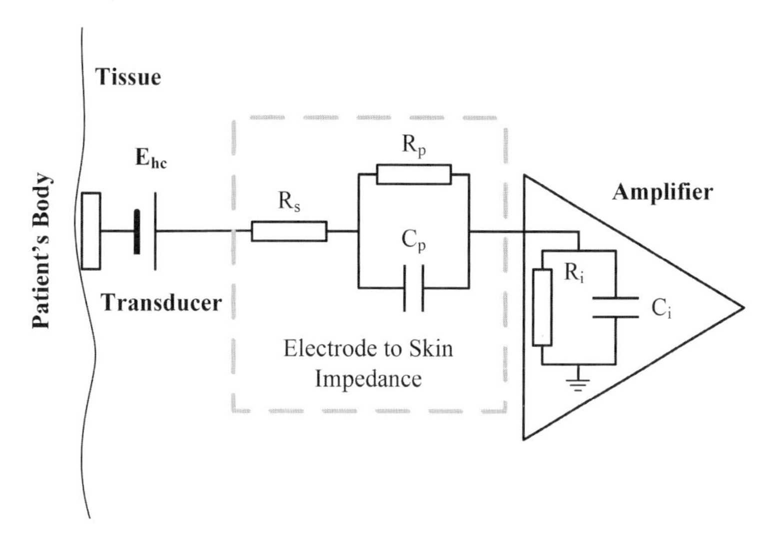

FIGURE 6-5b Equivalent electrode-skin impedance.

Voltaic Cell

In this type of electrochemical cell, the chemical reaction can be separated into two half reactions or two half cells. The half cell is the portion of an electrochemical cell in which a half reaction takes place. **Figure 6-6** and **Figure 6-7** explain the process of voltaic and electrolytic cells.

In **Figure 6-6,** there are two electrodes and two half cells of a voltaic cell that are connected with a conductive bridge. The two electrodes are zinc and copper and the bridge is a salt bridge. When an external circuit, such as a light bulb, connects these two electrodes, the electric circuit is complete (with no break). The chemical reactions now occur. The zinc half cell consists of the zinc electrode and the zinc sulfate solution as an electrolyte; the half-cell reaction can be explained as:

$$Zn(s) = Zn^{2+}(aq) + 2 \times e^-$$

In this half reaction, the solid zinc metal Zn(s) breaks down into ions and electrons. The two positive ions $Zn^{2+}(aq)$ enter the solution, leaving two electrons on the zinc metal. Similarly, the copper metal has the half-cell reaction, and the positive copper ions enter the copper sulfate solution leaving two electrons on the copper metal.

$$Cu(s) = Cu^{2+}(aq) + 2 \times e^-$$

These two half cells now are connected by a salt bridge, which is a tube of electrolytic gel that allows the flow of charged ions of the zinc and copper from one half cell to another.

As zinc tends to lose more electrons than copper, and more electrons now reach to the copper metal once the external circuit is complete, the zinc electrode is more positive compared to the copper electrode. The zinc electrode is now considered the anode and the copper electrode is the cathode.

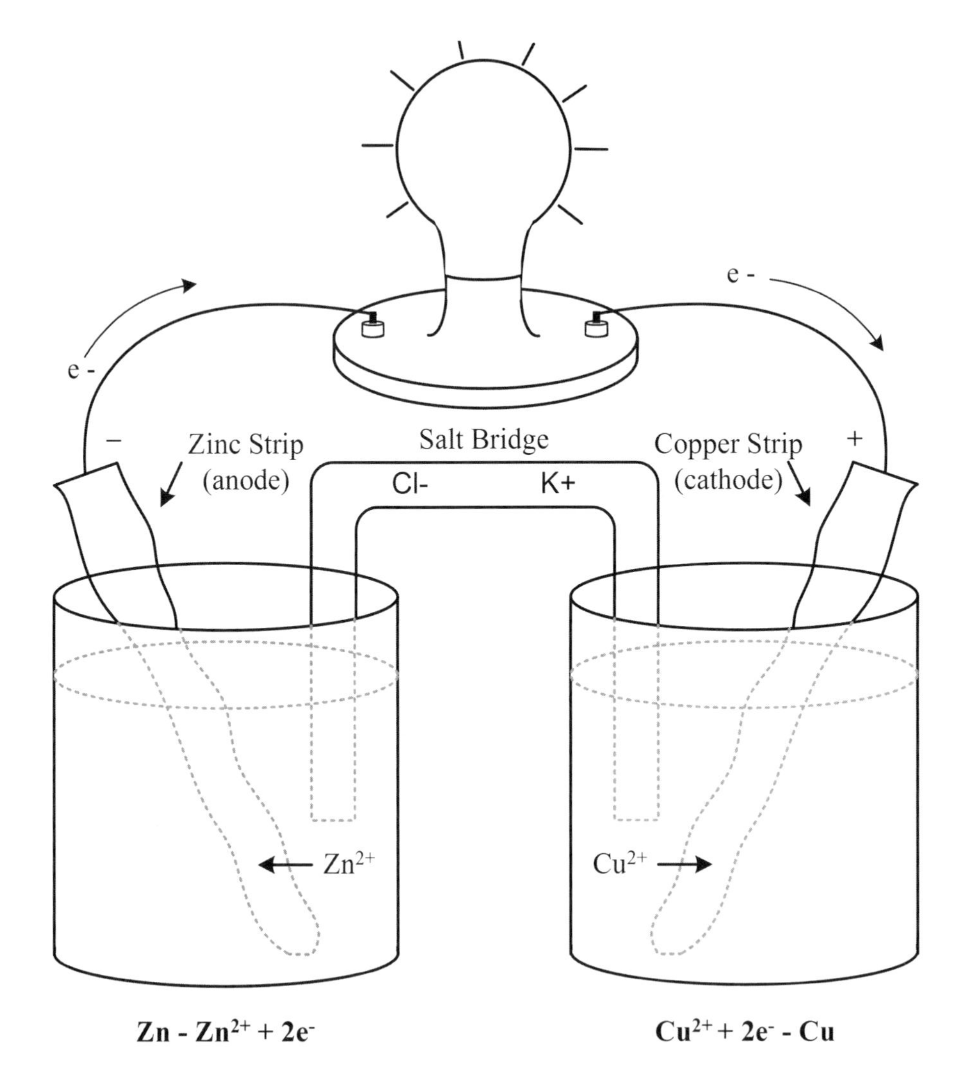

FIGURE 6-6 A voltaic cell.

The two half-cell reactions combine as follows:

$$Zn(s) = Zn^{2+}(aq) + 2 \times e^-$$

zinc ions into the solution, oxidation reaction,
= loss of electrons

$$Cu^{2+}(aq) + 2 \times e^- = Cu(s)$$

copper ions from the solution, reduction reaction,
= gain of electrons

The overall reaction is then:

$$Zn(s) + Cu^{2+}(aq) = Zn^{2+}(aq) + Cu(s)$$

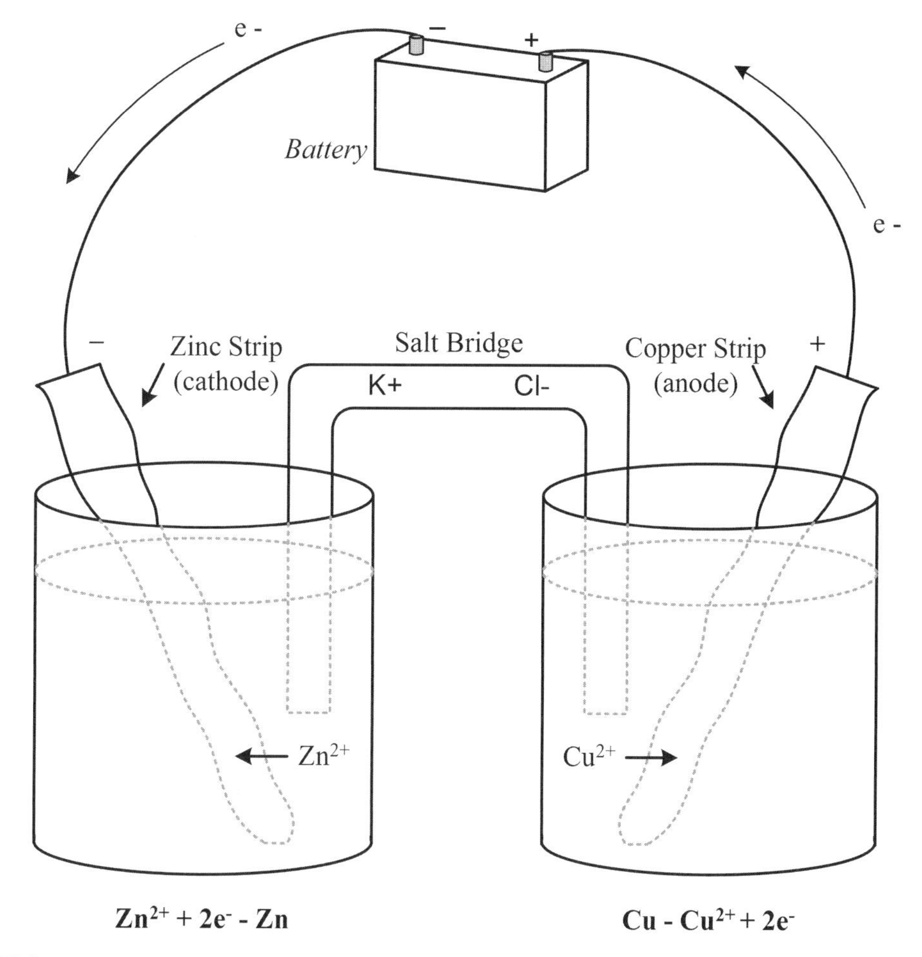

FIGURE 6-7 An electrolytic cell.

As electrons are lost at the zinc electrode, the reaction is called "oxidation" and as the electrons are gained at the copper electrode, the reaction is called "reduction."

If we connect a voltmeter instead of a light bulb, the voltmeter then reads the difference of these two half-cell potentials. Between zinc and copper electrodes, this difference will be $(-0.762) - (0.337) = -1.099$ V. The half-cell potentials for various metals and electrodes are given in **Figure 6-8**. The zinc and copper half-cell potentials are -0.762 V and $+0.337$ V, respectively.

Electrolytic Cell

Just as with a voltaic cell, we can determine the half-cell reactions when the external circuit is connected to an external voltage source as shown in **Figure 6-7**. The overall reaction will then be:

$$Zn^{2+}(aq) + Cu(s) = Zn(s) + Cu^{2+}(aq)$$

Electrode Reaction	E_{hc}(volts)	Electrode Reaction	E_{hc}(volts)
Li ⇆ Li +	-3.045	V ⇆ V^3 +	-0.876
Rb ⇆ Rb +	-2.925	Zn ⇆ Zn^3 +	-0.762
K ⇆ K +	-2.925	Cr ⇆ Cr^3 +	-0.740
Cs ⇆ Cs +	-2.923	Ga ⇆ Ga^2 +	-0.530
Ra ⇆ Ra^3 +	-2.920	Fe ⇆ Fe^3 +	-0.440
Ba ⇆ Ba^3 +	-2.900	Cd ⇆ Cd^2 +	-0.402
Sr ⇆ Sr^3 +	-2.890	In ⇆ In^2 +	-0.342
Ca ⇆ Ca^2 +	-2.870	Tl ⇆ Tl +	-0.336
Na ⇆ Na +	-2.714	Mn ⇆ Mn^3 +	-0.283
La ⇆ La^3 +	-2.520	Co ⇆ Co^2 +	-0.277
Mg ⇆ Mg^3 +	-2.370	Ni ⇆ Ni^2 +	-0.250
Am ⇆ Am^3 +	-2.320	Mo ⇆ Mo^3 +	-0.200
Pu ⇆ Pu^3 +	-2.070	Ge ⇆ Ge^4 +	-0.150
Th ⇆ Th^4 +	-1.900	Sn ⇆ Sn^2 +	-0.136
Np ⇆ Np^3 +	-1.860	Pb ⇆ Pb^3 +	-0.126
Bc ⇆ Bc^2 +	-1.850	Fe ⇆ Fe^3 +	-0.036
U ⇆ U^3 +	-1.800	D_3 ⇆ D +	-0.003
Hf ⇆ Hf^4 +	-1.700	H_3 ⇆ H +	0.000
Al ⇆ Al^3 +	-1.660	Cu ⇆ Cu^2 +	+ 0.337
Ti ⇆ Ti^3 +	-1.630	Cu ⇆ Cu +	+ 0.521
Zr ⇆ Zr^4 +	-1.530	Hg ⇆ $Hg_2{}^2$ +	+ 0.789
U ⇆ U^4 +	-1.500	Ag ⇆ Ag +	+ 0.799
Np ⇆ Np^4 +	-1.354	Rb ⇆ Rb^3 +	+ 0.800
Pu ⇆ Pu^4 +	-1.280	Hg ⇆ Hg^2 +	+ 0.857
Ti ⇆ Ti^4 +	-1.210	Pd ⇆ Pd^3 +	+ 0.987
V ⇆ V^2 +	-1.180	Ir ⇆ Ir^3 +	+ 1.000
Mn ⇆ Mn^2 +	-1.180	Pt ⇆ Pt^2 +	+ 1.190
Nb ⇆ Nb^3 +	-1.100	Au ⇆ Au^3 +	+ 1.500
Cr ⇆ Cr^2 +	-0.913	Au ⇆ Au +	+ 1.680

FIGURE 6-8 A table of half-cell potentials.

The oxidation occurs at the copper electrode and the reduction at the zinc electrode. The anode is now copper. The external voltage source drives the chemical reaction and the electron flow is reversed from copper to zinc.

6.4 GOLDMAN EQUATION AND NERNST EQUATION

The diffusion process for the sodium and potassium ion concentrations at the membrane generates a membrane potential similar to half-cell potentials in a battery. A high concentration of potassium appears on the outside of the cell at rest and then changes when the action potential starts. The Goldman equation relates these concentration changes, resulting in a membrane potential from inside to outside of the cell at a specific temperature.

$$V_m = -(kT/Q) \times \ln((P_K \times [K^+]_I + P_{Na} \times [Na^+]_I)/(P_K \times [K^+]_O + P_{Na} \times [Na^+]_O))$$

where

k = Boltzmann's constant Q = electron charge T = temperature
P_K and P_{Na} are the permeabilities of potassium and sodium, respectively
$[K^+]$ and $[Na^+]$ are the concentrations of potassium and sodium ions inside and outside of the cell

This relationship of the concentration, permeability, and temperature in the Goldman equation is the basis of understanding the transducer behavior in biomedical applications.

The Goldman equation reduces to a simplified Nernst equation when the sodium permeability is assumed to be zero.

Then,

$$V_m = -(kT/Q) \times \ln([K^+]_I/[K^+]_O)$$

Primarily, the resting potential in a cell is caused by the potassium concentration difference between inside and outside of the cell given by the Nernst equation. The result is approximately −94 mV. When the action potential propagates, the cell is referred to as depolarized. The −94 mV can change rapidly to a maximum of approximately 60 mV.

6.5 MODEL OF BIOMEDICAL ELECTRODE

Just as any electric wire has uniformly distributed internal resistance and inductance, an electrode also has uniformly distributed (not lumped) internal resistance if not inductance. We can model an electrode as its behavior exhibits voltage and current distribution.

From the previous discussion, we know now that the interface between a metal and an electrolyte starts a chemical reaction that produces a half-cell potential. The model should include the following:

1. A capacitance across the surface of the electrode and the electrolyte exists. At the interface, the tendency is for metallic electrode ions to enter the solution. There is also a tendency for the ions in the electrolyte to combine with the metallic electrode. A charge distribution occurs at the interface, as shown in **Figure 6-9.** There are two layers of charges, as shown in the figure, called a "double-layer," and this separation creates a capacitive effect between the electrolyte-electrode interface.
2. As there is finite current that flows through this interface, we must include a series resistance in the model.
3. The half-cell potential blocks current flow; this must be considered.
4. As the capacitor is a DC block, and the interface for biomedical electrode allows a DC current to flow, we must add another resistance to bypass this capacitor in parallel for the DC current.

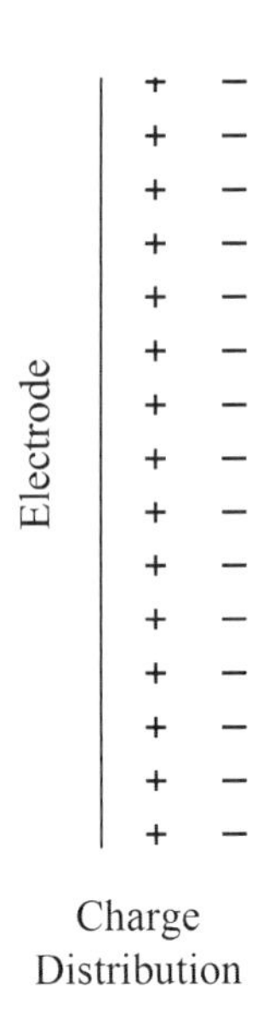

FIGURE 6-9 Charge distribution.

5. As the frequency decreases to 0 Hz, the electrolyte impedance increases. However, for higher frequencies, the capacitor creates a path for current to flow.
6. The magnitude of resistances and the capacitor depends up several factors: the diameter of the electrode, the metal type, the type of electrolyte, the condition of the surface, and the charge distribution.

The result of above discussion helps us to create a model of an electrode as shown in **Figure 6-10a** and **Figure 6-10b.** R_F is in parallel with the series combination of R and C, and the half-cell potential is in series to this combination. The positivity of the half-cell potential is towards the electrode. See **Figure 6-11** for a two-electrode model.

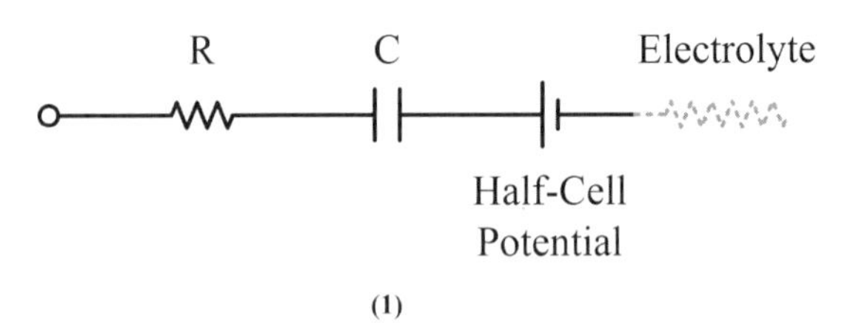

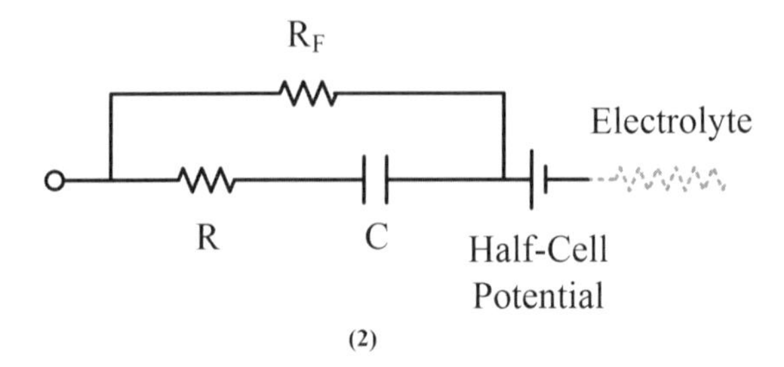

FIGURE 6-10a An electrode model.

FIGURE 6-10b An electrode model.

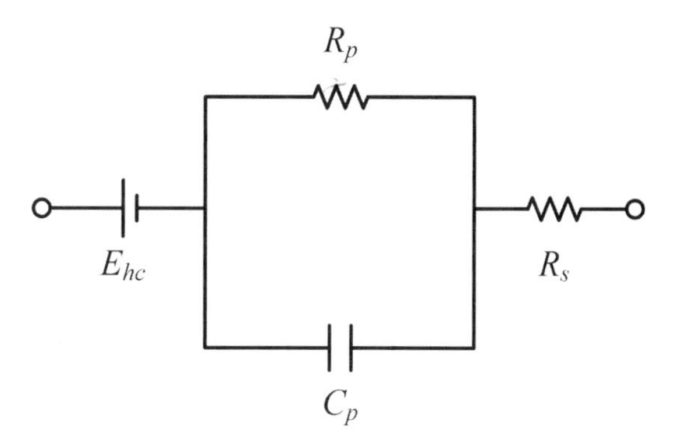

E_{hc} - half-cell potential
C_p - electrode capacitance
R_p - leakage resistance
R_s - series electrolyte and skin resistance

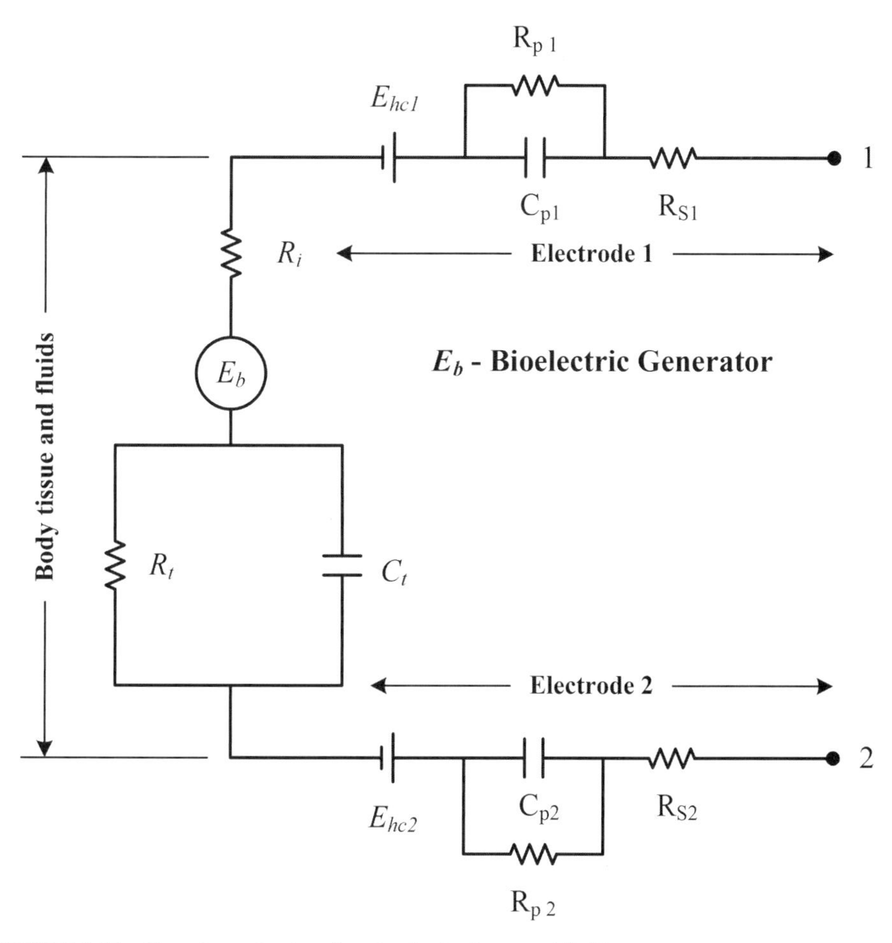

FIGURE 6-11 Two electrodes interfaced to body tissue and fluids.

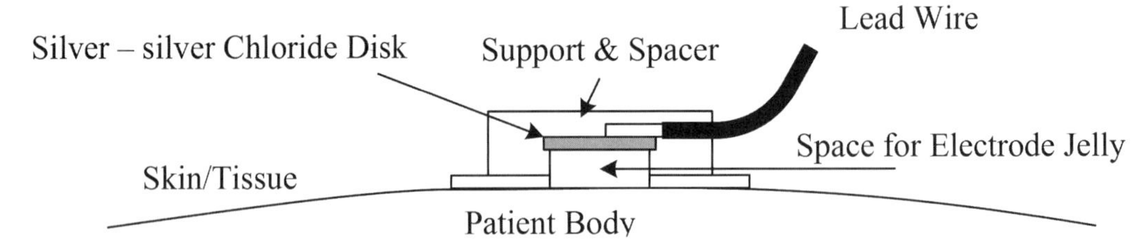

FIGURE 6-12a Silver/silver chloride electrode.

6.6 SILVER/SILVER CHLORIDE REFERENCE ELECTRODE

The silver/silver chloride (Ag/AgCl) is considered a stable reference electrode. **Figure 6-12a** and **Figure 6-12b** show the connection of the Ag/AgCl interface and an example of the Ag/AgCl electrode. The body of the electrode is a Vycor glass tube and the silver wire is the conductor that connects to the filling solution through plastic or a Teflon cap. The typical solution is either potassium chloride (KCl) or sodium chloride (NaCl). The concentration of these two solutions is reproducible when the temperature changes and the effect of the water evaporation is minimal on the concentration. Another example is given in **Figure 6-12c** for an Ag/AgCl electrode.

FIGURE 6-12b A view of a silver/silver chloride electrode.

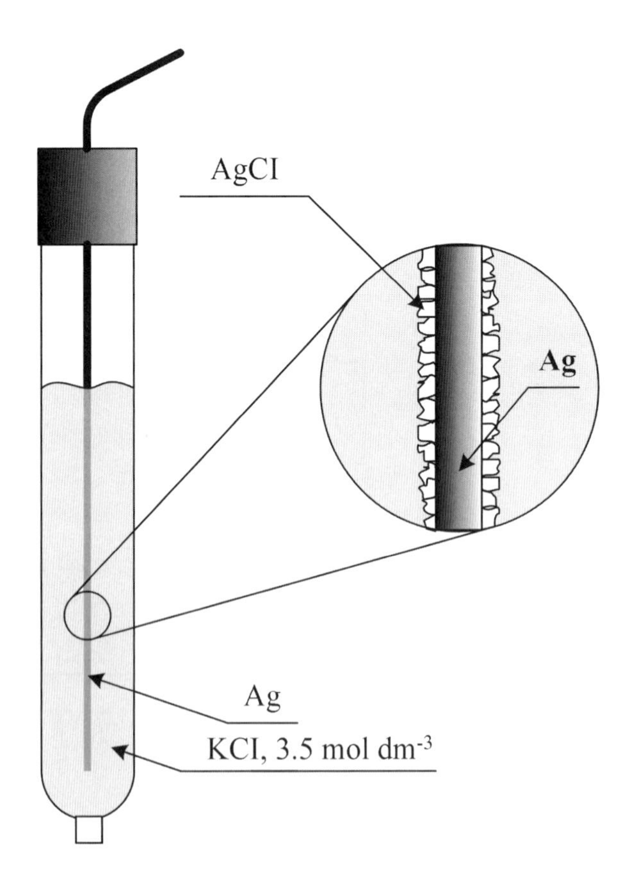

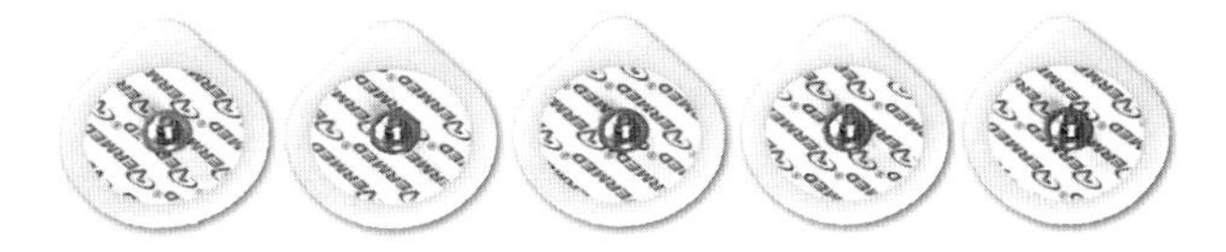

FIGURE 6-12c A photo of silver/silver chloride button electrodes.

6.7 TYPES OF ELECTRODES

Polarizable or Nonpolarizable

In polarizable electrodes, there is no movement of ions across the skin-electrode interface. See **Figure 6-13a, Figure 6-13b,** and **Figure 6-13c.** A DC signal cannot be detected, but is useful for higher frequency signals. Neither gel nor paste is needed at the interface and this type can be used for a long period of time. One of the disadvantages is that it is sensitive to motion artifacts.

In nonpolarizable electrodes, the ions move across the skin-electrode interface. The electrode then detects a DC signal. Gel or paste is necessary between the skin and the electrode surface. Long-term usage is not possible, but it is insensitive to motion artifacts.

Electrode Shapes: Button or Bar Types

Typically, button-shaped electrodes are used in hospitals, but the bar-shaped electrode is used at the wrist or ankle for evoked-potential or electrical stimulation tests.

Electrode Configurations: Monopolar, Bipolar

This states the polarity of the voltage signal: monopolar configuration generates only positive or negative signals, whereas the bipolar configuration can generate positive and negative signal deviations. The placement of the electrodes is what determines these kinds of signals.

Skin-surface Electrodes

In obtaining bioelectric potentials from the surface of the body, there are electrodes in various sizes and types. A larger size of surface electrode is usually used in ECG measurements and the smaller sizes can be used for EEG and EMG measurements.

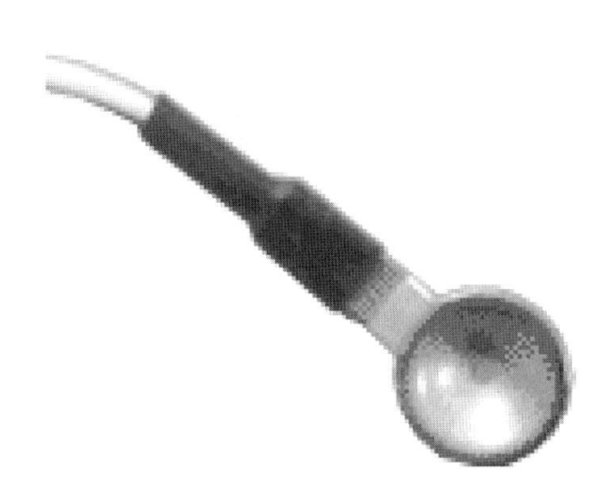

FIGURE 6-13a A surface electrode.

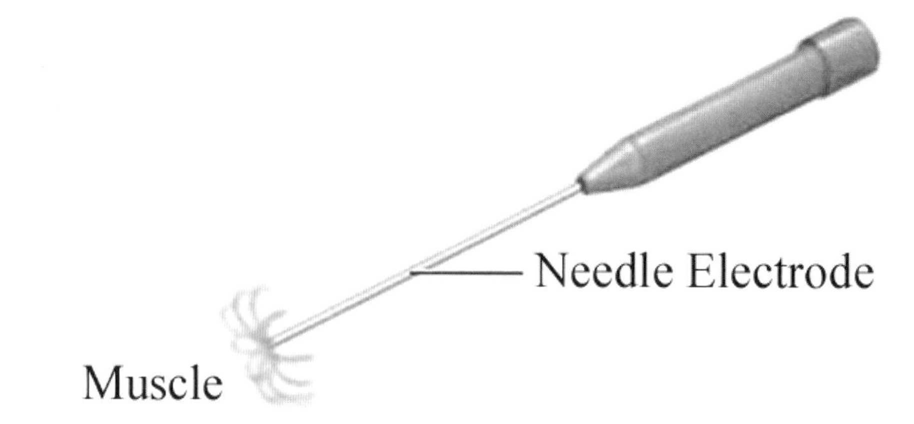

FIGURE 6-13b A needle electrode.

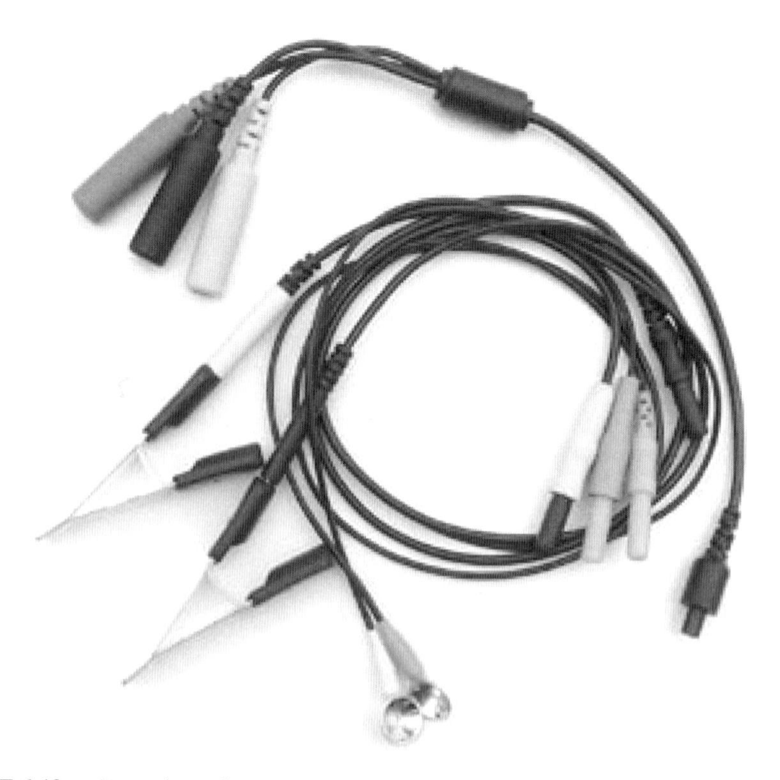

FIGURE 6-13c A cup electrode.

Earlier electrodes were sensitive to electrode movement, created large impedances at the skin surface, and used to be held by adhesive tape.

The floating type of surface electrode eliminates the electrode movement issue by avoiding any direct contact of the metal with the skin and, therefore, the likelihood of slippage. An electrolyte gel or paste makes a conductive path between metal and skin. These floating types are attached to the skin by adhesive collars or rings.

Needle Electrodes

In EEG studies, needle electrodes are used on the scalp, just beneath the surface of the skin, but not inserted into the brain. These types of electrodes reduce interface impedances and the motion artifacts.

Cup Electrodes

Cup-shaped electrodes are specially designed for clinical EEG, electrophysiology (EP), and polysomnography (PSG) examinations.

6.8 CLASSIFICATION OF SENSORS AND TRANSDUCERS

We can classify sensors and transducers in two ways: by the physical property that they use for conversion or the function that they perform. A piezoelectric transducer can be used for pressure measurement; a piezoelectric transducer exhibits piezoelectric property, but it can also be considered as a pressure transducer because its function is to measure pressure.

One way to look at a sensor is to consider all of its properties, particularly stimulus, material, application field, conversion mechanism, and the physical phenomenon. The physical property of a sensor must be altered by an external stimulus, thereby producing an electric signal or modifying an external electric signal. If the classification of sensors is based upon the stimulus, then the types of stimuli are:

Mechanical: position, force, pressure, strain, mass, density, compliance

Electric: current, voltage, conductivity

Magnetic: magnetic field, permeability

Optical: wave velocity, refractive index, absorption, reflectivity

Thermal: temperature, specific heat, thermal conductivity

Acoustic: wave velocity, wave polarization

6.9 PERFORMANCE CHARACTERISTICS OF ELECTRODES, SENSORS, AND TRANSDUCERS

Next, we will discuss the parameters that characterize electrodes, sensors, and transducers in terms of their performances such as sensitivity, accuracy, reproducibility, hysteresis, resolution, and the frequency response. The user can compare different types of sensors based on these parameters and then decide which one to use.

Sensitivity

Sensitivity is defined as the change in the output divided by the corresponding change in the input. When comparing transducers, you need to find out how sensitive one transducer's output is over the other with the changes in the input-sensing variable. For example, if the output changes to 2 V due to the temperature change of 2° F in a temperature transducer, then the sensitivity is defined as 1 V/° F. Some transducers may be too sensitive if the output changes with minimal change in the input. In some applications, this type of sensitivity is considered a positive quality.

$$\text{Sensitivity of a transducer or electrode} = (\text{change in output})/(\text{change in input})$$

As an example, thermocouple sensitivity can be given as 37.4 μV/° C if it measures over a range of −270 to 1,372° C by outputting −6.548 to 54.874 mV (courtesy of National Instruments). The calculation can be shown as follows:

$$[54.874 - (-6.548)]/[1372 - (-270)] = 0.0374 \text{ mV/° C} = 37.4 \text{ μV/° C}$$

Static and Dynamic Errors

Static error is the difference between a measured value and an actual value. In static versus dynamic, the measured value does not change with time in static measurements, but the measured value does change in the dynamic measurements. Consequently, the dynamic error changes with time. In general, error = measured value − actual value.

Accuracy

Accuracy is an important parameter in the measurement of the transducer or electrode output. How accurate is the output? Can we compare the output of this transducer with the output from a standard or reference transducer under the same conditions?

Accuracy refers to how close the output measurement is to the true value.

$$\text{Accuracy} = [(\text{measured output} - \text{actual output})/(\text{actual output})] \times 100$$

This parameter is in percent and it can be a positive or a negative value.

Hysteresis

Hysteresis refers to a transducer that is not able to repeat the data in the opposite direction of operation. For example, if the resistance of a sensor were decreasing with an increase in the temperature around it, would it follow the same result of data points when the temperature decreases? Actually, it should not matter whether the temperature is increasing or decreasing. When data is plotted in each direction for the temperature example, the graphs look like those in **Figure 6-14a.** In one graph, the direction is downward for increasing temperature, and in the next graph, the direction is upward for decreasing temperature. This is called a hysteresis loop of the sensor. If the loop is wider, then the sensor may not be useful because the changes in sensing a variable (like temperature, pressure, etc.) should be negligible with respect to time and any direction (ascending or descending). Most sensors have some form of hysteresis loop.

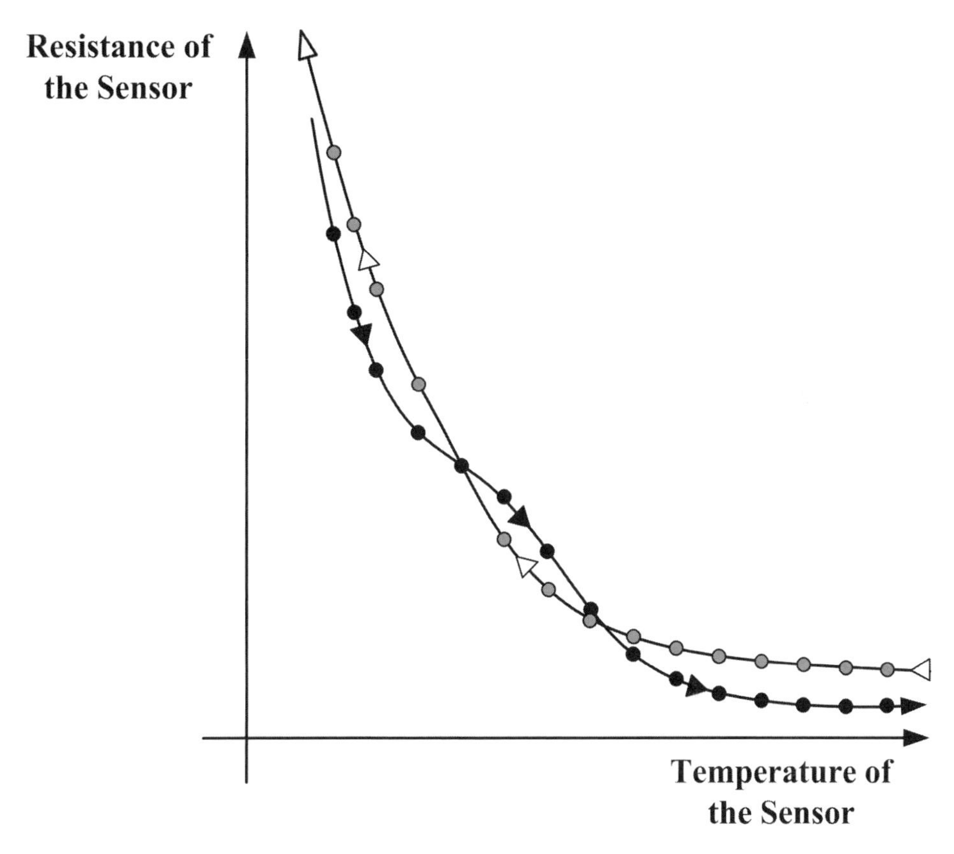

FIGURE 6-14a Hysteresis graph for temperature sensor.

Frequency Response

How does a sensor or transducer respond to a changing input signal of varying frequencies? The manufacturer provides the specification of the response to a range of frequencies. This range is called the bandwidth. The larger the bandwidth, the more likely the operation of the sensor may be considered adequate in some cases. In normal operation, the bandwidth (i.e., frequency response) is flat. This is shown in **Figure 6-14b** for two sensors. Sensor 2 has a wider bandwidth than sensor 1.

Numerically, the bandwidth (i.e., range of frequencies) is taken at 0.707 of the max (flat) gain. In the figure, the max gain is 10, and 0.707 of it is approximately 7. The bandwidth is shown for sensor 1. It is given as (7 kHz − 0.1 kHz).

Reproducibility

Reproducibility refers to a transducer's ability to produce identical output values repeatedly at different times under the same conditions for the same input. This is beyond the transducer's limits of accuracy and sensitivity. The equation or formula for reproducibility is not defined because no device, machine, or transducer can be relied upon to repeat the same output every time.

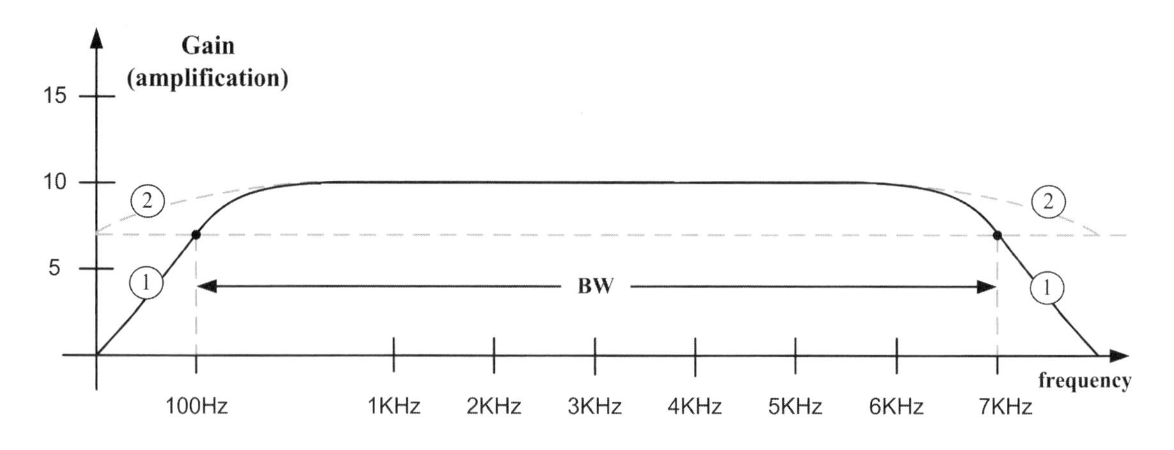

FIGURE 6-14b Frequency response of sensors.

Resolution

Before we define resolution, we should discuss the range for the output variable of a transducer. We know that there is a minimum output value and a maximum output value. In a way, the output varies from the lower range limit to the upper range limit. We can describe this change in the lower to upper limit as span of the range. The resolution is the smallest step of the output that is meaningful and measurable over its range. Resolution represents the smallest change that the data acquisition (DAQ) board can detect. For a temperature sensor, if the output varies from 1 V to 10 V when the input changes from 10° F to 40° F, then

$$\text{Span of the output} = 10\ \text{V} - 1\ \text{V} = 9\ \text{V}$$
$$\text{Span of the input} = 40°\ \text{F} = 10°\ \text{F} = 30°\ \text{F}$$
$$\text{Resolution of the output} = 9\ \text{V}/30°\ \text{F} = 0.3\ \text{V}/°\ \text{F}$$

If we line up the input of 10° F with the 1 V output, then for 11° F, the output will be 1.3 V. For 12° F, the output will be 0.3 V more (or 1.6 V), and so on.

6.10 PRESSURE TRANSDUCERS

Pressure is generally defined as force per unit area. Although this definition is correct when referring to pressure as the force exerted by one solid object on another, pressure is also used when referring to liquids or gases. In medicine, most pressure measurement is in the range of 50 to 1,000 mm Hg; considering that atmospheric pressure is 760 mm Hg, the pressure measurement in medical equipment is low pressure. We will discuss two types of pressure transducers in this section: the metal strain gauge and the linear variable differential transformer (LVDT).

Metal Strain Gauges

When a fine wire is stretched or compressed, its electric resistance changes. By measuring the change in the resistance, we can determine the amount of stretching or compression. Therefore, in determining small displacements, such as stretching or compressing a metal bar under some kind of load, we use the technology of metal strain gauge transducers. Here, the input to the transducer is displacement, and the output of the transducer is electrical resistance. In a voltage divider network, this change in electrical resistance implies a change in voltage.

Figure 6-15a, Figure 6-15b, and **Figure 6-15c** show a metal strain gauge made of a thin metal deposited in a special pattern on a backing material. For example, the gauge wire is mounted on a metal bar shown in **Figure 6-15a.** When the metal bar is compressed or stretched, the gauge wire is also affected in the same way, and both follow the stretching or compression in the same direction.

We can define a relationship between the resistance change and the displacement change by a gauge factor GF.

$$GF = \frac{(\Delta R/R)}{(\Delta L/L)}$$

where $\Delta R/R$ = fractional change in resistance
$\Delta L/L$ = fractional change in length

The gauge wire is affected in a "sensitive direction" as shown in **Figure 6-15b,** but not in the "insensitive direction." **Figure 6-15c** shows the placement of a dummy gauge and an active gauge in a balanced bridge circuit. The dummy gauge is not affected by stretching or compression but will react to any temperature changes and is used for temperature compensation in the bridge. The output of the bridge is due to the stretching or compression of the active gauge.

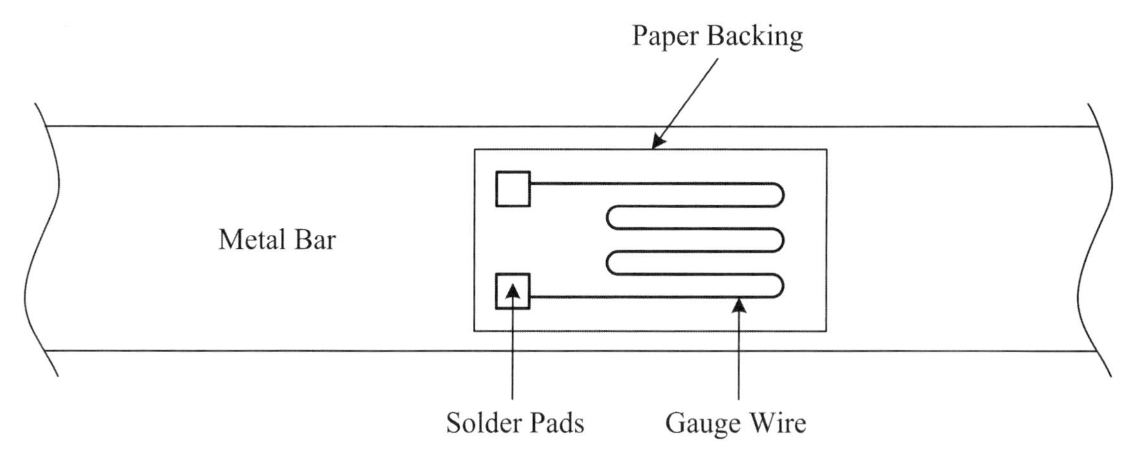

FIGURE 6-15a A simple metal gauge.

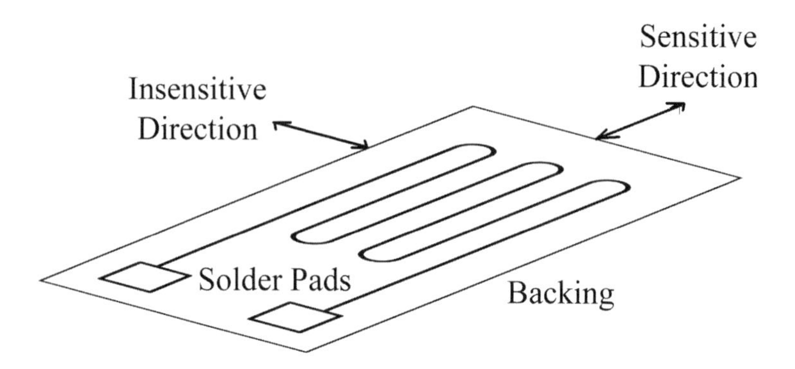

FIGURE 6-15b Backing material of a metal gauge.

Linear Variable Differential Transformer

Another method for converting a displacement into electrical signal is with a linear variable differential transformer (LVDT). The displacement can be determined as a change in the DC voltage at the secondary of a transformer when the iron core is proportionally displaced or moved.

A transformer has primary and secondary coils, and an iron core magnetically interfaces the primary voltage signal to be developed at the secondary in an equal or step-up

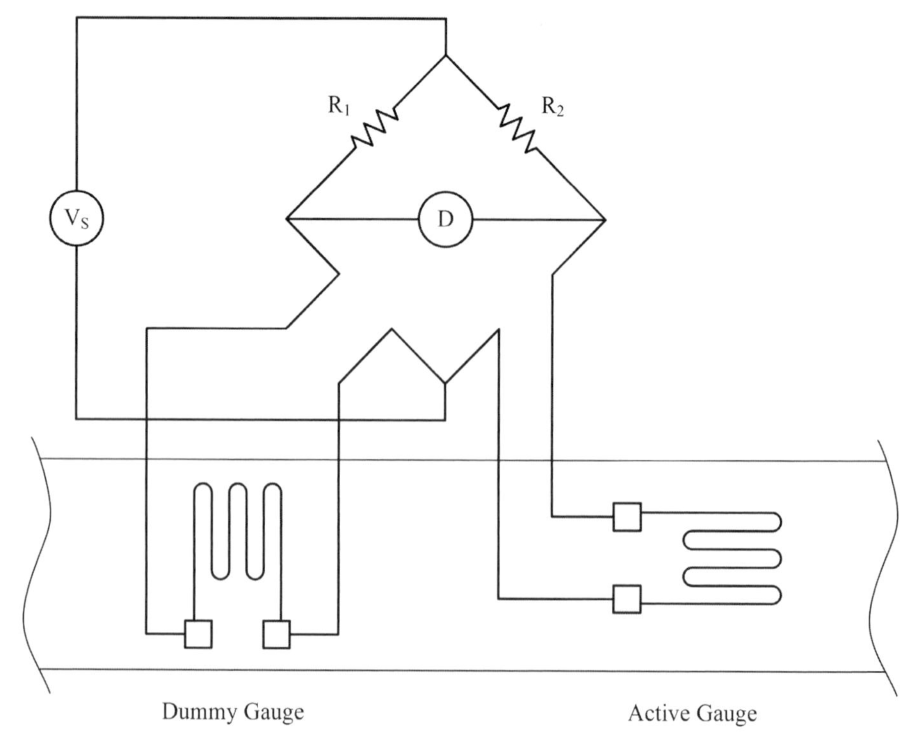

FIGURE 6-15c A balanced bridge circuit with a metal gauge.

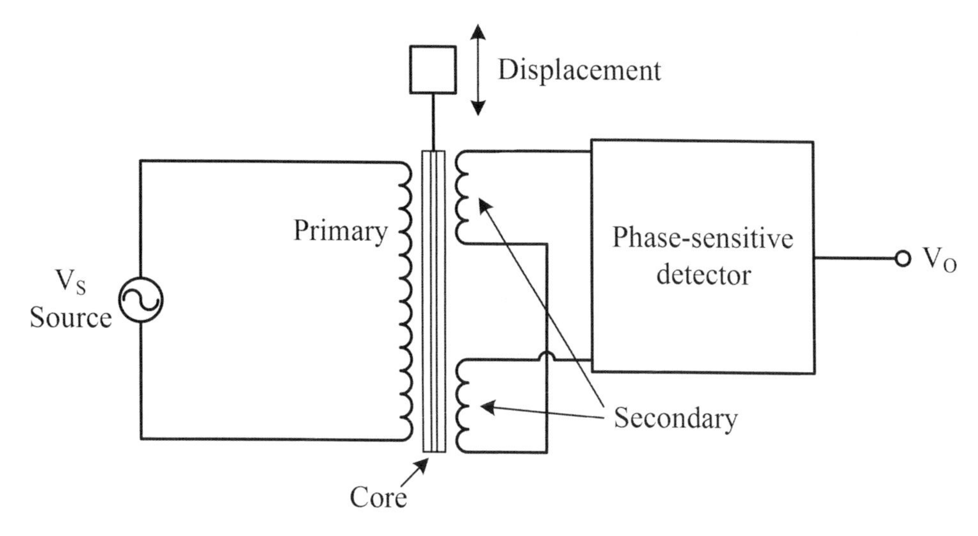

FIGURE 6-16a A simple LVDT transducer.

or step-down manner. The secondary voltage is called an induced voltage. **Figure 6-16a** shows a transformer with primary and secondary windings, and also the displacement input connected to the iron core. The core moves freely in and out of the coil windings. Notice that the secondary is split into two opposite coil windings.

When the core is in the middle, the total output voltage of the secondary is zero because the secondary coil voltage at A cancels the identical, but opposite, secondary coil voltage at B. However, the total output will be positive or negative other than the zero volts when the core is displaced in either direction. For example, if the core is moved upward, voltage A will be larger than voltage B, and the total output will be (A − B), the difference of the two voltages.

The phase-sensitive detector circuit compares the magnitude and phase of voltages A and B and generates a DC output. The result is linear and the polarity suggests the displacement direction. A linear variable differential transformer is used in medical pressure transducers because it can detect small displacements and the output is linear. **Figure 6-16b** and **Figure 6-16c** show simple circuits of LVDT.

As the core moves between the primary and secondary coils, the output voltage is detected sown in **Figure 6-16b**. An oscillator and an amplifier with a RC phase shift network are shown in **Figure 6-16c**. A DC output is held across a capacitor.

6.11 FLOW TRANSDUCERS

Flow transducers measure the flow of gases, liquids, or solids. Mathematically, flow can be given as:

$$Q = (\text{area})(\text{velocity})$$

The venturi-meter, thermal velocity probe, electromagnetic, and ultrasonic types of transducers measure the mean velocity of the flow. The flow rate calculation then depends on the accuracy of a cross-sectional area of the vessel.

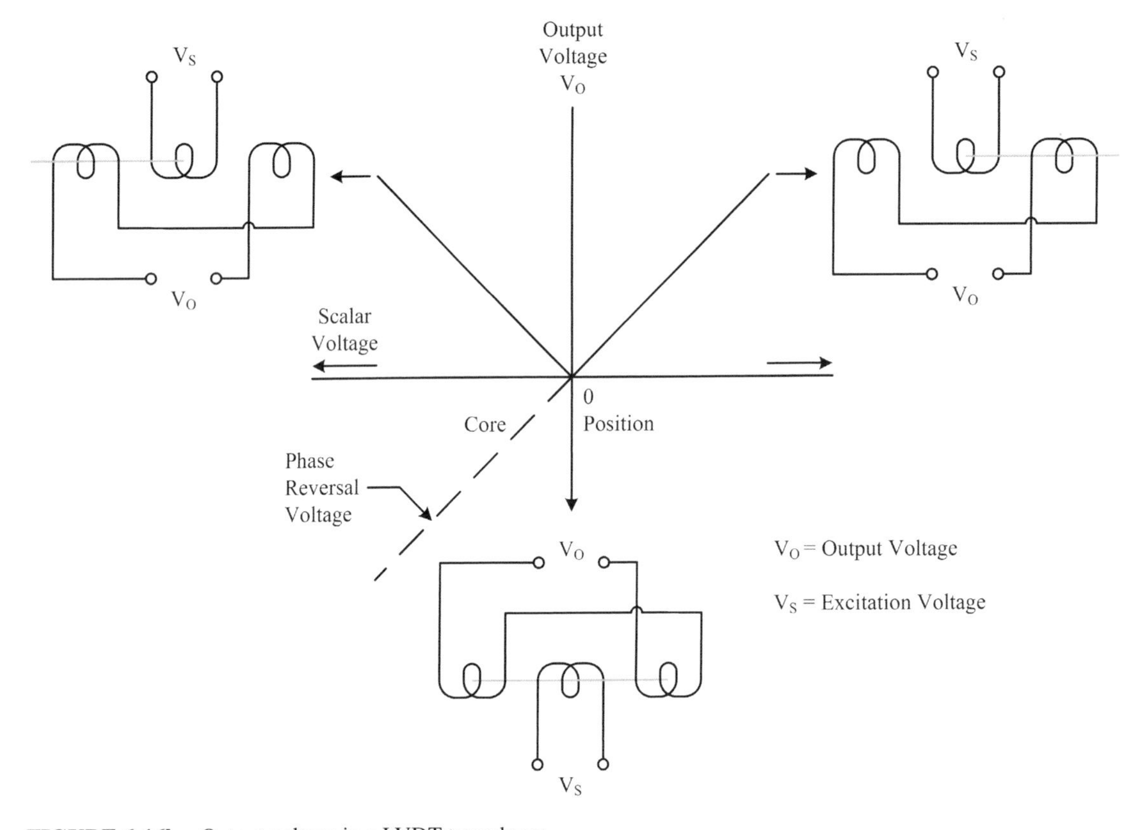

FIGURE 6-16b Output voltage in a LVDT transducer.

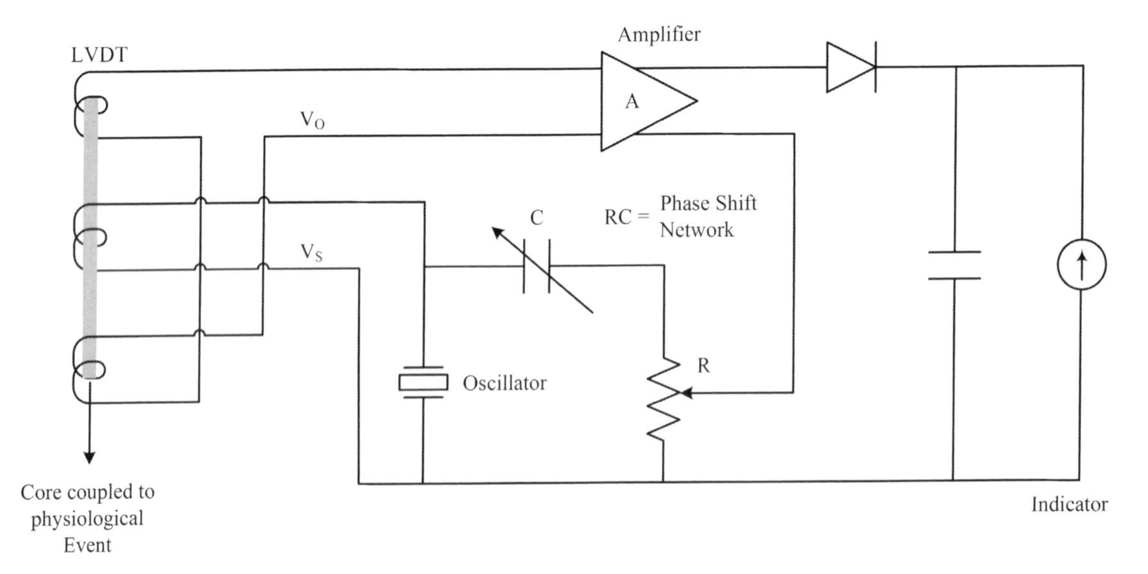

FIGURE 6-16c LVDT in an amplifier circuit.

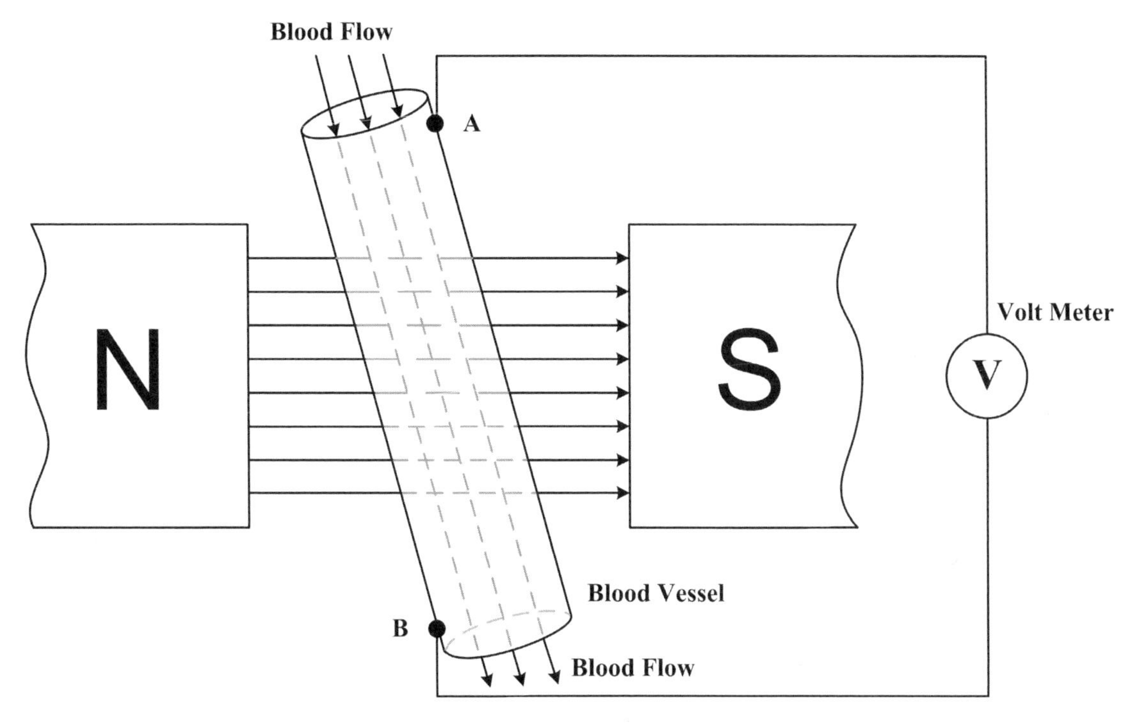

FIGURE 6-17 A simple flow transducer.

In an electromagnetic flow meter, a DC magnetic field is created around a blood vessel and electrodes are placed on the two sides of the vessel perpendicular to the magnetic lines of force. This is shown in **Figure 6-17** when the blood flows through the vessel. Electrical voltage proportional to the rate of flow is generated between the two electrodes. The pulsatile changes in flow as well as steady flow can be detected by the changes in voltages. Actually, the voltage indicates the mean velocity and the flow is then calculated with the consideration of the cross-sectional area of the vessel. The pickup voltages are in the microvolt range.

6.12 TEMPERATURE TRANSDUCERS

Here, we introduce three types of temperature transducers: the resistance temperature detector (RTD), the thermistor, and the thermocouple. Resistance temperature detectors or thermistors do not generate a voltage by themselves until they are connected to a voltage divider network. Resistance temperature detectors or thermistors are like resistors and their resistance changes with temperature. The typical range of the temperature measurement in the human body is approximately 98.6° F or 37° C; when the human body is unable to regulate its temperature, it suffers from hyperthermia (above-normal body temperature) or hypothermia (below-normal body temperature). Temperature transducers are used in applications such as blood flow, respiration, or skin temperature measurements.

Resistance Temperature Detector

The metal wire resistance increases with temperature in these kinds of transducers. Typically, the RTD transducer consists of a small coil of nickel or platinum wire protected by a stainless steel sheath. The manufacturer of RTDs provides a table or graph of resistance versus temperature. These are not linear except in small ranges at different spans.

For example, a 100 Ω platinum RTD can have a range of −200° to 850° C, a resolution of 0.2 to 0.4 Ω/° C, an accuracy of ±0.6° at 100° C, and a temperature coefficient of 0.4 in percent/° C at 25° C. An equation is provided by the RTD manufacturer:

$$R(T) = R(T_0) \times [1 + \alpha_0(T - T_0)]$$

where T = temperature at which the resistance is desired

T_0 = midpoint of valid temperature range

α_0 = temperature coefficient (i.e., fractional change in temperature per unit of temperature at T_0)

R(T) = resistance at T predicted and $R(T_0)$ = resistance at T_0 from the RTD table

Two-, three-, and four-lead RTDs connect to instrumentation to help engineer for optimum accuracy and cost. The four-lead RTD is usually expensive, but offers the most accuracy.

Thermistor

Thermistors are semiconductors that exhibit negative or positive temperature coefficient of resistance. This means that as temperature increases, the electrical resistances start to decrease. The characteristic is nonlinear, but for a very small range of temperatures, the graph is linear. A thermistor's negative temperature coefficient graph is shown in **Figure 6-18a.**

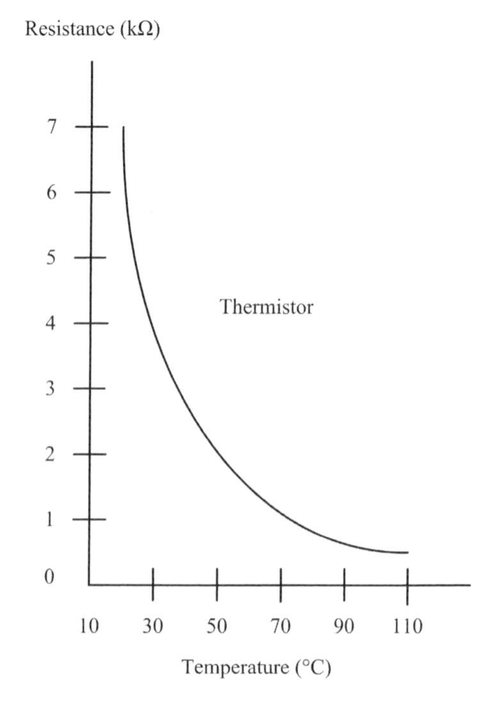

FIGURE 6-18a A thermistor temperature graph.

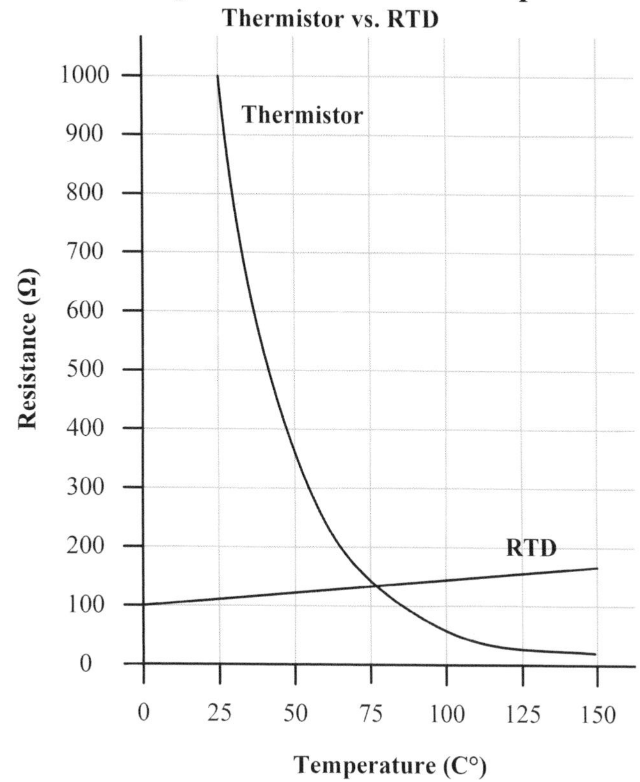

FIGURE 6-18b Thermistor versus RTD.

The change in semiconductor resistance with temperature can be deduced using the tables provided by the manufacturer. In addition, a thermistor is provided with a dissipation constant in mW/° C specifying the self-heating due to the current passed through the transducer. The equation for a thermistor is given as:

$$R_T = R_0 \times \exp\left[\beta \times \left(\frac{1}{T} - \frac{1}{T_0}\right)\right]$$

where R_T = resistance of the thermistor at temperature T in degrees kelvin
R_0 = resistance of the thermistor at the reference temperature T_0 in degrees kelvin
β = material constant in degrees kelvin

A comparative resistance graph between a thermistor and an RTD is shown in **Figure 6-18b**. RTD is linear and its resistance (compared to that of a thermistor) is low between 0° C to 75° C.

Thermocouple

This type of transducer converts a temperature reading into a voltage reading. A thermocouple is created when two dissimilar metals touch and a small open-circuit voltage is produced as a function of temperature at the contact point. This effect is called a Seebeck effect, which is a combination of the Peltier and Kelvin effects. This process is shown in **Figure 6-19a, Figure 6-19b,** and **Figure 6-19c.**

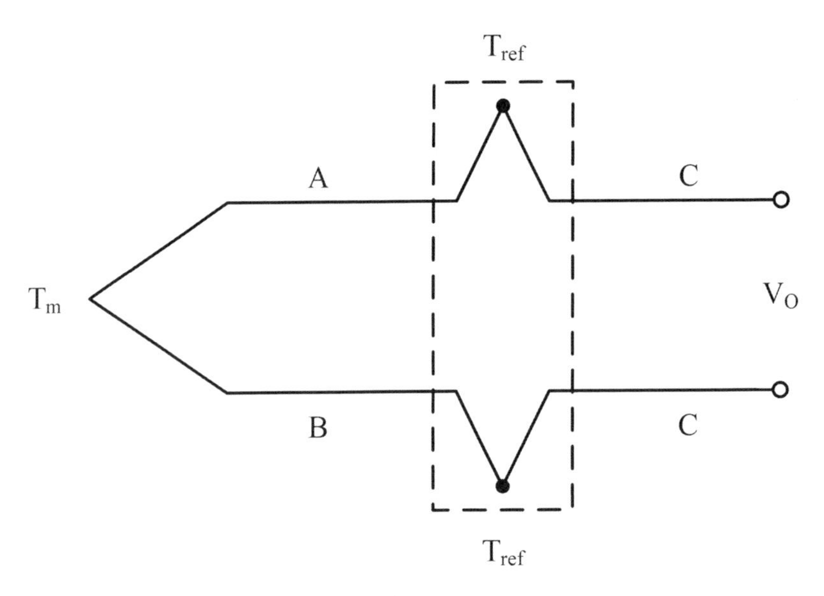

FIGURE 6-19a A simple thermocouple transducer.

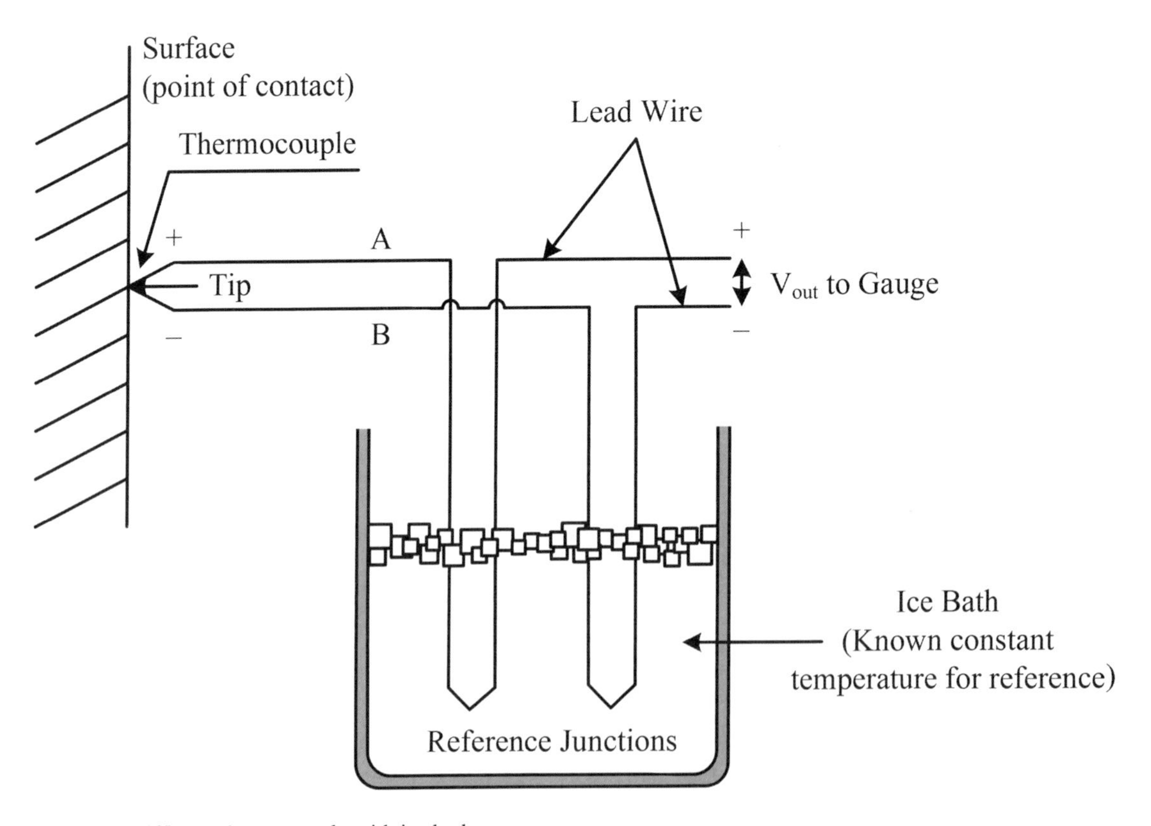

FIGURE 6-19b A thermocouple with ice bath.

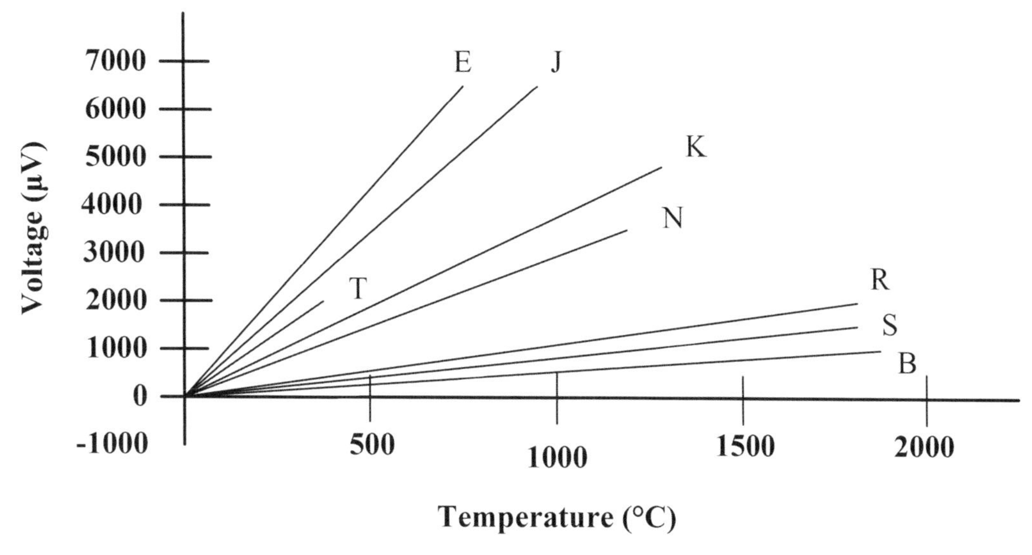

FIGURE 6-19c Graphs of thermocouple types.

The Peltier effect states that a small voltage exists at the contact point of two unlike metals and this voltage is temperature dependent, whereas kelvin effect states the presence of a small voltage along any conductor having a temperature difference across its two ends.

Thermocouples are designated by a single letter such as J, K, or T and the difference is due to metallic compositions. Type J is iron-constantan, Type K is chromel-alumel, and Type T is copper-constantan. The first named material is a positive potential terminal. **Figure 6-20** shows a table for the Type J thermocouple of National Instruments. The temperature of the contact point is given in the leftmost column in degrees centigrade, and the top row indicates the temperature increments from the leftmost column temperatures. The generated thermocouple voltage is given in each row for that temperature.

For example, when the contact point is at $-50°$ C, the thermocouple voltage is -2.43 V, but it is -2.89 V when the contact temperature is $-40°$ C.

The Type E thermocouple is chromel-constantan; Type N is nicrosel-nisil; types R, S, and B are platinum-rhodium, with varying rhodium percentages in the alloy for each conductor.

6.13 OPTICAL TRANSDUCERS

Optical measurements do not require direct physical contact. Therefore, they avoid any disturbance of the system being measured. We can measure distance with the time it takes for a pulse of light to reflect from an object. Similarly, to measure level, one can use the light reflected from the surface. A photoconductive cell is a common type of optical transducer that uses the reflection of light to detect the distance or level.

Type J: Iron - Constantan

	0	5.00	10.00	15.00	20.00	25.00	30.00	35.00
-150	-6.50	-6.66	-6.82	-6.97	-7.12	-7.27	-7.40	-7.54
-100	-4.63	-4.83	-5.03	-5.23	-5.42	-5.61	-5.80	-6.16
-50	-2.43	-2.66	-2.89	-3.12	-3.34	-3.56	-3.78	-4.00
-0	0.00	-0.25	-0.50	-0.75	-1.00	-1.24	-1.48	-1.72
+0	0.00	0.25	0.50	0.75	1.02	1.28	1.54	1.80
50	2.58	2.85	3.11	3.38	3.65	3.92	4.19	4.46
100	5.27	5.24	5.81	6.08	6.36	6.63	6.90	7.18
150	8.00	8.28	8.56	8.84	9.11	9.39	9.67	9.95
200	10.78	11.00	11.34	11.62	11.89	12.17	12.45	12.73
250	13.56	13.84	14.12	14.39	14.67	14.94	15.22	15.00
300	16.33	16.60	16.86	17.15	17.43	17.71	17.98	18.26
350	19.09	19.37	19.64	19.92	20.20	20.47	20.75	21.02
400	21.85	22.13	22.40	22.68	22.95	23.23	23.50	23.78
450	24.61	24.88	25.16	25.44	25.72	25.99	26.27	26.55
500	27.39	27.67	27.95	28.23	28.52	28.80	29.08	29.37
550	30.22	30.51	30.80	31.08	31.37	31.66	31.95	32.24
600	33.11	33.41	44.70	33.99	34.29	34.58	34.88	35.18
650	36.08	36.38	36.69	36.99	37.30	37.60	37.91	38.22
700	39.15	39.47	39.78	40.10	40.41	40.73	41.05	41.36

FIGURE 6-20 A thermocouple table.

The cadmium sulfide (CdS) is the most common type of a photoconductive cell. Its resistance changes with the intensity of light striking the cell. Primarily, the resistance decreases with increasing light intensity in a nonlinear manner.

EXAMPLE An RTD has $\alpha_0 = 0.0035/° \text{C}$ at $T_0 = 50° \text{C}$ and resistance $R(T_0) = 300\ \Omega$. Determine resistance at 80° C.

Using the RTD equation:

$$R(80° \text{C}) = 300[1+0.0035(80 - 50)]\ \Omega$$

■

EXAMPLE A strain gauge of 120 Ω (nominal) resistance with a gauge factor GF = 2 is mounted on a rod. The 5 m rod stretches by only 2 mm under a heavy stress. Find the change in resistance.

$GF = (\Delta R/R)/(\Delta L/L)$ = fractional change in resistance/fractional change in length

Therefore, the change in resistance $\Delta R = GF \times R \times \Delta L/L = 2 \times 120 \times (2\ \text{mm}/5\ \text{m}) = 0.096\ \Omega$.

■

EXAMPLE The ion concentrations and permeabilities of the membrane are given. Determine the following:

Membrane potential from inside to outside the cell at 310 K

Potassium concentration 11 mmol/liter inside and 146 mmol/liter outside

Sodium concentration 150 mmol/liter inside and 4 mmol/liter outside

Potassium permeability 2×10^{-6} cm/second

Sodium permeability 2×10^{-8} cm/second

Using the Goldman equation:

$$\text{Where } (K \times T)/Q = (1.38 \times 10^{-23} \text{ joules/kelvin} \times 310 \text{ kelvin})/(1.602 \times 10^{-19} \text{ coulomb}) = 0.0267 \text{ joule/coulomb}$$

$$V_m = -0.0267 \ln [(2 \times 10^{-6} \times 11 + 2 \times 10^{-8} \times 150)/(2 \times 10^{-6} \times 146 + 2 \times 10^{-8} \times 4)] \text{ volts}$$

■

SUMMARY

- In acquiring any biomedical signal, an electrode or a transducer is essential.
- An electrode is a solid electric conductor through which an electric current enters or leaves an electrolytic cell. A sensor is a part of a transducer and senses a stimulus such as heat, light, or pressure.
- The strain gauge and the LVDT are pressure sensors, while the RTD, the thermistor, and the thermocouple are temperature sensors.
- A strain gauge determines the amount of strain (change in dimensions) on a material when a force is applied. Metal foil gauges are the most commonly used types. The resulting dimension change creates a change in the electrical resistance.
- An LVDT provides an output voltage that is proportional to the displacement of the sample through the iron core of the transformer.
- In RTDs or thermistors, resistance varies with temperature, while in thermocouples, the voltage varies with temperature due to dissimilar metals being fused together.

MEDICAL TERMINOLOGY

Accuracy: the degree of conformity to a measured or calculated quantity to its actual value.

Cup electrode: a device for measuring the human electroencephalogram (EEG). The electrode provides a large signal to noise ratio, making it ideal for small amplitude flash stimuli.

Electrode: an electrical conductor used to make contact with a nonmetallic part of a circuit. This includes biological contact.

Needle electrode: device that is placed subcutaneously to measure or cause electrical activity in the tissue beneath.

Reference electrode: an electrode that has a stable and well-known electrode potential. Reference electrodes are used to measure electrochemical potential.

Sensitivity: the ability of a device to detect minute changes of any measured medium.

Surface electrode: a small device that is attached to the skin to measure or cause electrical activity in the tissue beneath.

Transducer: a device that converts a signal from one form to another, usually electrical, electronic, or electromechanical energy for purposes including measurement or information transfer.

QUIZ

1. Surface electrodes can measure EMG, and ____________________ can measure EEG.
2. Sensitivity means the change in the output due to the change in input. However, the resolution means ____________________.
   a) How accurate the output is.
   b) The smallest change in the output detectable.
   c) The same output again and again for the same input.
   d) None of the above.
3. A half-cell potential of silver is 800 mV, and the half-cell potential of gold is 2 V. If silver and gold electrodes are placed in the same electrolyte, what is the voltmeter reading between the two electrodes? The black cable of the voltmeter is connected to the gold electrode.
   a) −2.8 V
   b) −1.2 V
   c) 1.2 V
   d) None of the above.
4. A thermistor is connected to a voltage divider network driven by a 5 V power supply. The thermistor resistance is 100 Ω at 70° F and the value of the other resistor is 200 Ω. How much voltage is across the other resistor?
   a) 1.67 V
   b) −1.67 V
   c) 2.67 V
   d) 3.33 V
5. A pressure transducer is connected in a balanced bridge network driven by a 10 V power supply. Determine the resistance of the transducer when all other resistors in the bridge are balanced to 100 Ω and the output of the bridge network is 2 V.
   a) 42.86 Ω
   b) 25 Ω
   c) 233.33 Ω
   d) a or c

6. An eight-bit A/D converter has an input voltage span of 2 V to 6 V; its resolution is:
   a) 0.0156 V/step.
   b) 0.0234 V/step.
   c) 0.5 V/step.
   d) None of the above.
7. A semiconductor temperature transducer is:
   a) RTD.
   b) Thermocouple.
   c) Thermistor.
   d) None of the above.
8. Transducer A has a resolution of 0.1 V/° F, transducer B has a resolution of 0.2 V/° F, and transducer C has a resolution of 0.01 V/° F. Which transducer is considered the best under normal conditions?
   a) Transducer C.
   b) Transducer A.
   c) Transducer B.
   d) None of the above.
9. Hysteresis is:
   a) The value of the output for a given input in a transducer.
   b) A characteristic of magnets.
   c) The maximum difference in output for any given input when the value is measured first with increasing, and then with decreasing input signals.
   d) None of the above.
10. The main reason of using Ag/AgCl electrode in acquiring a biosignal is:

    ____.

PROBLEMS

1. An RTD has $\alpha = 0.004°$ C and $R = 300\ \Omega$ at 30° C. Determine the resistance at 0° C and 60° C.
2. Using the thermocouple table in **Figure 6-20,** find the voltage of a type J thermocouple with a 0° C reference if the measurement temperature is $-50°$ C and 320° C.
3. A strain gauge has a $GF = 2.1$ and $R = 115\ \Omega$. Calculate the resistance if the tension (strain) is 0.0005.
4. A transducer outputs a voltage V_o with a range of 4 V to 11 V. Design an op-amp amplifier circuit that converts this V_o range into an output V_{out} range of 0 V to 6 V.
5. Design a voltage divider and/or an amplifier circuit that provides 0 V to 5 V as its output when the light intensity measured by a CdS photocell detector varies from 5 W/m^2 to

10 W/m^2. Acquire a typical CdS photocell graph (resistance versus light intensity) from the Internet to help solve this problem.

6. A red blood cell has the following ionic concentrations: $[K^+]_I = 140$ mmol/liter, $[Na^+]_I = 20$ mmol/liter, $[K^+]_O = 10$ mmol/liter, $[Na^+]_O = 160$ mmol/liter. In addition, the permeability of sodium is 2.2×10^{-8} cm/s and the permeability of potassium is 2×10^{-6} cm/s. Calculate the cell voltage from inside to outside at a temperature of 38° C.

7. An RTD is used for R_4 in a bridge circuit, shown in **Figure 6-21**. The RTD has R(22° C) = 400 Ω and $\alpha_0 = 0.004$/° C. The bridge has $R_1 = 4$ kΩ, $R_2 = 1$ kΩ, and R_3 is a 10 kΩ potentiometer. The source voltage is 10 V DC. If the bridge nulls, that is, is balanced at $R_3 = 1.5$ kΩ, determine the temperature. Also, determine the RTD temperature when the output voltage V_o is 10 mV with the bridge unbalanced.

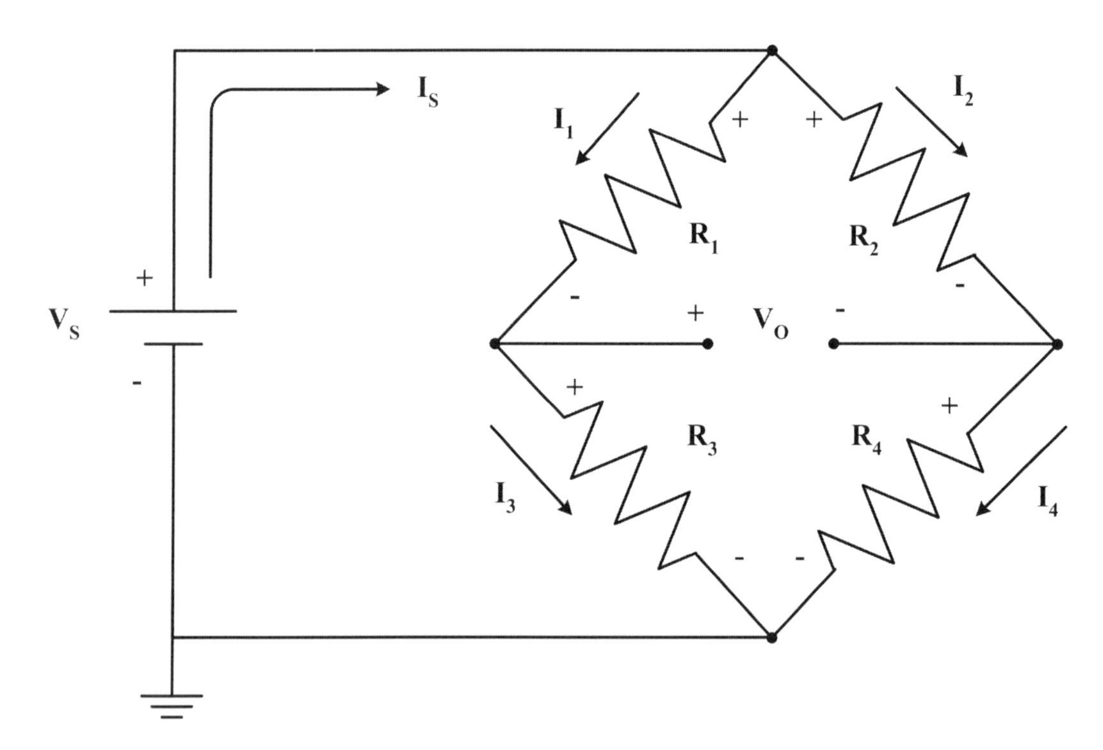

FIGURE 6-21

8. A voltage divider network has a 10 kΩ resistor and a thermistor. The source voltage is 10 V and the output is taken across the thermistor and the ground. The thermistor's temperature graph is shown in **Figure 6-18a.** Plot the output voltage versus temperature from 30° C to 80° C. Is the result linear? How does it compare to the graph shown in **Figure 6-18a** between the resistance and the temperature?

9. A thermistor graph is typically nonlinear. Design a circuit to make the thermistor behave in a linear fashion within a temperature range.

10. Discuss a typical LVDT in terms of linearity, sensitivity, resolution, normal frequency range and voltage, impedance, and phase angle, the core characteristics. You may use the Internet in your research.
11. Determine the total change in length for a strain indicator wire in a strain gauge when GF = 3, original wire resistance = 0.5 Ω, final strained wire resistance = 0.7 Ω, pre-strained wire length = 50 mm.
12. Aluminum and silver electrodes are placed in an electrolytic solution and are connected through an ammeter. Determine the current when the resistance of the electrolytic solution is 1.2 kΩ.
13. A blood vessel has a diameter of 0.8 cm and the blood flow rate is 10 cm/second. A magnetic flow probe surrounds the blood vessel when the magnetic field is 1×10^{-5} weber/meter^2. Calculate the voltage induced in the probe.
14. Determine the resistance of a thermistor at 100° F, when the resistance of the thermistor is 3 kΩ at 10° C. Given β = 3,200.
15. The resistance of a thermistor at 15°C is 350 Ω. The thermistor β is 5,000. Calculate the temperature of the thermistor when the resistance is doubled.

CASE STUDY

Based in California, Merit Sensors Systems designs piezoresistive pressure sensors for medical applications. A case study of this company will provide insight into piezoresistive technology (PRT), its design limitations, calibration techniques, and medical usage.

RESEARCH TOPIC

Biosensors are used in various applications for better resolution, sensitivity, and miniaturization. Discuss the types, characteristics, and the physics of these sensors. These sensors use antibodies, DNA probes, and enzymes as the biologically responsive material. Discuss also the associated electronic circuits.

CHAPTER 7

Instrumentation in Diagnostic Cardiology

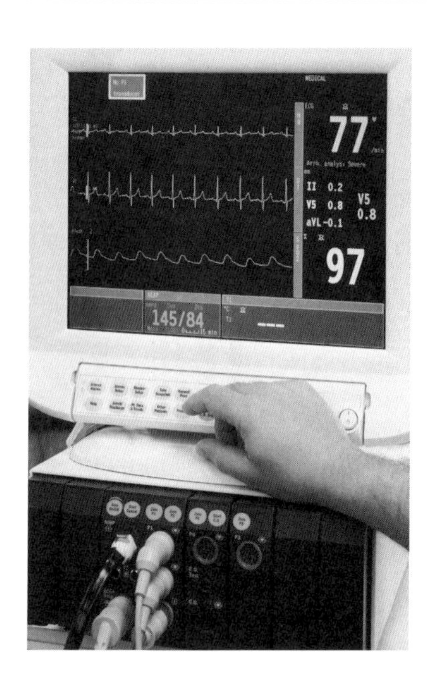

CHAPTER OUTLINE

OBJECTIVES

The objective of this chapter is to describe to the reader the basics of the ECG signal, the ECG electrodes, and the electronic circuits of the ECG machines.

Upon completion of this chapter, the reader will be able to:

- Sketch a normal ECG signal with proper labels.
- Explain depolarization and repolarization of the heart.
- Describe three abnormal ECG signals.
- Describe the components of an ECG machine.

INTERNET WEB SITES

www.escardio.org (European Society of Cardiology)
www.biores.org (Biomedical Research Directory)
www.cardiologyonline.com (International Academy of Cardiology)
www.cardiologyshop.com (Cardiology Shop)
www.heartmonitoring.net (National Cardiac Monitoring Center)
www.conmed.com (ConMed Corporation)
www.vermed.com (The Medical Sensor Company)

INTRODUCTION

Electrophysiology, or the study of electrical activity of the heart, is a diagnostic tool used by physicians to determine medical treatment of an abnormally functioning heart. Abnormalities may include "skipped" heartbeats, arrhythmias, or damage to the heart muscles or heart valves. Often, a patient's primary care physician or cardiologist will request an electrophysiological study of a patient's heart; however, sometimes the patient is sent directly from a hospital emergency room to an electrophysiology lab for testing.

The most common diagnostic tool used in cardiology is an electrocardiogram (ECG). Other types include an echocardiogram, heart catheterization, and a phonocardiogram. This chapter focuses on patient preparation for an ECG, the ECG monitoring electrodes, placement of electrodes, normal and abnormal ECG recordings, and the various types of ECG machines.

7.1 THE HEART AND THE ECG

The electrocardiogram (ECG) is a recording of the electrical activity of the heart. Each heartbeat is initiated by the excitation (depolarization) and recovery (polarization) phases of this electrical activity.

An ECG recording, or trace, shows the various phases of the electrical activity above or below a baseline—that is, a positive voltage above a baseline and a negative voltage below a baseline. The ECG records the activity of the sinoatrial (SA) node to the atrioventricular (AV) node, into the His-Purkinje bundle, then into the ventricular bundles, and finally out to the ventricles.

The cardiac impulse originates at the SA node, and then spreads through the atria. **Figure 7-1** shows the electrical system of the heart and the directions of the impulse from the SA node. The speed of the impulse is slow until it reaches the AV node, and then it spreads rapidly through the His-Purkinje bundle to the surface of the ventricles. The impulse travels to AV node, right atrium, or left atrium in less than 0.1 second; however, it can take approximately 0.2 second to reach the surface of the ventricles and the apex of the heart.

The heart contracts as the electrical impulse travels through the heart's conduction system. Each contraction is one heartbeat, and the atria contract before the ventricles. The process of blood flow is such that the blood empties into the ventricles before the ventricles contract.

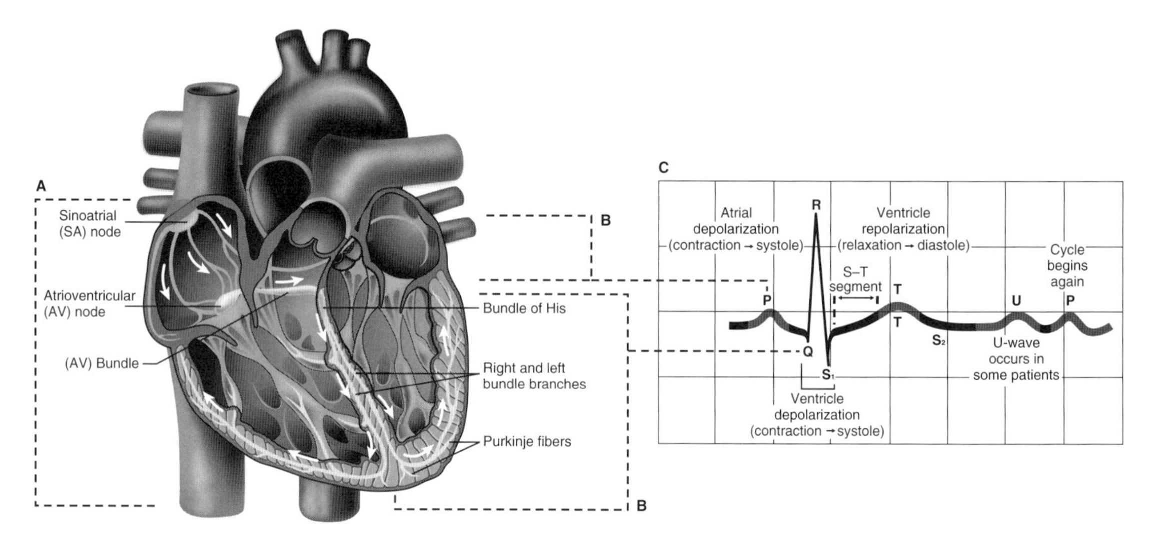

FIGURE 7-1 The heart and normal sinus rhythm.

An ECG machine records this trace when the patient is connected to the machine with 10 electrodes: one electrode is applied to each ankle and wrist and six electrodes are applied to the chest area over the heart. The electrodes and the wire connections are sometimes called electric leads or channels.

7.2 ECG SIGNAL: DEPOLARIZATION AND REPOLARIZATION

The anatomical differences of the atria and ventricles contribute to the depolarization and the repolarization in such a way that differentiable deflections in millivolts can be recorded as ECG signal from the surface of the heart. **Figure 7-2** shows the depolarization and repolarization processes in a cardiac muscle fiber. The normal negative potential inside the fiber is lost and changes to positive potential as the electrical stimulus wave passes from one end of the fiber to the other end. This is the depolarization process, and the fiber becomes slightly positive inside and negative outside. It is an advancing wave of positive charges within the myocardial cells of the fiber. The left electrode is in the area of negativity where it touches the outside of the fiber, while the right electrode is in the area of positivity and the meter reads a positive potential.

The maximum positive potential is when the depolarization wave has reached the middle of the fiber. The potential returns to zero value when both electrodes are at equal negative value. This completes the depolarization along the complete fiber. Next, the repolarization process takes place and the opposite of the previous polarity starts building up from the left to the right end of the fiber. The meter reads a negative potential and is at the most negative value when the right electrode is halfway negative and the left electrode is halfway positive.

Finally, the repolarization wave reaches to the extreme right end of the fiber, and both electrodes are then in positive areas and the meter reads a zero potential.

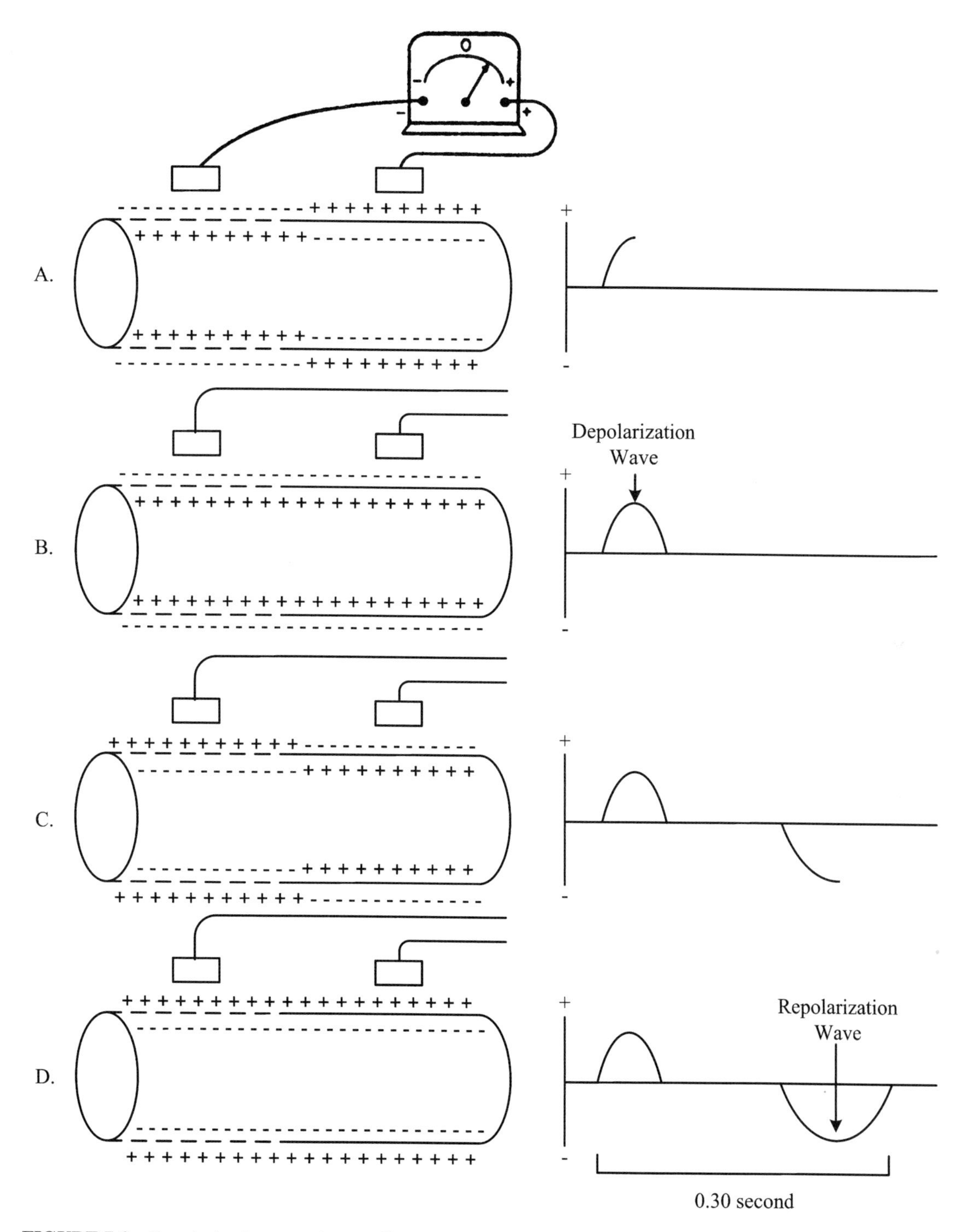

FIGURE 7-2 Depolarization wave in a cardiac muscle fiber.

Inside the myocardial cell, there is a resting potential of −90 mV. This resting potential is due to the inequality of sodium and potassium concentrations across the cell membrane. Normally, the depolarization follows a specific path from the SA node to the conduction system of the atria, then to the AV node, the bundle branches, and to the ventricles. This depolarization path occurs consistently and uniformly. When a wave of positive depolarization approaches the positive electrode, the ECG inscribes a positive signal; when the wave moves away from the positive electrode, the ECG then inscribes a negative signal. In this way, the instrument generates an ECG tracing that records the electrical activity of the heart. Each segment of the ECG tracing represents the different stages of the cardiac cycle of depolarization and repolarization.

The electrical conduction through the heart produces a normal ECG signal trace, as shown in Figure 7-1. This trace is from a healthy heart. The normal ECG is composed of a P wave, a QRS complex, and a T wave. The complex has three separate waves: the Q wave, the R wave, and the S wave.

With the transmission of the depolarization wave, also called the cardiac impulse, the P wave is caused due to the depolarization of the atria prior to their contraction, and the QRS complex is caused when ventricles depolarize prior to their contraction. Therefore, the P wave and the QRS complex both are generated and recorded due to the depolarization spread through atria and ventricles.

As the ventricles start to recover with the repolarization of the ventricles, the T wave is recorded. It is merely 0.25 to 0.30 second after the depolarization.

7.3 PATIENT NEEDING AN ECG

Many reasons exist for a physician to recommend an ECG recording for a patient. Some of the most common patient complaints that may alert a physician to a heart problem are:

1. **Chest pain**

   There are various reasons for chest pain. Though not always due to cardiac disease, chest discomfort related to angina is a common symptom of a heart problem and should be examined.

2. **Fatigue**

   Often patients complain of feeling unusually tired. This may be caused by inadequate cardiac output or excessive demand for the cardiac output due to cardiovascular disease. Inadequate cardiac output can be caused by ischemic heart disease, valve defects, cardiac lesions, heart block, constriction of the artery, or tachycardia. Fever and hyperthyroidism may be contributing factors for the excessive demand of the cardiac output.

3. **Palpitations**

   Heart palpitations are an abnormal beating of the heart when excited by exertion, strong emotion, or disease. They can be slow beats due to bradycardia or heart block, or rapid beats due to tachycardia or atrial fibrillation.

4. **High blood pressure (hypertension)**

   This may be a symptom of an underlying heart condition.

5. **Swelling**

   In certain areas of the body, this may be caused by edema triggered by a heart condition.

7.4 INFORMATION GAINED FROM THE ECG

The following is a list of information that can be acquired from an ECG recording:

- Heart rate
- Heart rhythm
- Abnormalities in how electrical impulse spreads across the heart
- Indication of coronary artery disease
- Indication of prior heart attack
- Indication of thickening of the heart muscle

7.5 ECG LEADS

The word "lead" in the standard ECG system can mean a wire connecting the patient to the ECG machine; however, the lead in an ECG can also be the electrical picture or trace of the heart. Typically, a maximum of twelve traces are possible with ten electrodes placed on the limbs and the chest. Four electrodes connect to the patient's limbs: the right arm (RA), left arm (LA), right leg (RL), and left leg (LL). The remaining six electrodes are connected to different areas on the chest. These electrodes are then joined to the ECG machine by cables or wires.

For the 12-lead ECG, three are bipolar limb leads: lead I, lead II, and lead III. The other three limb leads are unipolar leads: aVR lead, aVL lead, and aVF lead. The remaining six chest leads are bipolar leads: V_1, V_2, V_3, V_4, V_5, and V_6. The chest electrodes are placed at separate points on the anterior surface of the chest. The six standard limb leads trace the heart in a vertical plane from the sides or the feet, whereas the six chest leads trace the heart in a horizontal plane from the front and the left side.

Figure 7-3 through **Figure 7-5** show the various configurations of the ECG lead system. The ECG meter records the potential difference between any two electrodes and the voltage amplitude as shown is small, in the mV range. For amplification, the electrodes and their leads are connected to a differential amplifier or an instrumentation amplifier. The right leg (RL) lead is always connected to the amplifier ground.

Lead I

The right arm electrode is connected to the negative terminal of the ECG meter and the left arm electrode is connected to the positive terminal. When the point where the right arm electrode connects to the chest is negative with respect to the point where the left arm electrode connects to the chest, the meter reads a positive value of the voltage above the zero baseline voltage. When the opposite is true, the ECG will read a negative value of the voltage below the baseline voltage.

As both electrodes in lead I are at some potential, with the direction of the lead being from the electrode at lower potential to the one at higher potential, lead I is also called a bipolar lead.

Lead II

In this recording, the negative terminal is still connected to the right arm electrode, but, additionally, the left leg electrode is connected to the positive terminal. Therefore, the recording is positive if the right arm electrode is negative with respect to the left leg electrode.

Lead III

In the lead III configuration, the negative terminal of the ECG meter is connected to the left arm electrode and the positive terminal is connected to the left leg electrode. The recording is positive when the left arm electrode is negative with respect to the left leg electrode.

In addition to lead I, lead II and lead III are also called bipolar leads and the reference ground electrode is connected to the right leg.

Einthoven's Triangle

Einthoven's triangle is a diagram illustrating the apices of a triangle made by the polarities from the two arms and the left leg surrounding the heart. The upper two apices of the triangle electrically connect the two arms through the heart, whereas the lower apex connects the left leg to the right or left arm through the heart. Einthoven's law states that the sum of voltages in any two ECG leads equals the voltage in the remaining lead. The law assumes that the polarities may be positive or negative at different leads at any time when summed.

FIGURE 7-3a Limb leads: lead I, II, and III.

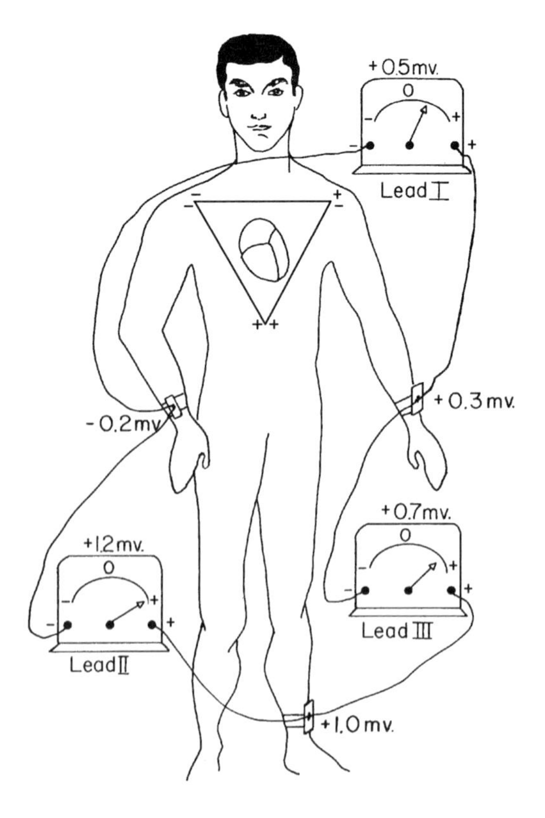

FIGURE 7-3b ECG signals: lead I, II, and III.

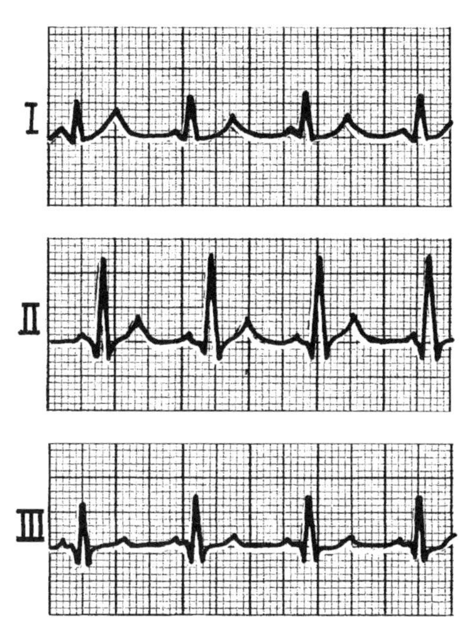

When the electrodes are placed correctly and the leads recorded simultaneously, the voltage in lead II should equal the sum of the voltages in lead I and lead III. In other words, if the R wave in lead II is not equal to the sum of lead I and lead III, the lead wires (the electrodes) are not placed appropriately.

Augmented Limb Leads aVR, aVL, and aVF

In this system, the leads are derived from the same three electrodes as lead I, lead II, and lead III, but view the heart from different angles. The two limb electrodes are connected to the negative terminal of the ECG meter and the third limb electrode is connected to the positive terminal. The result of the two limb electrodes connected together means that the negative terminal electrode is at zero potential (likened to the "neutral" of a wall socket) and the positive terminal electrode becomes the "exploring electrode" or a unipolar lead.

When the right arm electrode is connected to the positive terminal, this lead is the aVR lead; similarly, if the left arm electrode is connected to the positive terminal, it is called the aVL lead; and when the left leg (the foot) electrode is connected to the positive terminal, the lead is called the aVF lead.

The term "augmented" means amplified or large voltage at the positive electrode when compared to the negative electrode. The aVR lead (the augmented vector right) has the positive electrode on the right arm. The negative electrode is a combination of the left arm electrode and the left leg electrode, which "augments" the voltage or the signal strength of the positive electrode on the right arm.

Each augmented lead records the potential of the heart on the side nearest to the respective limb. For example, if the ECG meter reads a negative potential in the aVR lead system, then the side of the heart nearest to the right arm is negative compared to the remainder of the heart.

FIGURE 7-4a Augmented limb leads.

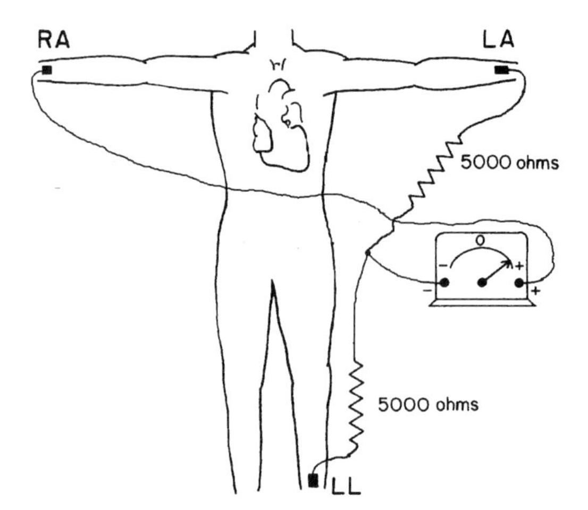

FIGURE 7-4b ECG signals: augmented limb leads.

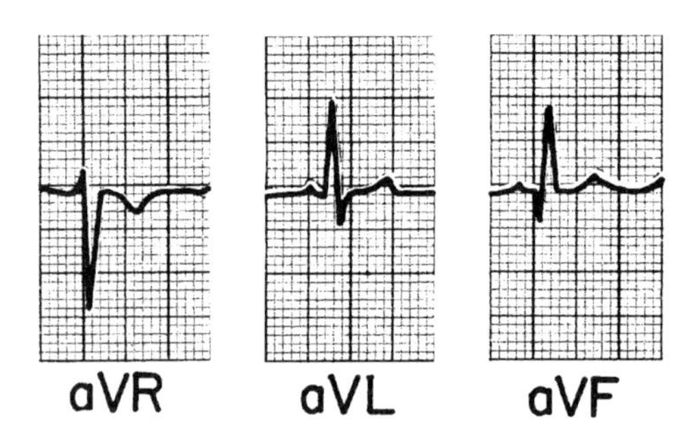

Chest Leads V_1, V_2, V_3, V_4, V_5, and V_6

In this system, the negative terminal of the ECG meter is connected to the right arm, left arm, and left leg electrodes, and the positive terminal is connected to one of the six chest electrodes. The standard chest leads V_1, V_2, V_3, V_4, V_5, and V_6 are recorded from the anterior chest wall, the chest electrode being placed respectively at the six points illustrated in Figure 7-5a.

The chest electrodes are also called the precordial unipolar leads, placed directly over the heart. These electrodes encircle the precordium and they provide information about the anterior, posterior, right, and left depolarization vectors. The chest leads are unipolar leads, as they explore the potential on various chest locations when all three limb electrodes are connected together as a negative electrode at about zero potential. Also, because of the proximity to the heart, the chest leads do not require augmentation.

The placement of the precordial electrodes are given as:

- V_1 Fourth intercostal space at the right sternal border
- V_2 Fourth intercostal space at the left sternal border
- V_3 Midway between V_2 and V_4
- V_4 Fifth intercostal space at the midclavicular line
- V_5 Fifth intercostal space (same level as V_4) at the left anterior axillary line
- V_6 Fifth intercostal space (same level as V_4) at the left midaxillary line

Figure 7-6 shows a 12-lead ECG. To obtain a 12-lead ECG, four wires are attached to each of the limbs and six wires are placed around the chest. This totals 10 wires; however, 12 "leads" or pictures are achieved.

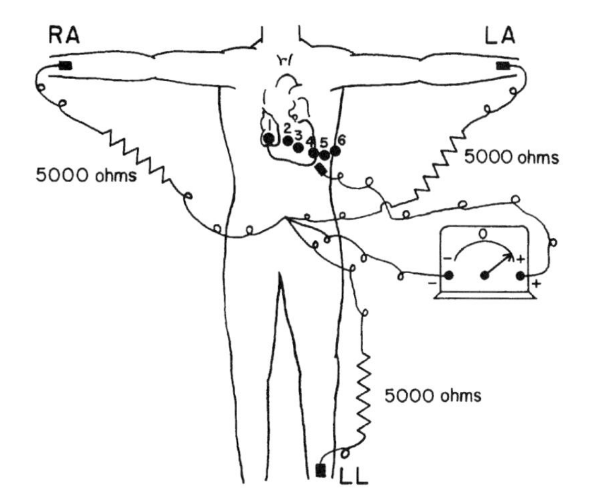

FIGURE 7-5a Chest leads.

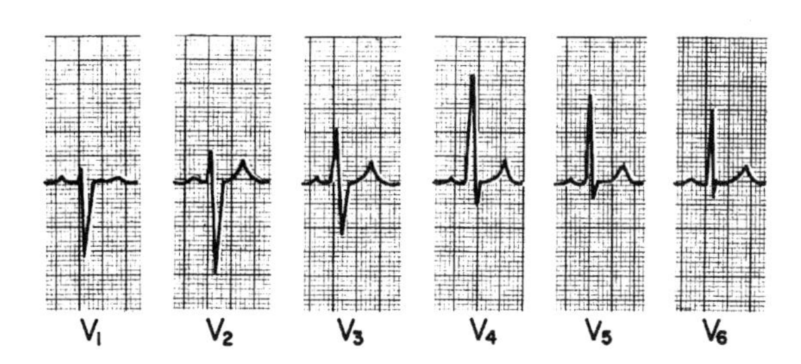

FIGURE 7-5b ECG signals: chest leads.

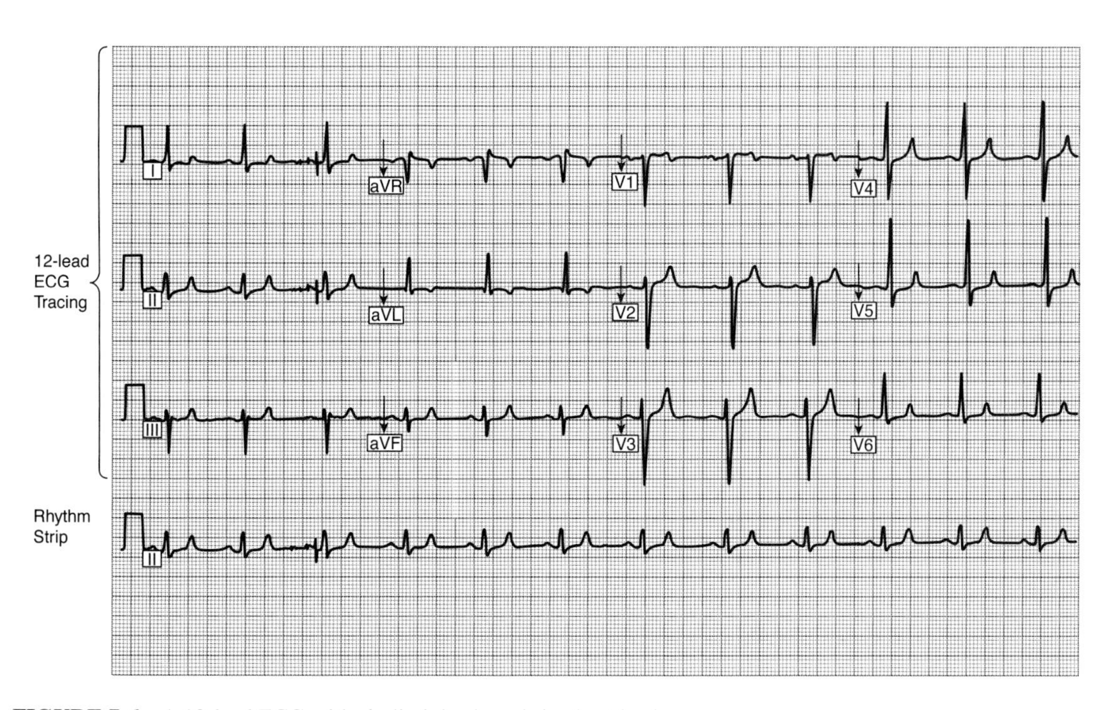

FIGURE 7-6 A 12-lead ECG with six limb leads and six chest leads.

7.6 VECTORCARDIOGRAPHY

Vectorcardiography makes it simple to visualize the electrical axis of the heart. By plotting the vectors of the lead voltages, a resultant mean QRS axis can be determined. This determination will indicate the mean axis of total ventricular depolarization. The average direction of the spread of depolarization wave through ventricles as seen from the front is also called the cardiac axis, and it is useful to know whether the flow of depolarization is in a normal direction. The axis is derived from the QRS complex as seen in leads I, II, and III.

Figure 7-7a shows the directions of the axes of different limb leads, three standard leads, and three unipolar leads. Each lead is actually a pair of electrodes connected to the body on opposite sides of the heart, and the direction from the negative to the positive electrode is called the axis of the lead. For lead I, the two electrodes are placed horizontally on the two arms; the axis of lead I is 0° with the positive electrode to the left.

In recording lead II, electrodes are placed on the right arm and the left leg; the direction of this lead is then approximately 60°.

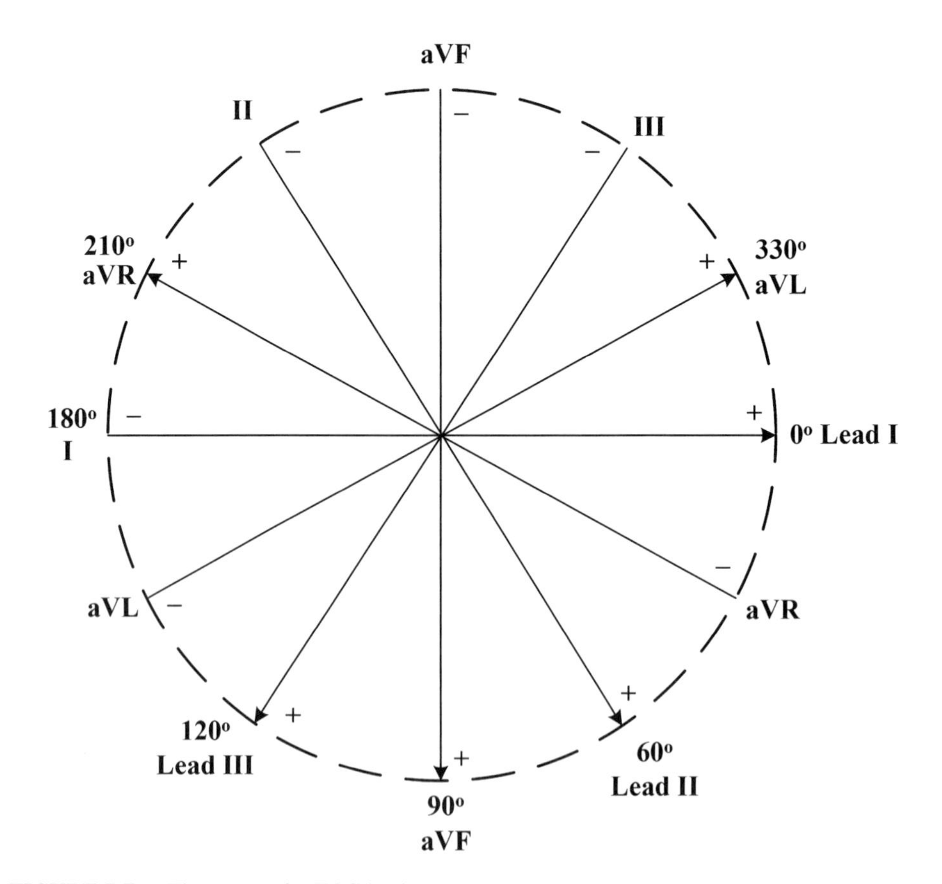

FIGURE 7-7a The vectors for ECG leads.

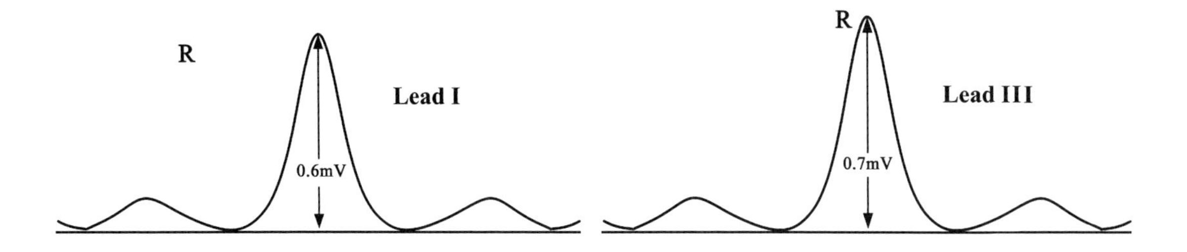

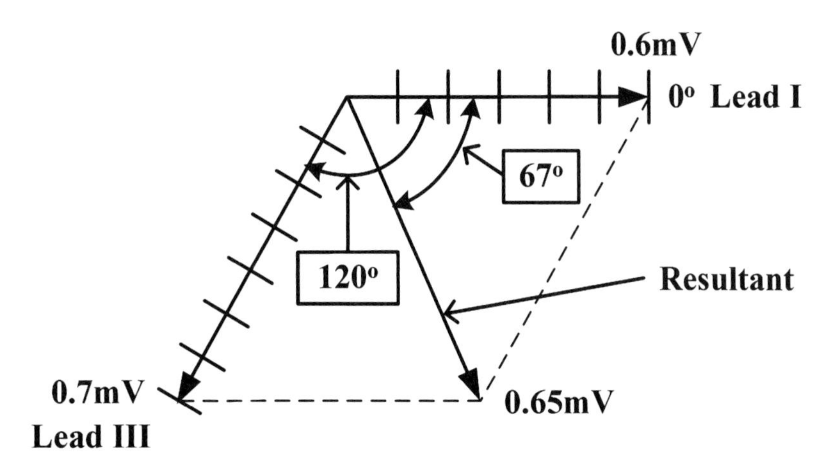

FIGURE 7-7b An example of cardiac axis.

In normal conditions, the mean QRS axis is between −30° and +90°. It also depends on the selection of leads. In abnormal conditions, such as light ventricular hypertrophy, the QRS axis angle may shift between 90° and 180°, or it may shift between −30° and −90° in left arterial blockage.

As an example of vectorcardiography, if the R-wave amplitude in lead I is 0.6 mV and in lead III the R-wave amplitude is 0.7 mV, then the resultant mean QRS axis is in the direction of 67° as shown in **Figure 7-7b**, and the heart depolarization wave is as shown in **Figure 7-7c.**

Vectorcardiography is not commonly used, but it provides continuous recording of the electrical activity of the heart and plotting of vectors using two or three leads.

7.7 NORMAL AND ABNORMAL ECG SIGNALS

The ECG signal consists of the "P-QRS-T complex" and reveals information about normal or abnormal cardiac rhythms. The P-QRS-T complex is composed of the P, Q, R, S, and T waves and the ECG baseline areas between the waves. The areas are then termed intervals, durations, and segments. The intervals are the distances between waves, durations are the time taken by the waves, and the segments are the ECG baselines between waves.

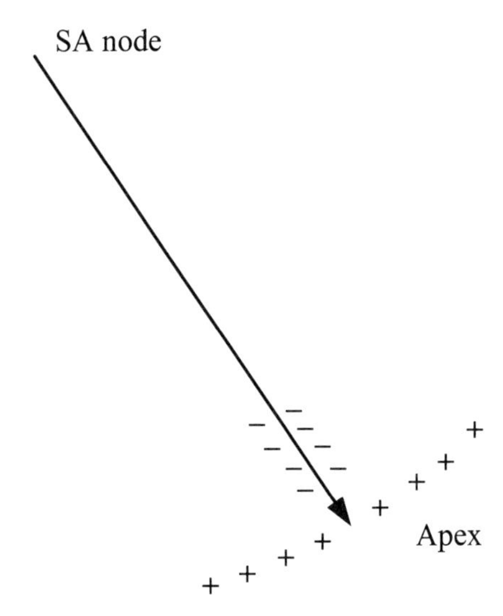

FIGURE 7-7c Vector resultant for the example in Figure 7-7b.

The PR interval is measured from the beginning of the P wave until the start of the QRS complex (normal PR interval is 0.12 to 0.20 seconds), whereas the QT interval is measured from the beginning of the QRS complex until the end of the T wave (normal QT interval is 0.4 second for the heart rate of 60 beats per minute). The QRS duration is measured from the start of the QRS complex to the end of the QRS complex and normally it is less than 0.12 second.

The ST segment is the portion of the ECG baseline between the end of the QRS complex and the start of the T wave and is approximately 0.12 second for a normal heart.

The values of the intervals, durations, and segments indicate the condition of the heart. The following two sections detail how to determine these intervals and discuss abnormal ECG signals and related heart conditions.

Determination of Heart Rate and ECG Intervals

The ECG prints out onto a paper with gridlines. The vertical lines on a standard ECG paper have one-millimeter (1 mm) rules with darker vertical lines every five millimeters (5 mm). This is the time axis. The ECG paper moves at a constant speed of 25 mm per second. Five large boxes of 5 mm each equal 25 mm, or one second of time. Therefore, one 5-mm box represents 0.20 second, and the single box of 1 mm width then represents one-fifth of 0.20 second, or 0.04 second (see **Figure 7-8a** and **Figure 7-8b**).

For the horizontal lines in the vertical direction, ECG paper represents the ECG signal amplitude in volts. Each small box of 1 mm in height represents 0.10 mV. One large vertical box of 5 mm is equal to 0.5 mV. Two large vertical boxes are then 1 mV. The calibration standard is 1 mV for exactly 10 mm deflection in the vertical direction. The standardization is checked and recorded before ECG signal is taken.

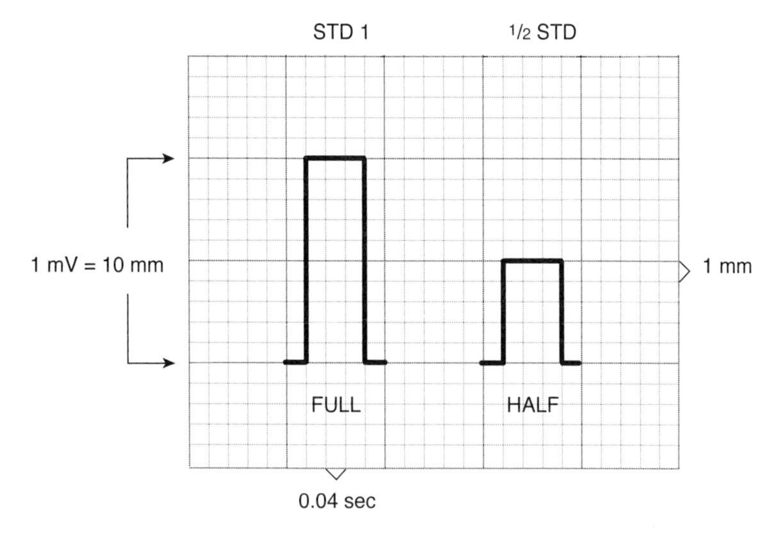

FIGURE 7-8a ECG standardization scale.

The normal heart rates can be estimated by measuring the interval between two adjacent QRS complexes.

For the atrial rate, the interval between two adjacent P waves is estimated. Similarly, two QRS complex intervals indicate the ventricular rate and a pacemaker spike interval indicates the pacemaker rate.

The heart rate can be calculated as:

$$\text{Heart Rate} = \frac{60}{\text{Mean R to R interval}} = \text{beats/minute}$$

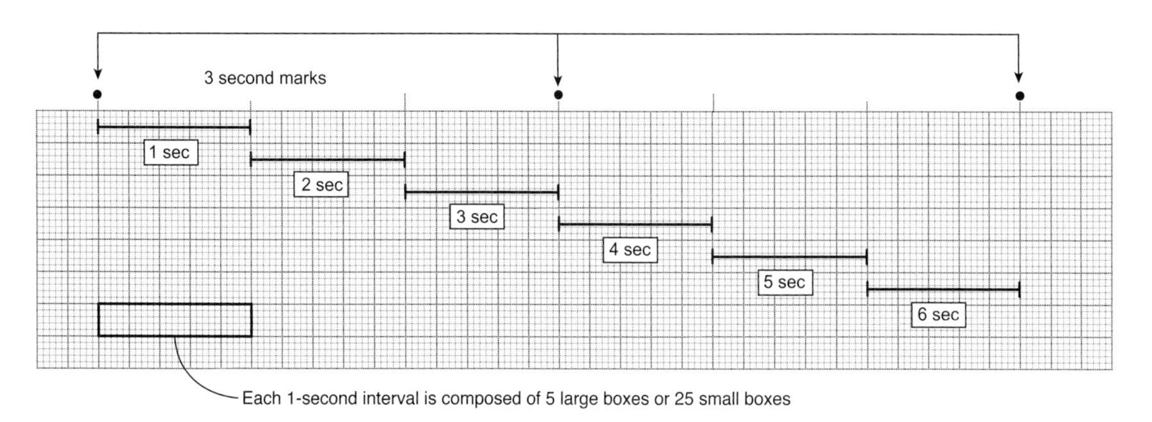

FIGURE 7-8b ECG intervals.

Figure 7-8c shows the various segments and the time intervals. The electrocardiographer measures these time intervals with a caliper at the beginning and end of the wave, or interval, and considers that each box represents 0.04 second per millimeter. If we count the number of large square boxes between two consecutive QRS complexes, the heart rate is determined. For example:

- One large square determines the heart rate is 300 beats per minute (bpm)
- Two large squares determines the heart rate is 150 bpm
- Three large squares determines the heart rate is 100 bpm
- Four large squares determines the heart rate is 75 bpm
- Five large squares determines the heart rate is 60 bpm
- Six large squares determines the heart rate is 50 bpm
- Seven large squares determines the heart rate is 42 bpm

The normal ECG signal and a series of abnormal ECG signals are shown in **Figure 7-9a** through **Figure 7-9k**.

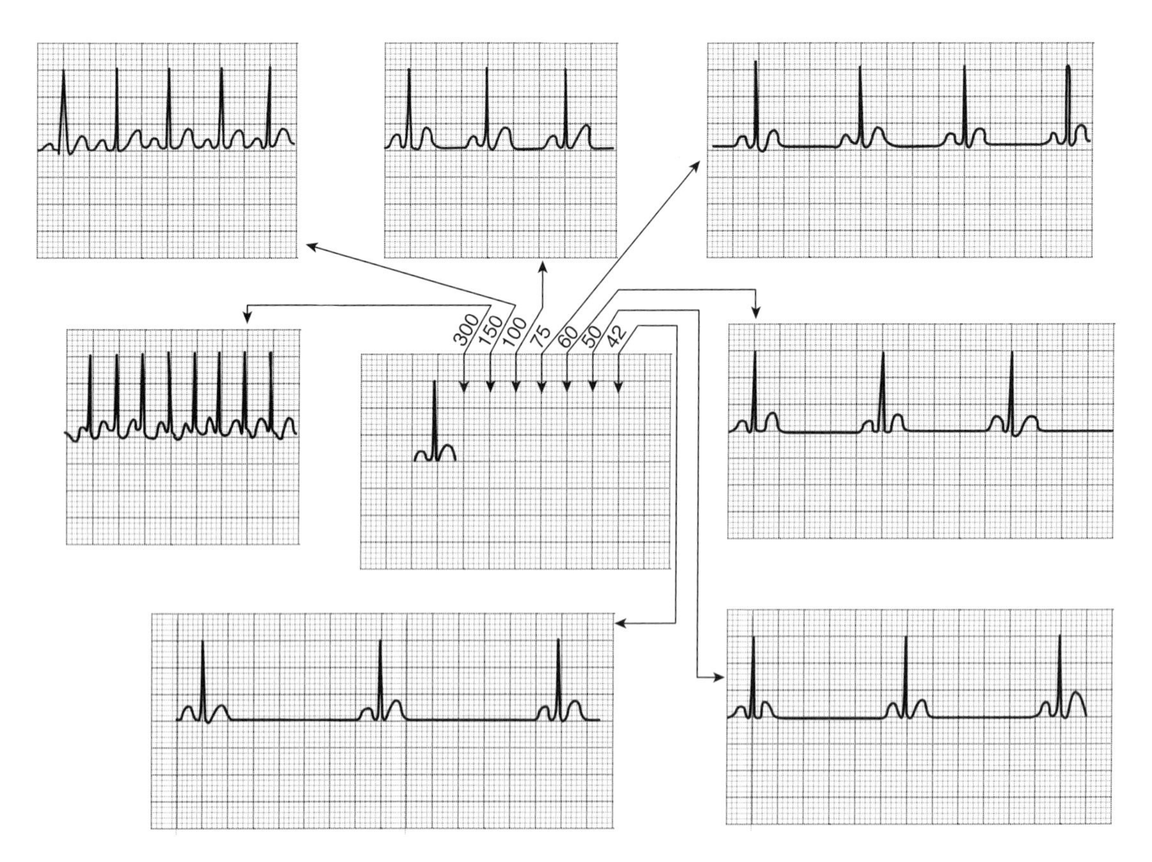

FIGURE 7-8c Cardiac cycle rates determined by the number of large ECG boxes.

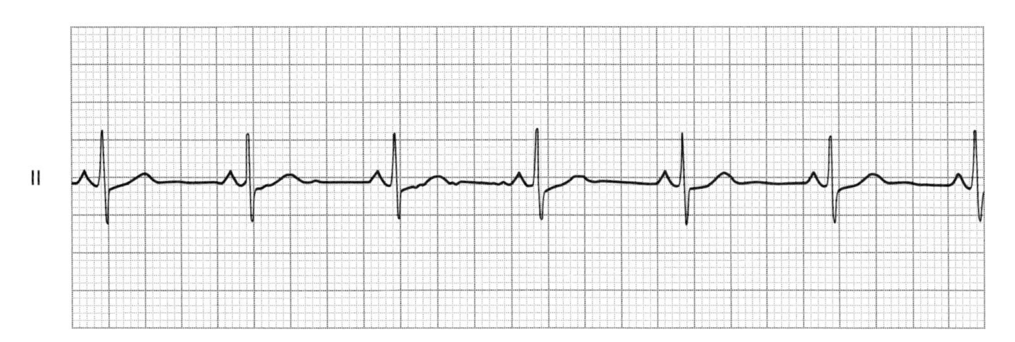

FIGURE 7-9a Normal sinus rhythm.

Normal Sinus Rhythm

The rhythm of a healthy heart is called normal sinus rhythm. The heart rate in this rhythm is between 60 and 100 bpm. The three deflections of P, QRS, and T follow in this order and can be differentiated. The QRS complexes have the same size and the QRS duration is less than 0.2 second. The AV conduction ratio is 1:1 for one P wave to each QRS complex. In this normal condition, the SA node triggers the cardiac activation and the electrical impulse follows the usual conduction path.

Abnormal ECG Signal

1. **Sinus tachycardia**

   When the resting heart rate is higher than 100 bpm, the condition is called sinus tachycardia. The upper limit is 150 bpm. The ECG trace will still show the normal P-QRS-T pattern; however, the heart rate is higher than normal. The P waves and the preceding T waves appear close together. Possible reasons may be physical exertion or mental stress. It may be due also to congestive heart failure.

2. **Sinus bradycardia**

   When the sinus rhythm is less than 60 bpm, the condition is called sinus bradycardia. The P waves, QRS complexes, T waves, and the AV conduction are all normal. The rhythm is regular but the rate is less than normal. The most common cause of sinus

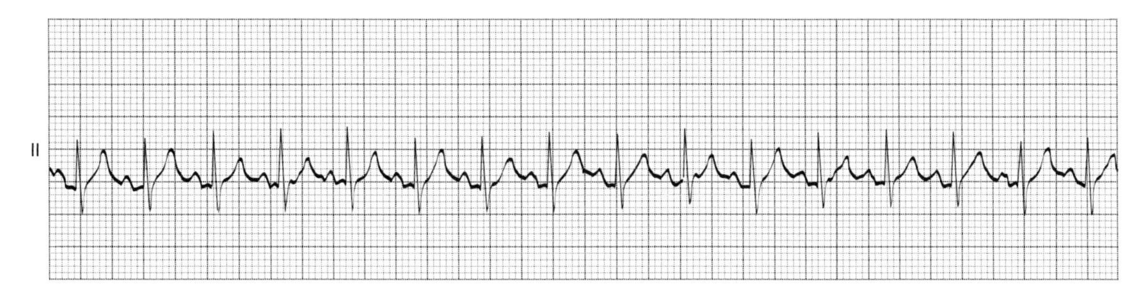

FIGURE 7-9b Sinus tachycardia.

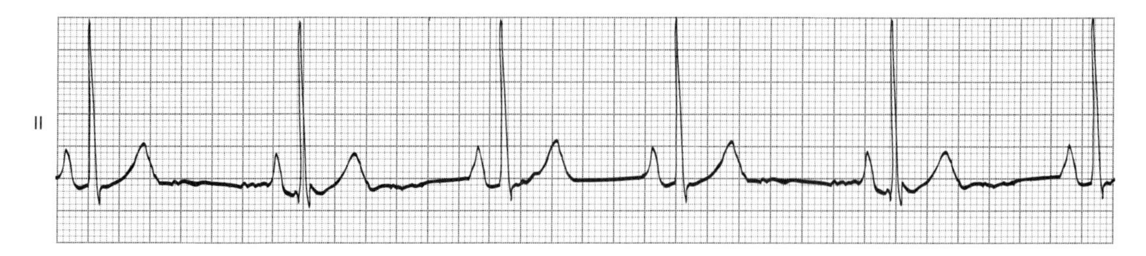

FIGURE 7-9c Sinus bradycardia.

bradycardia is increased vagal (parasympathetic) tone, hypothermia, or increased intracranial pressure.

3. **Sinus arrhythmia**

   In this condition, the rhythm of the heart rate is irregular. Notice that P-P interval or R-R interval is not the same every time, as it is in tachycardia or bradycardia. When the longest P-P or R-R interval exceeds the shortest interval by 0.16 second, this condition is called sinus arrhythmia. The AV conduction and the rate are normal in sinus arrhythmia. One of the reasons for this condition is that the vagus nerve may not be properly activating the SA node during respiration. During inspiration, this nerve is more active so that the SA node increases the heart rate. However, during expiration, its effect on the SA node is to slow down the heart rate.

   Notice also the P-P time is proportionally greater than the complete cardiac activation cycle of P-QRS-T. The main time interval change is between the T wave and the next P wave. Generally, the pulse rate of the SA node is affected by factors external to the heart, but the cardiac conduction cycle velocity is dependent on the internal condition of the heart.

4. **Atrial flutter**

   Atrial flutter occurs when the interval between the end of the T wave and the beginning of the P wave disappears. Multiple atrial flutter occurrences are seen between QRS complexes. The heart rate is elevated to 220 to 300 bpm. The AV node is activated by every second or every third atrial impulse and the AV conduction can reach 3:1 or 4:1. The condition may be due to mitral or tricuspid stenosis or hyperthyroidism.

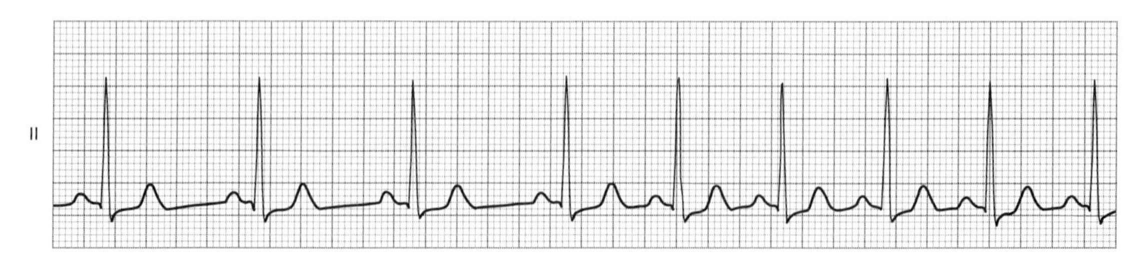

FIGURE 7-9d Sinus arrhythmia.

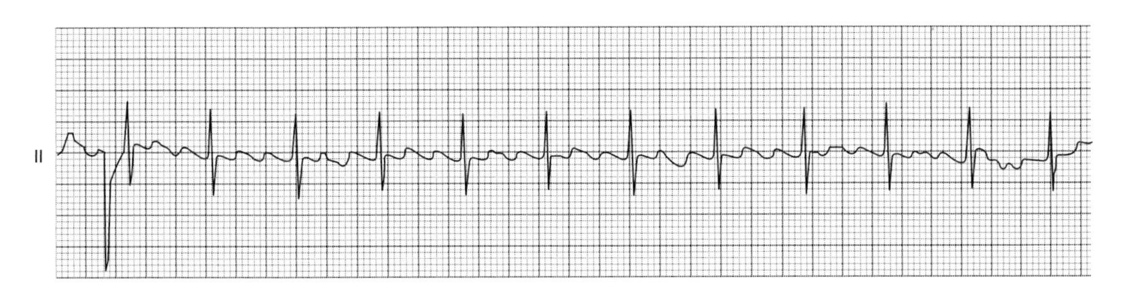

FIGURE 7-9e Atrial flutter.

5. **Atrial fibrillation**

   Atrial fibrillation occurs when the ECG trace has irregular fluctuations in the baseline due to hyperthyroidism, rheumatic disease, or pericarditis. The AV conduction is random, the QRS complexes are narrow and the ventricular rhythm is irregular.

6. **Ventricular fibrillation**

   In ventricular fibrillation, an ECG shows irregular fluctuations of ventricular depolarization without clear ORS complexes. The atrial, ventricular, and AV relationships are all absent. The major causes of ventricular fibrillation are myocardial ischemia or infarction, hypothermia, or electrolyte disorders. This serious condition results in unconsciousness and can lead to death within minutes. It can be stopped only with the use of an external defibrillator.

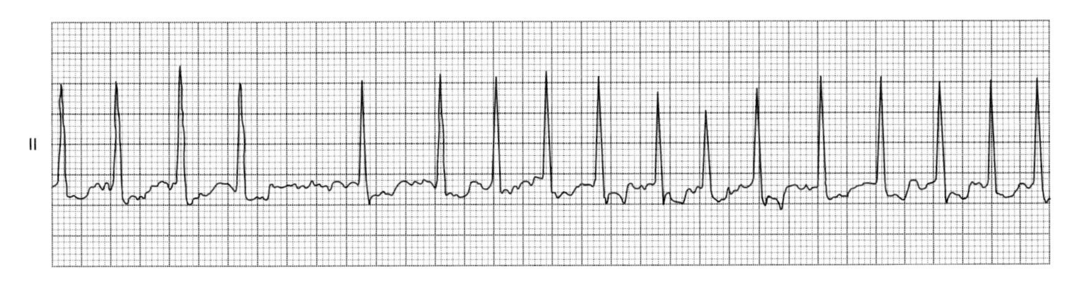

FIGURE 7-9f Atrial fibrillation.

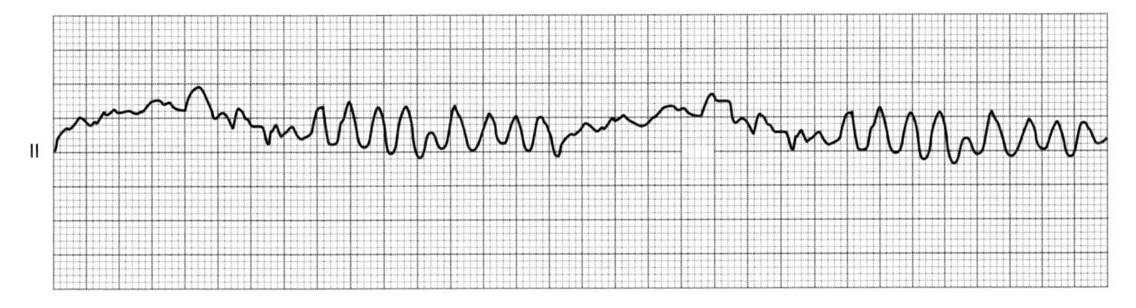

FIGURE 7-9g Ventricular fibrillation.

7. **Ventricular tachycardia**

Ventricular tachycardia is a serious dysrhythmia and can deteriorate into ventricular fibrillation. The QRS complexes are wide and distorted and the P waves are hard to detect. The condition is present when three or more successive premature ventricular complexes (PVCs) are occurring at a rate greater than 100 bpm. Premature ventricular complex is an early and extra depolarization wave and is taller than the sinus rhythms.

8. **AV block**

First-degree AV block is the condition when the PR interval is over 0.2 second. This condition involves delayed AV conduction after atrial depolarization, which leads to delayed ventricular depolarization. The blockage site is either in the AV node or in the common AV bundle. The most common cause is degenerative fibrosis or myocardial inflammation.

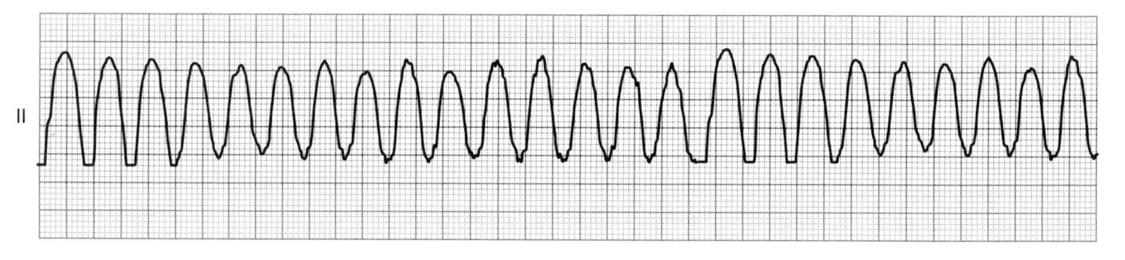

FIGURE 7-9h Ventricular tachycardia.

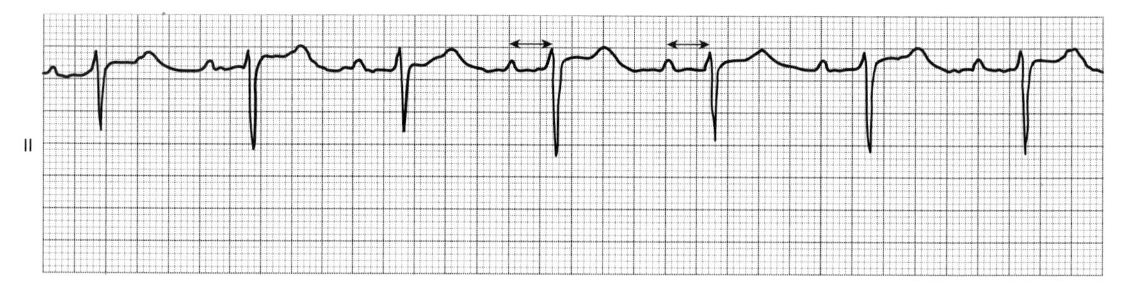

FIGURE 7-9i First-degree AV block.

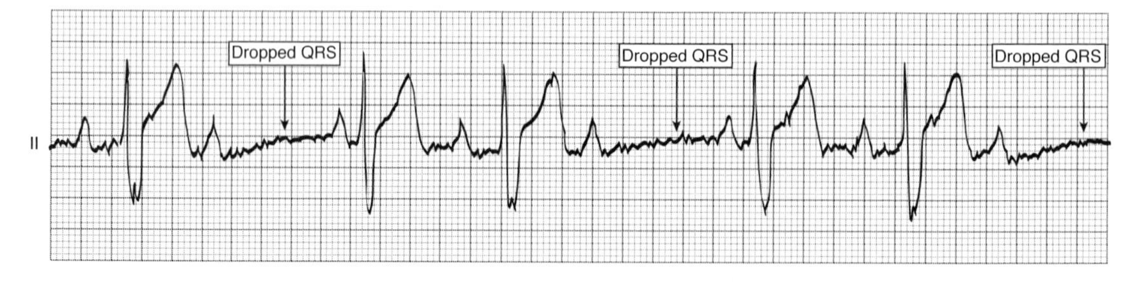

FIGURE 7-9j Second-degree AV block.

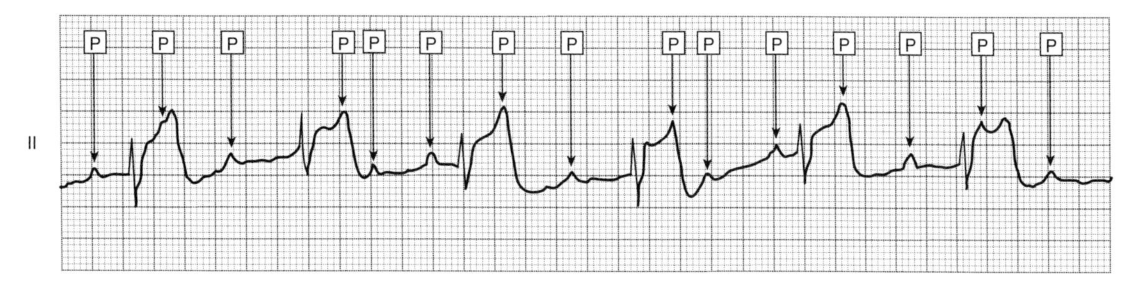

FIGURE 7-9k Third-degree AV block.

If the QRS complex is absent after the P wave, it is considered a second-degree AV block. There is a progressive PR interval prolongation and the RR intervals become shorter as the PR intervals increase. The causes are increased parasympathetic (vagal) tone or acute myocardial infarction.

In a third-degree AV block, there is no synchronization between the P wave and the QRS complex. This is a serious condition, as the AV heart block is complete or third-degree. Some P waves can be seen within the T waves or ST segments. The causes are due to advanced heart disease such as myocardial infarction, congenital heart, or inflammation of the myocardium.

7.8 NOISY OR POOR QUALITY ECG TRACES

The ECG technician is trained to ensure that the ECG shows acceptable traces before the patient is taken off the ECG leads. Poor quality, or noisy, traces cannot be used for evaluation by the physician or cardiologist. **Figure 7-10** shows a few examples of unacceptable ECG signals with noise. The noise or artifacts shown in the figure are caused by patient or cable movement, shivering or seizures, and electrical 60 Hz interference. If not corrected, the artifacts make the ECG traces more difficult to interpret. There are several other reasons why noise appears in an ECG trace. For example:

- Poor patient preparation
- Environmental interference such as disturbance or noise around the ECG machine or the ECG machine is too close to transformers or large metal conductors carrying a 60-Hz signal
- Defective electrodes or poor electrode-skin contact or interface
- Defective lead wires or ECG cables
- Electrode misplacement on the body
- Faulty acquisition module, computer system, or instrumentation error
- Uncorrected lead systems—an effect of the inhomogeneity of the thorax
- Blood resistivity or variation in respiration
- Variations in conductivity and geometrical parameters on the electrocardiogram

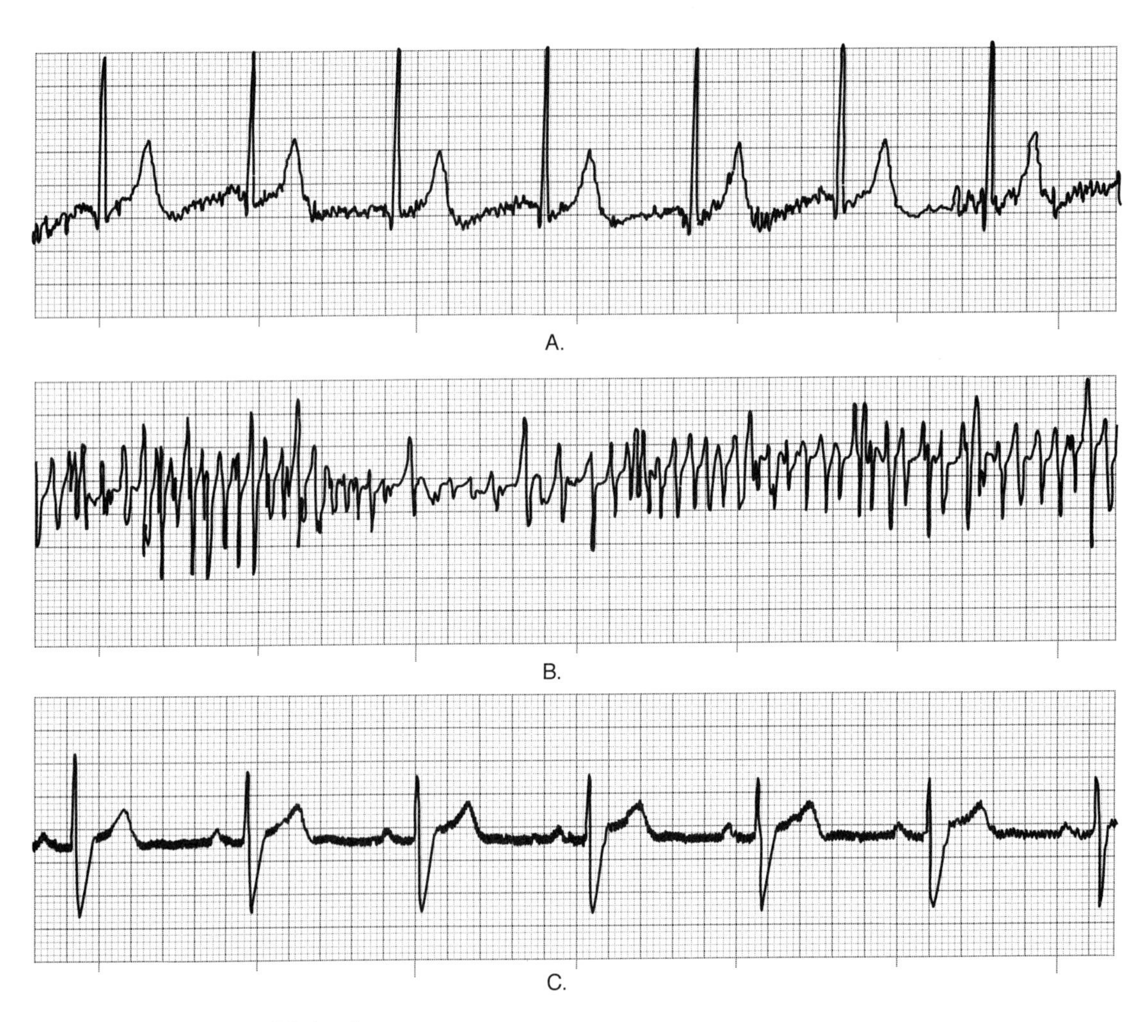

FIGURE 7-10 Noisy ECG signals.

7.9 SIMPLE GUIDELINES IN TAKING AN ECG

There are specific guidelines that technicians, cardiologists, and physicians must follow when conducting an ECG test. For example:

- The health care provider conducting the test must be competently trained. Appropriate continuing professional development to maintain the competence must be ensured
- The procedure must be thoroughly explained to the patient
- The patient must sign a consent form
- The equipment must be working properly, regularly maintained, and checked for safety
- Proper electrodes, jellies, and other accessories must be used and a supply of disposable electrodes must be maintained

EXAMPLE *On an ECG monitor, leads I and III display poor quality waveforms. Which electrode and/or lead cable is suspected to be bad?*

It is obvious that lead II is working because it shows a good ECG signal. That means the electrodes and cables connected to the LL and RA configurations are properly adjusted. By process of elimination, we can determine the LA electrode to be the cause of the problem.

■

EXAMPLE *We want to convert an R wave into a rectangular pulse. What type of circuit could be used?*

First, we need to amplify the R wave, and then feed it to a voltage comparator. The amplified R wave is compared with zero or a small voltage at the input of the comparator. This results the R wave into a rectangular wave.

■

EXAMPLE *In obtaining quality ECG readings, the minimum bandwidth of the ECG recording machine should be: (a) DC to 100 Hz; (b) DC to 1,000 Hz; (c) 0.05 to 100 Hz; or (d) 1 to 100 Hz?*

The answer is (c). Good-quality ECG signal typically has 0.05 Hz to 100 Hz bandwidth.

■

EXAMPLE *Determine which ECG trace in Figure 7-11a through Figure 7-11d is sinus rhythm, sinus arrhythmia, sinus tachycardia, and sinus bradycardia. Explain why.*

The following will help you make your determinations. In sinus rhythms, P waves are supposed to be upright and before the QRS complex. Additionally, the duration of QRS is 0.1 second and the PR interval is about 0.12 to 0.2 second. Moreover, the regular rhythm is 60 to 100 bmp.

In sinus arrhythmias, the irregular heartbeat repeats. The rate gradually slows and then gradually increases. Although the P wave is upright, the QRS complex duration is less than 0.1 second.

In sinus tachycardia, the rate is over 100 bpm, but the rhythms are regular. In sinus bradycardia, the rate is less than 60 bpm and the rhythms are regular. In this example, the sinus rhythm is shown in **Figure 7-11c,** arrhythmia is shown in **Figure 7-11b,** tachycardia is shown in **Figure 7-11a,** and bradycardia is shown in **Figure 7-11d.**

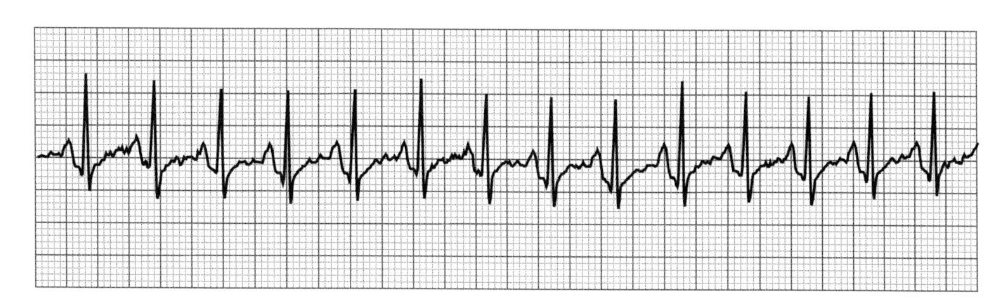

FIGURE 7-11a ECG signal.

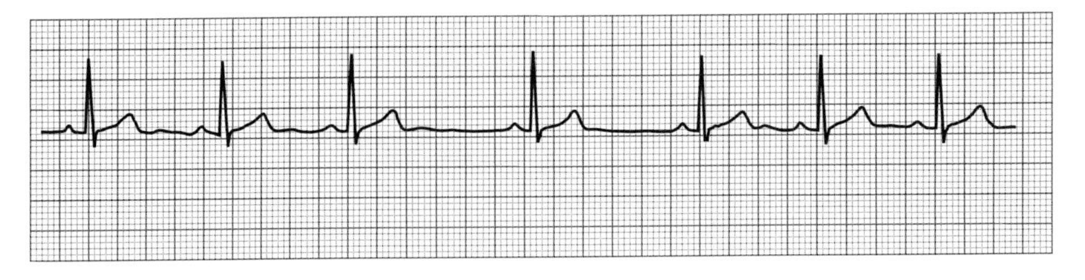

FIGURE 7-11b ECG signal.

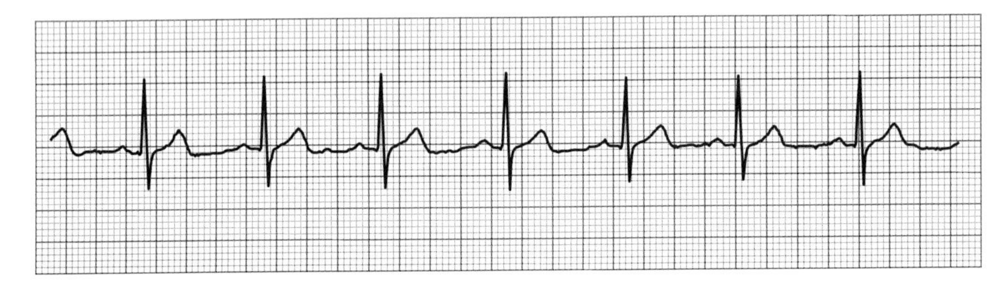

FIGURE 7-11c ECG signal.

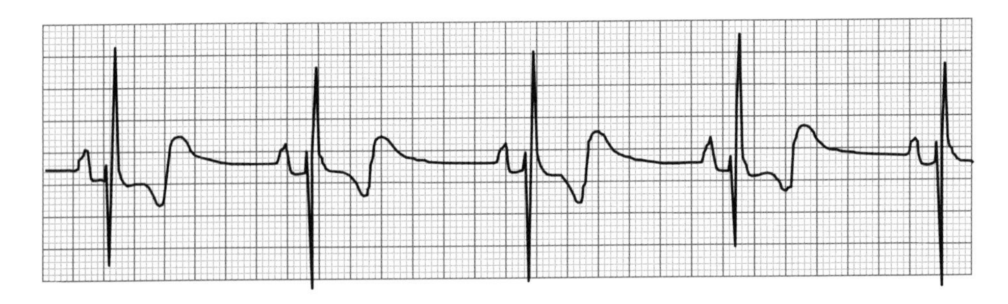

FIGURE 7-11d ECG signal.

7.10 BLOCK DIAGRAM OF AN ECG MACHINE

The block diagram in **Figure 7-12a** and **Figure 7-12b** (courtesy of Brentwood Medical Technology Corporation) provides the components of a simple ECG machine from the electrode-patient interface to the computer-monitor interface.

ECG electrodes and the electronic processors are key components in acquiring an ECG signal from the patient. The physician determines the number of ECG leads based on the patient's physiological condition. At least three leads are typical, but 5 or 12 leads can be used to detect more information about the patient's heart condition.

ECG Amplifiers and Circuit Analysis

An ECG signal level is a few millivolts and the circuit designer must accurately amplify it. **Figure 7-13** shows typical ECG amplifier circuit. Figure 7-13 is an ECG circuit with two inputs from RA and LA electrodes, and one output, V_{OUT}. The back-to-back diodes at

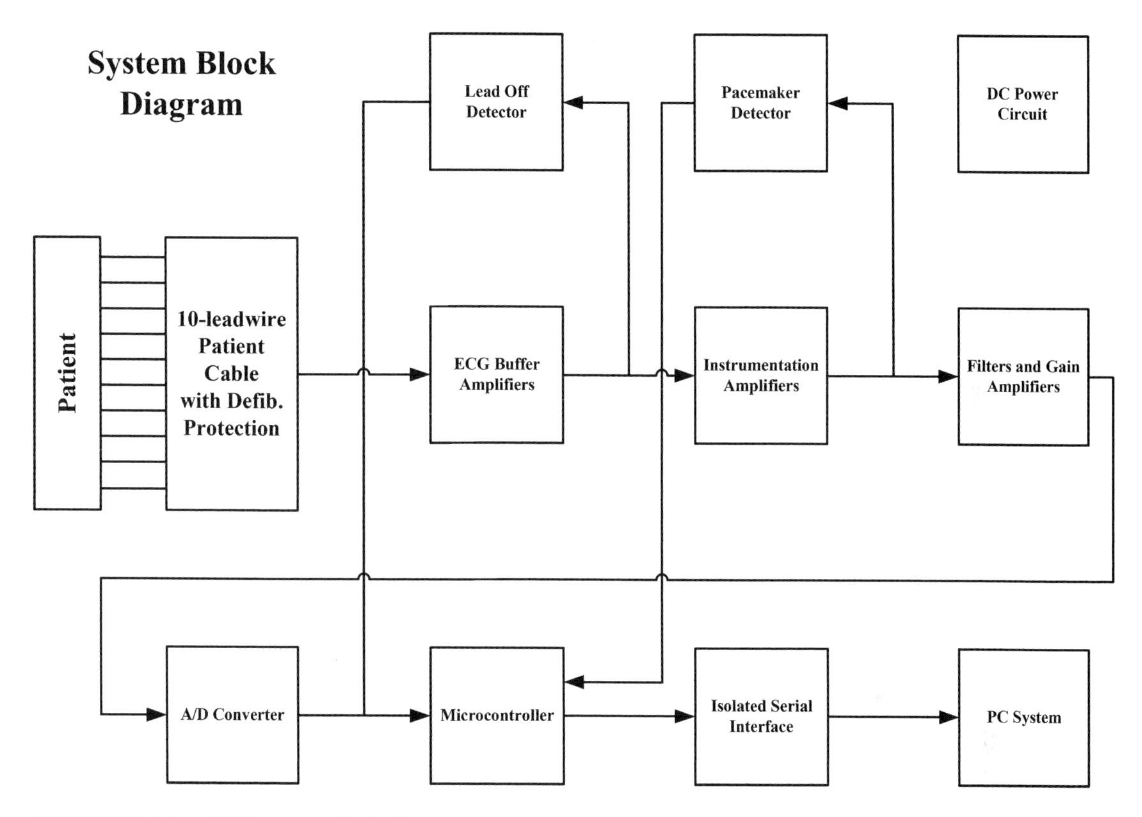

FIGURE 7-12a ECG system block diagram.

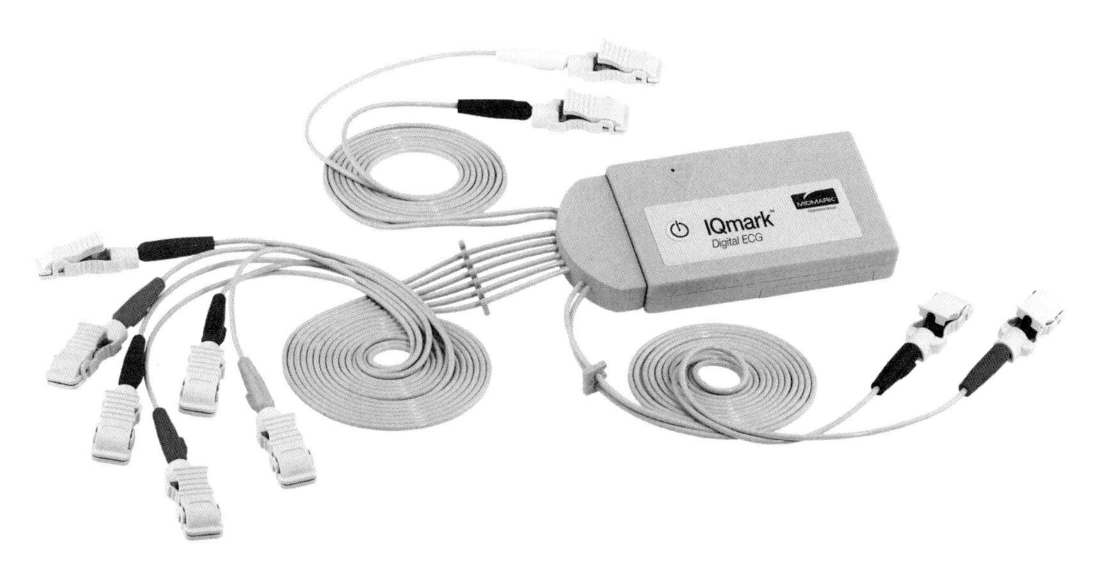

FIGURE 7-12b ECG leads courtesy of IQmark.

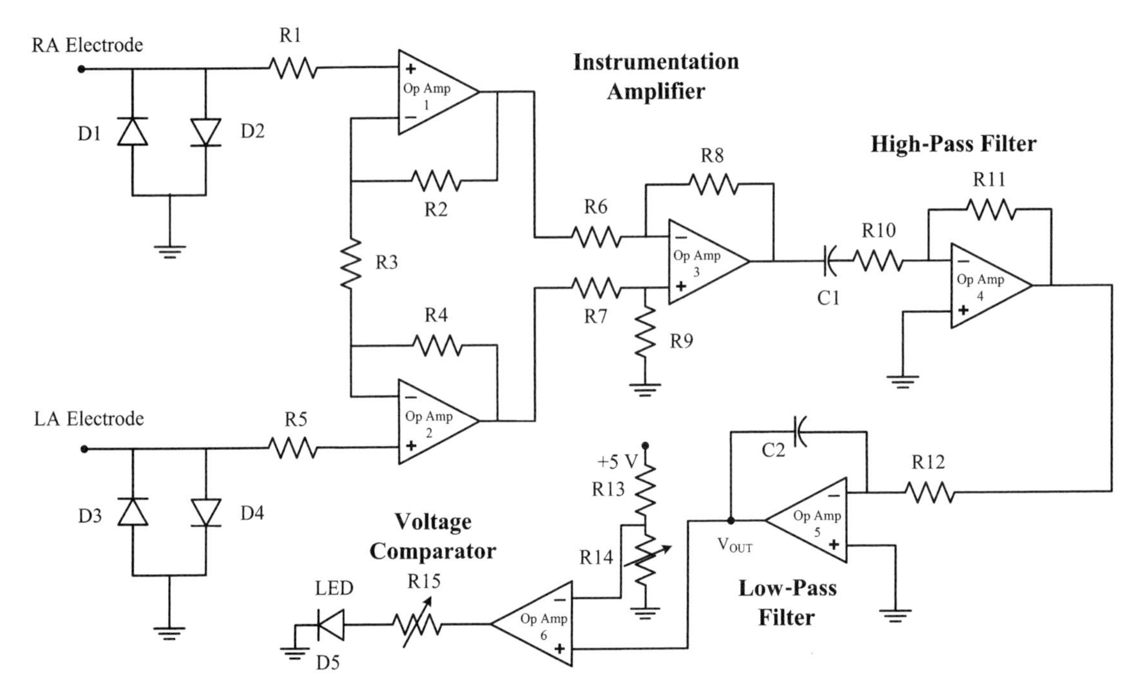

FIGURE 7-13 A simple ECG circuit.

two inputs are to hold the ECG signals in a small range of amplitudes between −0.7 V and 0.7 V. After the instrumentation amplifier, high-pass and low-pass filters process the amplified ECG signal for eliminating the DC offset and the 60 Hz noise, respectively. The output of the voltage comparator is connected to an LED to detect a large positive amplitude of the ECG signal.

Signal conditioning is required under some circumstances with an ECG signal, such as:

1. The magnitude of the R wave is less than 10 mV.
2. The frequency range of the ECG signal is 0.1 Hz to 250 Hz.
3. The magnitude of the noise is comparable to that of the ECG signal and to the electrode half-cell (DC) potential. Other than the ECG signal, ECG electrodes pick up the respiration noise (< 0.03 Hz), EMG noise (1 Hz to 5,000 Hz), 60 Hz noise due to power lines, and the baseline drift noise due to electrode movement.

To correct these problems, the following steps can be taken:

1. To enlarge the R wave, the ECG signal is amplified by several amplifiers. A total gain of 500 will enlarge the R wave to 5 V.
2. The low-frequency noise is removed by using a high-pass filter having a cutoff frequency lower than 1 Hz.
3. To reduce the 60 Hz noise, a low-pass filter is used with a cutoff frequency below 60 Hz.
4. A notch filter is used to notch out the 60 Hz noise.

In Figure 7-13, the ECG signal from the two leads (RA and LA) is amplified in the instrumentation amplifier and then filtered by the first-order high-pass and low-pass filters. The first-order high-pass or low-pass filter is designed by using the cutoff frequency needed for the ECG signal. The cutoff frequency is given as:

$$f_c = \frac{1}{2 \times \pi \times R \times C}$$

In Figure 7-13, the high-pass filter is $R = R_{11}$, $C = C_1$; the low-pass filter is $R = R_{12}$ and $C = C_2$. For the ECG signal, the high-pass cutoff is 0.5 Hz and the low-pass cutoff is 40 Hz.

A second-order high-pass filter as shown in **Figure 7-14a** can replace the first-order high-pass filter of Figure 7-13 for better control of low frequencies in the ECG signal.

The design procedure is:

$$\text{Pick } C_1\text{, then } C_2 = C_1$$

Calculate R_1 using the formula:

$$R_1 = \frac{1}{\sqrt{2}} \times \frac{1}{\pi \times C_1 \times f_c}$$

where f_c is the cutoff frequency of the high-pass filter

$$\text{Calculate } R_2 = 0.5 \times R_1$$

The values of R_1, R_2, C_1, and C_2 are computed based upon the cutoff frequency of 0.5 Hz.

A second-order low-pass filter is shown in **Figure 7-14b.** The design procedure is similar to the design procedure discussed for the high-pass filter. The value of the cutoff frequency is different in high-pass and low-pass filter design, however.

The value of the capacitor $C_2 = 2 \times C_1$ and the resistor $R_2 = R_1$, and the formula is:

$$R_1 = \frac{1}{2 \times \sqrt{2}} \times \frac{1}{\pi \times C_1 \times f_c}$$

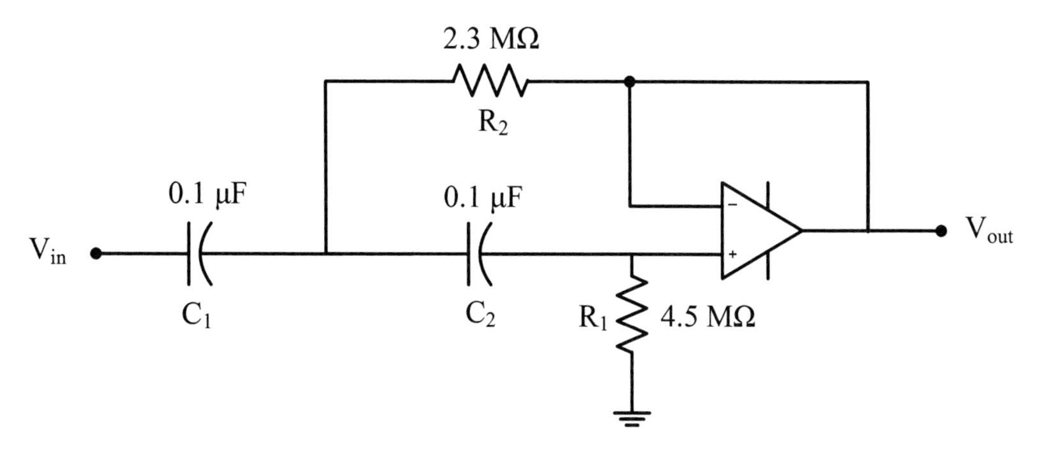

FIGURE 7-14a High-pass filter.

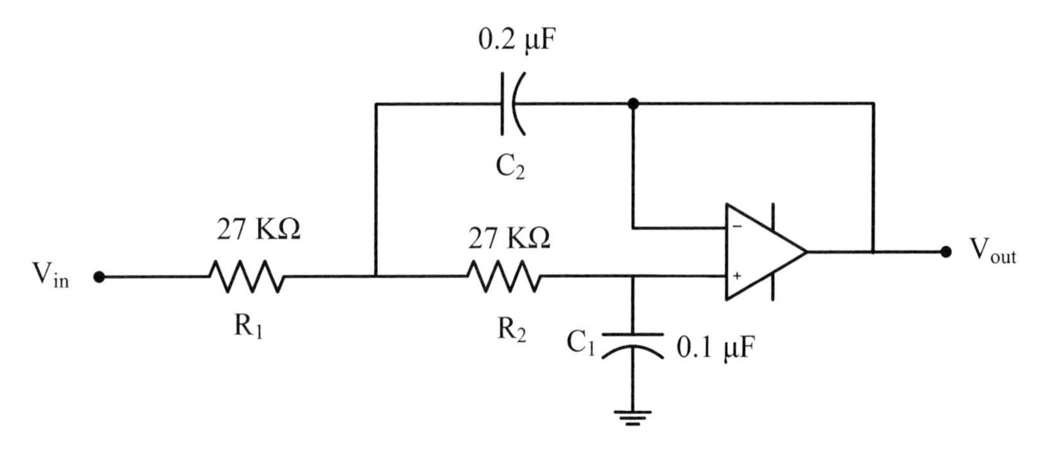

FIGURE 7-14b Low-pass filter.

The values of R_1, R_2, C_1, and C_2 are computed based upon the cutoff frequency of 40 Hz.

A recommended bandwidth of the processed ECG signal is shown in **Figure 7-14c.** A band-pass filter can be designed to pass the band of frequencies between cutoff frequencies while suppressing the bands below and above the pass band. A wide band-pass filter can be achieved by cascading low-pass and high-pass filters.

A band-stop or notch filter can be achieved by connecting the output of a band-pass filter and the input signal (same input as the input to the band-pass filter) to a two-input inverting summer. As the band-pass filter configuration is an inverting one, the inverting summer will generate a notched-out response. For notching out a 60 Hz from the ECG signal, a combination of a band-pass and the summer is recommended.

Figure 7-15 shows an ECG amplifier with the right leg drive op-amps OPA2604 to eliminate the common mode noise generated from the body. The two RA and LA signals entering the instrumentation amplifier INA118 are summed, inverted, and amplified in the right leg driver before it is fed to the electrode attached to the right leg. When the other electrodes pick up this inverted signal, ultimately the common mode noise will cancel out.

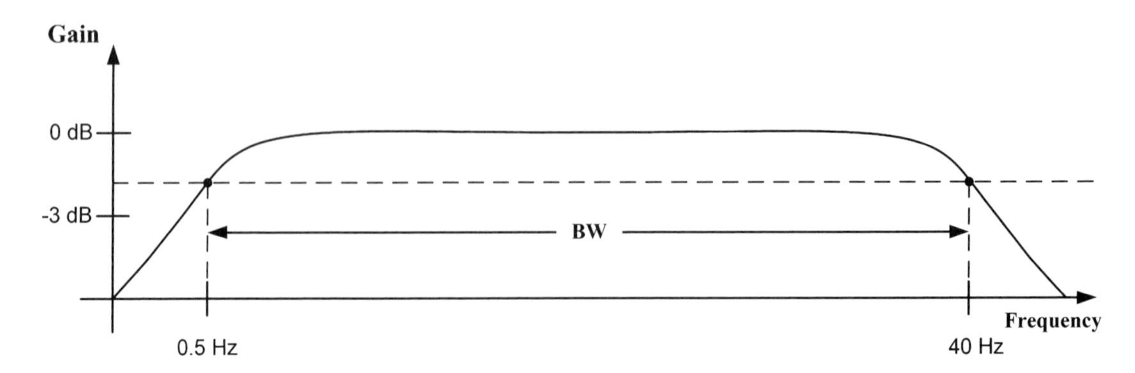

FIGURE 7–14c Bandwidth of the ECG signal.

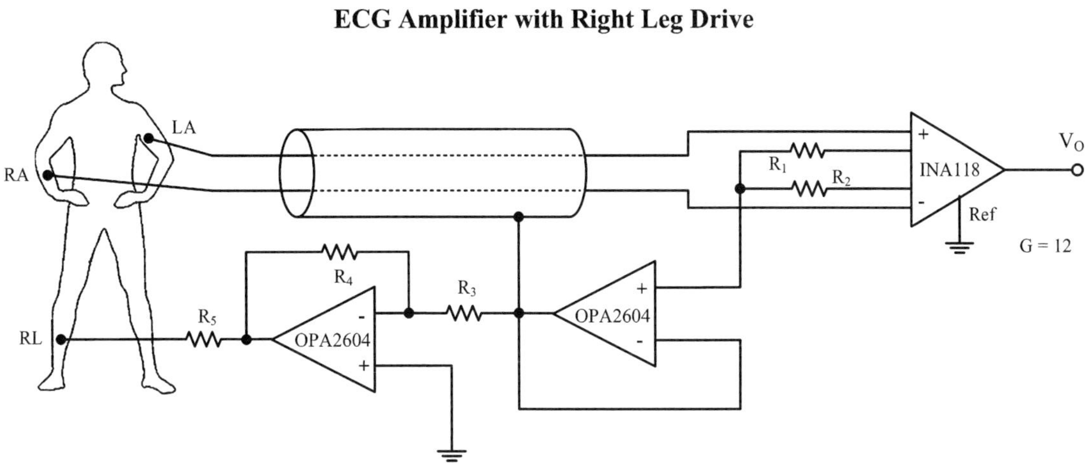

ECG Amplifier with Right Leg Drive

FIGURE 7-15 ECG amplifier with right leg drive.

Although the instrumentation amplifier cancels the common mode noise, the right leg drive circuit is an additional method. The amplified ECG signal is detected at V_O.

ECG Electrodes, Cables, and Accessories

An ECG electrode acts as an "electrical connector" between the patient's skin and the ECG cable. The cable can carry three or more electrodes from different parts of the body surface. Disposable electrodes attach to the color-coded wires of the cable. The other end of the cable connects to the electronic circuit board for signal processing. Similar to telephone cables with red, green, and black wires all in one cable, the ECG cable connects to the minimum of three electrodes with red, white, and black wires. In addition to its placement, color coding is used also to identify each electrode. The right arm (RA) is white, the left arm (LA) is black, the right leg (RL) is green, the left leg (LL) is red, and the chest is brown. The colors of the individual chest leads are V_1 (brown/red), V_2 (brown/yellow), V_3 (brown/green), V_4 (brown/blue), V_5 (brown/orange), and V_6 (brown/purple).

The processes of applying the ECG electrodes and making the actual recordings of the ECG signal take only a few moments. Proper leads and the placement of these leads are crucial in measuring the ECG signal. The ECG technician is trained and certified in acquiring the ECG data on the console port (monitor) or on the printer strip chart.

The ECG machine has several parts and accessories, such as cables, lead wires, electrode adapters, and stress harnesses. Some manufacturers use Series R, SRS, and FSR for three- or five-lead versions only. That means three or five ECG electrodes can be grouped in the cable. The D series uses more than three or five leads. Eight, 10, and 14 wires can be grouped in the D series. The cables are well shielded from motion artifacts and electrical interferences. Proper grounding is achieved to avoid any electrical shock to the patient.

For recording a 12-lead ECG, 5-lead ECG, or 3-lead ECG, the cables have color-coded 10 wires, 5 wires, or 3 wires, respectively. The five-lead ECG cable will provide limb leads and a choice of a chest lead, and a three-lead cable can give a choice of limb leads only.

7.11 ECG MACHINES AND MONITORS

A variety of ECG machines are used in hospitals and clinics. There are dedicated 3-channel to 12-channel ECG machines and patient monitors used not only for ECG monitoring but for monitoring blood pressure, respiration, temperature, and oxygen saturation in the blood as well. ECG machines may be portable. ECG machines are also called cardiac monitors, global ECG machines, interpretive ECG machines, ECG heart rate monitors, bedside monitors, and vital sign monitors. We will discuss one particular model of ECG machine, the MAC 5000, in the following section.

MAC 5000

Figure 7-16a through Figure 7-17 show the MAC 5000 machine. **Figure 7-16a** shows front and back views. This is the resting ECG analysis system made by GE Medical Systems. It looks like a laptop computer with a keyboard display monitor and disk drive slot. The

FIGURE 7-16a MAC 5000 ECG machine.

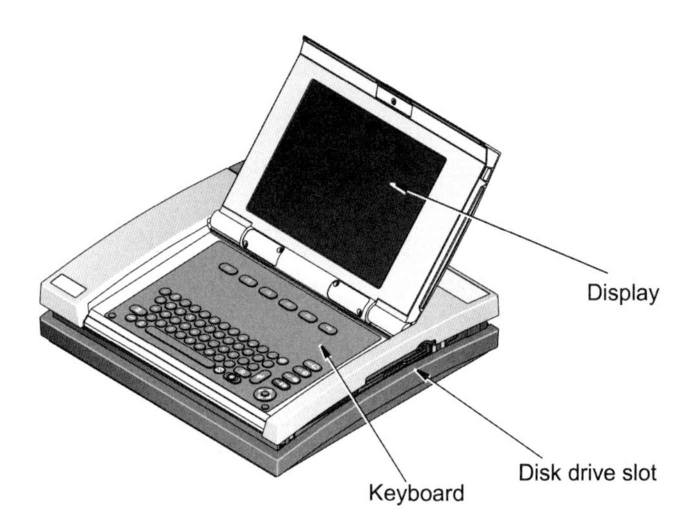

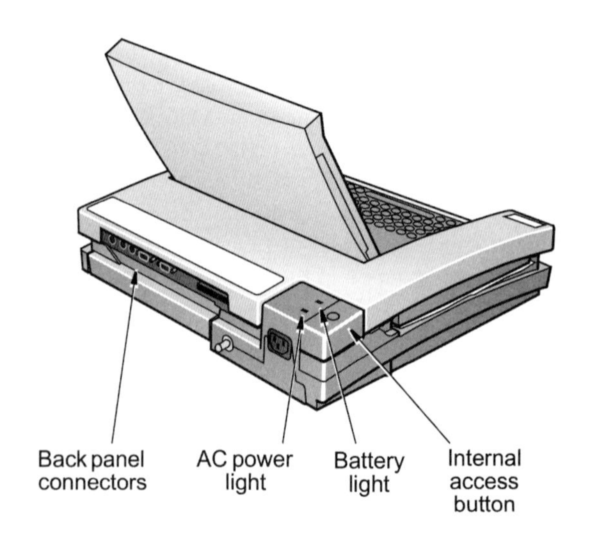

assembly block diagram is shown in **Figure 7-16b.** The CPU board contains circuitry for resting ECG analysis except for the power supply, acquisition module, keyboard, and display. The patient acquisition module connects to the CPU board with COM ports, analog I/O, and video-out connections. The MAC 5000 block diagram has more detailed information on the input and output processes. This is shown in **Figure 7-17.** All of the MAC 5000's proprietary hardware is contained in a single Xilinx field programmable gate array (FPGA) that contains boot ROM emulation, bus interface, bus controller, and interfaces to the acquisition module, EEPROM, and thermal printhead. The FPGA also has an audio beep generator and four pulse width modulation (PWM) analog outputs.

The system management and some I/O functions are implemented in preprogrammed 68HC05 microcontrollers. As referenced in Figure 7-17, "Curly" is responsible for configuring the FPGA and for loading the bootstrap program into the BootROM. "Shemp" scans the keyboard and "Larry" controls the paper drive motor and digitizes the analog inputs. "Moe" is responsible for controlling and monitoring the battery, power supplies, on/off key, and the system reset.

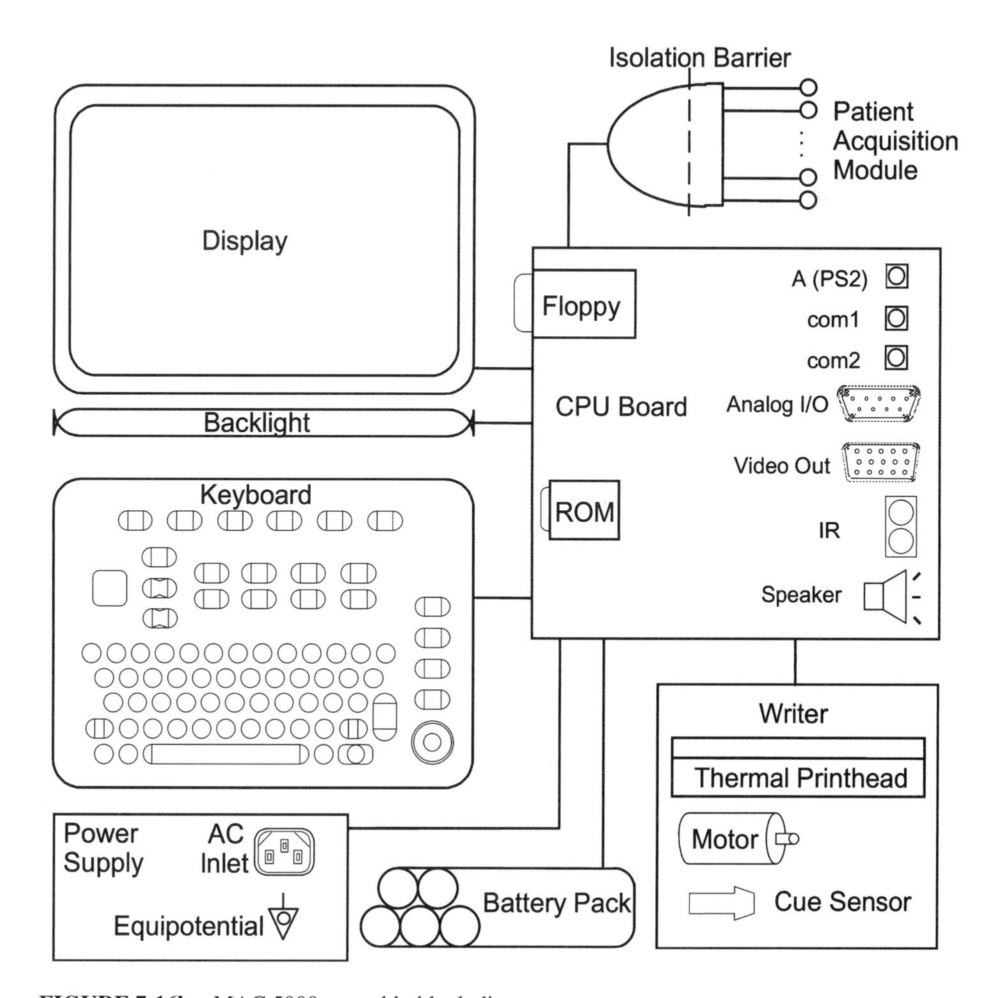

FIGURE 7-16b MAC 5000 assembly block diagram.

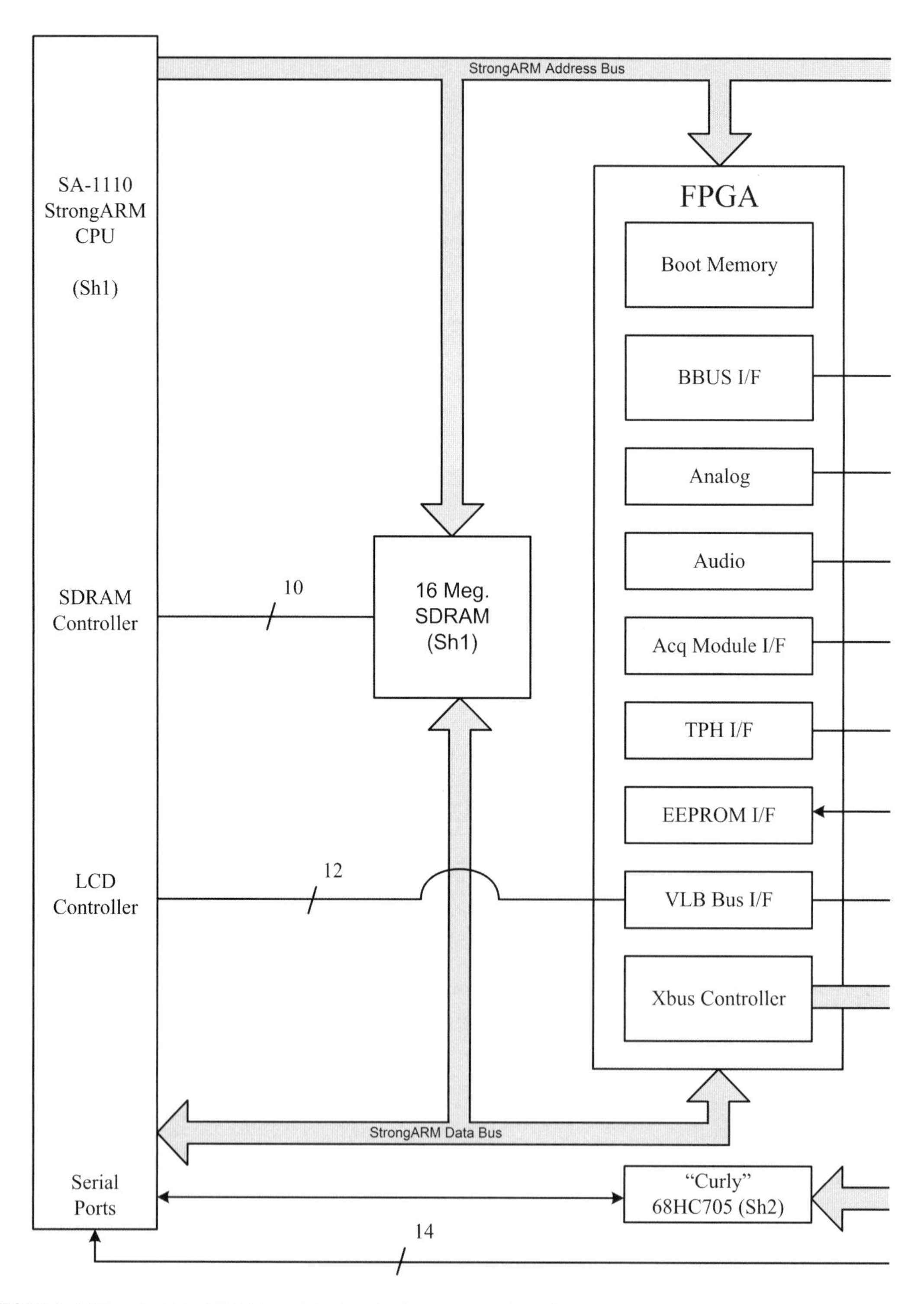

FIGURE 7-17 MAC 5000 ECG machine block diagram. (*continued*)

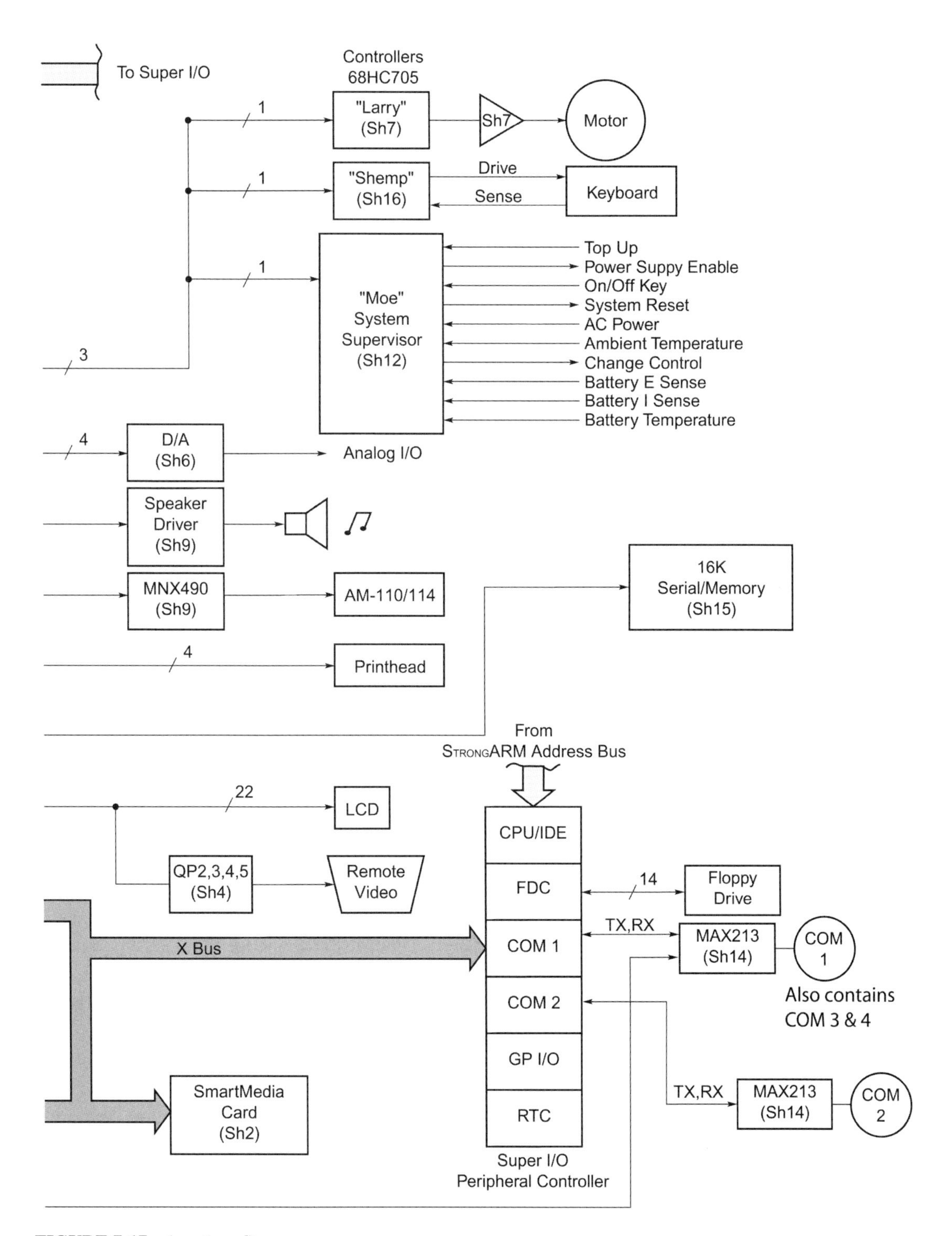

FIGURE 7-17 *(continued)*

MAC 5000 Detail Input/Output	
Display	Resolution 640 × 480 pixels
Instrument type	15 lead (14 channel)
Analysis frequency	500 samples/sec
Digital sampling rate	4,000 samples/sec/channel
Frequency response	−3dB @ 0.01 to 150 Hz
Common mode rejection	> 140 dB
Input impedance	> 10 MΩ @ 10 Hz
Patient leakage current	< 10 μA
Dynamic range	AC differential ± 5 mVDC offset ± 320 mV
Resolution	1.22 μV/LSB @ 500 samples/sec
Type of protection against electrical shock	Class 1 (internally powered)

7.12 HOLTER MONITOR

A Holter monitor is a portable tape recorder that records the electrical activity of the heart. The data is the ECG trace recorded over 24 to 48 hours. The three-channel ECG electrodes are positioned with adhesive on the patient's chest by the ECG technician and the cable is then connected to a tape recorder. The patient can place the tape recorder on the waist belt or on a shoulder strap for the next 24 to 48 hours. Today, wireless monitors are common. The ECG data is transmitted to a base station a few feet away or to a case on the patient's body. The data is processed at the base station and again transmitted to the necessary professional, usually in a doctor's office or clinic. This transmission may be through a cell tower for long distances. Noise and interference are greatly reduced in the wireless media.

Figure 7-18a and **Figure 7-18b** show the Marquette Holter recorder. It records two or three channels of continuous ECG data for up to 48 hours on a single cassette. On a separate channel, a digital timing track is simultaneously recorded. This channel can be electronically marked by the patient to identify symptomatic events or activities of which the cardiologist should be made aware.

Some of the characteristics of this recorder are as follows:

1. Three- or five-wire cable (modified V_5 and V_1 leads) positioned on the chest.
2. A Class III, type B equipment that is suitable for external application to the patient.
3. Automatic calibration is initiated when the recorder is turned on.
4. The signal test connectors and the Holter signal test cable for the ECG signal evaluation for the printouts are available.
5. The skin preparation list and the patient-hookup procedure for Holter recording are given.
6. The technical specifications list:

Maximum signal input level	100 mV (p-p)
Maximum electrode offset	± 300 mV DC
Input impedance (running)	10 mΩ minimum
Impedance (ground to case)	25 kΩ maximum
Resistance (ground lead to case)	130 kΩ, ± 5 percent
Minimum operable circuit voltage	4 V DC
Weight	16 ounces

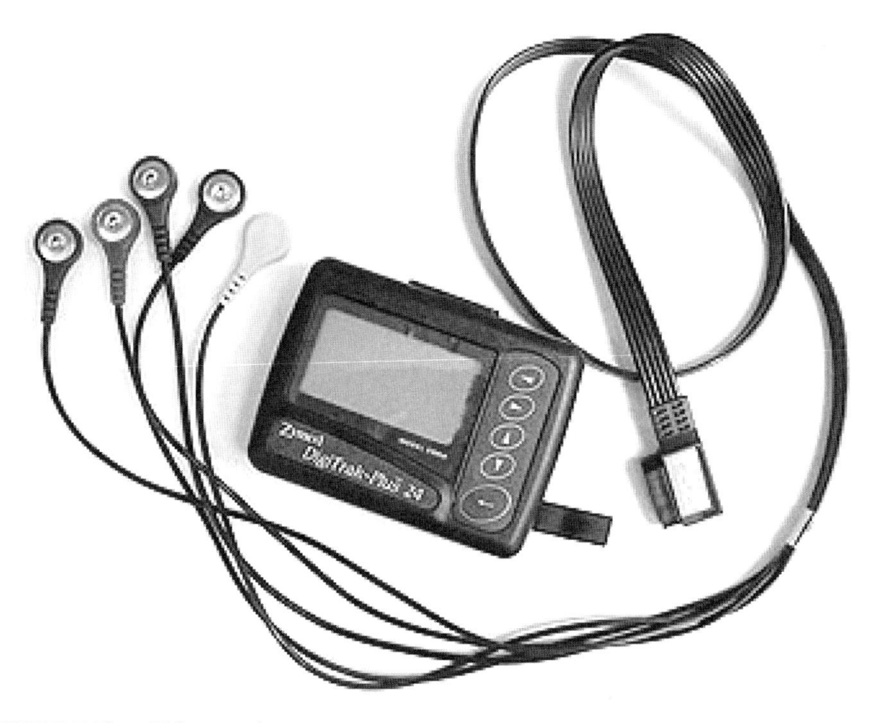

FIGURE 7-18a Holter monitor.

FIGURE 7-18b Holter monitor electrodes.

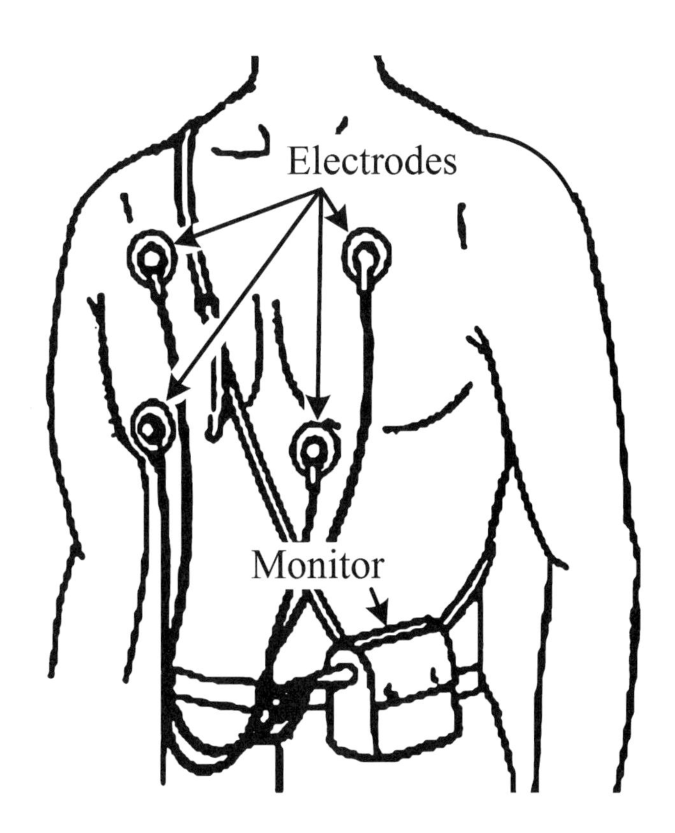

7.13 ECG SIMULATORS

An ECG simulator or multi-parameter patient simulator (with ECG feature) can help students interpret ECG signals prior to using ECG machines with patients. The unit can produce a wide variety of ECG simulations such as a complete P-QRS-T waveform at all rates, ECG, and square-wave outputs. **Figure 7-19** shows the PS-2210 patient simulator from BC Biomedical. The parameters of amplitude, rate, and arrhythmias are selectable. The unit can simulate 49 different arrhythmias. A special automatic mode is available to auto sequence through the entire range of waveforms. There are 10 patient lead connectors available on this unit. The PS-2210 unit includes simulation of ECG, respiration, blood pressure, temperature, and cardiac output. There are three separate electrically isolated sections: the main section contains ECG and respiration, the second section contains blood pressure, and the third section is temperature and cardiac output. A full remote operation via RS-232C interface is also included in the unit.

The LCD display provides information on the generated waveforms. All ECG leads have independently generated signals. The waveform parameters are selected from the keyboard. The ECG leads can also be used for the respiration signal and the respiration parameters can be entered from the keyboard.

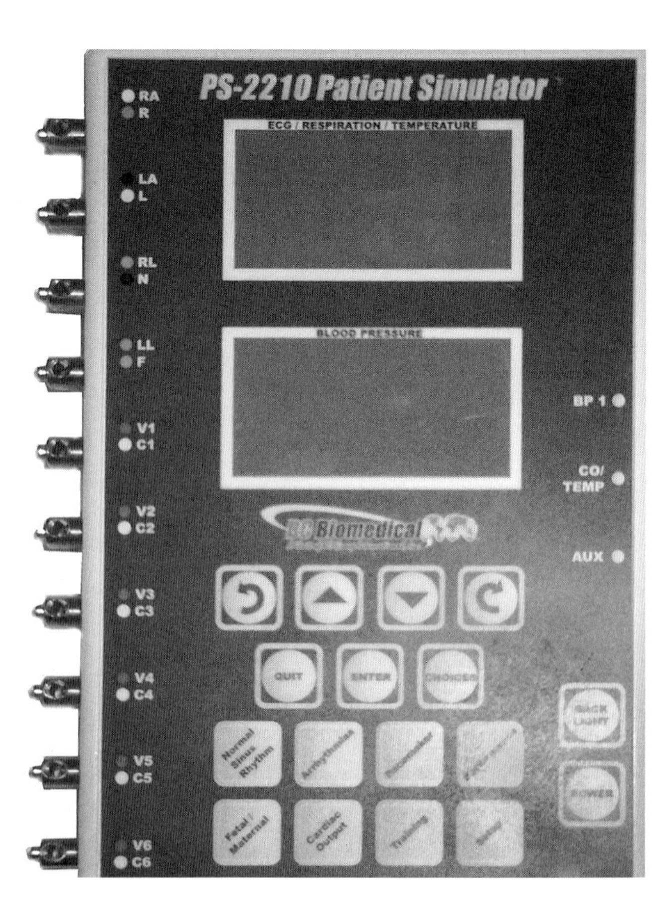

FIGURE 7-19 PS 2210 Patient Simulator.

Generally, a patient simulator generates biomedical signals similar to a live patient. Apart from training purposes, the importance of the simulator is to monitor and test ECG machines, blood pressure equipment, defibrillators, pacemakers, and other types of medical equipment.

SUMMARY

- An electrocardiogram (ECG) is the record, or trace, of the electrical activity of the cardiac muscle.
- In diagnostic cardiology, the ECG is used to record the signals of depolarization and repolarization of the heart.
- An ECG is recommended when the patient exhibits fatigue, chest pain, or palpitations of the heart and can show the abnormalities of conduction across the heart. It also can suggest coronary artery disease.
- Limb lead I is between the two arms, lead II and lead III are between the right or left arm and the left leg. The aVR, aVL, and aVF are the augmented leads and are derived from the same three electrodes as leads I, II, and III, but any two limb leads are connected to the negative terminal. V_1 to V_6 are chest leads. The right leg is always connected to ground.
- A general block diagram of an ECG machine and the various circuits in the ECG machine are part of the instrumentation. The circuit for signal conditioning includes the instrumentation amplifier, high- and low-pass filters, and a voltage comparator. The design of filter circuits uses the high cutoff frequency of 0.5 Hz and the low cutoff frequency of 40 Hz. The block diagram of the MAC 5000 shows the analog and digital interfaces to the CPU and to the FPGA array.
- Holter monitors are small portable devices to record ECG the entire time the patient is wearing it. Holter monitors record the heart rhythm continuously for 24 to 48 hours.
- ECG simulators generate normal and abnormal ECG signals for training purposes and to interface to ECG machines for diagnostics.

MEDICAL TERMINOLOGY

Angina: constriction of the heart causing a sense of suffocation and severe pain usually radiating down the left arm.

Arrhythmia: any deviation from the normal pattern of the heartbeat. This is also known as cardiac arrhythmia or dysrhythmia.

ECG leads: wires connected to pads that are placed on the chest and limbs. Leads are then attached to an electrocardiograph machine used to measure and record electrical activity in the heart.

Evoked potential (EP): a procedure used to detect an electrical response of a nerve cell or group of nerve cells by an external stimulus in order to identify neurological disorders.

Flutter: rapid heartbeat or vibration, as in an atrial or ventricular flutter of the heart.

Holter monitor: a small, portable monitoring device worn by an ambulatory patient to produce ECG recordings for 24 hours or more.

Palpitation: a pounding or rapid heartbeat with or without irregularity in rhythm; usually associated with emotional responses or heart disorders.

Phonocardiogram: a graphic recording of heart sounds and murmurs.

Second-degree block: increased parasympathetic (vagal) tone or acute (inferior wall) myocardial infarction (MI).

Third-degree block: advanced heart disease such as (anterior wall) myocardial infarction, congenital heart condition, or inflammation of myocardium. Anterior wall MIs cause permanent block while the block associated with the inferior wall MIs typically subsides in a week or two as the swelling diminishes.

Vectorcardiography: a method of recording of the direction and magnitude of the depolarization waves (over chest and limbs) by vectors that characterize the cardiac cycle.

QUIZ

1. True or False: The process of depolarization results in the stimulation of the cardiac cells.

   a) True. b) False.

2. The ______________________________ is the normal intrinsic pacemaker of the heart.

3. Match the ECG wave information with the appropriate action potential in the following columns:

____ QRS complex	a) depolarization of ventricles
____ P wave	b) repolarization of the ventricles
____ PR interval	c) travel time between SA node and AV node
____ QT interval	d) depolarization of the atria
____ T wave	e) cycle of ventricular depolarization/repolarization
____ ST segment	f) the resting period after ventricular depolarization

4. True or False: For the precordial lead monitoring, there are specific locations on the chest surface.

   a) True. b) False.

5. True or False: Diagnosis of arrhythmias depends mainly on the time relationships between the different waves of the cardiac cycle.

   a) True. b) False.

6. An ECG monitor usually has a frequency response of 0.05 Hz to about ________ Hz.

7. True or False: Electrode impedance increases with sweaty skin surfaces.

   a) True. b) False.

8. Generally, tachycardia has a range of __________________ bpm, whereas bradycardia has a range of __________________ bpm.

9. What part of the ECG signal is the most useful for determining heart rate?

   a) P wave. b) QRS complex. c) T wave. d) None of the above.

10. What happens when somebody is having heart palpitations?

    ____

PROBLEMS

1. For the given ECG diagram in **Figure 7-20,** determine the beats per minute, rhythm (regular, irregular, or absent), QRS duration, PR interval, and the ST segment and its interpretation.

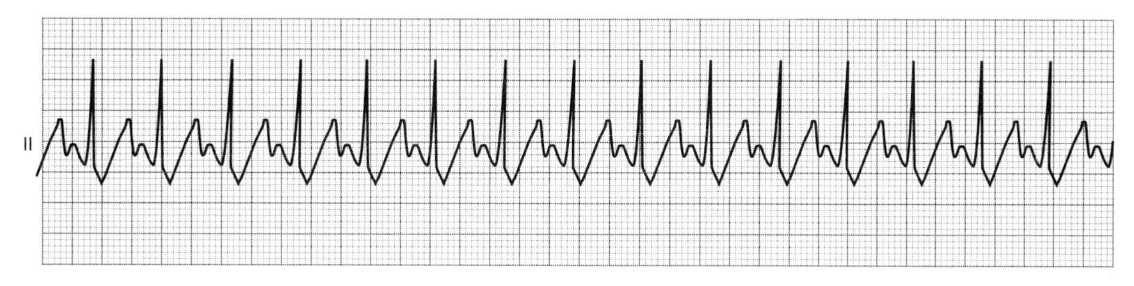

FIGURE 7-20 ECG signal.

2. For the ECG diagram in **Figure 7-21,** determine the interpretation of the given signal.

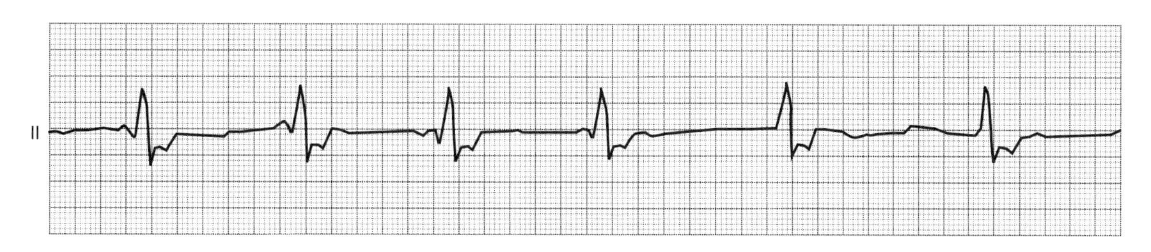

FIGURE 7-21 ECG signal.

3. **Figure 7-22** shows an ECG signal. Determine what kind of abnormality is indicated and provide your reasoning.

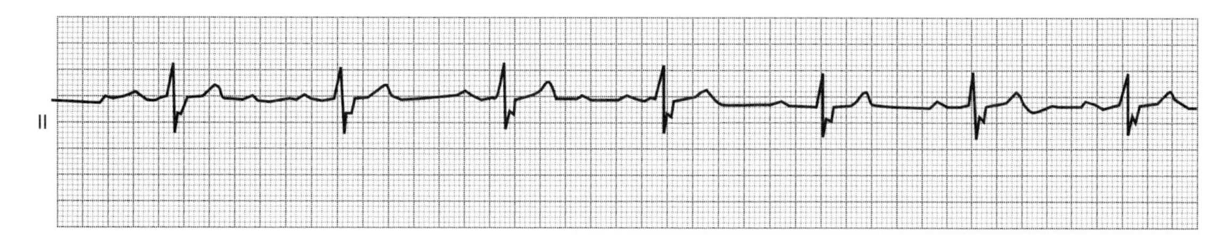

FIGURE 7-22 ECG signal.

4. Interpret the ECG signal shown in **Figure 7-23.**

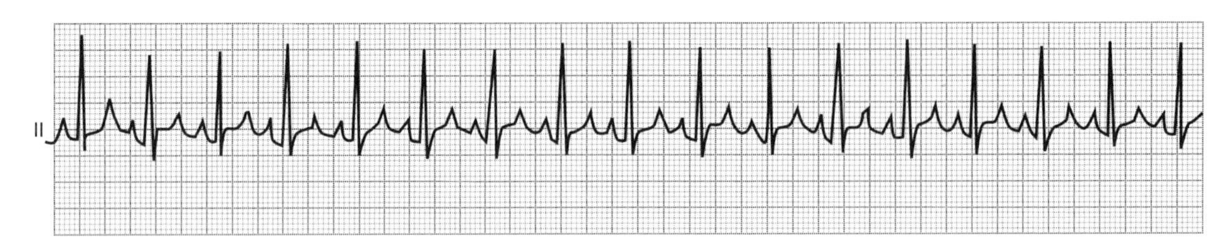

FIGURE 7-23 ECG signal.

5. Research the relationship between the cardiac vector and the ECG signal. Determine the cardiac vector when the R-wave amplitude for the three leads are given as: 0.5 mV lead I, 1.2 mV lead II, and 0.6 mV lead III.
6. Design a notch filter that can remove a 60 Hz noise signal from an ECG signal.
7. Explain how a differential amplifier can amplify the ECG signal while not amplifying the noise. Sketch how the patient is connected to the differential amplifier.
8. Draw a differential amplifier or instrumentation amplifier circuit to amplify a 3-, 5-, and 12-lead electrode ECG signal.
9. Identify the rationale behind ordering a 3-lead, 5-lead, or 12-lead ECG monitor by the attending physician. Apart from the cost, indicate other reasons for the decision.
10. Design an ECG circuit using a commercially available instrumentation amplifier chip such as AD624AD (Analog Devices Inc.) with a gain of 500 and a band-pass filter that will only pass the frequency band of 0.5 Hz to 50 Hz of the ECG spectrum.
11. Design an electronic circuit to determine the normal sinus rhythm in beats per minute by detecting the peaks of the R waves of an ECG signal. The design should include op-amps and the timer or counter circuit.
12. On choosing a threshold for the QRS complex to detect the heartbeat, explain how could you avoid a situation where the T wave is also large and exceeds this threshold. Design an electronic circuit to avoid the situation. A threshold is some percentage of the maximum value of the ECG signal.
13. Research the digital circuits of an ECG machine and indicate the type of microprocessor chips used.
14. Research digital signal processing techniques used in ECG monitors.
15. Show a block diagram of a patient simulator and identify its ECG section.

CASE STUDIES

1. Mike's cardiologist indicated that his mitral valve is defective and fails to close properly. Mike's lifestyle is excellent. He does not smoke and he exercises regularly. Mike takes regular heart medications prescribed by his doctor.

a) What type of ECG traces can be seen with Mike's condition?

b) What kind of medications might Mike take and why?

c) Are there differences in ECG traces for other types of valve defects, such as the tricuspid valve or the aortic valve?

RESEARCH TOPICS

1. Used as learning tools for BMETs, nurses, and other health care professionals, ECG simulators can generate normal and abnormal cardiac rhythms to test the professional's skills. Write a research paper that discusses a few case studies of ECG arrhythmias. Include comparisons with the simulated results.
2. Patients with kidney diseases often have some heart-related problems as well. Write a research paper on this subject and include an electrical model of the heart-kidney circuit.

CHAPTER 8

Defibrillators and Pacemakers

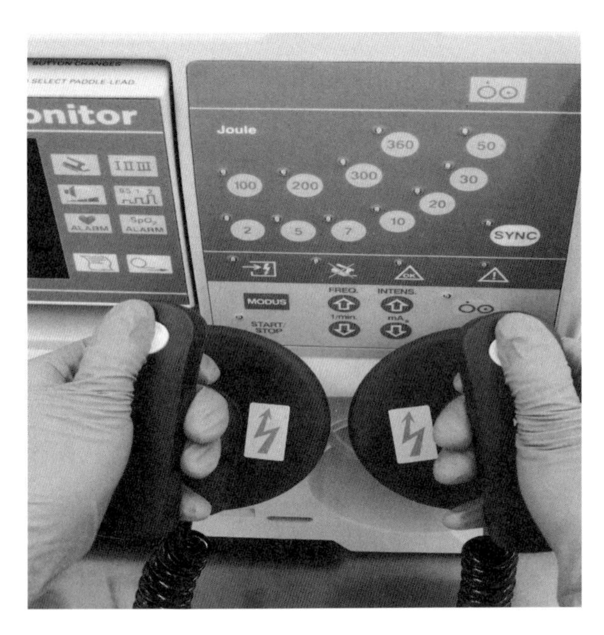

■ CHAPTER OUTLINE

■ OBJECTIVES

The objective of this chapter is to familiarize the reader with the theory and the electronic circuits of defibrillators and pacemakers. The use of a wide variety of these medical devices in and outside of the hospital environment is also discussed in this chapter.

Upon completion of this chapter, the reader will be able to:

- Define the defibrillator and pacemaker terminology.
- Compute the power and other parameters in defibrillators.
- Explain the components and the operation of the defibrillator circuit.
- Compare the differences of various defibrillators.
- Identify the components of a pacemaker.
- Identify the rationale of using various pacemakers.

■ INTERNET WEB SITES

http://www.nlm.nih.gov (National Library of Medicine National Institutes of Health)
http://www.medtronic.com (Medtronics)
http://www.guidant.com (Boston Scientific)
http://www.texasheartinstitute.org (St. Luke's Episcopal Hospital, Texas Medical Center, Houston)

■ INTRODUCTION

A defibrillator is a high-voltage electrical heart stimulator used to resuscitate heart attack victims. More than 200,000 people in the United States die each year from sudden heart attacks. The immediate initiation of cardiopulmonary resuscitation (CPR), quick response time of the EMS (emergency medical services) crew, and the rapid delivery of life-saving shock by the defibrillator are essential to saving these lives. Automatic external defibrillators (AEDs) can be implantable or external and have become integral devices in the medical and public communities.

Acting as a generator, the pacemaker allows physicians to maintain electrical stimulation to the heart in order to restore and stabilize normal rhythms. Just as a defibrillator, they can be implanted or used externally. Disturbances in the normal heart rhythm can arise from a variety of sources such as aging, hereditary defects, heart blocks, and even the side effects of cardiac drugs. This chapter will explain electronic circuits in defibrillators and pacemakers and the various types available from different manufacturers.

■

8.1 RATIONALE OF USING DEFIBRILLATORS

Several conditions of the heart are considered medical emergencies. The heart may go into ventricular fibrillation. Ventricular fibrillation in combination with arrhythmia is called pulseless ventricular tachycardia. When this occurs even for just a few seconds, blood circulation to the heart or to the brain stops and the person most likely will die. The heart will stop beating due to lack of pulse and blood pressure; this serious condition is known as cardiac arrest.

In ventricular fibrillation, the electrical activity in the ventricles is irregular, fast, and random, which affects the heart's pumping capability and the perfusion of blood to the brain. Ventricular tachycardia is an extremely rapid heartbeat; it can range from just over 100 beats per minute (bpm) to as fast as 250 bpm and can affect blood circulation and perfusion to the brain. If not treated aggressively, ventricular tachycardia may deteriorate into ventricular fibrillation.

The controlled electrical shock of defibrillation suppresses and potentially terminates ventricular fibrillation and ventricular tachycardia. This depolarizes the heart's electrical conduction system, a process that essentially resets and restarts the system, restoring it to its normal rhythm.

Figure 8-1 shows atrial fibrillation and **Figure 8-2a** and **Figure 8-2b** show abnormal ECG waveforms of ventricular tachycardia and ventricular fibrillation, respectively. In atrial fibrillation, there is no organized atrial contraction. The episodes of ventricular tachycardia progress into a sustained ventricular tachycardia and the P wave is not always visible. Ventricular fibrillation is a chaotic ventricular discharge and the ventricular depolarization, or contraction, is absent.

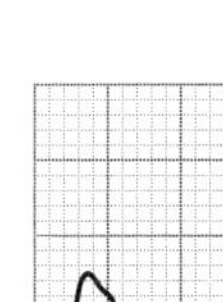

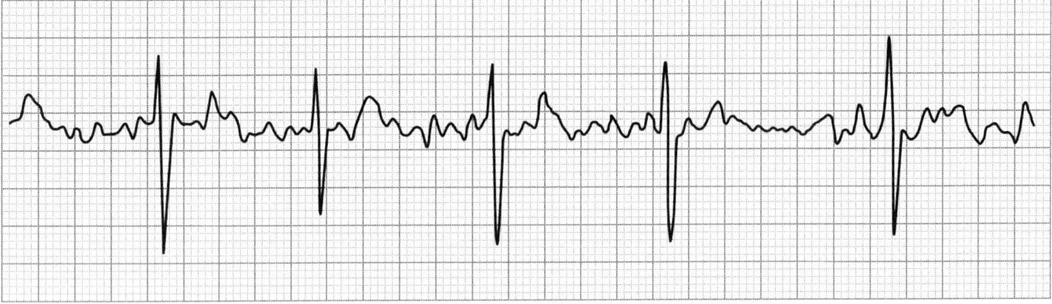

FIGURE 8-1 Atrial fibrillation.

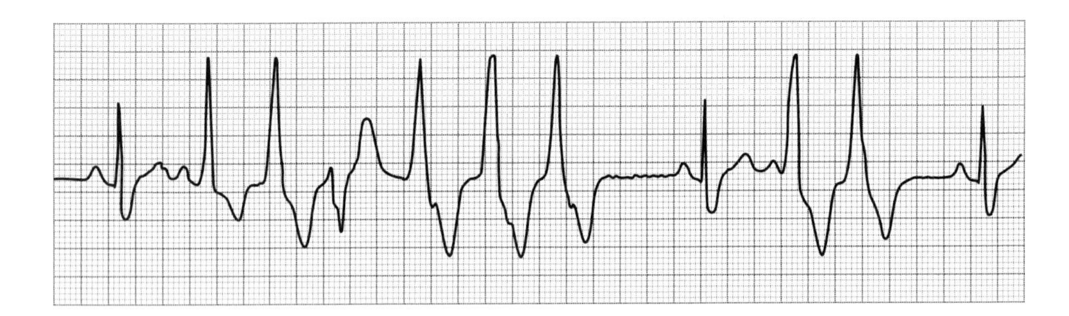

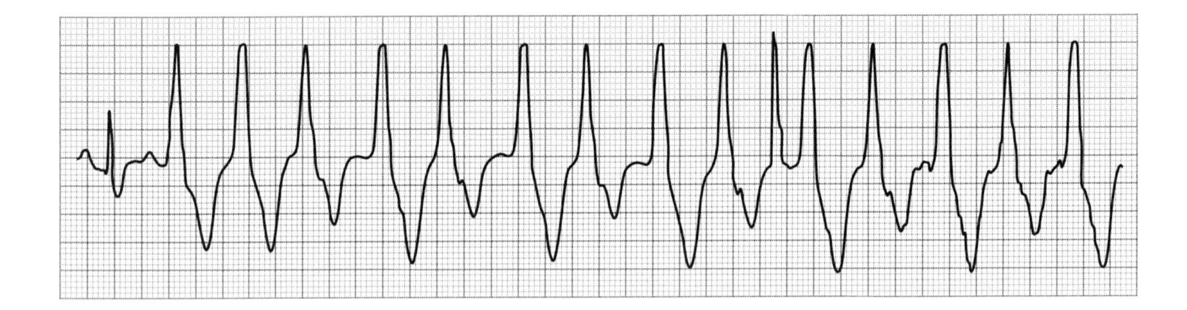

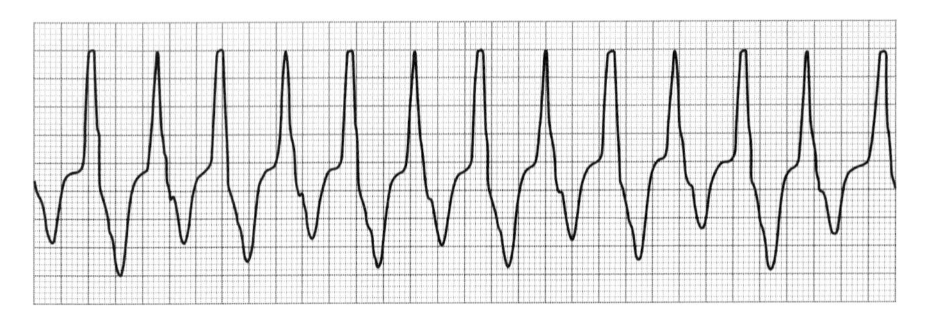

FIGURE 8-2a Ventricular tachycardia.

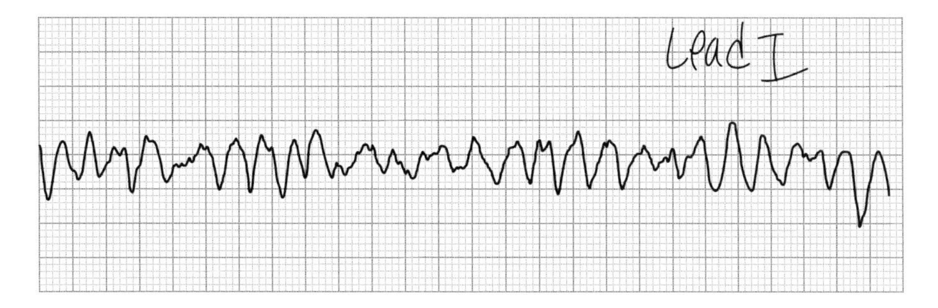

FIGURE 8-2b Ventricular fibrillation.

8.2 THEORY OF DEFIBRILLATOR CIRCUITS

A typical defibrillator must deliver a high amount of energy (in joules) to the heart, first by charging a large capacitor, and then by discharging it through an RLC circuit, two metal plates, and finally through the heart at approximately a 50-ohm load. **Figure 8-3** shows the block diagram of a typical defibrillator.

A simple schematic of a DC defibrillator is shown in **Figure 8-4a.** When the switch is in the charge position, the transformer output current flows through the diode and the source resistance R_s and charges the capacitor to the maximum peak value of V_p volts. In the circuit, the time constant of the circuit is ($R_s \times C$) seconds. The energy stored in the capacitor can be determined as:

$$= \frac{1}{2} \times C \times V_p^2 \text{ Joules}$$

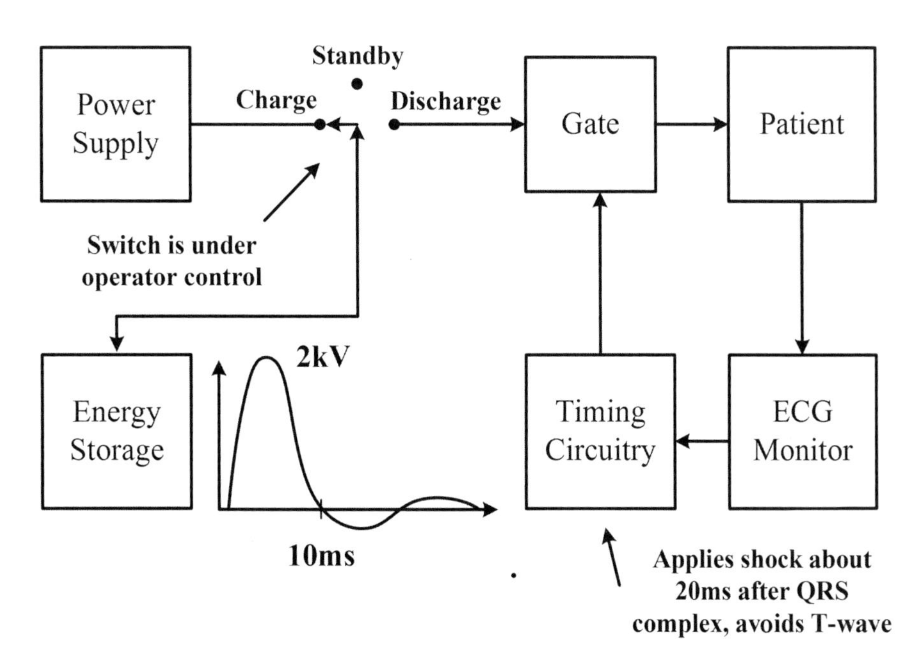

FIGURE 8-3 Block diagram of an external defibrillator.

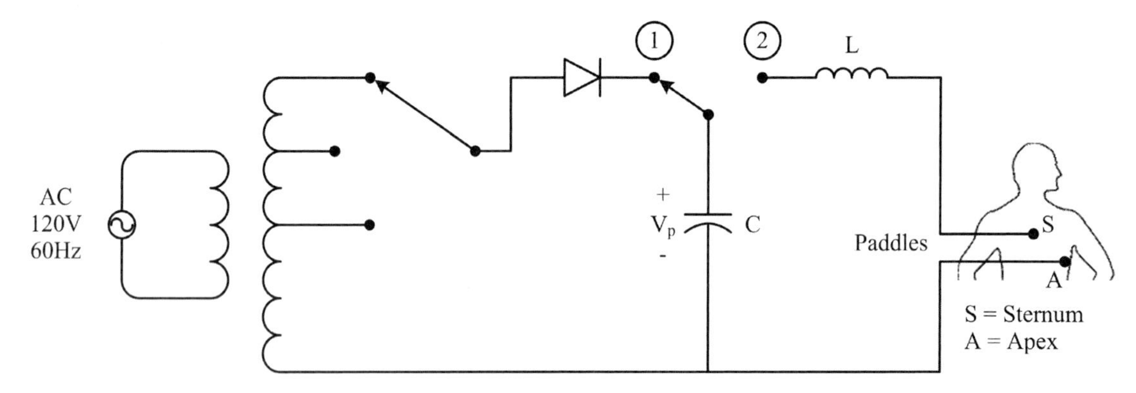

FIGURE 8-4a Defibrillator circuit for power calculation.

This energy is available for defibrillation; it can be varied by changing the output transformer's varactor setting.

In order to discharge the stored energy in the capacitor during fibrillation, flat electrodes called paddles are placed as follows: one on the right of the upper sternum (but below the clavicle) and one on the rib cage below the breast, wrapped toward the back (i.e., just above the apex of the heart). These paddles are called the sternum paddle and the apex paddle, respectively. (The sternum paddle should be placed to the side of the sternum because bone is not a good conductor of electricity.) When the paddles are positioned in this way, it is referred to as the "anterior-to-anterior" discharge position.

Another way of placing the paddles is in what is referred to as the "anterior-to-posterior" discharge position. In this position, one paddle is placed on the chest and the other is placed on the back. This allows the current to flow from the chest (anterior) to the back (posterior) by passing through the heart. Incorrect paddle placement will result in a large percentage of discharge current passing through non-cardiac tissue and thus will reduce the chances of successful defibrillation through failure to depolarize a critical mass of the myocardium.

In **Figure 8-4b,** the discharge circuit includes an inductor, the internal resistance of the defibrillator R_D, the electrode-skin resistance R_E, and the thorax (chest) resistance R_T.

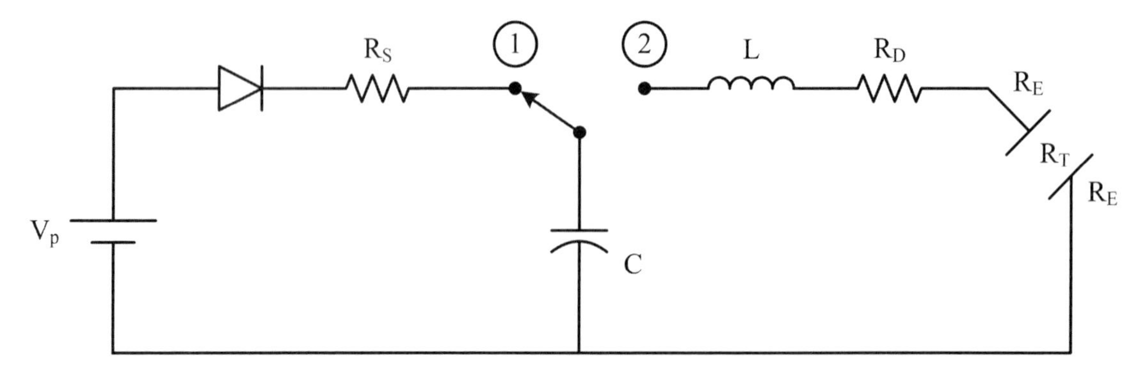

FIGURE 8-4b Resistance, capacitance, and inductance in the defibrillator circuit.

The discharge circuit resembles an RLC-series circuit and the actual energy delivered to the thorax can be calculated. We will neglect the inductance L at first and calculate the energy in joules. Later, we will include the inductance L in our calculation. The peak voltage V_p is constant for a short duration of T_D.

The total resistance in the circuit is given as:

$$R_{Total} = R_D + 2 \times R_E + R_T$$

Total available energy from the capacitor is:

$$W_C = \frac{1}{2} \times C \times V_p^2$$
$$= I_D^2 \times R_{Total} \times T_D$$

Where I_D is the defibrillator current in the discharge circuit, the current is given as:

$$I_D = \frac{V_p}{R_{Total}}$$

Apart from energy loss at the electrode-skin interface of each paddle, the energy delivered to the thorax is given as:

$$W_T = (I_D)^2 \times R_T \times T_D$$
$$W_T = (I_D)^2 \times (R_{Total} - 2 \times R_E - R_D) \times T_D$$

and the energy loss at each paddle is given as:

$$W_E = I_D^2 \times R_E \times T_D$$

If the inductor is placed in the circuit, then the delivered energy to the thorax is calculated using the Laplace transform. The initial voltage on the capacitor will be V_P and the circuit is analyzed as a step voltage response.

Using the Laplace transform (see **Figure 8-4c**), the voltage drop across R_T can be given as:

$$V_{R_T} = \frac{V_P \times \dfrac{R_T}{L}}{\left(s + \dfrac{R_{Total}}{2L}\right)^2 + \dfrac{1}{LC} - \left(\dfrac{R_{Total}}{2L}\right)^2}$$

This voltage can result in an overdamped, critically damped, or underdamped signal depending on the values of the capacitance, inductance, and resistance in the circuit. The conditions are:

overdamped when $\left(\dfrac{R_{Total}}{2L}\right) > \dfrac{1}{\sqrt{LC}}$,

critically damped when $\left(\dfrac{R_{Total}}{2L}\right) = \dfrac{1}{\sqrt{LC}}$,

and underdamped when $\left(\dfrac{R_{Total}}{2L}\right) < \dfrac{1}{\sqrt{LC}}$.

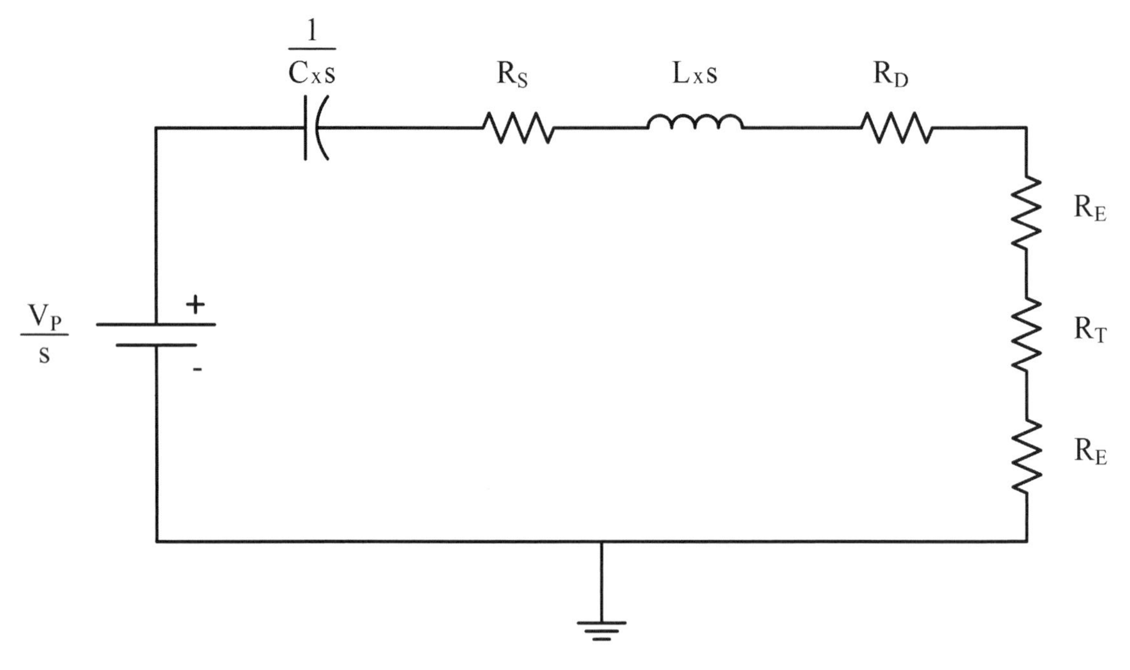

FIGURE 8-4c Laplace transformed defibrillator circuit.

Taking the inverse of the above equation, the underdamped signal in the time-domain is given as:

$$V_{R_T} = \frac{V_P \times R_T}{\omega L} \times e^{-(R_{Total}/2L)t} \times \sin wt$$

The resulting input and output voltages are shown in **Figure 8-4d.** The output is overdamped (indicated by "1"), then critically damped (indicated by "2"), and lastly the output is

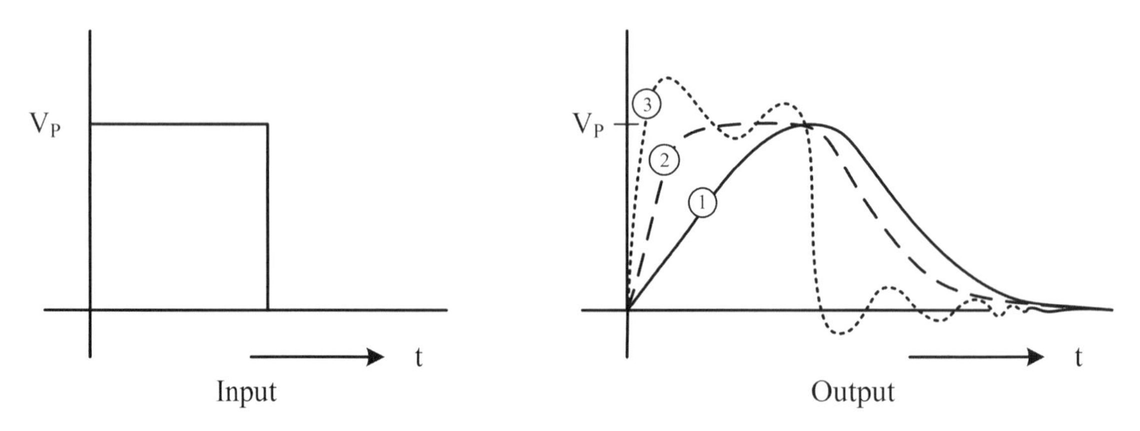

FIGURE 8-4d Input and output voltage waveforms in a defibrillator.

underdamped (indicated by "3"). These signals are produced by changing the time-constants of the defibrillator circuits.

EXERCISE Determine the available energy for a defibrillator when the defibrillator circuit has the following component values:

Internal resistance of the defibrillator = 12 ohms; skin-electrode resistance = 20 ohms; and the thorax resistance = 30 ohms. The ideal input square-wave pulse is 3,200 V for 4 msec duration.

Available energy $= (R_{Total} \times I_D^2 \times T_D) = V_P^2/R_{Total} \times T_D = 3200^2/82 \times 4 \text{ msec} = 499.51$ J ▪

EXERCISE Determine the defibrillator output signal with the same component values given in the previous exercise when the defibrillator inductance is 0.2 H and the capacitance is 20 μF.

$$R_{Total} = R_D + 2 \times R_E + R_T = 12\ \Omega + 2 \times 20\ \Omega + 30\ \Omega = 82\ \Omega$$

$$[(R_{Total}/2 \times L)^2 = (82/0.4)^2 = 42{,}025] < [1/(L \times C) = 1/(0.2 \times 20 \times 10^{-6}) = 250{,}000]$$

This results in an underdamped signal. Thereby, the result can be written as:

$$\text{Defibrillator output signal} = \left(\frac{(V_P \times R_{Total})}{(\omega \times L)}\right) e^{-(R_{Total}/2L)t} \times \sin wt$$

$$\text{where } \omega = \left[\left(\frac{1}{L \times C}\right) - \left(\frac{R_{Total}}{2 \times L}\right)^2\right]^{\frac{1}{2}}$$

▪

8.3 TYPES OF DEFIBRILLATORS

Figure 8-5a to **Figure 8-7** show the automatic external defibrillator (AED) machine and related concepts. Several hospitals in the United States are equipped with M-series monophasic and biphasic defibrillators. The portable units combine the defibrillator, ECG, noninvasive transcutaneous pacing (NTP), and other patient monitoring functions.

The buttons and switches on the front panel of the units are used for various operations including the display of the ECG. The various types of defibrillator operations and monitoring are:

- Manual defibrillation
- Advisory defibrillation
- Automated external defibrillation
- Synchronized cardioversion
- NTP
- ECG monitoring

Figure 8-5a shows the components of an AED unit. It consists of two large electrodes (pads), leads (cables), and a rechargeable battery source. The current flow between the

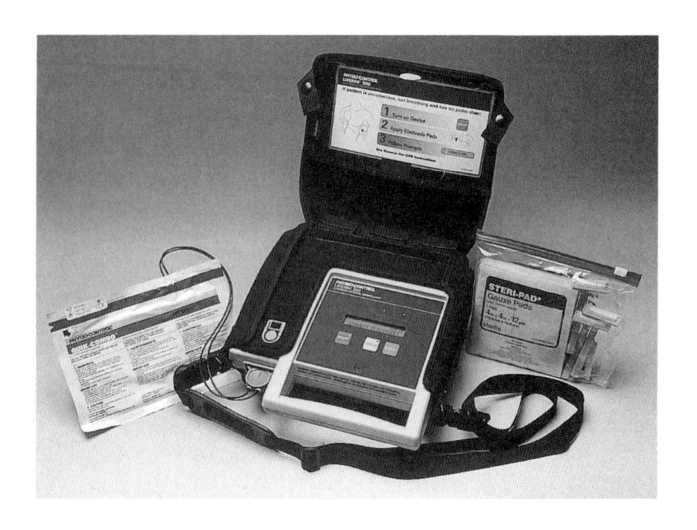

FIGURE 8-5a The automated external defibrillator (AED).

pads is either monophasic, biphasic, or triphasic. The placement of pads and the voltage waveforms are shown in **Figure 8-5b** and **Figure 8-5c.**

Figure 8-6 shows a block diagram of a biphasic unit. The system microprocessor in the main PCB board controls the charging and discharging of the capacitor. The patient's ECG, blood oxygen saturation, and blood pressure are continuously monitored before the shock button is pressed by the Emergency Medical Technician (EMT). The relay assembly with its biphasic bridge circuit delivers the brief but powerful shock of thousands of volts. The bridge enables the voltage to be applied to the chest in either direction. By changing the time duration of the positive and negative pulses, the energy delivered to the patient can

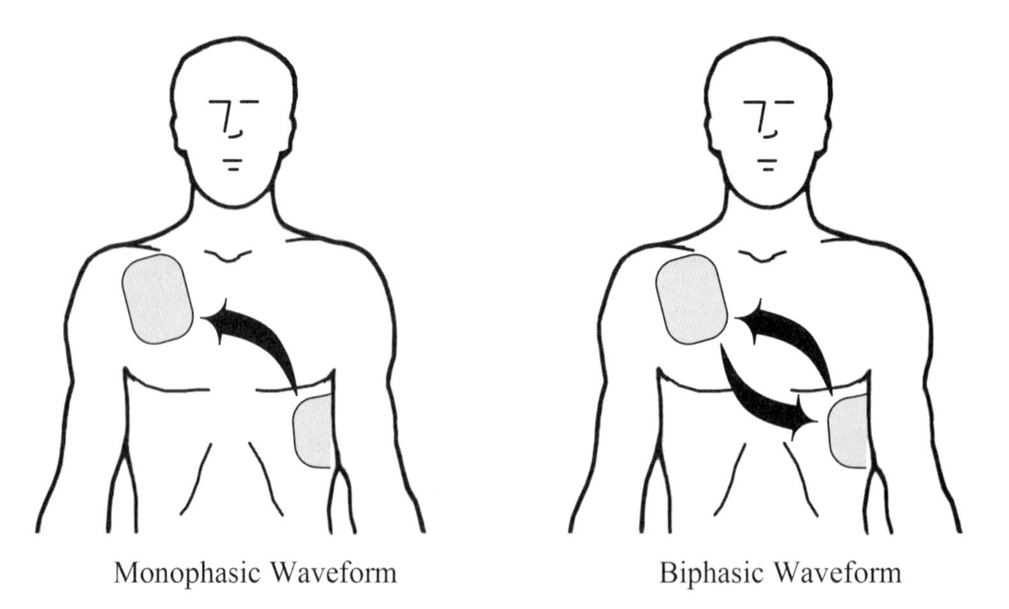

FIGURE 8-5b Position of monophasic and biphasic electrodes in a defibrillator.

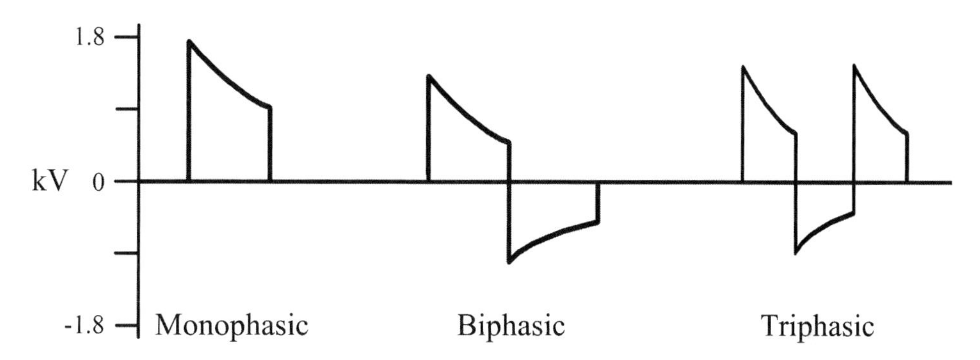

FIGURE 8-5c External defibrillator waveforms.

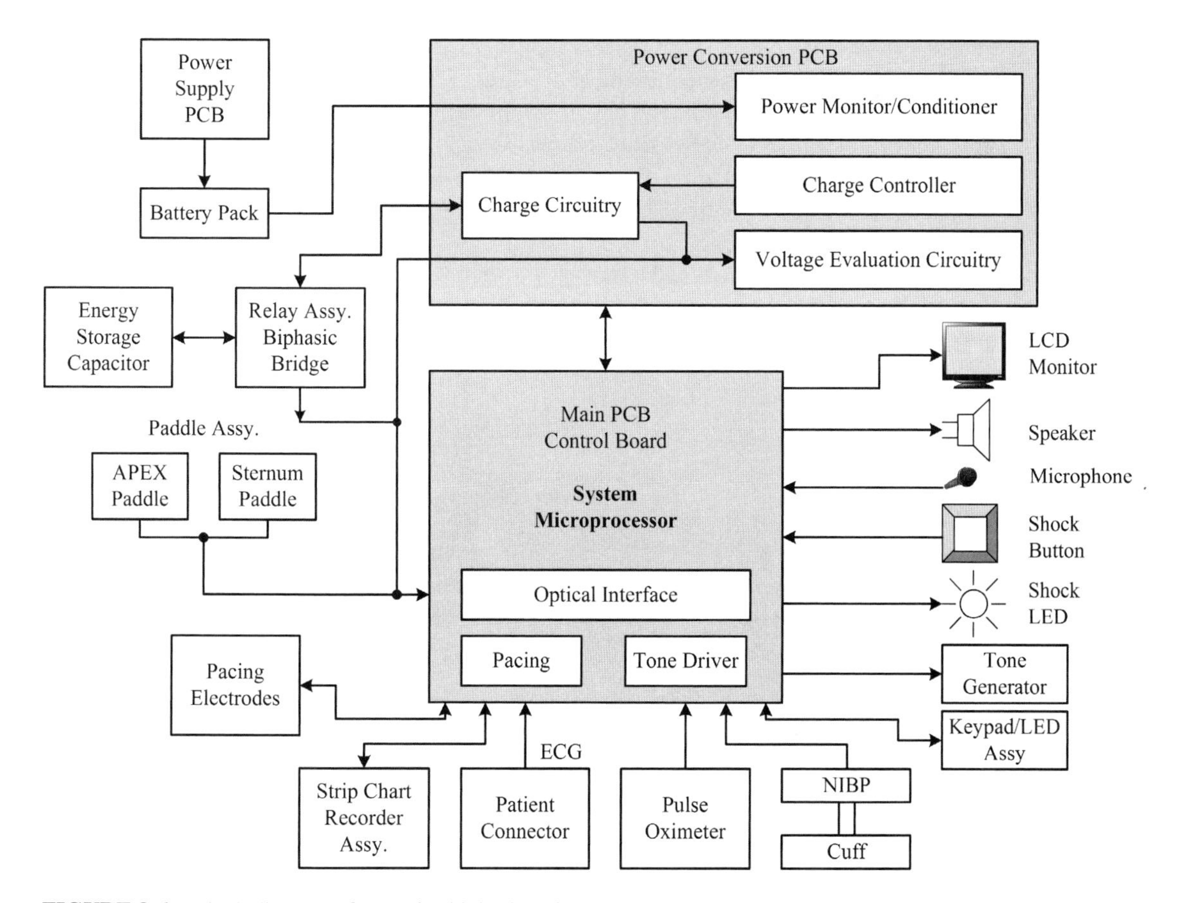

FIGURE 8-6 Block diagram of M-series biphasic unit.

be controlled. Because the current defibrillates the heart, the patient impedance changes the shape of the current waveform.

The biphasic waveform delivers the same amount of energy to every patient, but the shape of the waveform changes to provide the effectiveness for defibrillating the patient at each impedance value. The initial voltage remains the same, but the peak current depends on the patient impedance. The slope (tilt) and the time duration are adjusted for different patient impedances in order to maintain approximately 150 J for each shock. For example, for a 50-ohm patient, the current may start at 35 A and reduce to 10 A in 4 msec, whereas, for a 125-ohm patient, the current may start at 20 A and reduce to 5 A in 12 msec.

Generally, biphasic-waveform shocks are more effective than monophasic shocks in terminating ventricular fibrillation. In some cases, low-power triphasic-waveform shocks of equal duration are more effective than biphasic-waveform shocks of equal duration in terminating ventricular fibrillation.

Triphasic waveforms are composed with the polarity of the second pulse reversed (i.e., positive, negative, and positive). The first pulse acts as a "conditioning pre-pulse," the second pulse as an "exciting" or "defibrillating" pulse, and the third pulse acts as a "healing post-pulse," which ameliorates dysfunction caused by the first two pulses.

Most AEDs are equipped with primary and secondary batteries that must be adequately charged (some batteries may not need recharging for years). **Figure 8-7a** shows a rechargeable battery unit.

Figure 8-7b shows the placement of the defibrillator pads on the body. The pads are placed in anterior-to-anterior and anterior-to-posterior positions. The operation of the AED is shown in **Figure 8-7c.** The EMT follows the appropriate operation steps to perform an external defibrillation when a patient is in cardiac arrest. The round of shocks is only performed when the patient's pulse does not return.

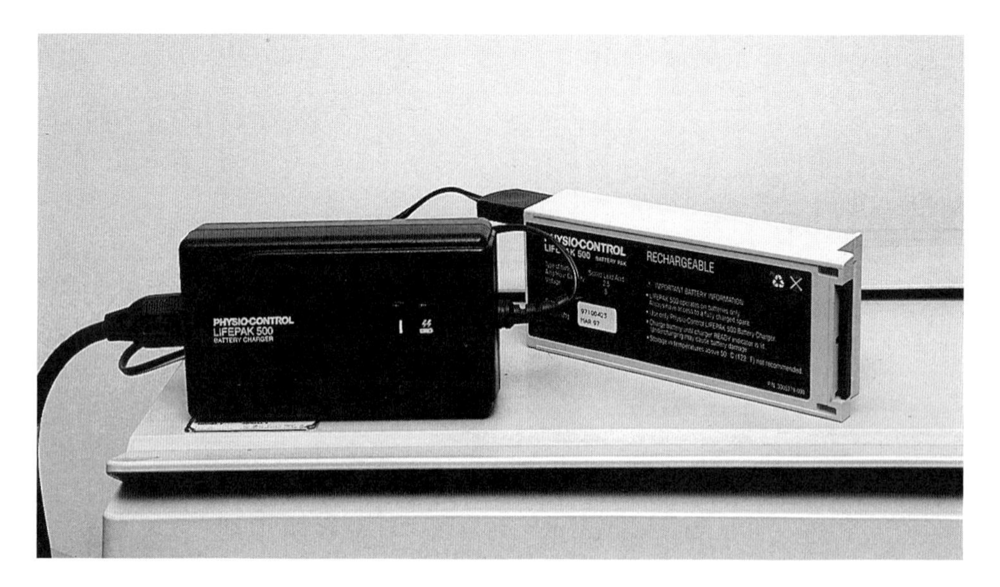

FIGURE 8-7a Rechargeable battery in AED.

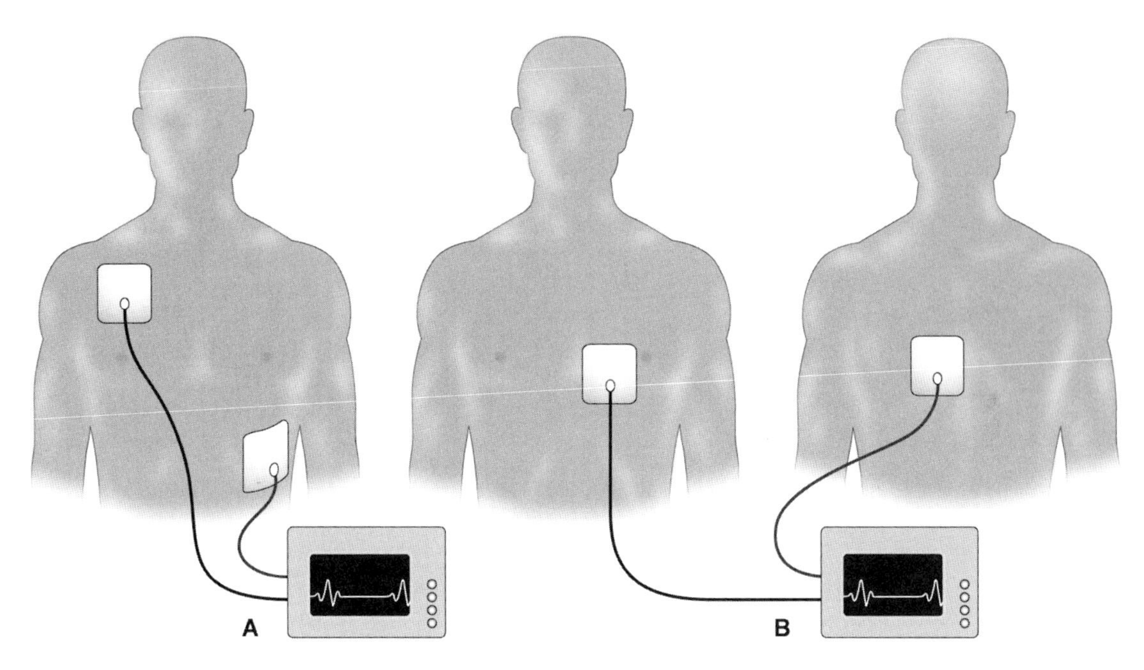

FIGURE 8-7b AED pads.

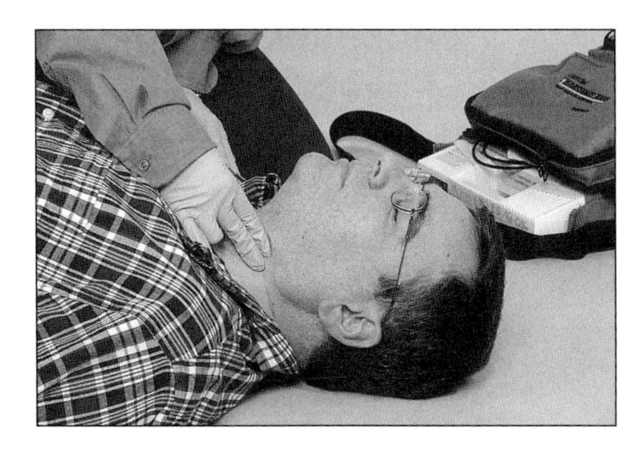

STEP 1 The EMT must confirm that the patient is in cardiac arrest.

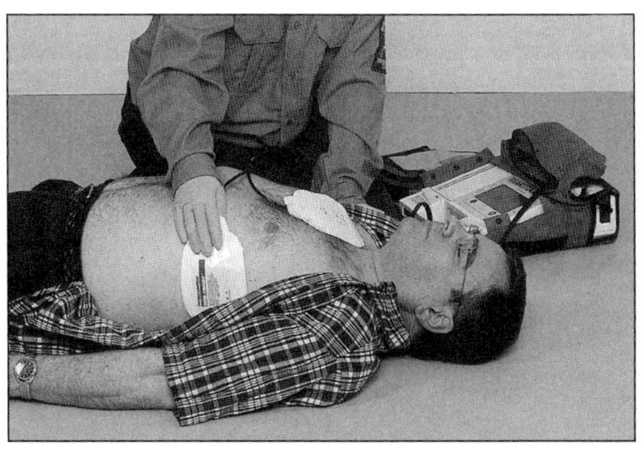

STEP 2 The EMT applies the electrode pads to the anterior chest wall, one to the apex of the heart at the lower left rib cage and the other to the right sternal border below the clavicle.

FIGURE 8-7c Operation steps of an AED. (*continued*)

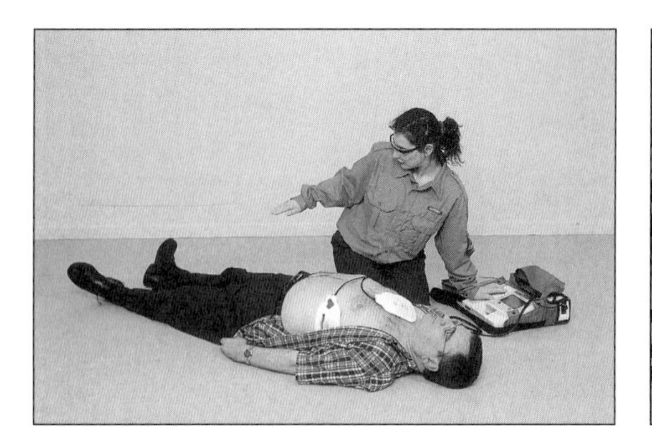

STEP 3 The EMT then turns the power on the AED while calling *"all clear."* The EMT must ensure that no one is touching the patient.

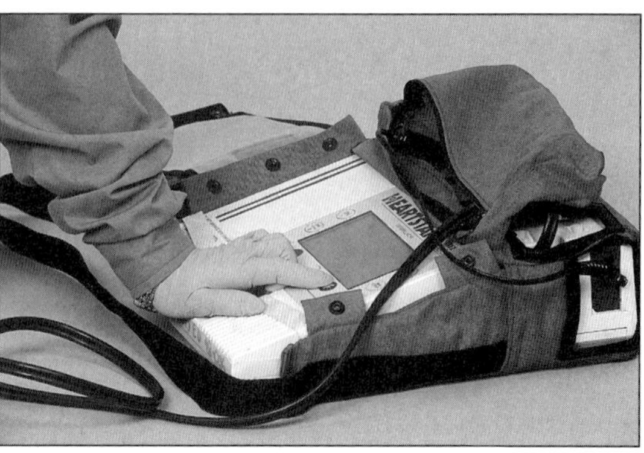

STEP 4 The EMT then presses the *analyze* button and presses the *shock* button, as advised. Again, the EMT must ensure that no one is touching the patient.

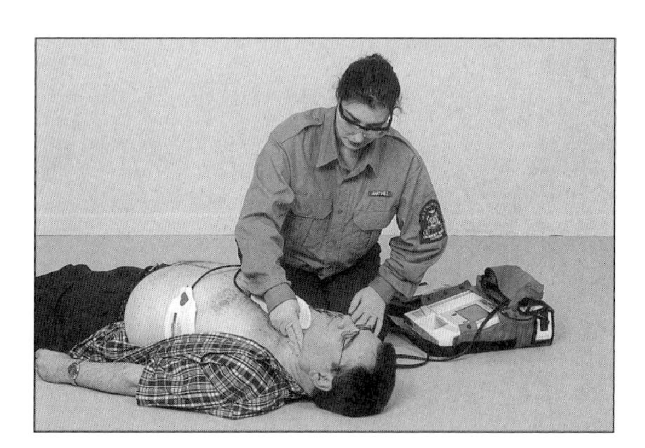

STEP 5 After the series of shocks has been performed, the EMT must check for the presence or absence of a pulse. If the pulse is absent, then CPR must be continued for another minute. If the patient's pulse returns, then the EMT checks for breathing. If the patient's pulse does not return, then another round of shocks may be indicated.

FIGURE 8-7c *(continued)*

AED Technical Specifications

The following table provides specifications of a portable, lightweight, battery-operated automated external defibrillator to treat patients requiring basic and optional advanced cardiac life support.

Weight (complete unit excluding batteries)	5 pounds (lb)
Safety	Must comply with IEC 601-1 for leakage currents
ECG signal	0.5 Hz to 40 Hz frequency response, via disposable defibrillation electrodes, LCD display
Optional manual mode (low energy)	Settings 5 joules (J) to 50 J
Optional manual mode (high energy)	Settings 70 J, 100 J, 150 J, 200 J, 300 J, 360 J
Basic AED mode	200 J, 300 J, 360 J
Charging time	360 J in 8 seconds
Rechargeable nickel metal hydride battery system	80 shocks at 360 J/150 minutes of monitoring
Non-rechargeable lithium battery system	200 shocks at 360 J/360 minutes of monitoring
Prompts	13-volume adjustable audible prompts 13-text prompts on LCD display
Biphasic waveform	Truncated exponential
Paddle (adult size)	8–9 cm diameter

Implantable Cardioverter Defibrillator (ICD)

Some heart rhythm disorders, such as premature ventricular complexes (PVC), ventricular tachycardia, and recurrent fibrillation, are considered ventricular dysrhythmias. A physician may choose to surgically implant into the patient an implantable cardioverter defibrillator (ICD). This device detects these disorders and automatically delivers shocks to terminate such rhythm disorders. **Figure 8-8** shows where the ICD is surgically implanted onto the patient's chest wall.

The ICD detects any irregularities using a microprocessor chip, similar to pacemaker technology. The other components of the device are the cardioverter/defibrillator generator, ventricular lead electrode, and the cardioversion electrode. One electrode is affixed into the muscle of the right ventricle and the other is affixed to the surface of the superior vena cava.

Upon detection of any irregularity, the device delivers a series of low-energy electrical discharges (<1 J). If the device determines this insufficient, it delivers a series of high-energy discharges (between 1 J and 25 J). The implantation cost of this device is relatively high, but it is remarkably effective.

Cardioverters

In some types of arrhythmias, it is necessary to avoid delivering the shock during the T wave when the ventricles refract. Otherwise, ventricular fibrillation may occur. A cardioverter

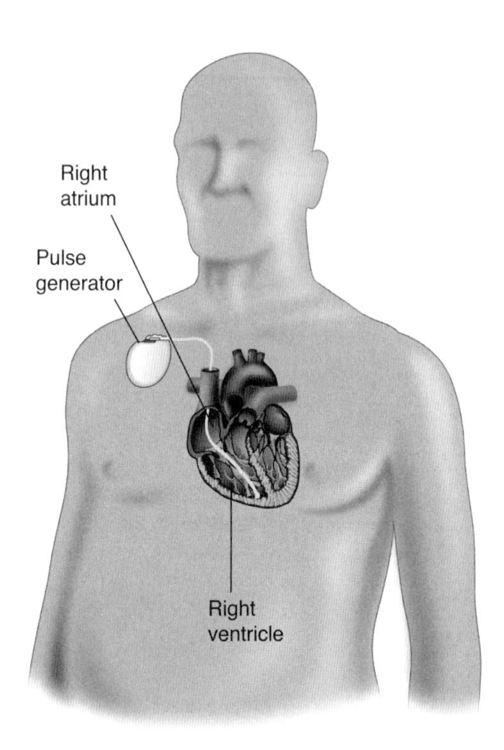

FIGURE 8-8 An automatic implantable cardioverter defibrillator.

device ensures that the delivery of shock pulses is timed immediately after the R wave and before the start of the T wave.

On AEDs, the switch has two positions: one for the defibrillator mode and one for the cardioverter mode. The circuit can discriminate the R wave over other waves. Even though R waves have larger amplitude, the slope of the R wave is different from the T wave. Based on the amplitude and the slope, the shock is delivered approximately 30 msec after the peak of the R wave.

8.4 SAFETY ISSUES IN DEFIBRILLATORS

Delivery of the defibrillator shock is provided by trained personnel. The steps are as follows: 1) prepare the paddles, 2) apply paddles to the body, 3) charge the defibrillator, and 4) deliver the shock. The AED uses voice prompts. They are generally as follows: 1) *attach pads;* 2) *stand clear;* 3) *press "shock";* 4) *check pads;* 5) *check pulse;* 6) *check patient;* 7) *if no pulse, perform CPR;* 8) *press "analyze";* and 9) *no shock advised.*

In addition to these prompts, the following conditions are possible on the *press analyze* display:

- when the unit is charged but no shock is delivered
- 70 seconds after completion of an analysis
- 70 seconds after delivery of the third shock in the three-analyses sequence

The *no shock advised* display appears when the ECG analysis determines that a normal rhythm is detected. Following the *press shock* display, all persons around the patient are prompted to *stand clear* prior to the defibrillator discharge. No one should be touching the bed, the patient, or any equipment connected to the patient. The patient's body should not be touching the bed frame or any metal objects. In some AEDs, a tone will sound continuously for 10 seconds, followed by an intermittent beeping for 5 seconds. The shock must be delivered within this 15-seconds interval; otherwise, the defibrillator will disarm itself.

8.5 THEORY OF PACEMAKERS

A pacemaker allows people with an irregular heart rate to lead a healthier and more normal lifestyle. The electric current generated from the pacemaker stimulates the heart causing proper contractions. This stimulation improves cardiac output, which helps to regulate oxygen intake.

A pacemaker is used in patients whose heart's electrical system, or "spark plug," is not functioning normally. This "spark plug" is actually the SA node, located in the right atrium. The normal sequence of the impulse travel through the heart muscle can be explained as follows:

The electrical impulse travels through the right and left atria when this SA node "fires." This signals both of these chambers to contract. The blood is then pumped into the ventricles. The impulse then travels to the AV node into the ventricles and signals the ventricles to contract. Blood is then pumped to the lungs and throughout the body. The contraction of the heart chambers is called the sinus rhythm. This process occurs 60 to 80 times every minute. The SA node is the heart's own natural pacemaker—a normal heart follows the sinus rhythm continuously without any physiological interruption.

Generally, the indication for pacemaker placement is a slow heart rate or a defect in the electrical conduction system of the heart. Lightheadedness (dizziness) and the loss of consciousness (fainting) are some of the symptoms in patients with slow heart rates. Partial or complete heart block may slow down the heart rate also.

A pacemaker device can take over the role of the heart's own natural pacemaker. The artificial pacemaker can be either an external pacemaker or a temporary or permanent internal (implanted) pacemaker.

8.6 TYPES OF PACEMAKERS

The pacemaker's primary function is pacing the heart; its secondary function is sensing for intrinsic signals. Pacemakers are designed to use one of three different response types: asynchronous (fixed rate), inhibited (the pacemaker does not generate output in the presence of a sensed cardiac activity), or triggered (the pacemaker generates output in response to a sensed cardiac activity). The inhibited-response and triggered-response pacemakers are called "demand" type pacemakers, in which a pacing pulse is only delivered when demanded by the heart. Typically, demand pacemakers sense the atrial rate and apply stimuli only during periods when the atrial rate falls below the desired pacing rate. Pacemakers can be categorized in several ways: they can be defined with a code of three letters or they can be unipolar, bipolar, single-chamber, or dual-chamber pacemakers. First, we will discuss the codes used to define different types of pacemakers.

The following letters are used in the code:

- A (Atrial)
- V (Ventricular)
- D (Dual [both] chambers)

- I (Inhibited)
- T (Triggered)
- O (Not applicable)
- R (Rate responsive)

The codes used to define different types of pacemakers consist of a series of five letters, the first three of which are usually emphasized. In the order of their placement in the code, letters 1 to 5 indicate: 1) chamber(s) paced; 2) chamber(s) sensed; 3) mode of response; 4) rate modulation programmability; and 5) the anti-tachycardia and anti-arrhythmia function(s). The following text provides several examples of these codes.

VVI

This type of pacemaker paces the ventricle as well as sensing it, but the pacemaker's response is inhibited, or limited to a specific range of sensory input from the ventricle. This means that the pacemaker will pace the ventricle if there is a need. For this reason, this type of pacemaker is known as a "demand" pacemaker. These types are typically used after bypass surgeries.

VOO

This type of pacemaker paces the ventricle, but since it does not sense the ventricles, there is no response to sensory input. The pacemaker fires at a fixed rate. This type of pacing is achieved after bypass surgery with a handheld external pacemaker.

DVI

This type of pacemaker paces both (dual) the atrium and the ventricle, though it senses the ventricle only, and its response to sense is inhibited.

DDD

Both chambers are paced and both chambers are sensed and the pacemaker responds to sensory input from both chambers. This type is most commonly used in dual-chamber pacing and is the most expensive.

VVIR

The ventricle is paced and sensed, and the pacemaker's response to sensory input is inhibited. However, the difference between the **VVIR** type and the **VVI** type is that the **VVIR** is rate responsive. That means that the patient's physical activity can change the rate of the pacing.

Based on the heart condition, the physician decides the type of pacemaker the patient needs and sets the minimum heart rate programmed on the selected pacemaker. Once the pacemaker senses that the heart rate is below the set rate, it generates an electrical impulse that travels to the heart chamber through the pacemaker lead. The impulse then causes the heart muscle to contract, and the proper heart rate is restored.

Figure 8-9a shows the upper chest area where the pacemaker is surgically implanted. This is the most common method and is called the endocardial approach, or transvenous approach. The surgery is performed under local anesthesia and takes only a couple of hours.

The pacemaker and its leads are inserted through the chest skin. The pacemaker stays in a pocket under the upper chest skin, whereas the leads are inserted into the veins and guided to reach the heart chambers and the heart muscle. The fluoroscopy machine guides in visualizing the lead insertion and its movement through the vein.

There is another method, shown in **Figure 8-9a**, which is called the epicardial approach. In this method, the pacemaker is placed under the skin in the abdomen. The leads are then attached to the heart muscle under general anesthesia. The recovery time is longer in this method compared to the endocardial approach.

They can also be defined as dual-chamber or biventricular pacemakers. In a dual-chamber pacemaker, one lead reaches to the right atrium and another reaches to the right

FIGURE 8-9a Placement of a pacemaker.

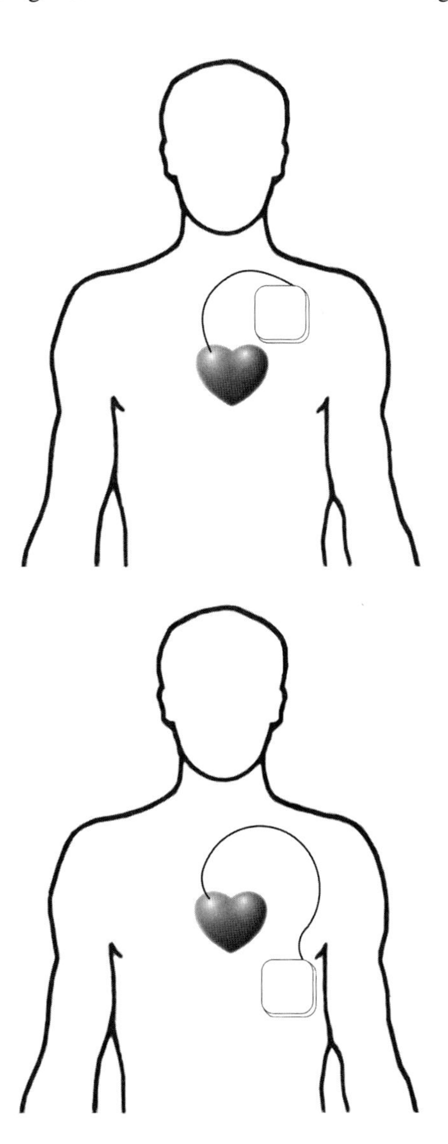

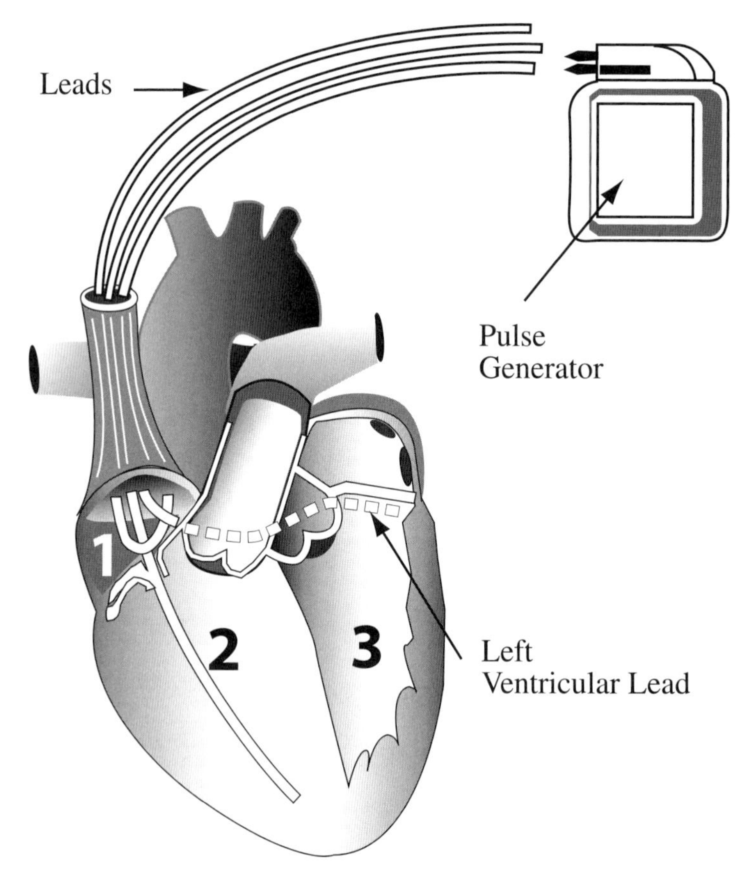

FIGURE 8-9b Pacemaker wires to the heart.

ventricle. In a biventricular pacemaker, there are three leads reaching to the heart chambers: one lead to the right atrium, the second to the right ventricle, and the third reaches to the left ventricle via the coronary sinus vein. This is shown in **Figure 8-9b.**

8.7 PACEMAKER CIRCUIT

A pacemaker has three components:

1. **Pacemaker electronic circuit:**

   This is kept in a small metal case and the circuit is connected to a battery. The circuit generates the impulses at a specific time.

2. **Pacing leads:**

   These insulated wires carry the impulses to the heart.

3. **Programmer:**

   This is kept in the hospital or clinic to program the pacemaker and to adjust the settings of impulse amplitudes and the frequency. The programmer is a specialized computer with a hardware and software interface.

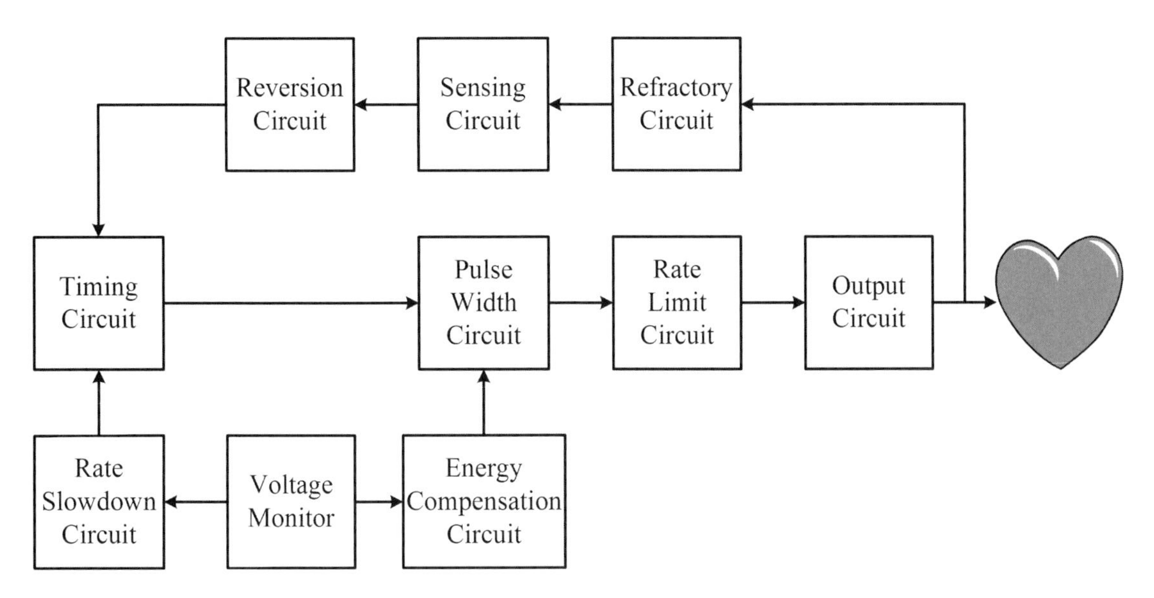

FIGURE 8-10a Block diagram of a pacemaker.

A block diagram of a pacemaker is given in **Figure 8-10a.**

The timing circuit determines the pacing rate of the impulse, whereas the pulse width circuit determines the duration of the impulse. Additionally, the rate limit circuit limits the pacing rate so as not to exceed 120 pulses per minute. An output circuit delivers the impulse to the heart after amplifying the impulse signal. Later, after a certain delay in the refractory circuit, the R wave is sensed and the timing circuit is adjusted by the reversion circuit for the delivery of the next impulse to the heart. The voltage monitor circuit checks the battery voltage and signals to the rate slowdown circuit and energy compensation circuit when battery voltage drops to a threshold voltage. The rate slowdown circuit restricts the current to the timing circuit, thereby decreasing the number of pulses delivered, while the energy compensation circuit increases the duration of each pulse. Together, these three circuits ensure that an adequate amount of stimulation energy reaches the heart at all times.

8.8 TECHNICAL SPECIFICATION OF A PACEMAKER

Several different types of pacemakers are manufactured in the United States. The following table lists some common technical specifications of pacemakers.

Pacing modes	VVI, VVT, VVO, AAI, AAT, AOO, OFF
Basic pacing rates	Between 30 bpm and 120 bpm
Pulse widths	Between 0.122 msec and 1.952 msec, in steps of 0.122 msec
Refractory periods	Between 203 msec and 438 msec, in steps of 15.625 msec

(*Continued*)

Sensitivities	Between 0.5 mV and 4.0 mV, in steps of 0.5 mV
Hysteresis	Between 0% and 20%, in steps of 5%
Electrical configuration for pacing	Monopolar/bipolar
Electrical configuration for sensing	Monopolar/bipolar
Maximum rate in tachycardia treatment	Between 60 bpm and 150 bpm
Battery chemistry	Lithium-iodide
Initial voltage	2.8 V
Maximum available capacity	1.66 ampere-hours (Ah)
Mass	38 g
Case material	Titanium
Electrode material	Titanium coated with iridium oxide (located at the tip of the lead)
Lead body	Polyurethane
Means of attachment	Titanium alloy screws

Pacemaker Calculations

The energy delivered by the pacemaker in pulses to the heart depends on the magnitude and width of each pulse and the duration between the pulses. As shown in **Figure 8-10b,** V_P is the magnitude of the stimulus voltage, τ_P is the pulse width, and T is the time duration between pulses. The energy delivered by the pacemaker during each pulse is then given as:

$$W_P = I_P^2 \times R_H \times \tau_P + (I_P \times R_H) \times I_D \times T$$

where

$$I_P = \frac{V_P}{R_H}$$

R_H = Electrode-heart resistance

I_D = Battery drain current when the pulse is off

The energy is measured in joules. The battery drain current is low compared with the magnitude of the pulse current.

We can also calculate the lifetime (in years) of a pacemaker battery if we know of the magnitude of the pulse, pulse width, time between pulses (i.e., period of the pulse), drain current, electrode-heart resistance, and the battery current rating in ampere-hours (Ah).

First, we calculate the energy in joules stored in a pacemaker battery:

$$\text{Battery energy in joules} = (\text{current rating in ampere-hours}) \times (\text{pulse amplitude in volts}) \times 3{,}600 \text{ seconds per hour}$$

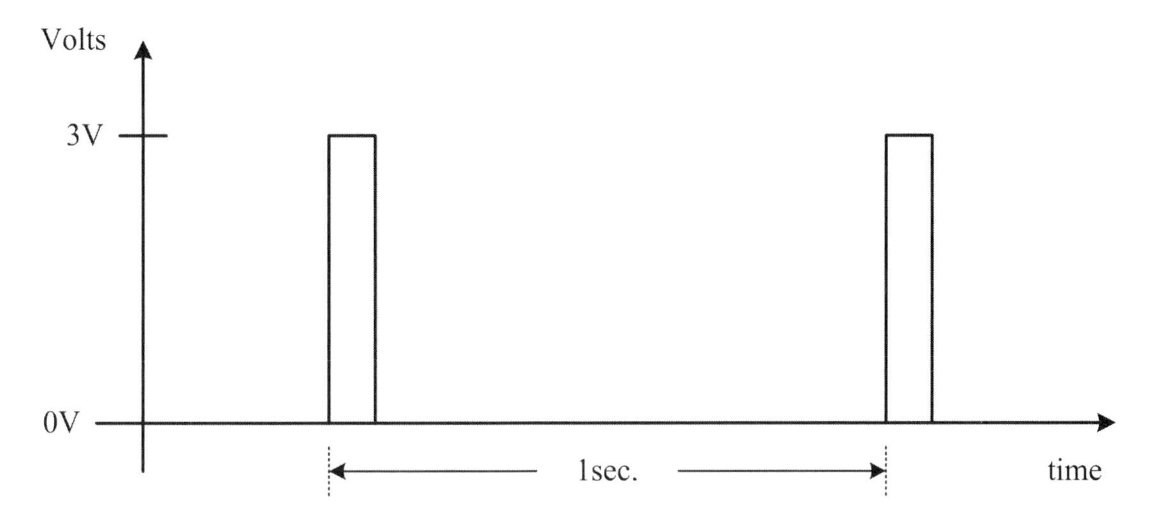

FIGURE 8-10b An ideal pacemaker signal.

Because the dimensions of the volts and amperes are joules/coulomb and coulombs/second, respectively, the resulting unit of battery energy is in joules.

Next, we calculate the battery lifetime in years:

$$\text{Battery lifetime in years} = \frac{(\text{battery energy in joules})}{(\text{energy per pulse in joules})} \times \frac{(\text{pulse period in seconds})}{(3{,}600 \times 24 \times 365)}$$

8.9 DEFIBRILLATOR AND PACEMAKER SIMULATORS

A patient simulator performs tests on defibrillators, pacemakers, and several other types of medical devices and measures and reports various performance parameters of these equipments and devices. It can report the output energy, voltage, current charge time, and discharge time of a defibrillator. In pacemakers, it can measure and report peak current, pulse width, and the refractory periods.

A patient simulator can simulate the human body with a resistance of 50 ohms. When a defibrillator is connected to a patient simulator, a specified energy from the defibrillator discharges into the 50-ohm patient simulator load. These simulators also may be referred to as defibrillator analyzers or pacer analyzers. They combine the complete testing functions of a defibrillator tester, an external pacemaker analyzer, and a true 12-lead ECG arrhythmia simulator into one compact instrument.

SUMMARY

- A pacemaker regulates a patient's heartbeat and a defibrillator shocks the heart to return to normal rhythm. Both of them are essentially helping the heart to "come to its senses" in a way!

- Defibrillation is the treatment for life-threatening arrhythmias, ventricular fibrillation, and ventricular tachycardia. A defibrillator is a device that delivers a therapeutic dose of electrical energy to the affected heart. This depolarizes the heart, terminates the arrhythmias, and allows the normal sinus rhythm to be re-established.
- The defibrillator circuit consists of a large capacitor charge circuit and a discharge circuit. The charge circuit has a high-voltage transformer and a diode rectifier, while the discharge circuit has resistors, a large inductor, and two chest electrodes.
- Safety is always important in using defibrillators and similar equipment. The AED is equipped with such features as voice prompts, beepers, and LCD display for warning purposes.
- Nearly all pacemakers are implanted to treat a slow heartbeat. The pacemaker system includes the pacemaker itself and wires that connect the pacemaker to the heart. The pacemaker contains a battery and electronic circuits. Single-chamber pacemakers have only one wire connected to the heart, while dual-chamber pacemakers have wires connected to both the top and bottom chambers of the heart.

MEDICAL TERMINOLOGY

Automated external defibrillator (AED): electronic device that externally shocks the heart to re-establish normal cardiac rhythm.

Cardiac arrest: a sudden cessation of the heart's activity and failure of the heart to maintain functional circulation.

Cardiopulmonary resuscitation (CPR): a life-saving procedure consisting of artificial respiration and manual external cardiac compression.

Cardioverter: a machine used to administer an electric shock after approximately 30 microseconds of the R-wave peak. The machine is equipped with the synchronizer circuit in such a way to avoid shocking the patient into unintended serious arrhythmia or ventricular fibrillation.

Endocardial: situated or generated within the heart. For example, endocardial murmurs.

Implantable cardioverter defibrillator (ICD): a device used to shock the heart by utilizing leads implanted in the heart or on the surface. The leads are used to deliver electrical shocks, sense cardiac rhythm, and pace the heart to establish normal rhythm.

Pacing: setting the rate of, or regulating the speed of, something (e.g., a pacemaker).

Ventricular fibrillations: irregular, rapid, and ineffective contractions of the ventricles in the heart. A patient will have no heartbeat, no palpable pulse, no respiration, and no blood circulation leading to cardiac arrest if not reversed by electric defibrillation.

Ventricular tachycardia: a condition of abnormally accelerated ventricular rhythm in which the heart muscles contract in an irregularly rapid and uncoordinated manner. The condition is a complex rhythm on the ECG with a rate of 150 to 200 beats per minute.

QUIZ

1. Synchronized cardioversion is another type of electrical therapy used to treat arrhythmias other than ____________________.
2. Defibrillator paddles should not be placed over the sternum because bone is not a good ____________________.

3. During a vulnerable period represented by the T wave (on the ECG trace), an electrical stimulus could cause ________________.
4. A lithium-iodide battery in a pacemaker stores ________________ if the battery rating is 1 Ah with a terminal voltage of 1.5 V.
   a) 6,000 J b) 5,400 J c) 1.5 J d) None of the above
5. Defibrillators discharge a strong electrical current through the patient's heart and attempt to shock the ________________ to resume its control.
   a) AV node b) Bundle of HIS c) SA node d) Purkinje fibers
6. The implantable defibrillator can protect patients from severe ________________.
   a) Ventricular tachycardia b) Bradycardia
   c) Mitral valve prolapse d) None of the above
7. The defibrillator circuit is responsible for three major functions:
   a) Charging the high voltage capacitor
   b) Providing feedback on the high voltage capacitor's voltage level
   c) ________________
8. Five causes of ventricular fibrillation are:
   a) Hypothermia. b) Electrocution.
   c) ________________. d) ________________.
   e) ________________.
9. A defibrillator discharges to the chest 200 J, 300 J, and ________________.
10. Most patients with ICDs have been ________________ at least once from a ________________.

RESEARCH TOPICS

1. Collect data or information on electromagnetic interference on pacemakers, either the external type or internal type or ICDs. Hint: The interference may come from cell phones, CB radios, microwave ovens, or x-ray machines (in hospitals and/or airports).
2. Defibrillator failure may be catastrophic; it is essential to find the causes for these problems and provide recommendations to prevent future failures. Write a research paper to assess the failures covering a variety of defibrillators, both external and internal.

CASE STUDY

A case study is recommended on the Philips Heartstream AED. This defibrillator is widely used in and outside of hospitals. The study may include technical specifications and its comparison with other AEDs.

PROBLEMS

1. What part of an ECG signal is most useful for the heart rate calculation? Explain.

2. For an ideal square-wave defibrillator, determine the energy delivered to the patient (see **Figure 8-11**).

   Given: Skin-electrode resistance = 25 Ω
   Internal resistance of the defibrillator = 5 Ω
   Thorax resistance = 30 Ω

FIGURE 8-11 An ideal defibrillator voltage.

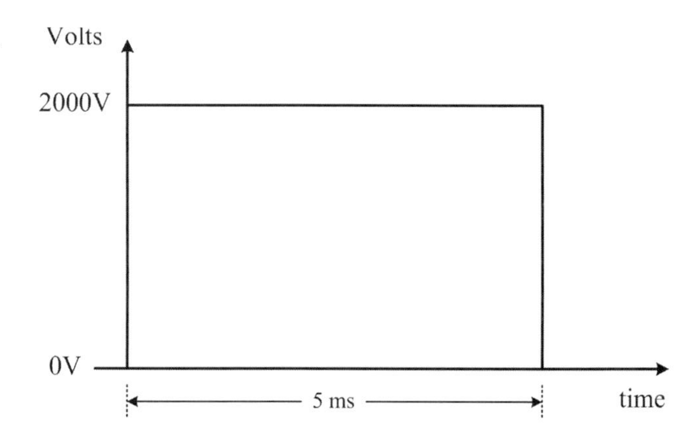

3. Given a situation when a fully charged defibrillator capacitor discharges through the chest, determine the current (peak) through the thorax and the voltage drop (peak) across the thorax.

   Where: L = Inductance of the defibrillator
   R_S = Internal resistance of the defibrillator
   R_E = Skin-electrode resistance/paddle
   R_T = Thorax resistance

   The charged voltage across the capacitor is 3,000 V. The value of the capacitor is 10 μF. Roughly sketch the voltage with respect to time. You may also use MATLAB, SIMULINK, or any other simulation software to plot the voltage (see **Figure 8-12**).

FIGURE 8-12 Defibrillator circuit values.

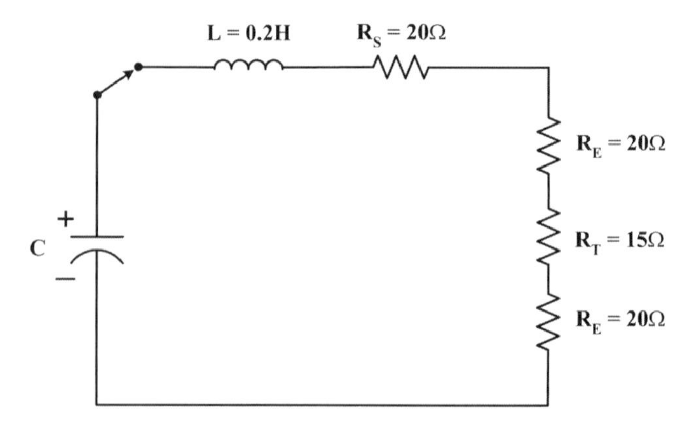

4. Determine the value of the capacitor when the circuit of Problem 3 becomes overdamped or critically damped. Compute the thorax voltage for the overdamped case.
5. Draw a flowchart starting when the patient is having either ventricular fibrillation or pulseless ventricular tachycardia until the patient receives the maximum defibrillation energy in joules.
6. In a certain defibrillator, a constant ideal voltage of 1,800 V is measured across the electrodes for 5 msec, and then the voltage drops to 0 V. The delivered energy is 200 J. Compute the energy delivered when the constant ideal voltage:

   a) drops to 900 V and the duration of the pulse remains 5 msec.

   b) drops to 900 V and the duration of the pulse is 10 msec.
7. Calculate the energy delivered by each pulse from a pacemaker from the given pulse signal as shown in **Figure 8-13**.

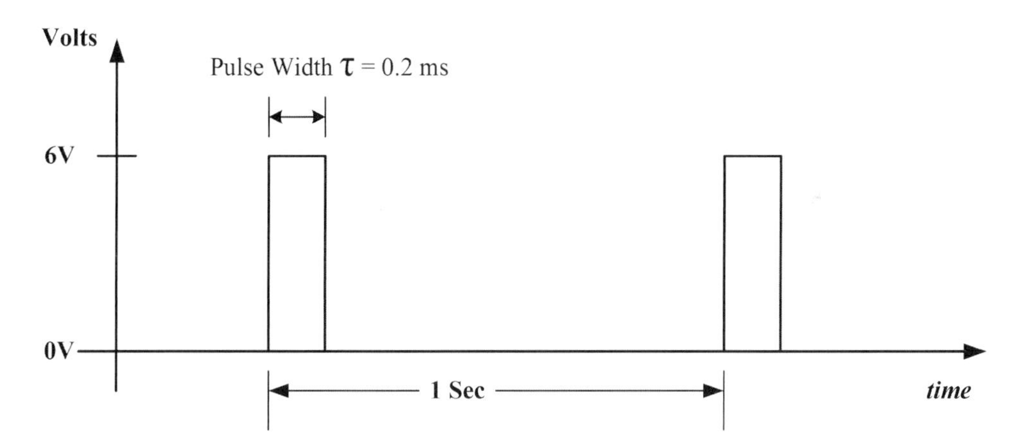

FIGURE 8-13 Pacemaker signal.

8. Design a pulse oscillator circuit for the pulse signal given in Problem 7.
9. Calculate the battery life in years when the pacemaker has the following characteristics:

   Battery ampere-hours (Ah) = 1.2; pulse voltage = 2 V; pulse width = 1 msec; pulse time period = 1 sec; electrode-heart resistance = 150 ohms; current drain on the battery = 1.3 μA.
10. A simple pacemaker is made with two multivibrators connected in series. The first one is an astable multivibrator, the second one is a monostable multivibrator. The output is taken from the monostable multivibrator. Discuss these two types of multivibrators and the rationale of them connected in series.
11. Design the circuit with op amps, resistors, and capacitors for a pacemaker operating with a pulse amplitude of 2 V to 10 V, a pulse width of 0.1 msec to 0.2 msec, and a pulse rate of 30 bpm to 150 bpm. You may use the Internet for this problem.

Instrumentation in Blood Circulation

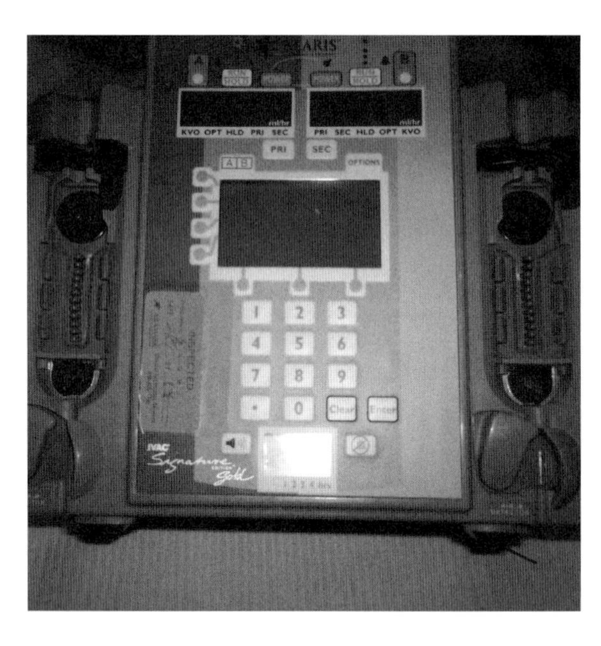

CHAPTER OUTLINE

OBJECTIVES

The objective of this chapter is to introduce the reader to the dynamics of blood circulation through the heart, the lungs, and the rest of the body. The reader will also learn the biomedical instrumentation used to measure blood pressure, blood flow, blood volume, oxygen delivery, and the corresponding electrical signals. Infusion pumps, their uses and varieties, and the process of catheterization are discussed at the end of the chapter to further familiarize the reader with biomedical instruments and their applications.

Upon completion of this chapter, the reader will be able to:

- Define cardiac output.
- Calculate mean arterial pressure.
- Calculate vascular resistance and compliance.

- Describe the differences among various types of sphygmomanometers.
- Describe the problems in pressure monitors.

INTERNET WEB SITES

http://www.hemodynamicsociety.org (Hemodynamic Society)
http://www.circ.ahajournals.org (American Heart Association, Journal Circulation)

INTRODUCTION

Understanding the behavior and nature of arterial blood flow is important in condition diagnoses and treatment decisions made by vascular physicians. For example, common conditions such as atherosclerosis occur when fatty material, such as cholesterol, is deposited along the walls of arteries, forming plaques and atheromas. This can cause stenosis, or narrowing, of the arteries, thus obstructing normal blood flow. Under such circumstances, not enough oxygen-carrying blood is carried to the areas of the body that need it. Stenosis can affect any part of the body. For example, if the brain is affected, a stroke may occur. When the heart is affected, it may result in angina chest pain or a heart attack. Stenosis is more likely to occur in smaller diameter blood vessels, as well as in portions of blood vessels that are very narrow and curved, since these are more susceptible to blockage from a buildup of plaque. Rapid blood flow, such as that found in the straight portions of blood vessels, creates a frictional force that can protect those areas against atherosclerosis, essentially "scrubbing" the vessel walls clean of potentially dangerous buildups.

This chapter introduces the blood flow related equations and the hemodynamic state as defined by the mean arterial pressure (MAP) and stroke index (SI, an indexed blood flow per beat), and emphasizes that every heartbeat is considered important for the patient's health.

With the advances in vascular technology and sonography, and the resulting decrease in the need for invasive procedures, the demand for Circulation Technologists and Cardiovascular Technologists in hospitals is increasing in the United States. These technologists operate, monitor, maintain, calibrate, and test diagnostic and therapeutic equipment such as heart-lung machines, intra-aortic balloon pumps, specialized catheters, and implanted devices.

9.1 PHYSICS OF PRESSURE AND FLOW

Fluid mechanics are the properties and movement of fluids when they are under the influence of a force. Of particular interest, not only to physicians but also to bioengineers, is the study of fluid mechanics as it applies to human blood circulation. The design of such devices as drug infusion pumps and artificial hearts, as well as such techniques as catheterization, are all influenced by the knowledge of fluid properties, pressure, and flow mechanics.

Consider a fluid flowing through a tube such as that shown in **Figure 9-1.** The pressure difference between the two ends will dictate the direction in which the fluid moves. The fluid will move to the right if pressure P_1 is larger than P_2. The pressure at each end depends on the force exerted on the fluid divided by the cross-sectional area of the tube. This pressure will increase in two ways at either end: either the exerted force has increased or the cross-sectional area of the tube has decreased.

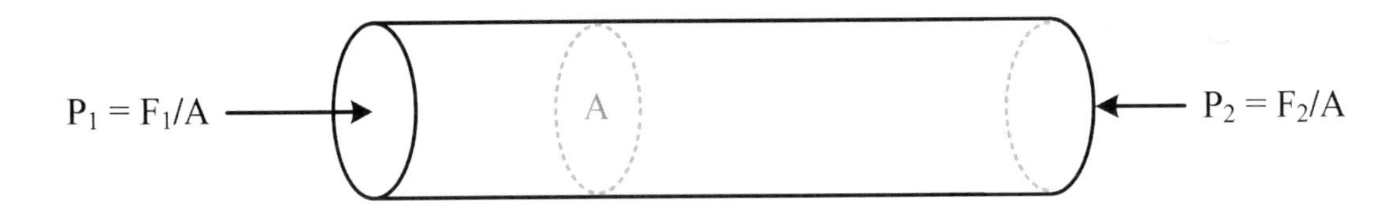

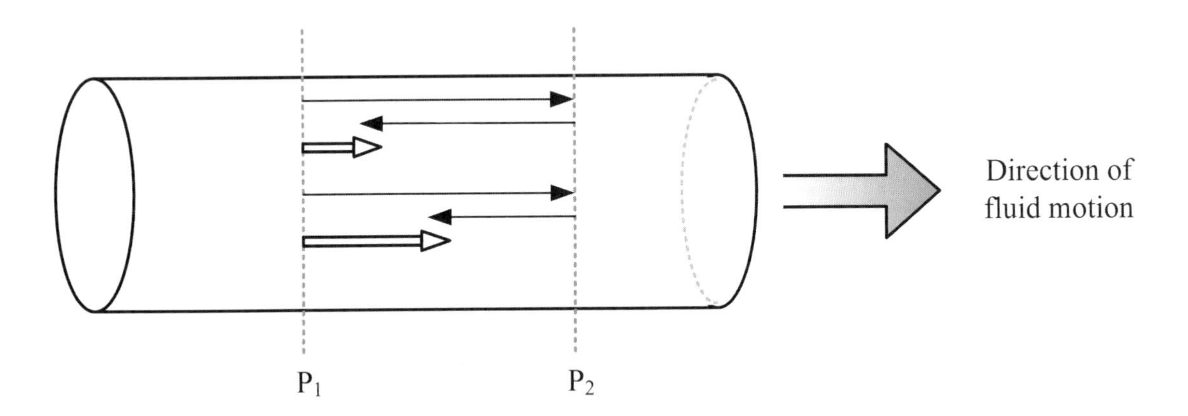

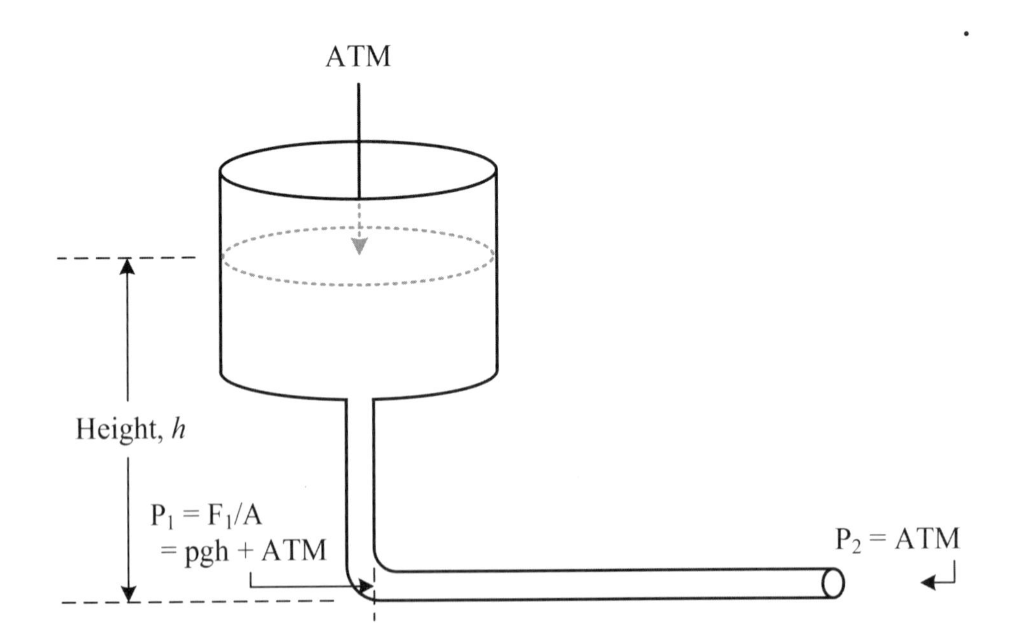

FIGURE 9-1 Fluid dynamics.

If a fluid is open to the atmosphere, the pressure it exerts at a given depth *h* is not determined by the shape of the vessel containing the fluid or by the amount of the fluid; the pressure is determined by the atmospheric pressure pushing down on the surface of the fluid. Moreover, if the fluid is viscous, more force will be needed to move the fluid. Friction develops between the moving fluid and the walls of the tube. The tube tends to resist fluid movement through it. Whether the force has increased or decreased at either end of the tube, the pressure difference is required for the flow of the fluid.

Therefore,

1. Pressure equals the exerted force on the fluid/cross-sectional area of the tube.

$$P = \frac{F}{A}$$

The unit of fluid pressure is given as millimeters of mercury (mm Hg) or Newtons per square meter (N/m^2).

2. Flow equals the pressure difference at each end of the tube/tubular resistance to the fluid.

$$Q = \frac{\Delta P}{R}$$

Where Q = flow rate in volume/time
ΔP = pressure difference in mm Hg
R = resistance to flow in mm Hg/volume/time

The movement of the fluid volume over time depends on the pressure difference and the tubular or peripheral resistance.

3. Flow is also defined in terms of cross-sectional area and the velocity of the fluid in the vessel.

$$Q = A \times V$$

Where A is the cross-sectional area and
V is the velocity of the fluid.

The unit of flow is cubic centimeters per second (cc/sec) or milliliters per second (ml/sec).

Now let's apply fluid mechanics to human blood circulation. The viscous fluid is the blood and the tube is the body's network of blood vessels. The pressure difference is created by the pumping action of the heart; this is the driving force for blood flow. (The principle of pressure difference can also be applied to cellular diffusion; the main difference is that instead of being driven by a difference in pressure, flow is driven by a difference in the concentrations of sodium and potassium in the cell endothelium.)

9.2 BLOOD CIRCULATION

Normal and Mean Arterial Pressures

Figure 9-2 shows normal ranges of blood pressure according to age. The ranges vary slightly due to the changing nervous and hormonal control mechanisms that occur with

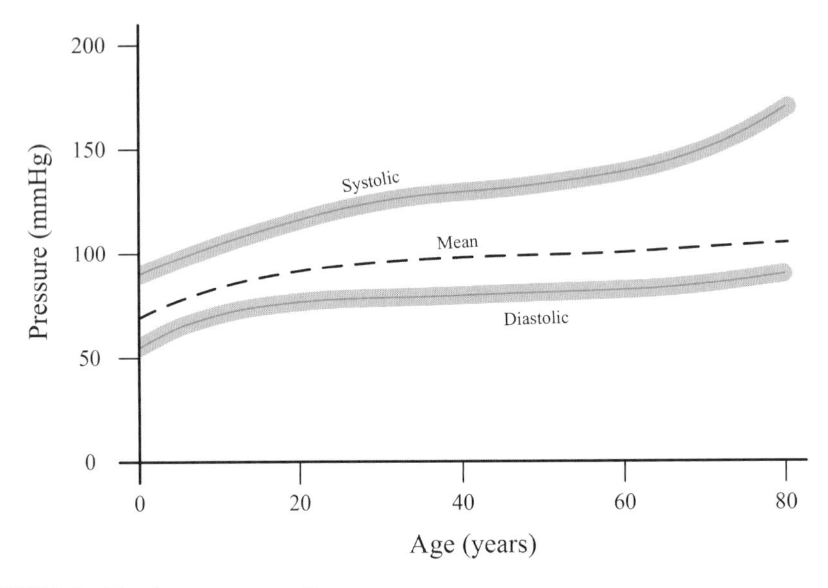

FIGURE 9-2 Blood pressure according to age.

aging; however, normal arterial pressure (systolic and diastolic) is 120/80 mm Hg in young adults. The MAP, therefore, is typically 100 mm Hg.

Blood pressure also varies within each heartbeat, but will stay, on average, within the normal range in a healthy person. **Figure 9-3** shows blood pressure in different portions

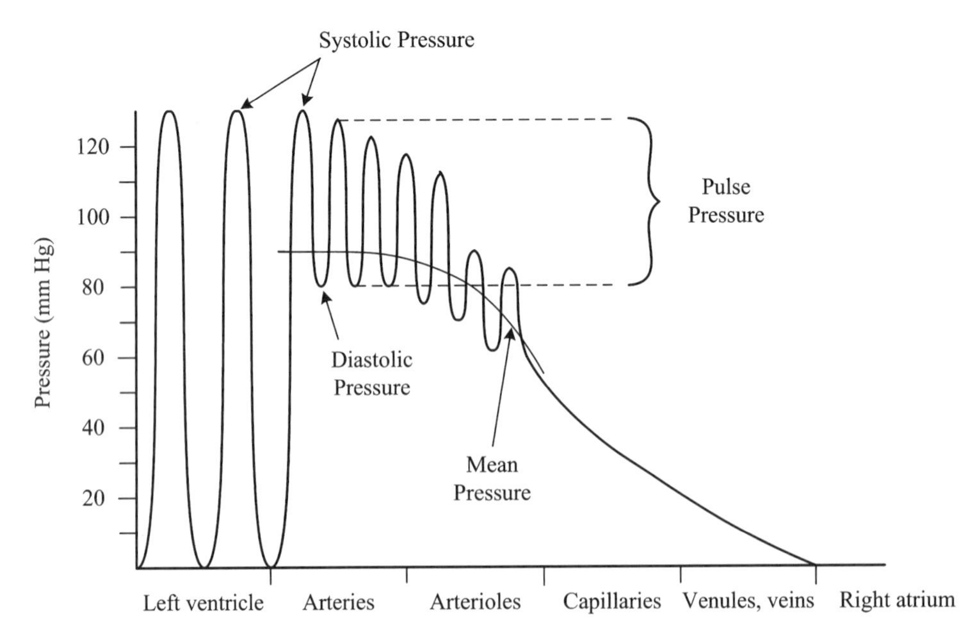

FIGURE 9-3 Blood pressure in systemic circulation.

of the systemic circulatory system. The following are some of the formulas for calculating blood pressure:

$$\text{MAP} = \text{Mean arterial pressure} = \text{diastolic pressure} + 1/3(\text{pulse pressure})$$
$$\text{Pulse pressure} = \text{systolic pressure} - \text{diastolic pressure}$$
$$\text{MAP } \alpha \text{ (cardiac output)(resistance of arterioles)}$$
$$\text{Also, MAP} = (\text{systolic pressure} + 2 \times \text{diastolic pressure})/3$$

Blood Flow Dynamics in Arteries, Capillaries, and Veins

The aorta and arteries are the larger blood vessels of the body, and the arterioles, veins, and capillaries are the smaller, or narrower, vessels. Therefore, because of their larger size, the aorta and arteries present less resistance to the blood flow through them. When the ventricle in the heart contracts (systole), blood is ejected into the aorta, from which it proceeds to the arterial vessels and the arterioles. As the blood vessels become progressively smaller, their resistance to blood flow increases, and the resulting slowdown of blood flow creates an excess of blood volume in the larger arterial vessels. The arteries then accommodate this extra blood volume by expanding when the arterioles slow down the flow. When the ventricle relaxes (diastole), the decrease in pressure allows the arterial walls to contract, thereby forcing the blood out to the arterioles. This elastic property of the arteries maintains constant blood flow through the circulatory system.

Alternatively, veins are collapsible vessels with lower pressure. The venous flow then depends on the negative transmural pressure (i.e., internal pressure – external pressure).

The pressure gradient ΔP is the pressure difference between the two ends of a blood vessel. It is measured in mm Hg units. The peripheral resistance unit (PRU) is the vascular resistance as the impediment to the blood flow through the vessel.

Blood flow can be defined as the quantity of blood passing a point in the circulation in a given period of time. It is expressed in milliliters per minute (ml/min) or liters per minute (l/min).

Another equation of the peripheral resistance can be given as

$$R = \frac{8 \times \eta \times 1}{\pi \times r^4}$$

Where η is the blood viscosity (in the unit of poises), l is the length of the vessel, and r is the radius of the vessel. Note that the resistance to flow increases proportionally to the increase in viscosity and to length. Flow is highly sensitive to the radius (i.e., the resistance is inversely proportional to the fourth power of the radius). Simply stated, slight change in the radius of the vessel greatly affects the resistance.

We can also investigate vessel connectivity in terms of series and parallel connections to each other. See **Figure 9-4** for the series and parallel connections of arteries and other vessels.

The total resistance accumulates in series connection; while, the total resistance decreases in the parallel connection.

$$\text{Total peripheral resistance in series} = R_1 + R_2 + R_3 + + +$$

In the parallel connection,

$$\text{Total peripheral resistance in parallel} = (1/R_1 + 1/R_2 + 1/R_3 + + +)^{-1}$$

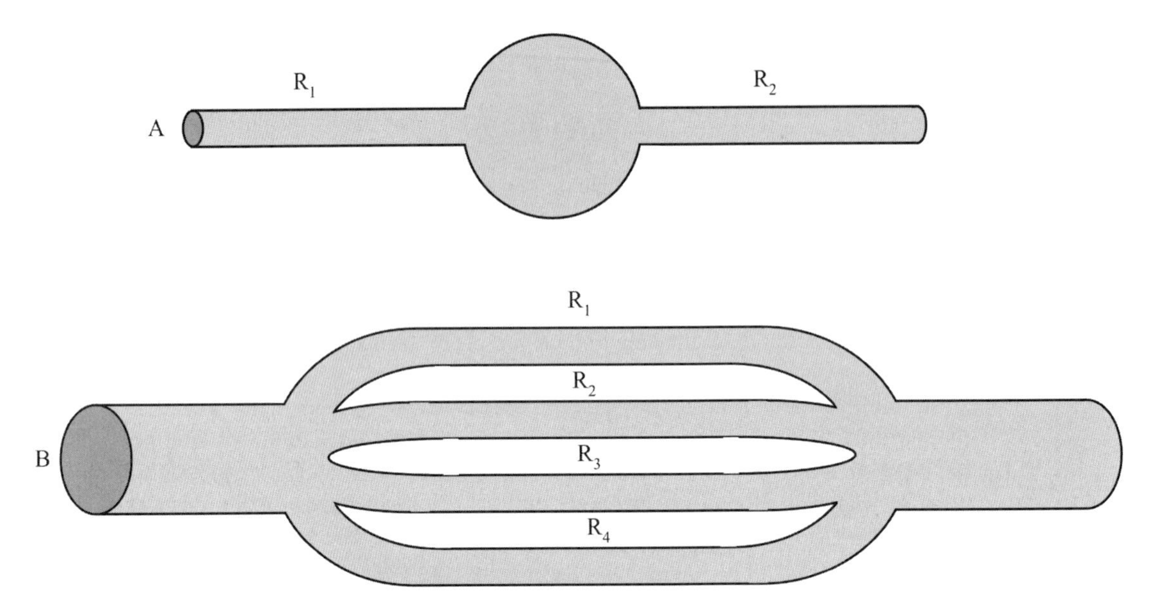

Figure 9-4 Peripheral resistances in blood vessels.

The total resistance is far less than any individual resistance of a single vessel and the blood flow rate will be higher in this connection than the flow in any single vessel.

Vascular Distensibility and Vascular Compliance

Blood vessels are distensible and compliant. That means that the diameter of the blood vessels change with the pressure changes throughout the circulatory system. This is called distensibility of the blood vessels. Additionally, the blood vessels can store more or less blood in a given segment of the circulation due to this distensibility. This is referred to as the compliant property of the vessels.

We can define these terms as:

Distensibility = (increase in volume)/(increase in pressure)/(original volume)

and

Compliance = (increase in volume)/(increase in pressure) = distensibility × volume

The veins are more compliant than the arteries due to the fact that they are more distensible and they have more volume to store the blood.

9.3 MODEL OF HEMODYNAMICS

A block diagram of the hemodynamic system is shown in **Figure 9-5.** The components of this block diagram include the heart, lungs, and peripheral circuit.

The laws and the properties of fluid dynamics apply to the blood circulation in arteries, capillaries, and veins. This includes the Bernoulli's law of flow through a tube of various cross-sectional areas and the phenomena of laminar and turbulent flow. This can also be

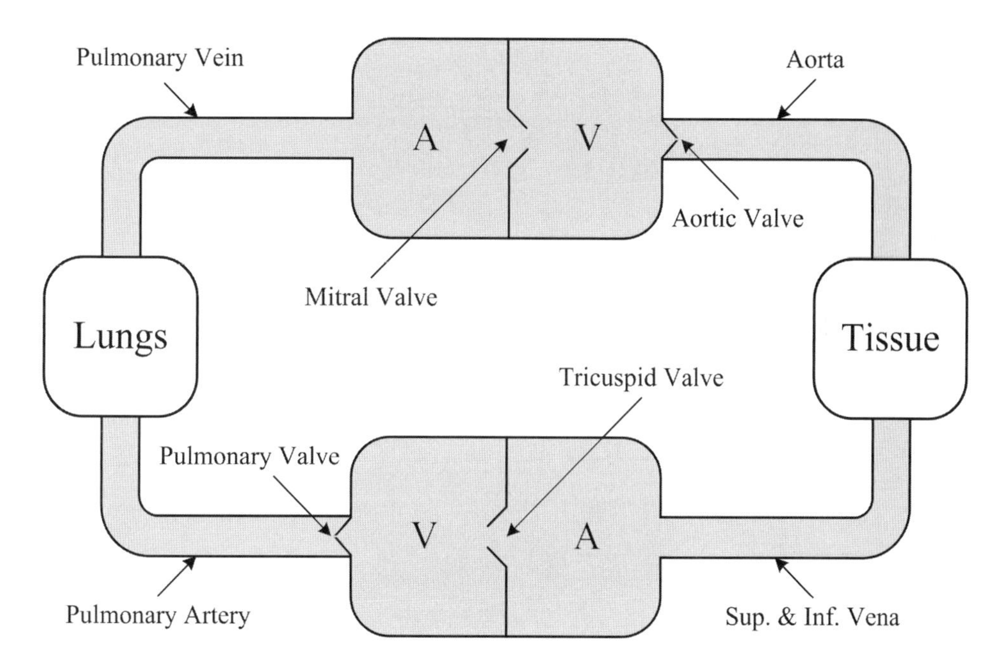

FIGURE 9-5 Blood circulation.

considered a fluid circuit with various points of pressure gradients with or without constrictions in the tube at several locations in the circuit.

In order to further understand blood circulation, we will look into a simulated tube (called a Bernoulli tube) circuit shown in **Figure 9-6.** A source bucket filled with water is placed at a higher point than the Bernoulli tube. Variable clamps are applied on the flow tube so that the flow rate can be controlled. The water exiting the Bernoulli tube is allowed to drain into a second outflow bucket. The return flow from this second bucket to the source bucket is maintained by a roller pump. The pressure at three points of the Bernoulli tube can be sensed by a strain gauge pressure transducer that is then connected to a pressure monitor.

The Bernoulli equation states that the total energy of the fluid at any point in a tube is assumed to be constant. The sum of the pressure, kinetic energy, and potential energy is equal at all three points of the Bernoulli tube.

A fluid can possess energy in three forms (if the temperature of the fluid is constant, thermal energy is not counted): as pressure, as kinetic energy, and as potential energy. These energies can be computed using the following formulas:

$$\text{Pressure} = \text{height of the fluid column multiplied by the density of the fluid}$$

$$\text{Kinetic energy} = \frac{1}{2} \times \rho \times V^2$$

$$\text{Potential energy} = \rho \times g \times h$$

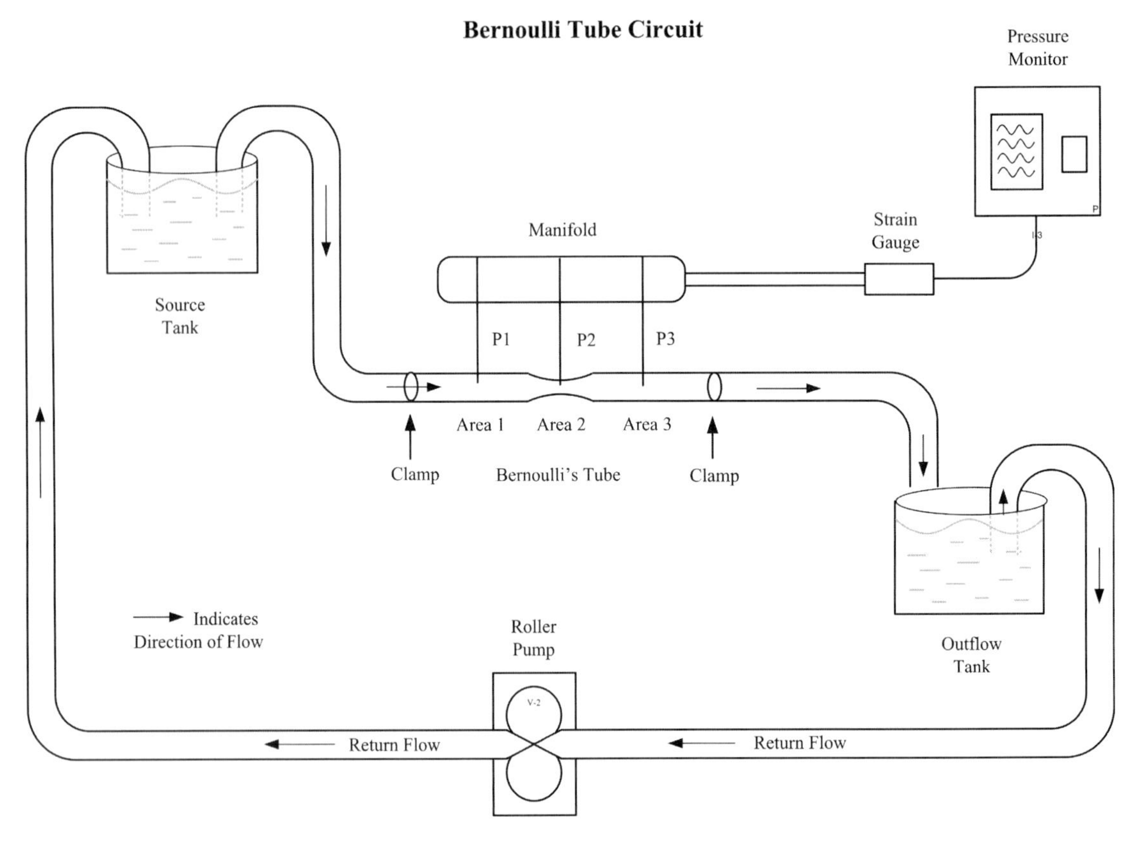

FIGURE 9-6 Bernoulli tube circuit.

where

$$V = \text{velocity of the fluid}$$

and

$$\rho = \text{density of the fluid and for water } \rho = 1 \times 10^3 \text{ kg/m}^3,$$
$$g = \text{gravitational force} = 9.8 \text{ m/sec}^2, \text{ and } h = \text{height}$$

As the levels of all points are equal from a reference point, the potential energy ρgh is constant (but never zero).

The Bernoulli equation can be written at all three points:

$$\text{Total energy} = P1 + \left(\frac{1}{2} \times \rho \times V1^2\right) + (\rho \times g \times h_1) =$$

$$P2 + \left(\frac{1}{2} \times \rho \times V2^2\right) + (\rho \times g \times h_2) =$$

$$P3 + \left(\frac{1}{2} \times \rho \times V3^2\right) + (\rho \times g \times h_3)$$

where P1, P2, and P3 are pressures; V1, V2, and V3 are velocities; and h_1, h_2, and h_3 are heights with respect to a reference point.

The flow is assumed to be constant at all three points and is written as an equation of continuity:

$$Q = A1 \times V1 = A2 \times V2 = A3 \times V3$$

where A1, A2, and A3 are cross-sectional areas and V1, V2, and V3 are velocities.

Using **Figure 9-6** as an example, with the meter-kilogram-second system of units (MKS), assume:

A1 = Area 1 initial inflow to the Bernoulli tube = 7.8×10^{-5} m^2

A2 = Area 2 constricted tube = 2.5×10^{-5} m^2

A3 = Area 3 outflow from the tube = 7.8×10^{-5} m^2, Q = the water flow rate = 5.5×10^{-6} m^3/sec, and the pressures are P1 = 1,730 N/m^2, P2 = 1,708.25 N/m^2, P3 = 1,730 N/m^2

We can calculate the fluid velocities at these points by dividing the flow rate by the areas.

Therefore,

V1 = 0.07 m/sec, V2 = 0.22 m/sec, V3 = 0.07 m/sec

$$\text{Total energy} = 1730 + \left(\frac{1}{2} \times 1000 \times 0.07^2\right) + \rho g h_1 =$$

$$1708.25 + \left(\frac{1}{2} \times 1000 \times 0.22^2\right) + \rho g h_2 =$$

$$1730 + \left(\frac{1}{2} \times 1000 \times 0.07^2\right) + \rho g h_3$$

The total energy results in 1,765 N/m^2. Note that 1 N/m^2 = 0.0075 mm Hg and the total energy of 1,765 N/m^2 is approximately 13 mm Hg.

As we start out with a certain section, the fluid velocity increases as the cross-sectional area decreases. The opposite is true when the fluid velocity decreases as the area increases. (Additionally, velocity also increases with higher flow rate.) For a constant flow, as the fluid passes through the smaller area, the pressure decreases and the velocity increases, which, in turn, increases the fluid's kinetic energy. However, in the larger area, pressure increases and velocity decreases, which, in turn, decreases the fluid's kinetic energy.

Ideally, at low flow rates, the pressure, velocity, and the kinetic energy will behave predictably, but when the flow rates are moderate or high, resistance due to the viscosity of the fluid and the geometry of the surrounding vessel (the tube's interior cross section) can affect the rate of flow and create what is called a turbulent flow.

The normal fluid flow in a vessel is a streamline or a laminar flow where the velocity of the flow in the center of the vessel is far greater than that toward the outer edges. The fluid molecules and layers in the laminar flow are capable of slipping over each other in the middle of the vessel. In turbulent flow, however, the fluid starts flowing in all directions, continually mixing within the vessel and forming eddy currents. The turbulent flow is defined by the Reynolds number (R_e) and is calculated as:

$$R_e = \frac{V \times \rho \times d}{\eta}$$

where V = fluid velocity, ρ = fluid density, d = diameter of the vessel, and η = fluid viscosity.

When the value of R_e is greater than 1,000, the flow is considered to be a turbulent flow.

This Bernoulli tube simulation can be translated in real blood flow circulation. In this case, the heart is the pump in the systemic circulation circuit.

9.4 CARDIAC OUTPUT

Cardiac output (CO) is the quantity of blood pumped by the left ventricle into the aorta each minute and is considered an important circulation parameter. Cardiac output is close to 5 l/min for a normal adult. It is affected by age, metabolism, surface area of the body, exercise, and oxygen consumption. In contrast, venous return is the quantity of blood flow from the veins into the right atrium. Ideally, taking all variables into consideration, it should be equal to the CO over a certain period of time.

Peripheral resistance of the vessels is an important factor in CO and the venous return. When the vessels dilate in the circulatory path, there is a notable increase in both CO and the venous return. We can relate venous return with the peripheral resistance as:

$$\text{Venous return} = \frac{(\text{arterial pressure} - \text{right atrial pressure})}{\text{total peripheral resistance}}$$

Cardiac output is also related to the heart rate and the stroke volume. For example, blood volume in each ventricle increases to approximately 130 ml during diastole (end-diastolic volume); however, it decreases by approximately 70 ml during systole (end-stroke volume). The remaining blood volume in each ventricle is approximately 60 ml. This is called the end-systolic volume (end-systolic volume = end-diastolic volume – end-stroke volume).

Therefore,

$$\text{Cardiac output} = (\text{end-stroke volume in ml/beat})(\text{heart rate in bpm}) \times 1/1{,}000$$

This process repeats with each contraction of the heart. Cardiac output is measured in liters per minute; therefore, given the aforementioned data, approximately 5 liters of blood is pumped per minute.

With strong contractions during systole, the end-systolic volume can fall to less than 70 ml, while the end-diastolic volume can increase to 200 ml (more than 130 ml difference) during diastole. The result may be that the stroke volume increases to more than double the normal values with this decreased end-systolic volume and the increased end-diastolic volume. In this case, the total CO increases.

EXAMPLE A patient has an 8 l/min CO. His pulmonary artery has a 14 mm diameter with a 20 mm Hg pressure. His left atrium pressure is 8 mm Hg. What is the patient's pulmonary vascular resistance? (Hint: Ignore kinetic energy and use a hybrid unit such as l/min and mm Hg.)

$$\text{Resistance} = \frac{\text{Pressure difference}}{\text{Flow}}$$

$$\text{Resistance} = \frac{20\text{ mm Hg} - 8\text{ mm Hg}}{8\text{ l/min}}$$

$$\text{Resistance} = \frac{12}{8} = 1.5\text{ mm Hg/l/min}$$

■

EXAMPLE

1. True or False: Fluid flow can be from an area of higher pressure to an area of lower pressure.

a) True

b) False

True. The flow of fluid is always from higher pressure to lower pressure.

■

9.5 PRESSURE MONITORS

Pressure monitors are biomedical devices used to measure various pressures in the body, most commonly the pressure of the blood flowing through the vessels. There are two techniques used to measure blood pressure: Invasive and noninvasive. The invasive technique is to insert a catheter into an artery. While catheterization is the most accurate form of monitoring blood pressure, it is not always practical. The more convenient techniques used are noninvasive instruments, such as sphygmomanometers (blood pressure monitors). These monitors are used in hospitals, clinics, emergency units, pharmacies, and even in the home. They may be manual or automated. For home use, electronic units are popular, but these units require regular calibration to ensure accurate measurement. The electronic devices are not recommended for patients with specific medical conditions who need regular and reliable blood pressure recordings.

The sphygmomanometer involves a method of listening to body sounds, called auscultatory measurement, with the Korotkoff sound as the main parameter. This device allows the user to detect pressure levels by listening through a stethoscope to the sound of the turbulent blood flow in the vessels.

This auscultatory technique employs a pneumatic (air) pressure cuff, hand pump, manometer (pressure gauge), and stethoscope. The sphygmomanometer uses the pressure cuff over the upper arm and the pressure gauge to indicate the pressure in the cuff. **Figure 9-7** shows a sphygmomanometer with an occluding bladder, rubber tubing, rubber bulb, stethoscope, and gauge. **Figure 9-8** shows the process of detecting blood pressure.

When the pneumatic cuff is placed over the upper arm and is pumped to a pressure that is greater than the systolic arterial pressure, the cuff pressure stops the blood flow to the lower arm. As the cuff pressure is slowly released and becomes slightly less than the systolic arterial pressure, the blood spurts from the compressed upper arm (underlying brachial artery) and creates noises known as Korotkoff sounds. The following describes the auscultatory method:

FIGURE 9-7 Sphygmomanometer.

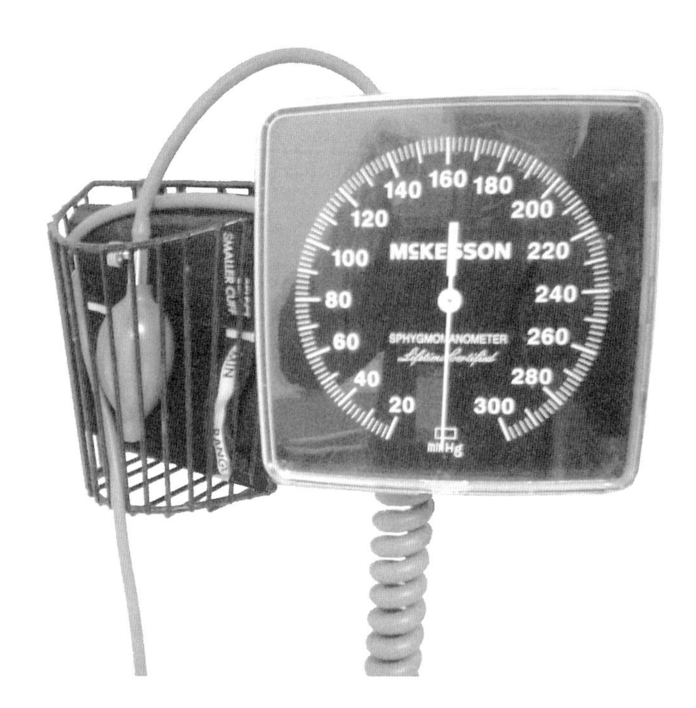

FIGURE 9-8 Process of blood pressure auscultatory measurement.

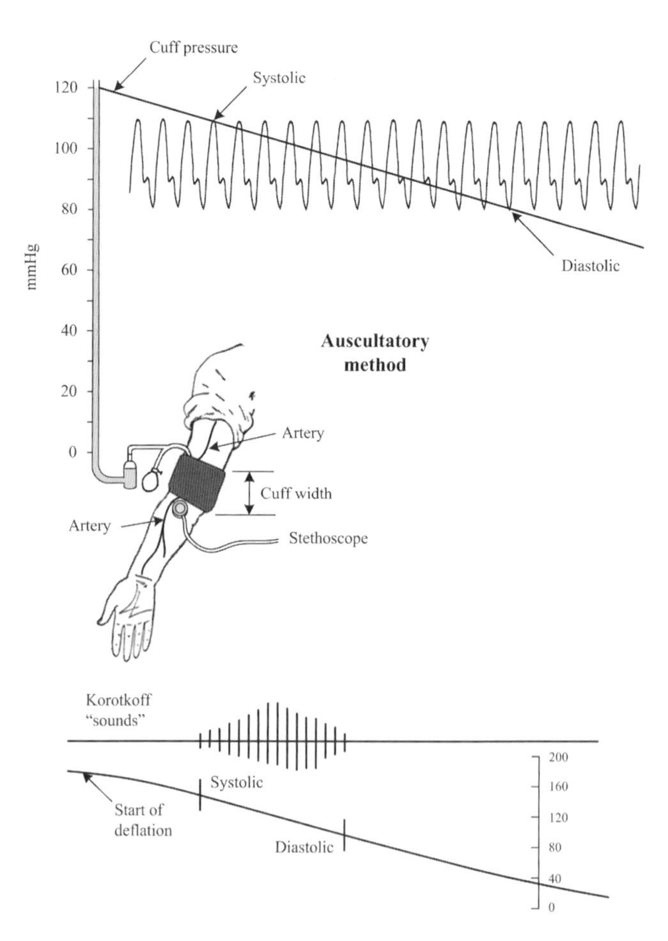

- The cuff is first inflated until the blood flow is stopped due to the compression of the brachial artery. With no flow, no sound is detected by the stethoscope.
- Next, the pressure in the cuff is slowly released. The flow in the brachial artery slowly builds up and the corresponding sound (the Korotkoff sound) is heard by the stethoscope.
- The first sound (heard when the blood flow begins) indicates systolic pressure and the last sound heard (before normal blood flow is restored) indicates diastolic pressure.

Korotkoff Sounds

There are five phases of Korotkoff sounds heard during cuff deflation:

Phase I: the onset of the sound is indicative of the systolic pressure. This is the first sound heard when the falling cuff pressure is slightly less than the systolic pressure. The sound is soft in the beginning of the measurement and increases in intensity.

Phase II: This is the phase of the murmur-like sound. It may fade quickly or may not be detected as the cuff pressure decreases.

Phase III: This is the phase of the "thumping" sound and is very loud.

Phase IV: This is close to the diastolic pressure and is a muffled sound.

Phase V: With the cuff pressure continually decreasing, this is the phase when the sound disappears completely. This is usually slightly below the diastolic pressure.

The measurement of blood pressure by auscultation is shown in **Figure 9-9.** The systolic and diastolic pressures are recorded by the technician as he or she listens for the first and the last sounds using the stethoscope.

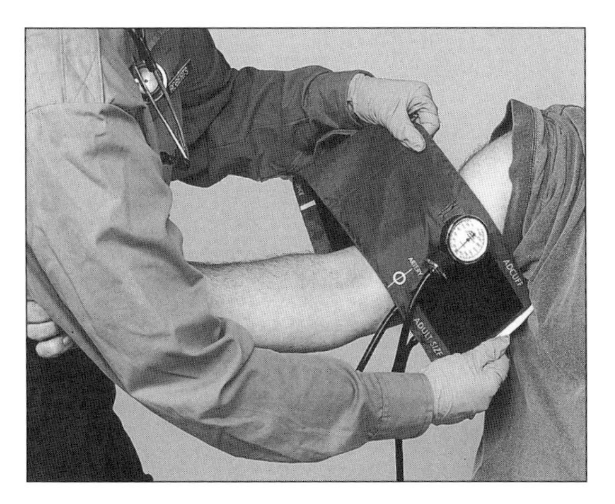

STEP 1 The EMT places the blood pressure cuff around the patient's upper arm snugly. The cuff should cover more than half but less than two-thirds of the length of the upper arm.

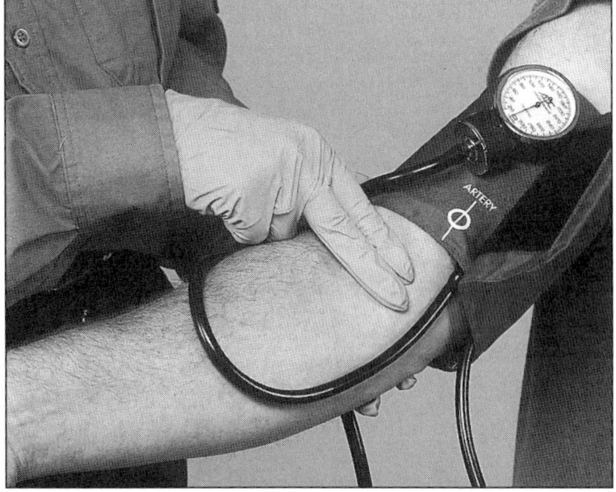

STEP 2 The EMT then finds the brachial pulse. The brachial pulse is usually found on the medial side of the elbow.

FIGURE 9-9 Steps in measuring blood pressure. *(continued)*

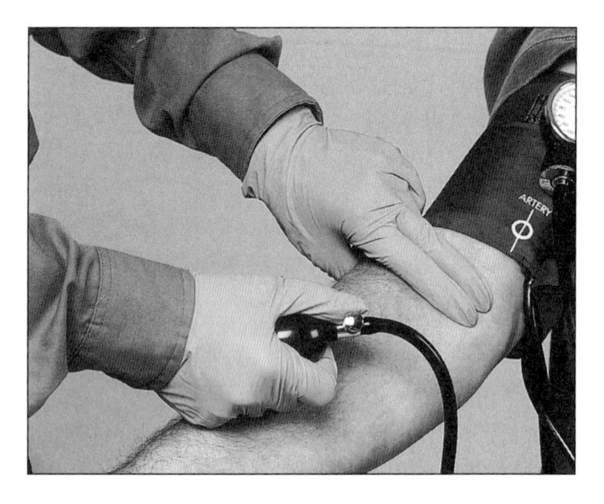

STEP 3 Next, the EMT closes the valve on the cuff and inflates the cuff until the brachial pulse is no longer felt, then continues inflating for 20 mm Hg higher.

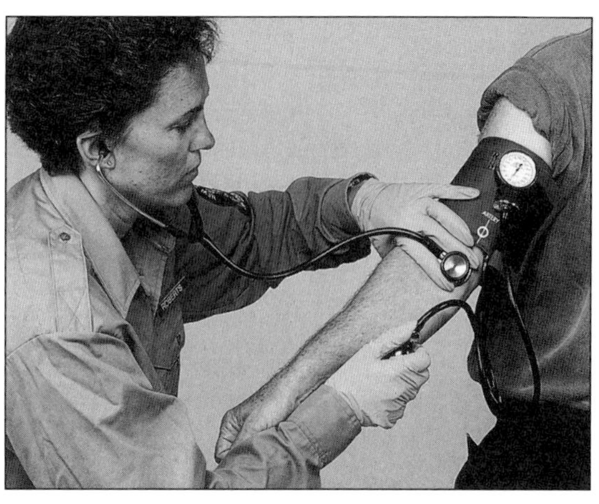

STEP 4 Then the EMT places the head of the stethoscope on the brachial pulse and the ear tips in the ears.

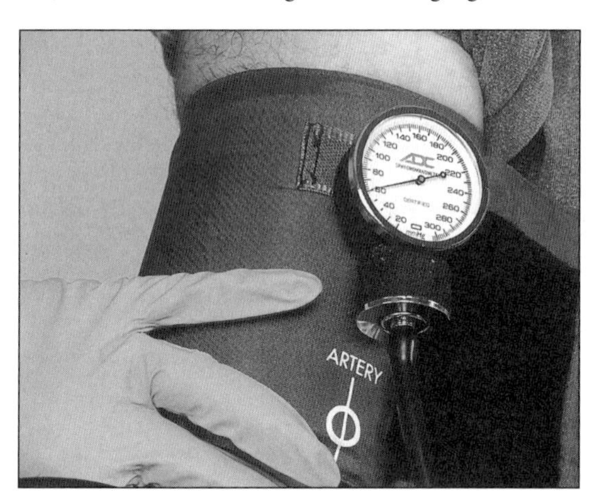

STEP 5 Slowly deflate the blood pressure cuff, at about 10 mm Hg a second, using the relief valve next to the bulb.

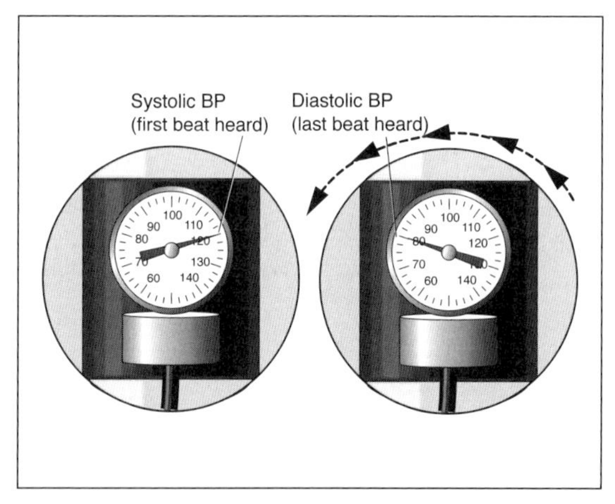

STEP 6 Note the systolic and the diastolic pressures.

FIGURE 9-9 (*continued*)

Automated Blood Pressure Equipment

There is a variety of biomedical devices used to measure arterial blood pressure noninvasively and automatically using either the auscultatory technique or another technique called oscillometric.

Auscultatory Method Noninvasive blood pressure measurement can be automated by replacing the hand pump with an automatic pump. This pump can be set to inflate the cuff when activated. The Korotkoff sounds can then be detected by a small microphone placed in the cuff. A microprocessor circuit with programmed software determines the blood pressure range.

Oscillometric Method Most automated blood pressure devices use an oscillometric method. This is an indirect method as no stethoscope is used and the cuff does not necessarily need to be wrapped over the brachial artery (it can be wrapped over another part of the arm, around the wrist, or even around the finger). In this method, a pressure sensor senses the amplitude changes in cuff pressure due to the opening of the artery and the start of the blood flow in the deflation phase. A tiny perturbation as an oscillation is superimposed on the existing cuff pressure during the deflation phase.

- Even before the bladder begins to deflate, a small amplitude of the oscillation is sensed.
- At the systolic pressure, the oscillation amplitude rises rapidly. It reaches maximum between the systolic and diastolic pressures.
- As the cuff pressure decreases, the oscillation amplitude also decreases.

In most blood pressure monitors used in hospitals, sophisticated sensors detect the pressures and the associated electronic circuit then displays the systolic and diastolic pressures. A menu tree in the monitor display allows all possible choices available in the menu structure. This is shown in **Figure 9-10.**

Blood pressure device calibration is recommended every 12 months. This is done by using a calibration kit, a digital manometer (calibrated to ± 0.5 mm Hg), and the inflation bulb pump. On selecting the noninvasive blood pressure (NIBP) mode from the service menu, the monitor displays the systolic and diastolic pressures. When pressure is applied with the pump, the monitor must agree with the readings on the digital manometer with a specified tolerance of ± 3 mm Hg. Overpressure occurs before 330 mm Hg. An adult blood pressure cuff wrapped around a semi-rigid cylinder may also be used in the calibration process.

Hospitals are usually equipped with several of these monitors, which are used to provide noninvasive measurements of blood pressure, pulse rate, temperature, and

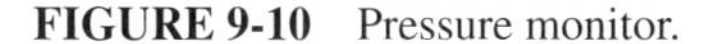

FIGURE 9-10 Pressure monitor.

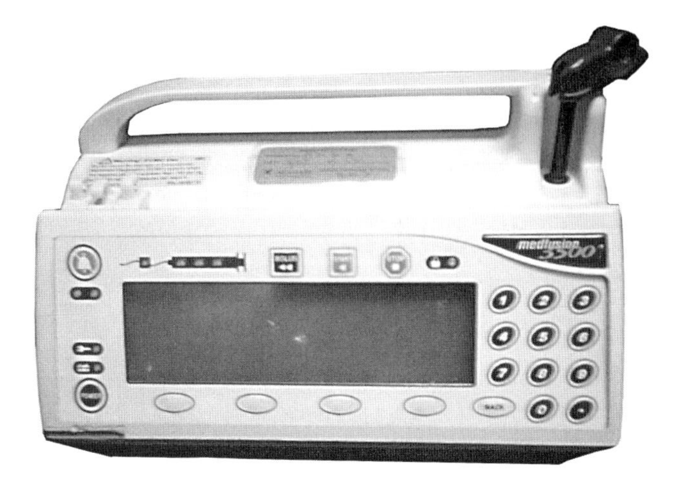

oxygen saturation. The blood pressure measurements include the systolic, diastolic, and the MAPs.

Typically, the front panel shows the displays of systolic pressure (120 mm Hg), diastolic pressure (70 mm Hg), MAP (95 mm Hg), temperature (36.9° C), pulse rate (70 bpm), and the oxygen saturation, or SPO_2 (90%).

In other displays, the alarms, interface messages, and the configuration options are indicated. The SPO_2 monitor artifact indicator light-emitting diode (LED), blood pressure cuff hose attachment, temperature probe cable attachment, and the SPO_2 sensor cable attachments are easy to locate. The rear panel is mostly the host communication serial port RS-232 or other type of a serial bus.

In NIBP monitoring, a pump inflates the cuff, two pressure transducers sense the blood pressure, and the pneumatic manifold (with two valves) deflate the cuff. The pneumatic system has an overpressure sensor built in to prevent overinflation. All controls are initiated by the main board that includes (minimally) 16-bit ADCs, several PROMs (programmable ROMs), RAMs, LED displays, and microprocessor chips. Usually, the inputs are on the left and the outputs are on the right. The primary microprocessor controls the patient interface and the secondary microprocessor controls the displays, alarm sound, and real-time clocks.

9.6 VITAL SIGNS MONITORS

Skilled clinicians use vital signs monitors for multi-parameter monitoring of ECG channels, respiration channels, invasive blood pressure (IBP), and NIBP channels. The vital signs can be monitored for neonatal, pediatric, and adult patients. These can be used at bedside or in ambulance transport and intra-facility monitors.

The NIBP channel indirectly measures arterial pressures using an inflatable cuff, while the IBP channel measures arterial, venous, and intracranial blood pressures using invasive transducers.

When the device is turned on, the NIBP channel is at a default inflation pressure based on the patient mode (adult pressure level is 160 mm Hg, pediatric pressure level is 120 mm Hg, and neonate pressure level is 90 mm Hg).

The following NIBP and IBP specifications are provided in vital signs monitors:

Noninvasive Blood Pressure	
Method	Oscillometric
Displayed pressure	Systolic, diastolic, and mean
Systolic range	Adult 30 mm Hg – 260 mm Hg
Diastolic range	Adult 20 mm Hg – 235 mm Hg
Turbocuff	Maximum measurements allowable in a five-minute period
Normal overpressure	Adult 280 mm Hg
Pulse rate	30 bpm – 220 bpm
Artifact filtering	Smartcuf® software

Invasive Blood Pressure	
Transducer type	Strain-gauge resistive bridge
Transducer excitation impedance	200 Ω to 2,000 Ω

(*continued*)

Invasive Blood Pressure (*continued*)	
Transducer sensitivity	5 μV/V/mm Hg
Excitation voltage	4.85 V pulsed DC at 181 Hz
Bandwidth	Digital filtered, DC to 20 Hz
Pressure	−30 mm Hg to 300 mm Hg
Pulse	25 bpm to 250 bpm

9.7 PATIENT SIMULATORS

The patient simulator such as MedSim300 simulates several dynamic blood pressure channels and CO. The characteristics of blood pressure and CO are as follows:

Output	−10 mm Hg to 300 mm Hg
Output sensitivity	5 μV/V or 40 μV/V
Accuracy	1% +1 mm of Hg full range at 80 bpm
CO injectate volume	10 cc
CO baseline temperature	36° C to 38° C
CO injectate temperature	2° C for a wide range of thermistors; varies from <1 kΩ to 95 kΩ
Rates	Dynamic pressures track normal and abnormal rates
Insulation	Electrically isolated from other outputs

9.8 FLOW INSTRUMENTATION

Flow is the motion of the fluid and the volumetric flow rate is the volume of the fluid transferred per unit of time. If we integrate the volume over a certain time, we can then determine the flow rate.

Magnetic Blood Flow Meter

Faraday's law of electromagnetic induction is applied to an electrical conductor that moves through a magnetic field. As blood behaves like a conductor, an alternating magnetic field is created across the blood vessel, and an electrode at the surface of the blood vessel detects a small induced voltage.

Doppler Ultrasound Blood Flow Meter

Either continuous or pulsed ultrasonic energy is transmitted and the returning echoes are picked up by a separate or same transducer. Frequency shifts due to blood flow (that is the movement of the reflected interfaces) are detected and recorded. The average velocity and the distance of the moving target can then be measured.

9.9 CARDIAC OUTPUT MEASUREMENT

Several direct and indirect methods are available to measure CO. Direct methods include dye dilution and thermodilution to measure changes in the blood; indirect methods include echocardiographic measurement and radionuclide imaging to find the stroke volume and compute CO.

Dilution Technique

The dilution technique includes two methods used to determine cardiac output. Dye dilution is a time-honored method based on how rapidly flowing blood dilutes a dye that has been injected into the pulmonary arterial circulation. The CO is measured as inversely proportional to the concentration of the dye when sampled at two points downstream of the injection site. Cardiac output increases as the concentration of dye in the blood decreases.

The contemporary dilution method is thermodilution. In thermodilution, a special thermistor-tipped catheter (Swan-Ganz catheter) is inserted from a peripheral vein into the pulmonary artery, as shown in **Figure 9-11a.** A cold saline solution of known temperature and volume is injected into the right atrium from a proximal catheter port. The injectate mixes with the blood as it passes through the ventricle and into the pulmonary artery, thus cooling the blood. The blood temperature is measured by a thermistor (a temperature sensory device) at the catheter tip, which lies within the pulmonary artery, and a computer is used to acquire the thermodilution profile. This computer calculates flow (CO from the

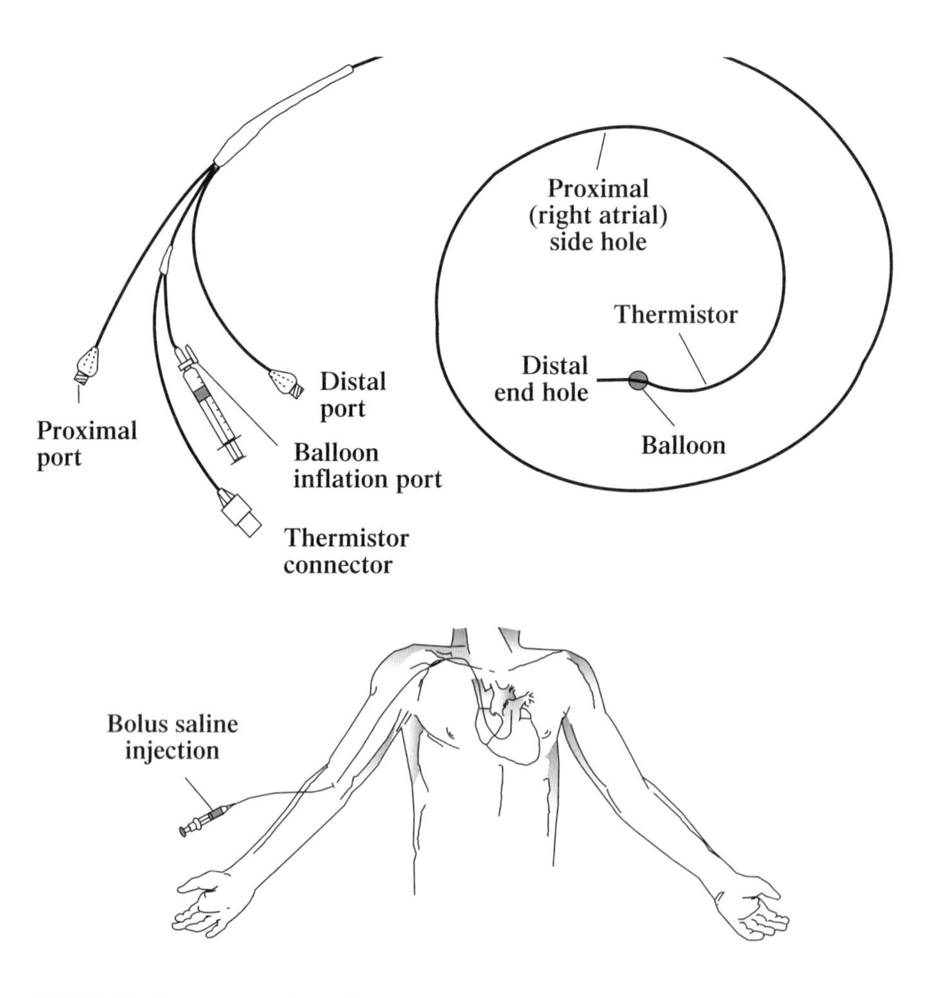

FIGURE 9-11a Catheter in cardiac output measurement.

right ventricle) using the blood temperature information and the temperature and volume of the injectate. Because CO changes with respiration, it is important to inject the saline at a consistent time during the respiratory cycle, usually at the end of expiration.

A block diagram of a CO monitor is shown in **Figure 9-11b.** The device's system consists of the CO board and the CO cables. The board has several amplifiers, voltage sources and regulators, an analog-to-digital converter, and a digital section with a microprocessor and digital signal processing.

There are two CO system cables: one cable connects to the thermistor, which is attached to the catheter; the second cable connects to the open bath temperature probe or injectate flow-through probe.

The CO measurement begins when the injectate (with a known temperature) is diluted with an unknown amount of blood inside the right ventricle. Cardiac output, stroke volume (SV), end-systolic volume (ESV), end-diastolic volume (EDV), and right ejection fraction (REF) are calculated by the algorithms and equations already stored in the erasable programmable read-only memory (EPROM).

Various parameter ranges are as follows:

Cardiac output range: 0.01 l/min to 19.99 l/min

Cardiac output accuracy: +/− 2 percent, or 0.2 l/min from the mean value, whichever is greater

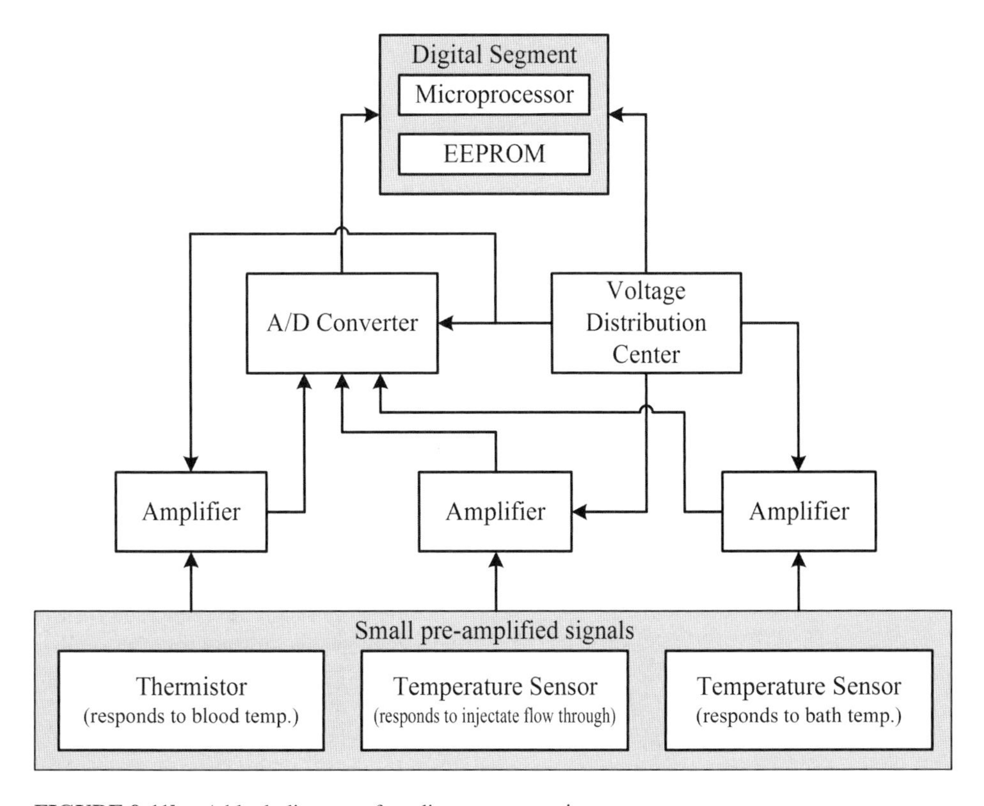

FIGURE 9-11b A block diagram of cardiac output monitor.

Injectate temperature range: 0.0° C to 27.0° C

Injectate accuracy: +/− 0.3° C

Blood temperature range: 17.5° C to 43.0° C

Blood temperature accuracy: +/− 0.5° C

The equation that governs the calculation of CO is given as:

$$CO = \frac{[V_i \times \rho_i \times C_i \times (T_b - T_i) \times 0.82 \times 60]}{[\rho_b \times C_b \times \text{Integrated value of the deflection curve} \times K]}$$

The formula is defined in **Figure 9-11c.**

EXAMPLE Find the CO in the thermodilution method if:

Injectate volume = 11 ml

Injectate temperature = 24° C

Blood temperature before injection = 37° C

Specific gravity of injectate (5% dextrose in water) = 1.05

Specific heat of injectate (5% dextrose in water) = 0.61

Specific gravity of blood = 1.06

Specific heat of blood = 0.9

Integrated value of the deflection = 80° C-seconds

Calibration factor = 0.01

FIGURE 9-11c Cardiac output equation.

$$CO = \frac{V_i \rho_i C_i (T_b - T_i) \bullet 0.82 \bullet 60}{\rho_b C_b \bullet \int_0^\infty \Delta D_b(t)dt \bullet K}$$

where

V_i = Volume of injectate (ml)

ρ_i = Specific gravity of injectate

ρ_b = Specific gravity of blood

C_i = Specific heat of injectate

C_b = Specific heat of blood

T_b = Initial temperature of blood (°C)

T_i = Initial temperature of injectate (°C)

0.82 = Empirical correction factor for indicator loss between end and tip of the catheter

60 = 60 seconds/minute

K = Calibration factor for the curve (°C/mm deflection)

$\int_0^\infty \Delta D_b(t)dt \bullet K$ = Area under the deflections-time curve registered following injection of the thermal indicator, in °C sec.

On substitution of the parameters in the aforementioned equation, the CO is:

CO = 5,904.48 ml/min (or 5.9 l/min)

The catheter commonly used to monitor CO in ICUs is the Swan-Ganz catheter (with the thermistor tip), which is introduced into the pulmonary artery. The temperature measured by a thermistor shows sequential changes in temperature with respect to time. The graph shown in **Figure 9-11d** is called a thermodilution curve. The integrated value of deflection is the area under this curve and is inversely related to the CO.

FIGURE 9-11d Thermodilution curve.

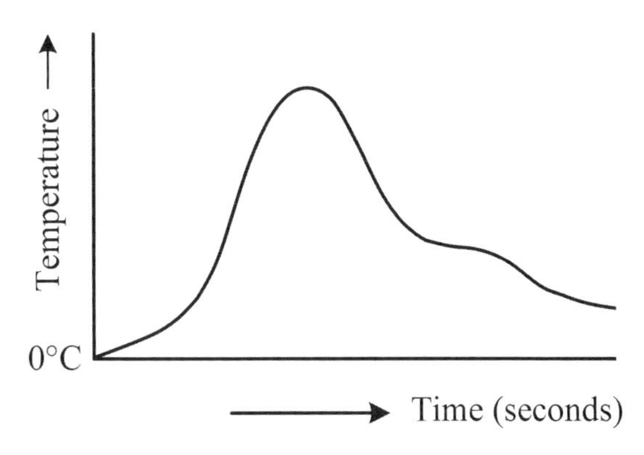

EXAMPLE True or False: In thermodilution CO, the area under the curve is proportional to the CO.

a) True

b) False

False. The area under the curve in the thermodilution method suggests that the temperature changes at the injectate site within a short period. The CO is higher when the temperature change is minimal and the area under the curve is small.

9.10 PLETHYSMOGRAPH

The instrument used for the detection of blood volume changes in the peripheral circulation is called a plethysmograph and the record of this change with respect to time is called a plethysmogram. The changes in the blood volume can be recorded for the whole body, in the chest area, or in any limb during respiration or blood flow. Several methods are used to measure blood volume changes:

1. Impedance plethysmograph: When two electrodes are placed on the skin surface and the electrical impedance is measured between them, the impedance varies due to blood volume changes in the tissue between these electrodes.
2. Photoplethysmograph: This technique utilizes the transmission or reflection of light through the blood volume changes.
3. Mercury plethysmograph: A strain gauge containing a small amount of mercury is used around the chest or limb to record the resistance changes due to the blood volume changes.

9.11 INFUSION PUMPS

Infusion therapy, or intravenous (IV) therapy, is the delivery of drugs, antibiotics, nutrients, and other fluids into the bloodstream via a catheter. An infusion pump is an important component of this delivery system. With at least 80 percent of hospital patients receiving some sort of IV therapy, physicians must decide carefully which type of infusion pump is best for each patient's treatment. Dose rates, patient safety, the type of patient (pediatric or adult), and single or multi-channel access are some of the criteria used by physicians to determine what type of infusion pump to use. Some types of pumps are the general-purpose infusion pumps (such as syringe, volumetric, and ambulatory pumps) and specialty infusion pumps (such as enteral feeding pumps, insulin, and implantable pumps).

The general-purpose infusion pumps are used in such applications as the delivery of basic fluids for hydration and the delivery of pain medications and antibiotics. The specialty infusion pumps are typically designed for the delivery of a particular type of fluid or medication. For example, enteral feeding pumps are used to reach the intestines; while, insulin pumps are used in the treatment of diabetic patients. We will discuss two types of pumps, the syringe and volumetric, in detail in the following sections.

Syringe

A syringe infusion pump uses a syringe plunger to pump saline, glucose, liquid drugs, and liquid nutrients into the body's bloodstream. The syringe containing the fluid is connected to a tube. This tube is connected to a needle that is inserted into a vein in the patient. An infusion pump pushes the syringe plunger, forcing the fluid through the tube and the needle and into the patient's body. The diameter of the syringe and the required flow rate determine the speed of the pump. The plastic syringes and infusion pumps are always matched so that fluid volume and delivery timing are accurate for each patient's treatment. For patient safety, syringe infusion pumps are equipped with alarms that signal any abnormalities in flow rate, total volume, or fluid pressure. **Figure 9-12** shows a photo of a syringe pump.

Volumetric

A volumetric infusion pump performs the same action as a syringe pump in that it delivers fluids to the body. However, a volumetric pump, also called a peristaltic pump, uses a bag of fluid that is hung above the pump and two tubes for the fluid to flow into the body. **Figure 9-13** is a photo of a common volumetric infusion pump. The fluid flows from the bag through the first tube and into the pump. The pump contains a series of rollers that rotate to "push" the fluid into the second tube. The fluid flows through the second tube and is delivered into the body via a needle. A health care provider monitors the flow rate and the volume of the fluid. This type of infusion pump is equipped with two alarms: one that detects the end of the fluid volume and another that detects the presence of air bubbles in the tubing. Air bubbles delivered into blood circulation can cause embolisms, or blockages in vessels. Embolisms can also cause damage to pulmonary circulation and can be life threatening. If the air bubble is large, it can even cause the heart to stop.

The volumetric infusion pumps such as Baxter's Colleague, the Medsystem III, and Cardinal Health's Alaris can have multiple infusion channels to distribute more than one fluid to the body at the same time. Multiple channels are particularly useful in ICUs, in the practice of oncology, and in the delivery of anesthesia to a patient when even slight errors

FIGURE 9-12 Photo of a syringe pump.

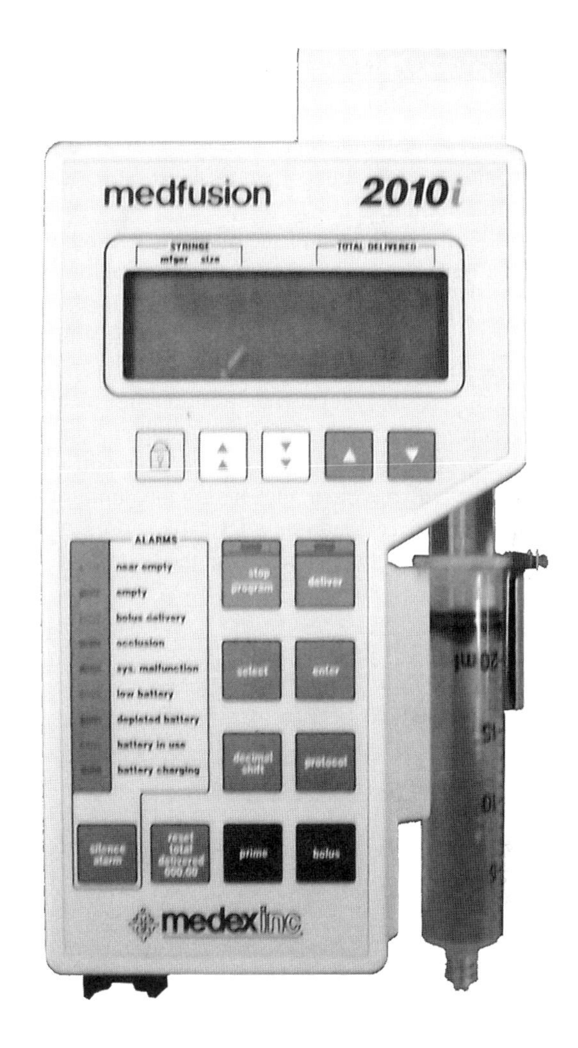

FIGURE 9-13 Photo of a volumetric infusion pump.

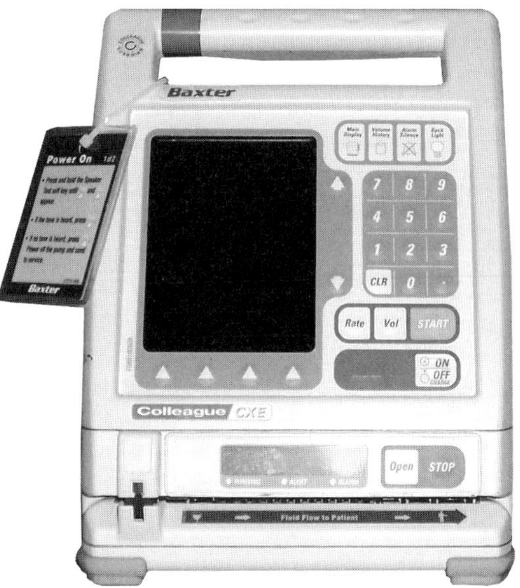

in medication levels and combinations can be fatal. Such specifications as flow rate, infusion volume, and correct dose for one or more patients can be programmed using up to 10 different formulas.

The diagram of the pumping mechanism of a volumetric infusion pump is shown in **Figure 9-14.** The main components of the pumping mechanism are the DC motor, encoder, valve actuator, and a cassette piston.

The fluid is delivered to the patient by a piston pump that is powered by a DC motor system. The cassette piston is moved back and forth by the pumping mechanism. The encoder on the cam shaft provides position information for the control of fluid delivery. The fill stroke and delivery stroke of the pumping chamber are part of the pumping mechanism.

The valves on this device are positioned such that the outlet valve is closed and the inlet valve is open, thus letting the pumping chamber fill by retracting the piston. Once the chamber is filled, the inlet valve closes and the outlet valve opens to deliver the fluid by advancing the piston toward the bottom of the chamber.

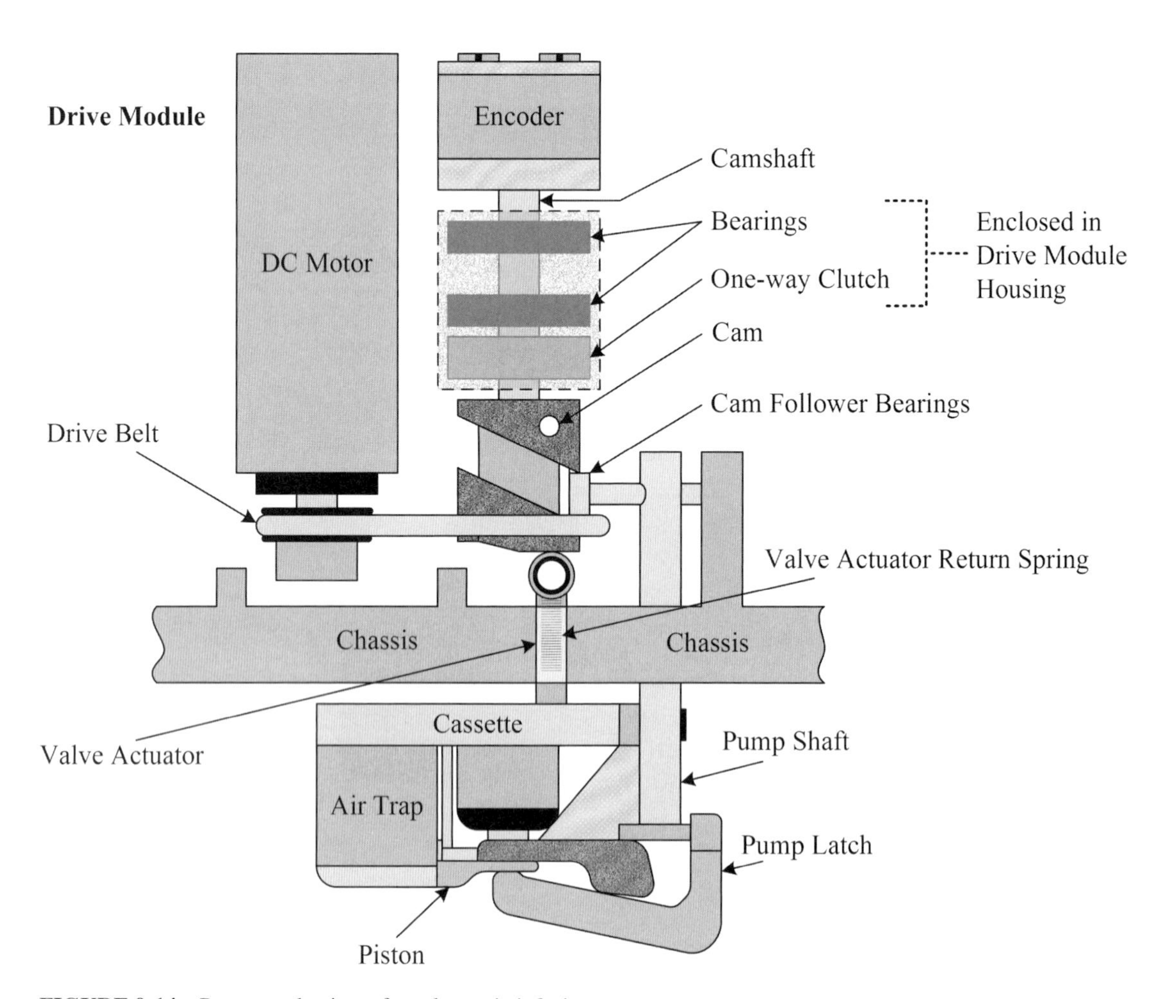

FIGURE 9-14 Pump mechanism of a volumetric infusion pump.

The device has a front panel and keypad with several setting options, such as the keep vein open (KVO) rate or intravenous (IV) delivery rate. The air-in-line sensors activate when bubbles of air are detected during infusion. Other sensors monitor the infusion process and can detect cassette placement or any occlusions in the line. Watchdog circuitry ensures that the microprocessor is properly executing the software steps. In addition to these settings, a list of drugs and dose rates can be programmed into the volumetric infusion device.

A monitor accompanying the device shows a graph with start-up curves and trumpet curves. The start-up curve represents the continuous flow rate versus the operating time during two-hour intervals from the beginning of the infusion. The trumpet curves show the accuracy over which fluid delivery is measured, although the accuracy is indicated during various periods during the delivery.

The volumetric infusion pumps use an electronic system that is a microprocessor-based integrated circuitry. Precision stepper motors with gear controls and lead-screws are used to move the piston.

Figure 9-15 shows a block diagram of electronic circuits in an infusion pump. The motor control and sensor interfaces receive instructions from the main combo I.C. and at least two stepper motors (as channel A and channel B) operate simultaneously with pulse width modulation (PWM) inputs. Each channel is activated for a different infusion task. The pressure sensor sends the digitized signal to the combo I.C. through an A/D converter. A

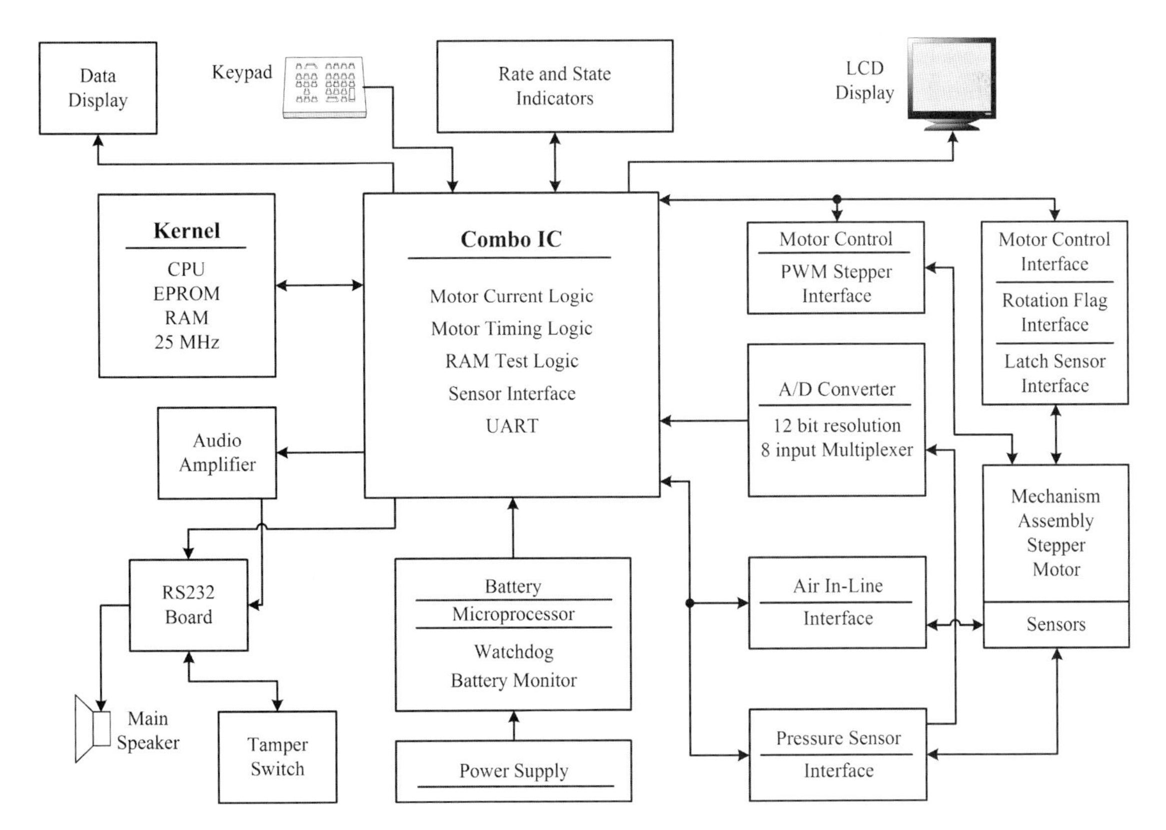

FIGURE 9-15 Block diagram of electronic circuits in an infusion pump.

tamper switch is used to sense any unauthorized tampering of the equipment and activates an alarm system. The CPU is driven by a 25 MHz crystal.

Procedure of Setting Up Infusion Therapy

1. The first step is to locate a healthy vein on the patient into which the needle will be inserted. The best veins are on the forearm or on the dorsum of the hand. Use a tourniquet and gentle tapping to plump the vein. Shave the area, if needed, prior to applying the tourniquet.
2. Using a syringe with a needle, insert the cannula in the vein. Remove the needle and the tourniquet, if used.
3. Set up the bag of fluid, fix the cannula securely, then start the fluid infusion.
4. Dispose of all the sharps.

9.12 CATHETERIZATION

A catheter is a thin flexible tube (**Figure 9-16a** shows the tubing in a cardiovascular catheterization). There are a variety of catheters used in patient health care such as Swan-Ganz pulmonary artery catheters, cardiac ablation catheters, double lumen catheters, vein infusion catheters, and intrathecal catheters. If placed in a vein, it is a channel to deliver medications or fluids. Blood can also be withdrawn through a catheter. Of course, when any catheter is used, proper protocols must always be followed to ensure minimal risk of injury or transferring of disease to the health care provider.

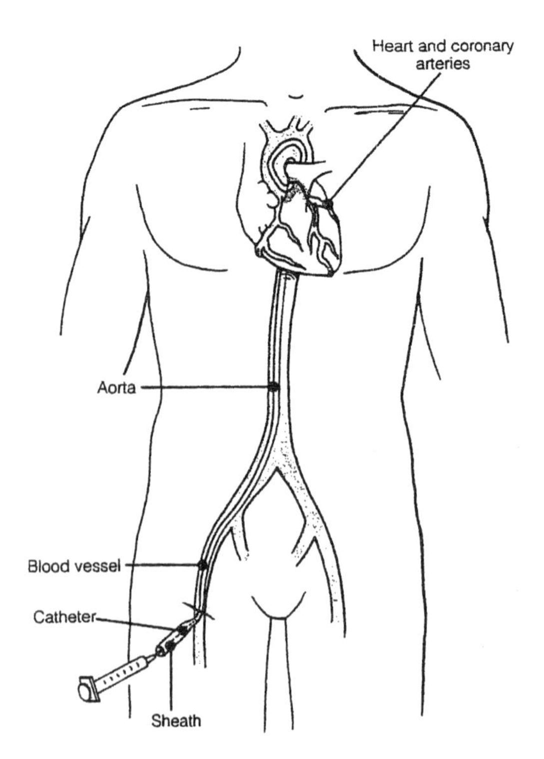

FIGURE 9-16a Cardiovascular catheterization.

Cardiovascular Catheterization

The first recorded insertion of a catheter into a human heart was in 1929 by Dr. Werner Forssmann. Ignoring his department chief's warnings, he placed a ureteral catheter into a vein in his right arm, threaded it to the right atrium of his heart, and walked upstairs to the x-ray department to document the procedure on film. Dr. Forssmann was awarded the Nobel Prize in Physiology or Medicine in 1956. Today, cardiovascular catheterization is used to measure pressure and flow, in angiography and angioplasty, and in the study of coronary thrombolysis. It is considered a safe procedure in diagnostic and therapeutic cardiac health.

Cardiovascular catheterization and angiography can provide a detailed assessment of the anatomy and physiology of the heart. In angiography, a cardiologist inserts an introductory sheath into a blood vessel in the arm or groin. The catheter is threaded into the blood vessel through this sheath and a guide wire then assists the catheter to reach the desired position in the heart. The guide wire is removed and a contrast solution is injected into the catheter. The contrast solution allows the images of the heart, blood vessels, and catheter to show on X-rays. The catheter is made of a radio-opaque material, which allows it to be visible in the x-ray images.

Cardiovascular catheterization is now a common procedure in the United States. **Figure 9-16b** is a table of estimated costs for various catheterization lab supplies. Note that the most expensive of these instruments are the dilatation catheters and the stents used to open blocked arteries.

Estimated Cost for Cardiovascular Lab Supplies:

Sheaths:	
Cordis Avanti sheath 6F	$ 11.15
Cordis Avanti sheath 7F	$ 10.80
Guidewires:	
Choice guidewire with/ICE	$ 124.50
Cordis Emerald Guidewire	$ 12.00
Daig Guide Right	$ 18.00
Coronary Artery Catheters:	
Cordis Judkins Right Coronary A Catheter	$ 10.50
Cordis Judkins Technique - Left Coronary	$ 18.00
Catheters for Angiography:	
Cordis Pig 145 Angiographic Catheter	$ 12.00
Cordis Plus TL Angiographic Catheter	$ 12.00
Specialized Catheters:	
Baxter Edwards Swan-Ganz Catheter	$ 63.00
Pacel Right Heart Curve Catheter	$ 108.00
Balloons of r Angioplasty:	
Ace PTCA Dilatation Catheter	$ 435.00
Cordis Valor PTCA Dilation Catheter	$ 412.50
Quantum Ranger PTCA Dilatation Catheter	$ 435.00
Coronary Stents:	
GRII Coronary Stent	$ 1890.00
Palmaz-Achatz Balloon Expandable Stent	$ 1837.50
Schneider Wall Stent	$ 1785.00

FIGURE 9-16b A cost table for cardiovascular catheterization lab supplies.

SUMMARY

- Biomedical instruments used to measure blood circulation include blood pressure monitors, cardiac output (CO) equipment, plethysmographs, and infusion pumps.
- Blood pressure is the pressure of the blood within the arteries and is recorded by two numbers—the systolic pressure amount and the diastolic pressure amount.
- The systolic pressure is measured after the heart contracts; the diastolic pressure is measured before the heart contracts.
- The pressure gradient in the blood vessels moves the blood as flow against the vascular resistance. Blood flow is pulsatile in large arteries; however, it is nonpulsatile in veins.
- Cardiac output is the amount of blood that is pumped by the heart per unit time and is measured in l/min. The amount of blood that is ejected from the heart in one contraction is called the stroke volume. The stroke volume multiplied by the heart rate is the CO.
- Given in this chapter is a model of hemodynamics in a Bernoulli tube circuit with kinetic and potential energies. The Bernoulli's equation states that in a steady flow, the sum of all forms of mechanical energy in a fluid (such as pressure, kinetic energy, and the potential energy) is the same at all points on the streamline in a vessel. Velocity of fluid flow in a given section increases when it moves from a region of higher pressure to a region of lower pressure. Consequently, highest velocity occurs where the pressure is lowest, and the lowest speed occurs where the pressure is highest.

MEDICAL TERMINOLOGY

Aneroid: using or containing no fluid. For example, an aneroid barometer utilizes atmospheric pressure instead of liquid mercury.

Auscultation: the act of listening to sounds within the body to ascertain the condition of the heart, pleura, abdomen, lungs, and other organs.

Cardiac output (CO): the volume of blood ejected from the left side of the heart, particularly the ventricle, in one minute. Cardiac output can be measured in volume of blood per unit time or in liters per minute.

Catheterization: insertion of a tubular device into a blood vessel, duct, hollow organ, or body cavity to inject or remove fluid for diagnostic or therapeutic purposes.

Hemodynamics: physiology involving the forces circulating blood through the body.

Infusion pump: device used to release certain amounts of a substance over a specified period of time. The pump can be driven mechanically, electrically, or osmotically to inject agents.

Intravenous (IV) therapy: administration of a liquid substance directly into a vein. The procedure can be continuous or intermittent depending on the prescribed treatment and is often the fastest delivery route for medications to the body. Also called infusion therapy.

Mean arterial pressure (MAP): describes the average value for arterial pressure in a person. Can be computed by systolic pressure + diastolic pressure divided by 2.

Perfusion: pumping of fluid, such as blood, through the vessels of an organ.

Sphygmomanometer: device used to measure arterial blood pressure composed of an inflatable cuff used to restrict blood flow and a mercury or manometer to determine pressure. The device is used to measure the pressure when blood flow starts and at what pressure blood flow is unimpeded.

Swan-Ganz catheter: flexible catheter containing a balloon near its tip that is inserted into the pulmonary artery to measure blood pressure. It is used to detect heart failure, monitor therapy, and evaluate the effects of drugs. This device is also known as a pulmonary artery catheter.

QUIZ

1. When the blood pressure of a patient is 150/95, his or her mean arterial pressure (MAP) is:

   a) 140. b) 113. c) 150. d) None of the above.

2. Invasive blood pressure measurement is a(n) ________________ method to measure blood pressure.

   a) Direct
   b) Indirect
   c) Both direct and indirect
   d) Neither direct nor indirect

3. Preload and after load relate to:

   ____

4. Determine your cardiac output (CO) if your pulse rate is 72 bpm and the stroke volume is 80 ml.

   a) 600 liters per minute (l/min)
   b) 5,760 l/min
   c) 6 l/min
   d) 5.76 l/min

5. The ratio of the maximum CO to the resting CO is called:

   a) Reserve. b) Capacity. c) Cardiac reserve. d) Cardiac capacity.

6. If a patient's pulmonary arterial pressure is given as 26/10 mm Hg, what could be the corresponding pressure (systolic/diastolic) at the right ventricle?

   a) 20/2 mm Hg b) 26/10 mm Hg c) 26/0 mm Hg d) 30/0 mm Hg

7. Which two main measurements are obtained by the cardiac output module of patient monitors?

   a) Inspired and end-tidal CO_2
   b) Blood and injectate temperatures
   c) Heart rate and blood pressure

8. The difference between pulse oxymetry and plethysmography is:

   ____

9. What range of frequencies can be expected in the normal blood pressure wave?

   a) 10 Hz to 25 Hz b) 0.5 Hz to 1 Hz c) 1 Hz to 5 Hz

10. True or False: A person's blood pressure increases when he or she stands up. Please provide the reason for your answer.

    a) True. The reason is ________________________________.

    b) False. The reason is ________________________________.

RESEARCH TOPICS

1. Statins (types of medication) are used in controlling cholesterol and triglycerides. Research indicates that blood pressure is also controlled by these medications. Write a research paper about this subject and consider the following guidelines:

   a) Discuss statins and their effect on the heart and circulation.

   b) Compare a variety of these medications in the paper.

   c) Include the opinions of regulatory agencies.

   d) Discuss how to prevent a future heart attack from occurring.

2. Write a research paper describing the design of the instrumentation devices used to monitor the blood pressure and femoral artery blood flow in an anesthetized animal prior to an operation. Include a block diagram.

3. Write a case study-based research paper discussing power infusers that are used to administer IV fluids in emergency situations. The research should include collected data of the power infuser's use in and around the hospital. An example device is the Infusion Dynamics Power Infuser by Zoll Medical. The research could site advantages and disadvantages of this device and provide data from case studies involving patients.

4. A doctor detected a heart murmur in a 35-year-old male patient. Through radioisotope imaging and an echocardiogram, the doctor diagnosed a leak in the patient's aortic valve. The valve was repaired properly and the patient's heart function improved. Write a research paper about this subject and consider the following guidelines:

   a) Discuss myocardial dysfunctions in patients.

   b) How does radioisotope imaging work on the heart function?

   c) What are the symptoms of a heart murmur?

5. Write a research paper discussing other types of heart disorders such as mitral regurgitation, congestive heart failure, mitral stenosis, and aortic stenosis. Include the dynamics of pressure, flow, volume, peripheral resistance, and capacitance in your paper.

CASE STUDIES

1. A 50-year-old male patient has been awakened for some time by heart palpitations just after drifting off to sleep. They occur during the day or night. During the palpitations, he suffers no sweating or irregular breathing. However, the patient does experience dry mouth, clenched jaws, and notices his body is unusually warm. He explains to a cardiologist that his daily routine includes heavy coffee or tea consumption, work and family stress, and that he tends to wear heavy clothing while sleeping. After examination, the physician found no apparent heart problems and the patient's stress test results were normal. Consider the following:

   a) The effects of caffeine on the patient's heart rate or heart sound.

   b) The effects that heavy clothing can have concerning heart palpitations.

   c) The effects of anxiety or stress on the heart.

   Investigate how these considerations can affect the heart and may contribute to cardiovascular diseases.

2. An 82-year-old female patient with a history of high blood pressure underwent catheterization to insert stents in her right atrium and left kidney in an effort to control her blood pressure. After the catheterization procedure and proper medications, her blood pressure stabilized. She did experience blood clots in her right leg, however, and received a filter as a precautionary measure. Eventually, her blood pressure began to increase and her condition returned. Examination showed the stents and filter to be performing appropriately. Consider the following:

   a) Does she need another catheterization procedure?

   b) Is it common to perform this procedure at her advanced age?

   c) Is this the only possible procedure? What other choices are possible? She takes a high dose (800 mg/day) of blood pressure medication. How much higher, if any, can the dosage be increased?

PROBLEMS

1. Discuss the advantages and disadvantages of the following (you may use the Internet):

   a) Various types of blood pressure transducers that can be implanted or placed in the blood flow through a catheter.

   b) Dyes and cold saline methods of CO measurements.

2. Tension in the wall of a blood vessel is given as:

   Tension in dynes/cm^2 = (radius of the vessel) $\times$ (internal pressure of the vessel)

   Determine the tension in the wall of a capillary vessel and of the aorta.

   Given: Radius of the capillary = 10 μm; radius of the aorta = 2 cm; internal pressure in the capillary = 20 mm Hg; internal pressure in the aorta = 108 mm Hg.

   1 mm Hg = 1,300 dynes/cm^2.

3. Define coronary artery disease (CAD) and discuss the causes and the various ways to detect the disease. Collect clinical data on this disease.

4. Determine the approximate mean arterial pressure (MAP) by integrating the pressure pulse shown in **Figure 9-17** given the conversion factor for pressure as 6.5 mm Hg/cm deflection. Also, draw the mean arterial pressure as a straight line over the shaded area.

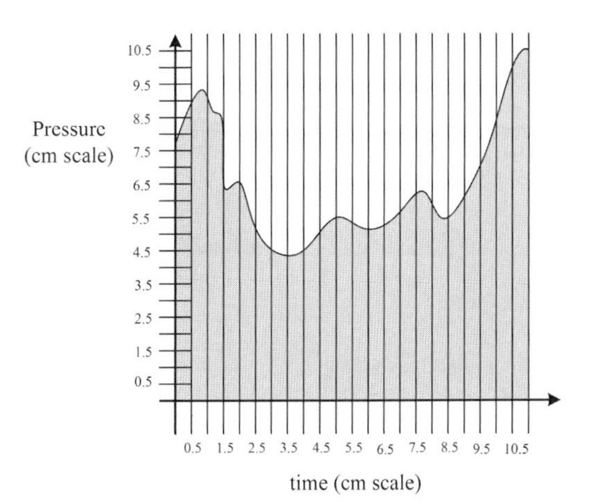

FIGURE 9-17 Pressure versus time graph.

Suggestion: Determine the total shaded area in cm^2; then, divide by the total time base (in cm). Finally, multiply by the deflection to provide the MAP in mm Hg. Each vertical line (i.e., the time scale) is separated by 0.5 cm. The pressure axis is given in 0.5 cm divisions. The nonlinear areas at the peaks can be approximated by right-angled triangles between two points and the remaining areas by rectangles.

5. What will be the blood flow in l/min if the injection rate of 4 mg/min results in a downstream concentration of 1 mg/l?
6. In the Bernoulli tube shown in **Figure 9-18,** is velocity $V_2 > V_3$? Also, is $P_1 < P_2$?

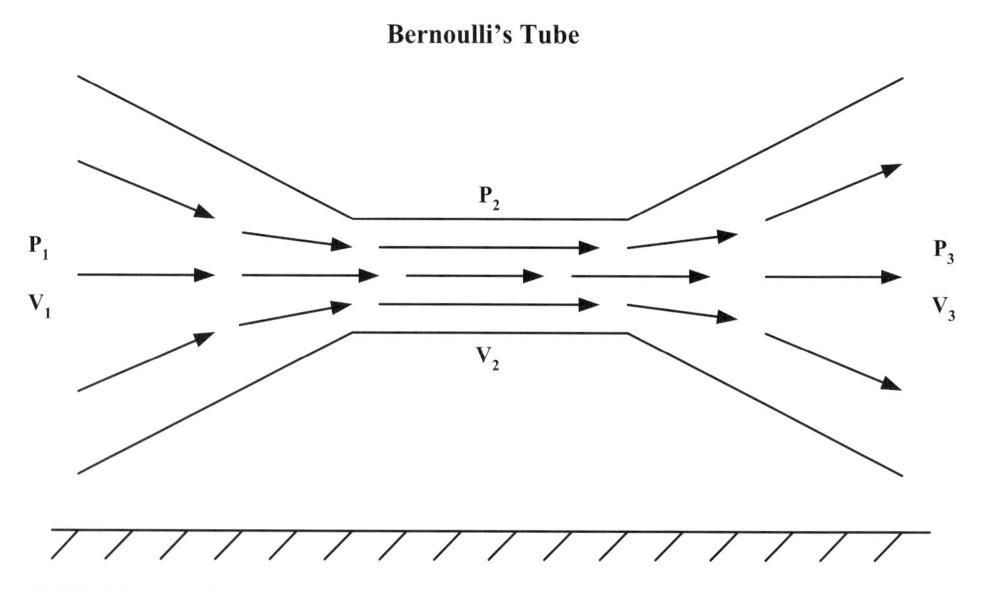

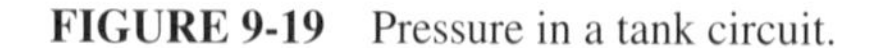

FIGURE 9-18 A Bernoulli tube.

7. As shown in **Figure 9-19,** find the pressure P_2.

   Given: Area of the reservoir is very large. Point 1 is at 20 m elevation, point 2 is at 15 m elevation, and point 3 is at 5 m elevation. Also, the cross-sectional area of 0.05 m^2 is the same at point 2 and point 3.

FIGURE 9-19 Pressure in a tank circuit.

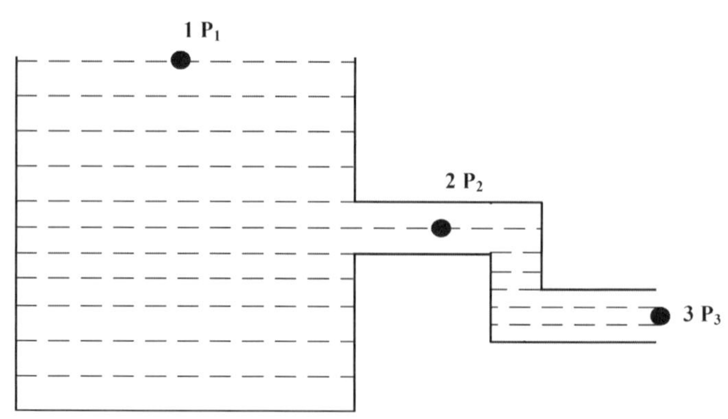

8. A pipeline of 0.2 m in diameter is flowing with water and ends in a constricted pipe of 0.1 m diameter. If the velocity in the 0.2 m section is 2 m/sec, find the velocity and the flow rate in the constricted section.
9. A patient has a 10 l/min CO. His PA has a 15 mm diameter with a 20 mm Hg pressure. His LA pressure is 8 mm Hg. Calculate the pulmonary vascular resistance.
10. A fluid-filled catheter is 100 cm long and has a diameter of 2 ml. Compute its resistance to the blood flow when the viscosity of blood is 0.0027 newton-seconds (N-s) per m^2.
11. Water flows through a constricted pipe at a uniform rate. At one point, the diameter of the pipe is 0.08 m and the pressure is 3×10^4 N/m^2. At another point, 0.5 m higher than the previous point, the diameter is 0.04 m and the pressure is 1.5×10^4 N/m^2. Calculate the velocities at the lower section and the upper section as well as the rate of the flow.
12. Find the CO using the thermodilution technique with the given parameters: injectate volume = 15 ml, blood temperature before injection = 37° C, injectate temperature = 23° C, post-injection temperature of the blood = 28° C after 12 seconds of injecting the cold saline, calibration factor = 0.02.

    Suggestion: consider the graph of temperature change in the blood as a straight line from 37° C to 28° C in 12 seconds and the area under the curve approximates a right-angled triangle.
13. Determine the Reynold's number when the water flows in a tube of 1 cm diameter with a velocity of 10 cm/sec. The density of water is 1 g/cm^3 and its viscosity is 0.01 dyne-sec/cm^2. One dyne is the force that imparts an acceleration of 1 cm/sec/sec to a mass of 1 g (that is, the unit of dyne is (g)(cm)/sec^2).

CHAPTER 10

Instrumentation in Extracorporeal Circulation and Cardiac Assist Devices

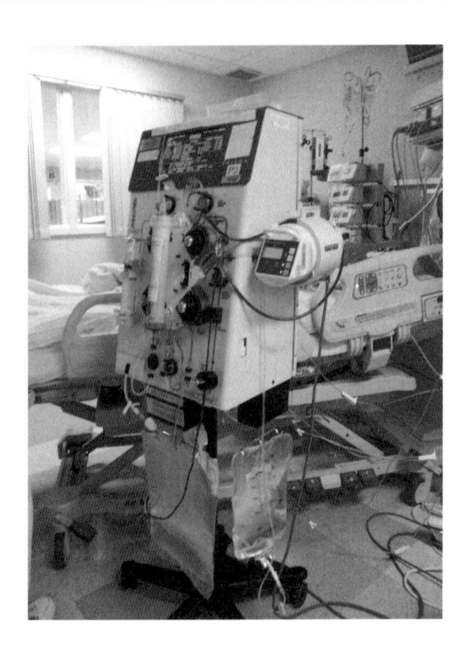

CHAPTER OUTLINE

OBJECTIVE

The objective of this chapter is to introduce to the reader extracorporeal (outside of the body) bioinstrumentation systems, designed to assist a patient's heart, lungs, and systemic blood circulation, and cardiac assist devices, designed to assist the heart in proper pumping of the blood through the body.

Upon completion of this chapter, the reader will be able to:

- Name several extracorporeal devices.
- Name the components of a dialysis machine.
- Discuss the processes of a heart-lung machine.
- Define apheresis and discuss the components of apheresis systems.
- Name two cardiac assist devices.
- Describe the function of ventricular assist devices and their applications.

INTERNET WEB SITES

http://www.circ.ahajournals.org (American Heart Association, Journal Circulation)
http://www.amsect.org (American Society of Extracorporeal Technology)
http://www.davita.com (Kidney disease and dialysis information source)
http://www.aami.org (Association for the Advancement of Medical Instrumentation)

INTRODUCTION

The term "extracorporeal treatment" is used to describe any sort of medical treatment that takes place outside the body, though not necessarily without some form of invasive procedure. Most extracorporeal treatments are related to the circulatory system and involve the removal and treatment of blood and then the subsequent return of that blood to the body.

Circulatory procedures classified as extracorporeal treatment include hemodialysis, apheresis, and cardiopulmonary bypass and assisted blood circulation, among others. All of these procedures involve the use of machinery to pump blood outside the body, process it, and then return it to the body. They are used to treat a variety of conditions. For example, hemodialysis is used to filter the blood during kidney failure, replacing the failing kidneys and filtering out harmful substances in the blood. Assisted blood circulation is used specifically in surgery to take over the duties of the heart for cardiac procedures.

Cardiac assist devices are mechanical devices that are used to partially or completely replace the function of a failing heart. Some cardiac assist devices are intended for short-term use, typically for patients recovering from heart attacks or heart surgery, while others are intended for long-term use (months to years and in some cases for life).

We discuss in this chapter several important extracorporeal treatments and their instrumentation: hemodialysis, apheresis, cardiopulmonary bypass (using the heart-lung machine), and extracorporeal membrane oxygenation. The two most common implantable cardiac assist devices discussed in this chapter are the ventricular assist device and the intra-aortic balloon pump.

10.1 EXTRACORPOREAL CIRCULATION PROCEDURES

Between the years of 1935 and 1954, John Gibbon, Clarence Dennis, and others pursued the development of a mechanical device to take over the function of the heart and lungs to permit surgical operations on the heart and great vessels. The entire project was stimulated by a patient with a lethal pulmonary embolism. Obviously, a machine that could be used to permit cardiopulmonary bypass for this problem could be used for cardiac surgery and a variety of other applications. Today, extracorporeal devices are used not only to maintain circulation in cardiac surgery, but also to cleanse the blood for malfunctioning kidneys, substitute for the pulmonary system by oxygenating blood, and administer life support for neonatal intensive care patients, among many other functions. In fact, extracorporeal devices are being used more frequently than ever before in modern hospitals. There are several explanations for this including improved devices that are less prone to complications and more convenient to use. In addition, we have a better understanding of the physiology of extracorporeal devices and can tailor their use to the needs of individual patients.

10.2 HEMODIALYSIS

Dialysis treatment replaces the function of the kidneys, which normally serve as the body's natural filtration system. When the kidneys fail to function properly, wastes can build up in the body, blood pressure can rise, and the body may stop making a sufficient supply of red blood cells. By using a blood filter and a chemical solution known as dialysate, the dialysis treatment removes waste products and excess fluids from the bloodstream, while maintaining the proper chemical balance of the blood. There are two types of dialysis treatments: peritoneal dialysis and hemodialysis. Peritoneal dialysis uses the membranous lining of the abdominal cavity to clean the blood. Hemodialysis is a treatment where the blood is cleansed outside the body and is then returned to the body. The extracorporeal instrument used in this treatment is called a hemodialysis machine.

Hemodialysis is the most frequently prescribed type of dialysis treatment in the United States. The treatment involves circulating the patient's blood outside of the body through an extracorporeal circuit (ECC), or dialysis circuit. Two needles are inserted into the patient's vein, or access site, and are attached to the ECC, which consists of plastic blood tubing, a filter known as a dialyzer (artificial kidney), and a dialysis machine that monitors and maintains blood flow and administers dialysate. Dialysate is a chemical bath that is used to draw waste products out of the blood.

Since the 1980s, the majority of hemodialysis treatments in the United States have been performed with hollow fiber dialyzers. A hollow fiber dialyzer is composed of thousands of tube-like hollow fiber strands encased in a clear plastic cylinder several inches in diameter. There are two compartments within the dialyzer (the blood compartment and the dialysate compartment). The membrane that separates these two compartments is semipermeable. This means that it allows the passage of certain-sized molecules across it, but prevents the passage of other, larger molecules. As blood is pushed through the blood compartment in one direction, suction or vacuum pressure pulls the dialysate through the dialysate compartment in a countercurrent, or opposite direction. These opposing pressures work to drain excess fluids out of the bloodstream and into the dialysate, a process called ultrafiltration. A second process called diffusion moves waste products in the blood across the membrane into the dialysate compartment, where they are carried out of the body. At the same time, electrolytes and other chemicals in the dialysate solution cross the membrane into the blood compartment. The purified, chemically balanced blood is then returned to the body.

Figure 10-1 shows the hemodialysis circuit. Note the large canister in the center of the image. This is the dialyzer, the main component of the dialysis machine.

Phoenix Hemodialysis Delivery System

A common type of hemodialysis machine used in hospitals is the Phoenix Hemodialysis Delivery System. **Figure 10-2a** shows a diagram of this complex machine (front view), while the accompanying **Figure 10-2b** lists each component of the device and its use. **Figure 10-3a** and **Figure 10-3b** provide rear views of the device, its components, and their uses.

Figure 10-4a is a block diagram of the main board of the Phoenix machine. Note that the device has five main circuit boards: the main board, hydraulic slave board, blood slave board, bio slave board, and protective slave board. The communication between the main board and the slave boards is through a serial peripheral interface (SPI) bus. The control

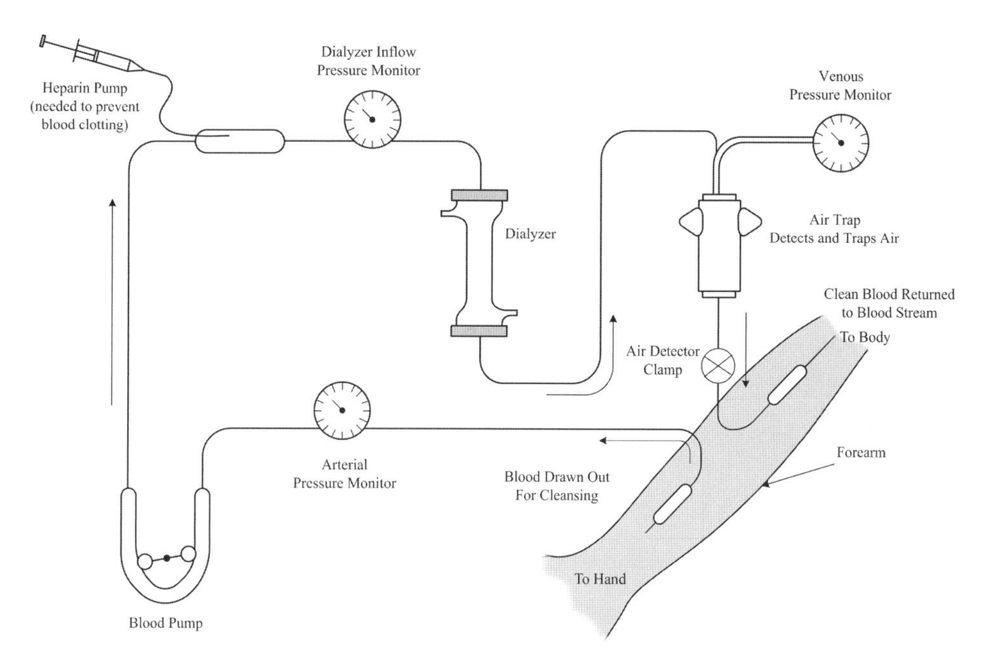

FIGURE 10-1 Hemodialysis circuit.

FIGURE 10-2a Phoenix Hemodialysis System (front view).

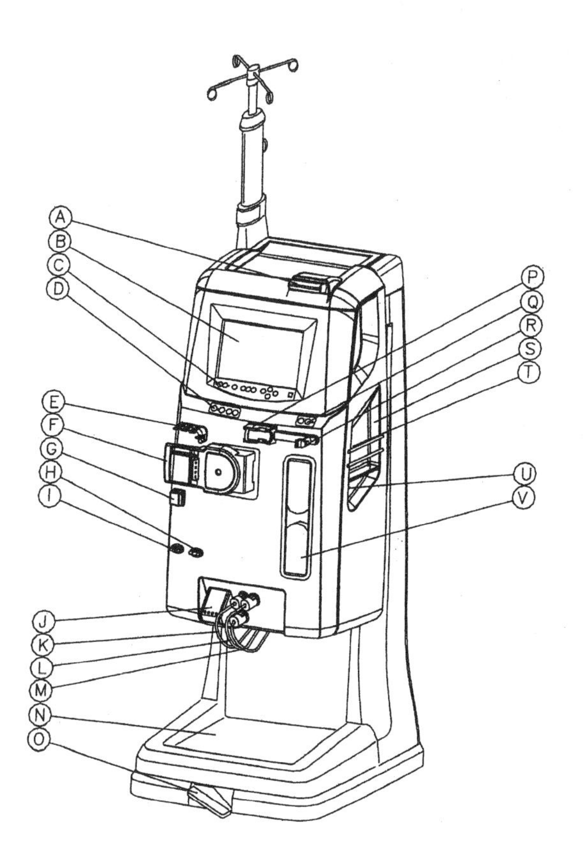

FIGURE 10-2b Listing of components in Figure 10-2a.

Front Panel Machine Components

(A)	**Patient Card Reader**	Reads the Patient Card.
(B)	**Display/ Touchscreen**	Allows the operator to communicate with the Phoenix machine via color screens and control buttons and vice versa.
(C)	**Main Keyboard**	The modification buttons can be used to access and modify the parameters. A dedicated button could be used to override the alarms.
(D)	**Blood Pump Keyboard**	Switches the blood pump on and off and regulates the speed.
(E)	**4-Position line clamp**	Plastic assembly that holds the four smaller lines extending from the arterial and venous chambers. The four thumb clamps are color coded for correct line placement, as follows: Green: heparin line; Red (right): arterial access line; Red (left): cartridge saline line; Blue: venous access line.
(F)	**Blood pump cover and cover latch**	Cover protects the blood pump from foreign objects; provides a track inside the cover to hold the pump segment of the Cartridge Blood Tubing Set. Latch keeps the blood pump cover closed during operation. The blood pump will not run unless the door is securely latched.
	Blood pump (behind the blood pump cover)	Pumps blood through the blood flowpath of the extracorporeal circuit.
(G)	**Air bubble detector housing**	The air bubble detector housing contains the ultrasonic sensor that detects macro and micro air in the fluid within the venous patient line. If macro or micro air is detected, the ! Air in Blood #4 alarm occurs (blood pump stops and venous line clamp closes). Also located in the housing are the optical patient sensor which detects the presence of blood in the tubing (when blood is detected the Protection Module is fully activated) and a position sensor which detects if blood tubing is inserted.
(H)	**Arterial line clip**	Secures arterial patient line to the machine.
	Arterial Line clamp	Optional Arterial line clamp (used for Single Needle dialysis)
(I)	**Venous line clamp**	Occlusive clamp that closes the venous patient line during certain red-light alarms and some self-tests, and when power is off. Prevents blood flow from going to the patient. The clamp assembly contains a position switch to ensure that the venous blood tubing is inserted into the clamp.
(J)	**WHO™ (Waste Handling Option)**	Used to discard unneeded saline solution during the blood circuit priming phase.
(K)	**Acid/Acetate line** (white/red connector) **and rinse port**	Connects to acid concentrate container (for bicarbonate dialysis) or acetate concentrate (for acetate dialysis). The acid/acetate line is connected to its rinse port during rinse and storage.
(L)	**Bicarbonate line** (blue connector) **and rinse port**	Connects to a bicarbonate concentrate container. The bicarbonate line is connected to its rinse port when a BiCart is in use, when the machine is used for acetate dialysis, and during rinse and storage.
(M)	**Disinfectant line** (yellow connector) **and rinse port**	Connects to a chemical container used during the machine chemical processes. During the main machine phases it must be connected to its rinse port.
(N)	**Concentrate container shelf**	Located on bottom front; holds containers of fluid concentrates needed for dialysis therapy.
(O)	**Locking brake**	Locks the casters so the machine will not move.
(P)	**Heparin syringe holder**	Holds the barrel of the heparin syringe.
(Q)	**Heparin Control Panel**	Allows the operator to regulate the heparin pump carriage position.
(R)	**Heparin syringe plunger clamp**	Holds the plunger of the heparin syringe. Moves to the left to push heparin into the blood flowpath at the specified rate.
	Heparin pump (inside machine)	Controls the rate of heparin delivery into the blood flowpath. Heparin can be delivered continuously or in bolus amounts.
	Blood leak detector (inside machine)	Infrared light detector that detects red blood cells in the fluid leaving the dialyzer. Blood indicates a leak or tear in the dialyzer membrane. If blood is detected, the Blood Leak alarm occurs (blood pump stops and venous line clamp closes).
(S)	**BPM cuff holder**	Houses the BPM cuff when not in use.
(T)	**Blood handling panel latch**	Secures the blood handling panel (middle third of front panel). The latch can be opened with a hex key or with the blood pump crank/panel latch key that is stored on the lack of the machine. Only service technicians should open the latch (to service internal components).
(U)	**Main power switch/circuit breaker**	Turns machine power ON and OFF. The label "I" means ON and the label "O" means OFF. The switch is also a circuit breaker and shuts off power in the event of an internal electrical overload. The breaker can be reset by turning the machine OFF, then ON.
(V)	**BiCart holder**	Holds a BiCart® column (powdered bicarbonate) for bicarbonate dialysis. The holder arms flip up and down so BiCart® can be inserted between them.
		Note: Bicarbonate concentrate pre mixed in a container can be used for bicarbonate dialysis instead of BiCart®, if desired.

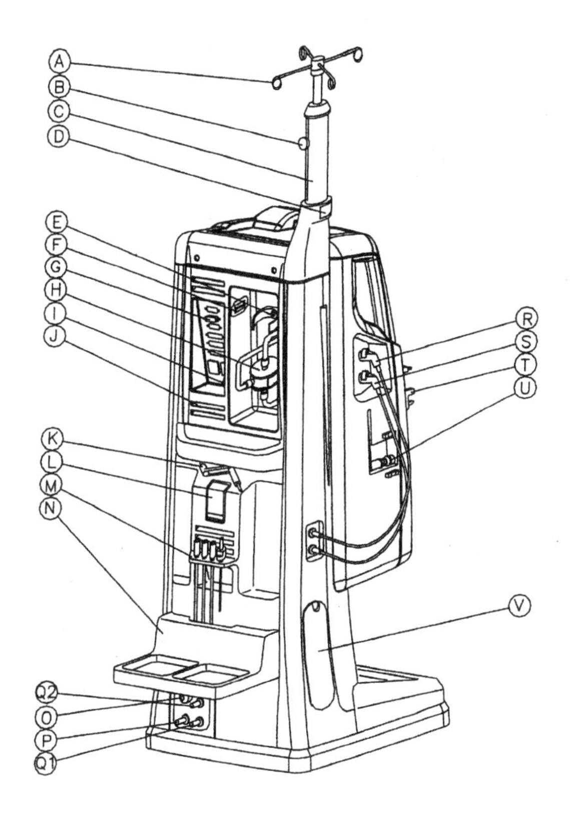

FIGURE 10-3a Phoenix Hemodialysis Delivery System (rear view).

FIGURE 10-3b Listing of components in Figure 10-3a.

Rear Machine Components

(A)	**Solution bag hooks**	Hold plastic bags of IV solutions for administration through the Cartridge Blood Tubing Set.
(B)	**IV pole adjustment knob**	Tightens to hold the IV pole in place at the desired height.
(C)	**IV pole**	Fits inside the machine for convenient placement of IV solutions.
(D)	**Status lights**	Illuminate to give a general indication of operating conditions.
	Yellow	A steady yellow light indicates that one or more alarms have been overridden.
		A flashing yellow light indicates a low priority alarm has occurred, for example, the machine is operating in Bypass or Minimum UFR. Immediate patient safety is not compromised, but the operator should investigate.
	Red	A flashing red light indicates a high priority alarm has occurred, for example the machine has detected air in the venous patient line or blood in the effluent line. A condition of possible patient or machine hazard exists; the operator should intervene immediately. A steady red light will be displayed in the event of a general safe state condition.
(E)	**Ultrafilter detection switch**	Detects the presence of the Diaclear Ultrafilter or its Hydraulic Bypass.
(F)	**Hour meter**	Accumulates hours of full power operation. Hours spent in low power are not counted on the meter.
		Depending on the machine version, the Hour Meter can be located either on the left side of the Ultrafilter Bypass Connector (as shown in the Figure) or in the Computer Interface Panel (see Figure 15.0 in the Section 15 – Specifications).
(G)	**Computer interface panel**	Provides ports for the machine options including connection to external networks.
(H)	**Ultrafilter bypass connector**	A connector which links the ultrafilter lines when the Diaclear Ultrafilter is not being used.
(I)	**BP tubing attachment site**	Connects luer lock on tubing of the machine BP Monitor Cuff to the internal electronic module.
(J)	**Air vents**	Provide continuous ventilation of interior components.

FIGURE 10-3b *(continued)*

(K)	**Blood pump crank**	Crank fits on the blood pump rotor, allowing manual blood return to the patient, if necessary.
(L)	**Cable holder** (for storage)	Holds the power cable when the machine is being moved or not being used.
(M)	**Wands holder**	Stores the wands and the conductivity sampler when they are not being used.
(N)	**Chemical container shelf**	Located on bottom right and left sides; holds containers of liquid chemicals needed for ADR procedures.
(O)	**Power cord**	For North American machines, the power cord is permanently attached. For non-North American machines, an IEC 320 connector at the power cord attachment site accepts most international style, 110-volt and 220-volt power cords.
(P)	**Inlet water hose**	Connects to the facility's dialysate water supply and carries water to the machine.
(Q1)	**Drain hose**	Connects to the facility's drainage system; carries away used dialysate, ultrafiltrate, and other waste fluids (main).
(Q2)	**Drain hose**	Connects to the facility's drainage system; carries away other waste fluids (secondary).
(R)	**Dialysate hose *From Dialyzer*** (red connector) **and bypass port**	Carries used dialysate from the dialyzer. During the hydraulics portion of pretreatment self-tests, ADR procedures, and storage, this hose must be connected to its bypass port.
(S)	**Dialysate hose *To Dialyzer*** (blue connector) **and bypass port**	Carries fresh dialysate to the dialyzer. During the hydraulics portion of pretreatment self-tests, ADR procedures, and storage, this hose must be connected to its bypass port.
(T)	**Cartridge holder**	Accepts the drip chamber portion of the blood tubing set and secures it in position with the cartridge clip (on the left) and the blood pump rotor (on the right). Has two sealing cones in the center for pressure monitoring. The red cone connects with the arterial chamber; the blue cone connects with the venous chamber.
(U)	**Dialyzer holder**	Holds the dialyzer. Consists of a movable holder arm and two grippers attached to the machine.
(V)	**Inlet Water Filter**	Depending on the machine version, the Inlet Water Filter can be located either on the left side of machine (as shown in the Figure) or inside the machine. The filter used are: Inlet Water Filter Standard (240 μ) or Deep Profile Filter (40 μ) code 6958821.

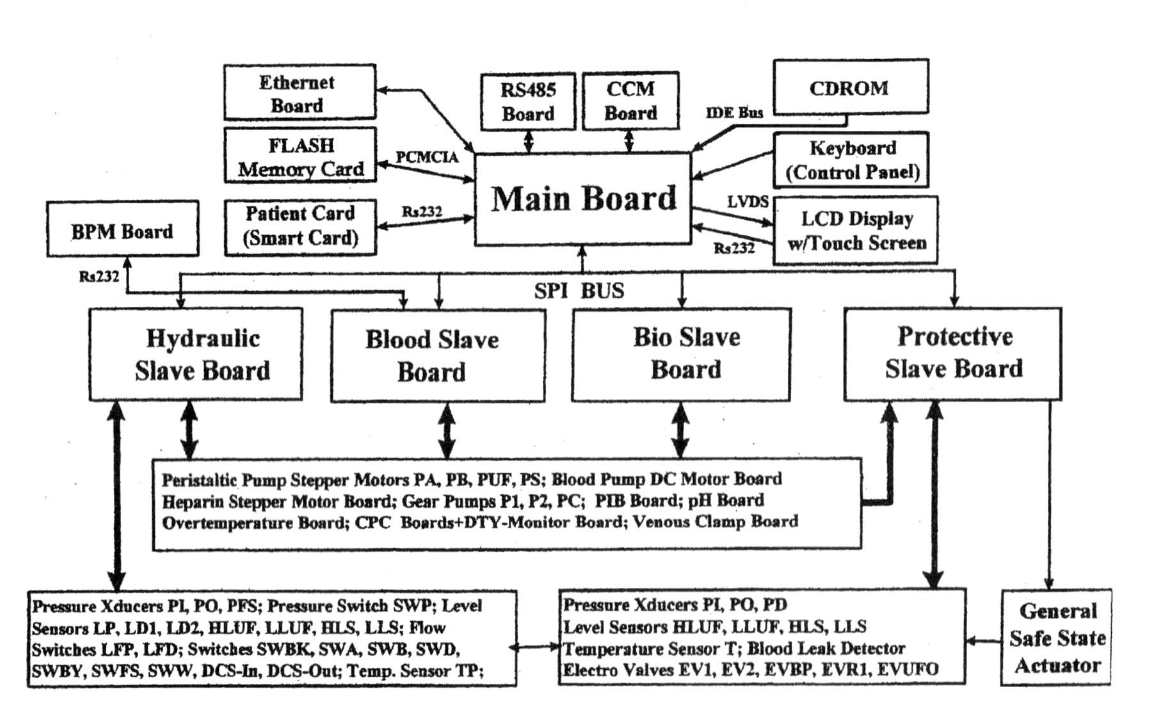

FIGURE 10-4a Block diagram of the main board of the Phoenix System.

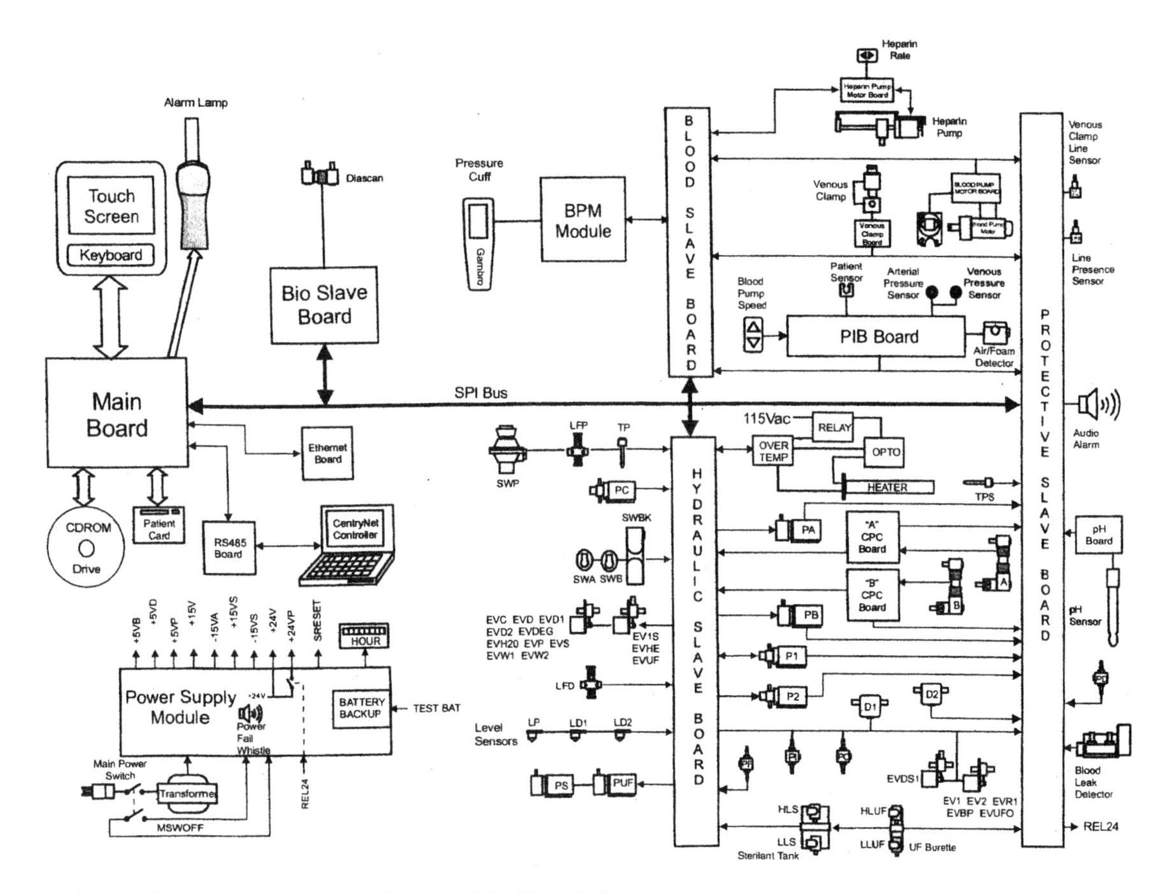

FIGURE 10-4b A detailed block diagram of the Phoenix System.

system in the Phoenix machine heats up the incoming water flow, de-aerates the water, mixes the water with concentrate, and stabilizes the dialysate solution. **Figure 10-4b** is a detailed system block diagram of the Phoenix machine.

After the dialysate is properly prepared, the temperature and conductivity of the solution is monitored. Ultrafiltration is controlled and the waste fluids are disposed. The waste-handling option (WHO) is to dispose waste fluid during the Phoenix blood tubing set priming. The waste is routed via Venturi, which supplies millimeters of mercury (mm Hg) pressure to draw waste fluids from the blood tubing set.

Dialysis Treatment Routine

Prior to performing this treatment on a patient, the dialysis machine must be prepared properly. The following are steps followed to ensure proper function of the device:

1. Firstly, the dialysis machine is rinsed thoroughly. This will eliminate any possibility of contamination in the machine. The rinsing may take about fifteen minutes and will clean the machine of bacteria, endotoxins, bleach, and any stale water remaining from the previous use.

2. The water treatment room requires safety checks to determine if the reverse-osmosis (RO) machine is working properly. The technician checks the water for its pH, calcium and magnesium hardness, temperature, conductivity, chlorine, and chloramines. These types of safety checks must meet the Association for the Advancement of Medical Instrumentation (AAMI) standards.
3. The next process is the dialysate preparation. This is the mixing of the baths (that is, the solution in which the blood is "washed"). The components of the dialysate are sodium bicarbonate and acid. The acidic balance of the bath is important. More acid in the preparation better controls the growth of any bacteria in the wash. The bicarbonate is made daily; otherwise, the bacteria will grow too quickly. The central delivery system will distribute the ingredients of the dialysate to the machines. Sometimes, five-gallon jugs of dialysate are used to wash the machines, as well.
4. The device is warmed up to a pre-set temperature of 37° C and brought up in conductivity of 13 mS (milli-Siemens) to 15 mS.
5. The device next performs a safety self-test. The safety features include high and low values of the following parameters: temperatures, conductivities, arterial pressures, venous pressures, and transmembrane pressures. The transmembrane pressure (TMP) is the pressure exerted on the semipermeable membrane of the dialyzer. In addition, the self-test is performed for blood and air leaks.
6. Next, the extracorporeal circuit is placed on the machine. The circuit consists of the dialyzer (artificial kidney), arterial blood line, venous blood line, and the saline line. Saline is circulated for about 15 minutes to allow for the removal of residual disinfectant ethylene-oxide and air bubbles.
7. The previous steps performed prior to the arrival of the patient. Upon arrival, the patient's standing and sitting blood pressures, pre-weight, breathing, and vascular access is recorded. If the patient has gained weight or if his or her blood pressure has changed, a weight goal in the range of 2 kg to 10 kg is determined.
8. Next, the patient is cannulated and a bolus of anticoagulant (such as porcine heparin) is given. Final checks are performed on the machine for temperature, pH, and conductivity, and the weight goal and treatment time is programmed into the machine. The patient is now ready for treatment, which can last up to approximately four hours.
9. The vital signs of the patient are monitored every 30 minutes. Additionally, the machine parameters are checked regularly during the treatment.
10. After treatment, the patient's blood is returned from the extracorporeal circuit and vital signs are monitored again. A post-weight is determined to see how much fluid has been removed. The patient is then released. The process is repeated as often as three times a week for some patients. There is no cure for kidney failure other than kidney transplant. Therefore, this type of life-saving treatment can be performed indefinitely, even for the rest of the patient's life.

10.3 APHERESIS SYSTEMS

Apheresis (a Greek word meaning, "to take away") is a medical treatment in which the blood of a donor or patient is passed through an apparatus that separates out one particular constituent and returns the remainder to the circulation. It is thus an extracorporeal treatment.

The various apheresis techniques may be used whenever the removed constituent is causing severe symptoms of disease. Generally, apheresis has to be performed often, and is an invasive process. It is therefore only employed if other means to control a particular disease have failed, or the symptoms are of such a nature that waiting for medication to become effective would cause suffering or risk of complications.

Depending on the substance that is being removed, different processes are employed in apheresis. If separation by weight is required, centrifugation is the most common method. Other methods involve absorption onto beads coated with an absorbent material and filtration.

The centrifugation method can be divided into two basic categories:

1. **Continuous-flow centrifugation**

   Continuous-flow centrifugation (CFC) historically required two venipunctures as "continuous" in this regard means the blood is collected, spun, and returned simultaneously. Newer systems can use a single venipuncture. The main advantage of this system is the low extracorporeal volume (calculated by volume of the apheresis chamber, the donor's hematocrit, and total blood volume of the donor) used in the procedure, which may be advantageous in the elderly and for children.

2. **Intermittent-flow centrifugation**

   Intermittent-flow centrifugation (IFC) works in cycles, taking blood, spinning/processing it, and then giving back the unnecessary parts to the donor in a bolus. The main advantage of this method is a single venipuncture site. To stop the blood from coagulating, anticoagulant is automatically mixed with the blood as it is pumped from the body into the apheresis machine.

Apheresis System

Figure 10-5a is a diagram of an apheresis system machine, such as a COBE® Spectra or Baxter unit, and its numerous components. This system of separating blood cells is automated and monitors the extracorporeal circuit. Common to most apheresis systems, it has a blood tubing set with a preconnected channel that spins blood in the centrifuge, separates the blood components, and routes the blood and replacement fluid.

The control panel for an apheresis system is shown in **Figure 10-5b.** The panel has a numeric keypad, display keys, miscellaneous keys, and a display screen. The keypad is used to enter numbers and YES/NO questions. The display keys are grouped as flow rates, volumes, and target values. The miscellaneous keys are at the bottom and the left side of the panel.

When manually controlled, the pump flow rates and centrifuge speeds (for anticoagulant and centrifuge) are adjustable. However, under automatic control, the software calculates the flow rates and the speed based on patient height, weight, and sex. A collect concentration monitor (CCM) based on optical sensing is used to count platelets and update the operator to make changes during the apheresis procedure. A flow diagram for collection and depletion procedures is shown in **Figure 10-5c.**

In addition to the acid citrate dextrose (ACD) and saline sets, there are sets for collections and depletions in the blood tubing. The plasma valve is activated by the centrifuge separation channel at the plasma port. The control port controls the activity of collection and depletions based on the inlet pump and the centrifuge pressure sensor.

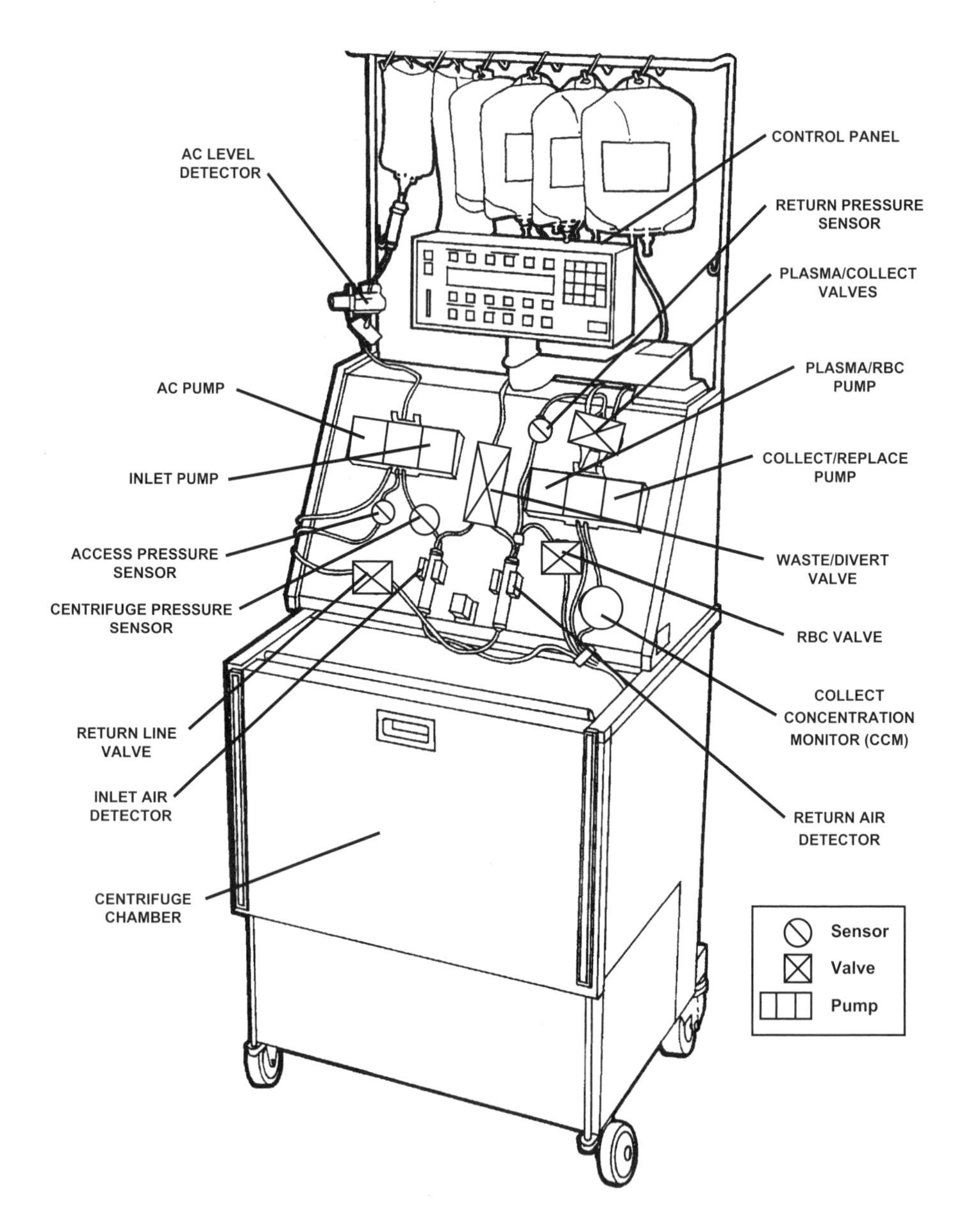

FIGURE 10-5a Apheresis system.

FIGURE 10-5b Display panel of an apheresis system machine.

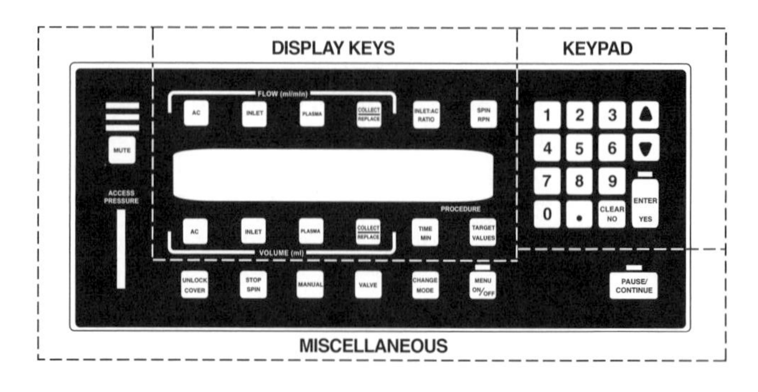

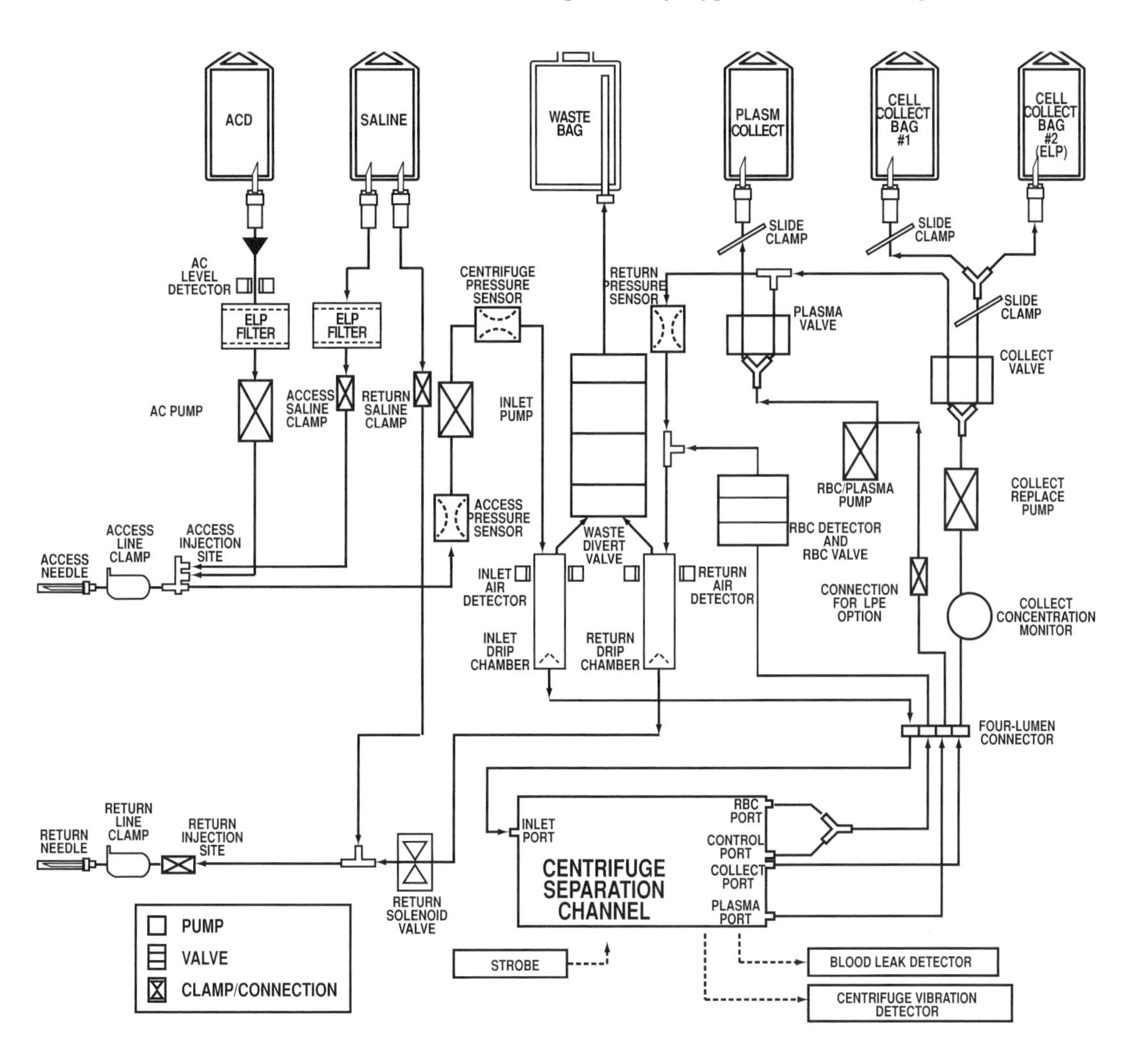

FIGURE 10-5c A flow diagram of the procedures in an apheresis machine.

10.4 CARDIOPULMONARY BYPASS AND HEART-LUNG MACHINES

Another form of extracorporeal circulation is the cardiopulmonary bypass (CPB). This technique temporarily takes over the function of the heart and lungs during surgery in order to maintain the circulation of blood and the oxygen content of the body. The CPB pump itself is often referred to as a heart-lung machine or simply the pump. Cardiopulmonary bypass pumps are operated by health professionals known as perfusionists in association with surgeons who connect the pump to the patient's body.

Cardiopulmonary bypass is commonly used in heart surgery because of the difficulty of operating on the beating heart. Cardiopulmonary bypass mechanically circulates and oxygenates blood for the body while bypassing the heart and lungs so that the surgeon works in a bloodless surgical field. The surgeon places a cannula in the right atrium, vena cava, or femoral vein to withdraw blood from the body. The cannula is connected to tubing filled with isotonic crystalloid solution. Venous blood that is removed from the body by the cannula is filtered, oxygenated, cooled or warmed, and then returned to the body. The cannula used to return oxygenated blood is usually inserted in the ascending aorta, but it may be inserted in the femoral artery. The patient is administered heparin to prevent clotting and protamine sulfate is given after to reverse effects of heparin. During the procedure, hypothermia is maintained (body temperature is usually kept at 82.4º F to 89.6º F). The blood is cooled during CPB and returned to the body. The cooled blood slows the body's basal metabolic rate, decreasing its demand for oxygen. Cooled blood usually has a higher viscosity, but the crystalloid solution used to prime the bypass tubing dilutes the blood. **Figure 10-6a** shows a simple block diagram of a cardiopulmonary bypass system. Refer to **Figure 10-6b** for a data sheet with technical details of a typical bypass machine.

Cardiopulmonary bypass machines are standard equipment in most cardiac operating rooms. Some of the more common surgeries for which CPB is used are:

- Coronary artery bypass surgery.
- Cardiac valve repair and/or replacement (aortic valve, mitral valve, tricuspid valve, pulmonic valve).
- Repair and/or palliation of congenital heart defects.

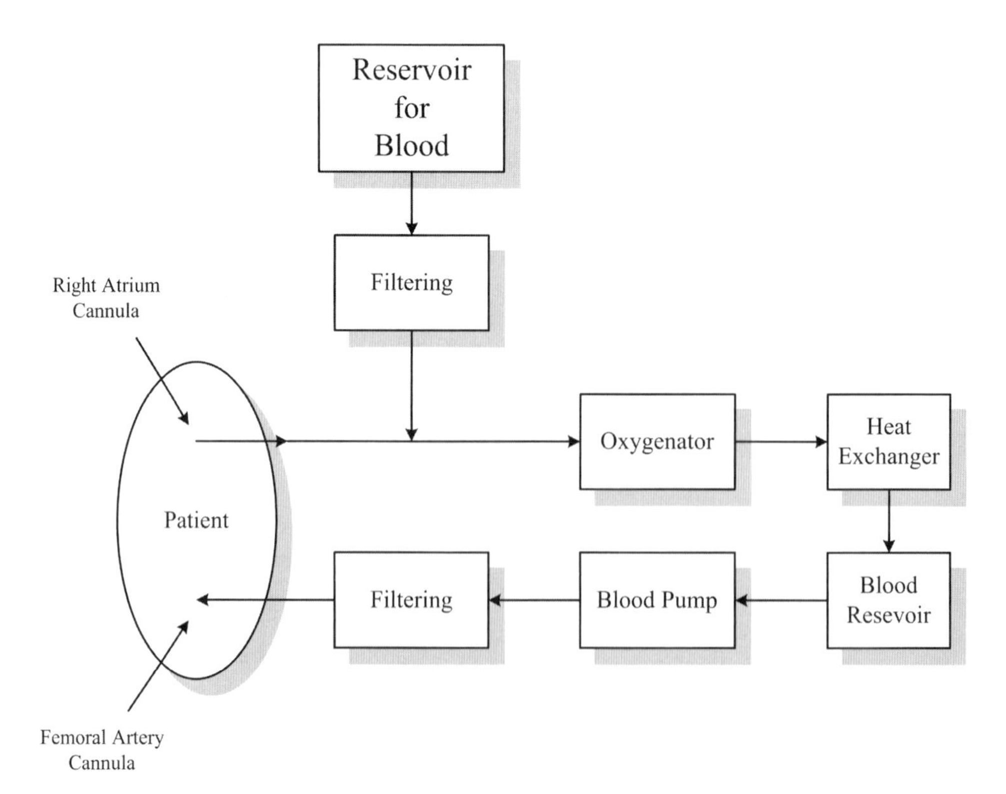

FIGURE 10-6a A block diagram of a cardiopulmonary bypass system.

- Transplantation (heart transplantation, lung transplantation, heart-lung transplantation).
- Repair of some large aneurysms (aortic aneurysms, cerebral aneurysms).
- Pulmonary thromboendarterectomy and pulmonary thrombectomy.

Emergency Power	2 x 12V batteries Automatic battery backup provides power to two pumps, all safety systems and accessories for 25 minutes. Switchover from main power to battery backup is automatic & immediate, providing uninterrupted power supply
Power Supply	Protected power cords from spills but easily accessible. Fully loaded current rating of 6 amps for 4 pump base.
Lighting	High intensity low voltage quartz Goose neck lamp. Power to the lamp is uninterrupted if a battery module is installed.
IV Poles & Accessories	Sturdy poles make it easy to mount monitors & additional equipment. Adjustable height Shelving Stopwatches (additional for Cobe)
Design	Solid stainless steel base.
Alarms	Ergonomically positioned

Power Consumption	*Biomedicus*	*SARNS 7000*	*SARNS 8000*	*COBE*
Pump Module	1.5 Amps	1/8 hp motor	Current rating: 0.7 Amps	150 watts typical 280 watts max 1.5 Amp circuit breaker
Base Leakage Current			6 Amps (4 pump base)	20 mA Max

FIGURE 10-6b Data sheet of a cardiopulmonary bypass machine.

Components of a Cardiopulmonary Bypass Machine

The CPB machine consists of several main functional components: the pump, the oxygenator/heat exchanger unit, and tubing, or cannulae. The pump and oxygenator remove oxygen-deprived blood from a patient's body and replace it with oxygen-rich blood through a series of tubing.

Pumps

Roller pump The pump console of a CPB is usually comprised of several rotating motor-driven pumps that peristaltically "massage" the tubing. This action gently propels the blood through the tubing. This is commonly referred to as a roller pump, or peristaltic pump.

Centrifugal pump Many CPB circuits now employ a centrifugal pump for the maintenance and control of blood flow during CPB. By altering the speed of revolution (RPM) of the pump head, blood flow is produced by centrifugal force. This type of pumping action is considered superior to the action of the roller pump by many because it is thought to produce less blood damage. A centrifugal pump is a rotodynamic pump that uses a rotating impeller to increase the pressure of a fluid.

Cardioplegia delivery pump As a CPB consists of a systemic circuit for oxygenating blood and reinfusing blood into a patient's body, a separate circuit for infusing cardioplegia to stop the heart and provide myocardial protection is necessary, as well. Cardioplegia is the intentional and temporary cessation of cardiac activity and is used primarily in cardiac bypass surgeries. The cardioplegia delivery pump delivers a high-potassium solution to the coronary vessels in order to provide intentional and temporary cessation of cardiac activity.

Emergency back-up pump The CPB contains an emergency back-up pump in order to provide continued treatment in case of mechanical failure.

Oxygenator The oxygenator is designed to transfer oxygen to infused blood and remove carbon dioxide from the venous blood. Oxygenators contain an integral heat exchanger, a metal coil that contacts the blood as it enters the oxygenator. Water passing through the coil alters the core temperature of the patient accordingly. Cardiac surgery was made possible by CPB using what is called bubble oxygenators, but membrane oxygenators have supplanted bubble oxygenators since the 1980s.

The oxygenator was first conceptualized in the seventeenth century by Robert Hooke and developed into practical extracorporeal oxygenators by French and German experimental physiologists in the nineteenth century. Bubble oxygenators have no intervening barrier between blood and oxygen; these are called "direct contact" oxygenators. Membrane oxygenators introduce a gas-permeable membrane between blood and oxygen that decreases the blood trauma of direct-contact oxygenators. Much work since the 1960s focused on overcoming the gas exchange handicap of the membrane barrier, leading to the development of high-performance microporous hollow-fiber oxygenators that eventually replaced direct-contact oxygenators in cardiac operating rooms.

Another type of oxygenator gaining favor recently is the heparin-coated blood oxygenator, which is believed to produce less systemic inflammation and decrease the propensity for blood to clot in the CPB circuit.

Cannulae The components of the CPB circuit are interconnected by a series of tubes made of silicone rubber or PVC (similar to a transparent garden hose) and cannulae. Multiple cannulae are sewn into the patient's body in a variety of locations, depending on the type of surgery. For example, a venous cannula removes the oxygen-deprived blood from a patient's body; an arterial cannula is used to infuse the oxygen-rich blood; and a cardioplegia cannula is sewn into the heart to deliver the cardioplegia solution used to stop the heartbeat.

10.5 EXTRACORPOREAL MEMBRANE OXYGENATION

In intensive care medicine, extracorporeal membrane oxygenation (ECMO) is an extracorporeal technique of providing both cardiac and respiratory support oxygen to patients whose heart and lungs are so severely diseased or damaged that they can no longer serve their function. This simplified form of CPB is most commonly used in neonatal intensive care units (NICUs) as life-support for newborns with serious birth defects or in pulmonary distress. It is also commonly used to oxygenate and maintain organ function for transplant recipients until new organs can be found.

To initiate ECMO, cannulae are placed in large blood vessels to provide access to the patient's blood. Anticoagulant drugs (usually heparin) are administered to prevent blood clotting. The ECMO machine continuously pumps blood from the patient through a "membrane oxygenator" that imitates the gas exchange process of the lungs, (i.e., it removes carbon dioxide and adds oxygen). Oxygenated blood is then returned to the patient. **Figure 10-7a**

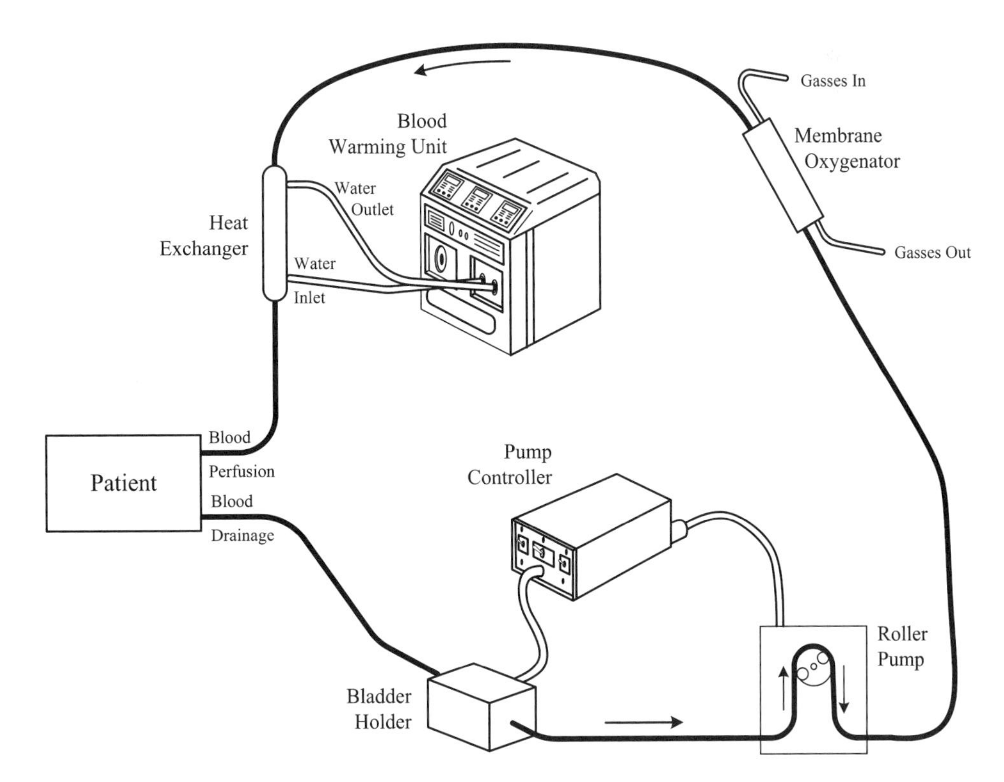

FIGURE 10-7a Seabrook Medical Systems, Inc., ECMO circuit system.

illustrates an EMCO circuit system developed by Seabrook Medical Systems, Inc. Refer to **Figure 10-7b** for detailed specifications of the Seabrook ECMO device.

There are several forms of ECMO, the two most common are veno-arterial (VA) and veno-venous (VV). In both modalities, blood drained from the venous system is oxygenated outside of the body. In VA ECMO, this blood is returned to the arterial system; in VV ECMO, the blood is returned to the venous system. In VV ECMO, no cardiac support is provided.

Veno-venous ECMO can provide sufficient oxygenation for several weeks, allowing diseased lungs to heal while the potential additional injury of aggressive mechanical ventilation is avoided. It therefore may be life saving for some patients. However, due to the high technical demands, cost, and risk of complications (such as bleeding under anticoagulant medication), ECMO is usually only considered as a last resource in therapy. In VA ECMO, patients whose cardiac function does not recover sufficiently to be weaned from ECMO may be bridged to a ventricular assist device (VAD) or transplant.

Management of the ECMO circuit is done by a team of ECMO specialists that includes ICU physicians, perfusionists, respiratory therapists, and registered nurses that have received training in this specialty.

Physical	
Size	9.75"W x 14"H x 11"D
Weight (Dry)	24 lbs.
Hose Length	48 Inches
Couplings	Quick-Connect
Case Material	Modified Polyphenylene Oxide Plastic
Case Color	Light Grey

Control System	
Type	Microprocessor-based,
Accuracy	± 0.1°C
Self-Calibrating	120 Second Intervals
Setpoint Display	7 Segment, 3 Digit
Water Temp. Disp.	7 Segment, 3 Digit
Blood Temp. Disp.	7 Segment, 3 Digit
Display Range (H_2O)	5° - 50°C
Display Range (Blood)	30° - 45°C

System Safety	
Reservoir Capacity	3 Quarts
Reservoir Fluid	Sterile Distilled Water
Fill Cap	Vented
Flow Rate (through Heat Exchanger)	2 to 3 GPM
Maximum Pressure	8.2 PSI

Heating System	
Setpoint Range	35° - 40°C
Heating Element	300 Watts, Cartridge type

Electrical System	
Voltage	115V, 60 Hz
Current	4.25 Amps
Circuit Breaker	7 Amps
Power Cord	3 Conductor, 16 AWG, 8' Long, w/Hospital Grade Plug
Leakage Current	Under 100 μA

System Safety	
Over Setpoint Alarm (Blood)	0.3°C above Setpoint
Over Setpoint Alarm (H_2O)	1°C above Setpoint
Under Setpoint Alarm (Blood)	0.3° Below Setpoint
Under Setpoint Alarm (H_2O)	1°C Below Setpoint
High Limit Alarm	43°C
Back-up High Limit Alarm	43° - 47°C
Add Water Alarm	Activates at "Add" on Reservoir

FIGURE 10-7b Specifications data sheet of the Seabrook ECMO.

10.6 VENTRICULAR ASSIST DEVICE

An implantable ventricular assist device (VAD) is a mechanical device that is used to partially or completely replace the function of a failing heart. Some VADs are intended for short-term use, typically for patients recovering from heart attacks or heart surgery, while others are intended for long-term use (for months or years and, in some cases, for life), typically for patients suffering from congestive heart failure. Ventricular assist devices need to be clearly distinguished from artificial hearts, which are designed to completely take over cardiac function and generally require the removal of the patient's heart.

Ventricular assist devices are designed to assist either the right ventricle (RVAD), the left ventricle (LVAD), or both ventricles (BiVAD). The choice of device depends on the underlying heart disease and the pulmonary arterial resistance, which determines the load on the right ventricle. Left ventricular assist devices are most commonly used; however, when pulmonary arterial resistance is high, right ventricular assist becomes necessary. Long-term VADs are normally used to keep a patient alive with a good quality of life while he or she awaits a heart transplant (referred to as a bridge to transplant). However, while LVADs are used as a bridge to recovery, they are sometimes used as destination therapy as well. **Figure 10-8** shows an illustration of an implanted VAD.

Most VADs operate on similar principles. A cannula is inserted into the apex of the appropriate ventricle. Blood passes through this to a pump and then through a tube to the aorta (in the case of an LVAD) or to the pulmonary artery (in the case of an RVAD). The pump is powered through a lead that connects it to a controller and power supply. In

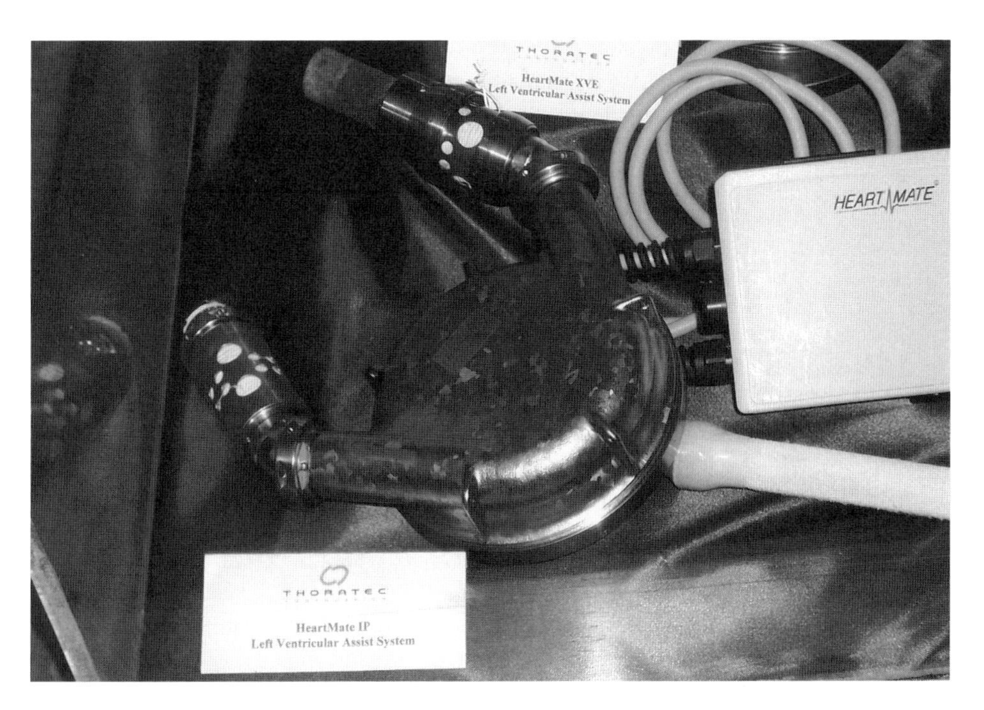

FIGURE 10-8 Implanted ventricular assist device.

some cases, there is also a tube to vent the pump to the outside air. Some devices, such as the Jarvik 2000, operate slightly differently—the pump is actually located inside the left ventricle and its outflow passes through the apex of the ventricle to a tube that leads to the aorta.

Major distinguishing features between the different VADs are the pump (which can vary substantially in method of operation, size, and placement), the controller, the materials used both for the pump and the associated tubes and cannulas, and the lead between the pump and the controller/power supply.

A newer class of percutaneous ventricular assist devices has been developed. These are typically introduced into the circulation by an interventional cardiologist using nonsurgical techniques, and may be used for short-term support of the left or right ventricles.

Pumps

Pumps used in VADs can be divided into two main categories: pulsatile pumps, which mimic the natural pulsing action of the heart; and continuous-flow pumps.

Pulsatile VADs use positive displacement pumps. In some of these pumps, the volume occupied by blood varies during the pumping cycle; and if the pump is contained inside the body, a vent tube to the outside air is required. The only three LVADs approved by the FDA for use in the United States are all pulsatile pumps. All were approved between 1994 and 1998, indicating the relative maturity of this technology.

Continuous-flow VADs normally use either centrifugal pumps or axial flow pump. Both types have a central rotor containing permanent magnets. Controlled electric currents running through coils contained in the pump housing apply forces to the magnets, which cause the rotors to rotate. In the centrifugal pumps, the rotors are shaped to accelerate the blood circumferentially; thus, they cause it to move toward the outer rim of the pump. In the axial flow pumps, the rotors are cylindrical with blades that are helical, causing the blood to be accelerated in the direction of the rotor's axis.

An important issue with continuous-flow pumps is the method used to suspend the rotor. Early versions used solid bearings; however, newer pumps (not all yet approved for use in the United States) use either electromagnetic or hydrodynamic suspension. These pumps contain only one moving part. Manufacturers claim that these methods of suspension not only virtually eliminate wear but also reduce damage to blood cells.

10.7 INTRA-AORTIC BALLOON PUMP

The intra-aortic balloon pump (IABP) is a mechanical device that is used to decrease myocardial oxygen demand while at the same time increasing cardiac output (CO). By increasing CO, it also increases coronary blood flow and, therefore, myocardial oxygen delivery. It consists of a cylindrical polyurethane balloon that sits in the aorta and counterpulsates. That is, it actively deflates in systole increasing forward blood flow by reducing after load; and, it actively inflates in diastole increasing blood flow to the coronary arteries.

These actions have the combined result of decreasing myocardial oxygen demand and increasing myocardial oxygen supply. The balloon is inflated during diastole by a computer-controlled mechanism, usually linked to either an ECG or a pressure transducer at the distal tip of the catheter; some IABPs allow for asynchronous counterpulsation at a set rate, though this setting is rarely used. The computer controls the flow of helium from a cylinder into and out of the balloon. Helium is used because its low viscosity allows it to travel quickly through the long connecting tubes, and has a lower risk of causing a harmful embolism should the balloon rupture while in use. More than 100,000 IABPs are inserted every year in the United States. They are most often used in open-heart operating rooms and in catheterization laboratories.

Figure 10-9a shows the balloon deflation and inflation and the location of the catheter and the balloon pump with respect to the heart. An IABP catheter with a large balloon wound tightly around the distal end is inserted at the femoral artery and a guide wire guides the balloon advancing slowly to a position just distal to the left of the subclavian artery. The guide wire is removed and the balloon is secured. The catheter is then attached to an oxygenator pump. The balloon is deflated during systole and inflated during diastole. **Figure 10-9a** shows the balloon collapsed and also fully inflated.

FIGURE 10-9a IABP procedure.

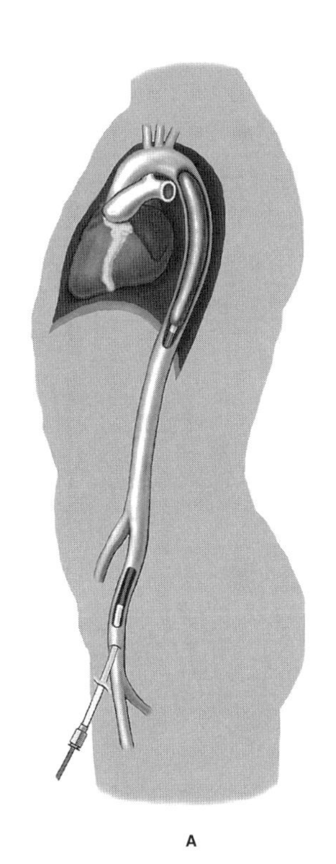

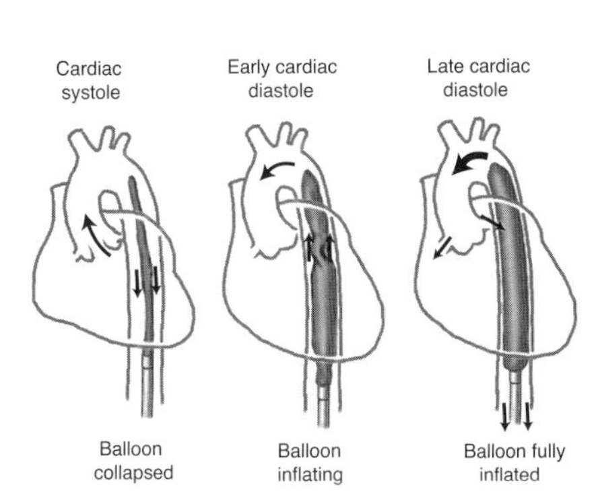

The IABP increases coronary perfusion (flow) via the augmentation of aortic diastolic pressure during diastole of the cardiac cycle. This is achieved by inflating the balloon at the dicrotic notch. Similarly, the IABP also decreases the left ventricular workload during systole by deflating the balloon just before the aortic valve opening, resulting in a decrease in end-diastolic and augmented systolic pressures. This decrease in pressures will help the heart to eject its blood volume with less oxygen demand.

Figure 10-9b shows the arterial pressure, ECG, and balloon inflation and deflation pressures (two different periods). It illustrates the effects of intra-aortic balloon therapy by showing the relationship among assisted and unassisted arterial pressure waveforms (top tracing), ECG triggering (middle waveform), and the changes in pressure within the balloon.

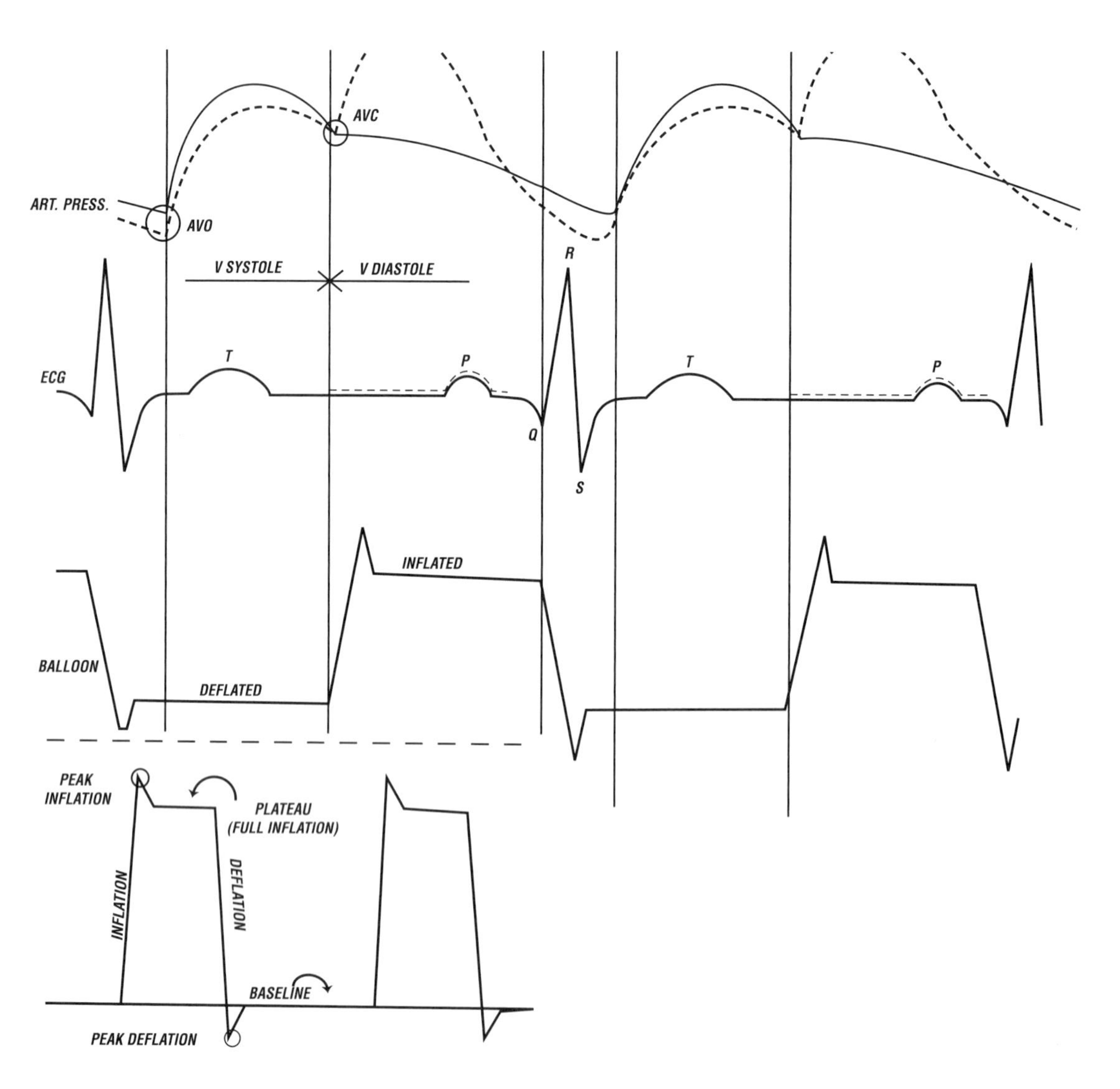

FIGURE 10-9b Blood pressure waveforms.

Inflation of the balloon may be triggered from the ECG waveform, the arterial wave, the pacer, or intrinsically. If ECG triggering is utilized, it is triggered via the R wave and is initially set to inflate the balloon in the middle of the T wave (diastole) and deflate just prior to the QRS complex (systole). ECG triggering is the most common method of activating the balloon pump.

Figure 10-10a shows the insertion of the balloon through the left common femoral artery through a short segment of a prosthetic vascular graft. In **Figure 10-10b,** the catheter

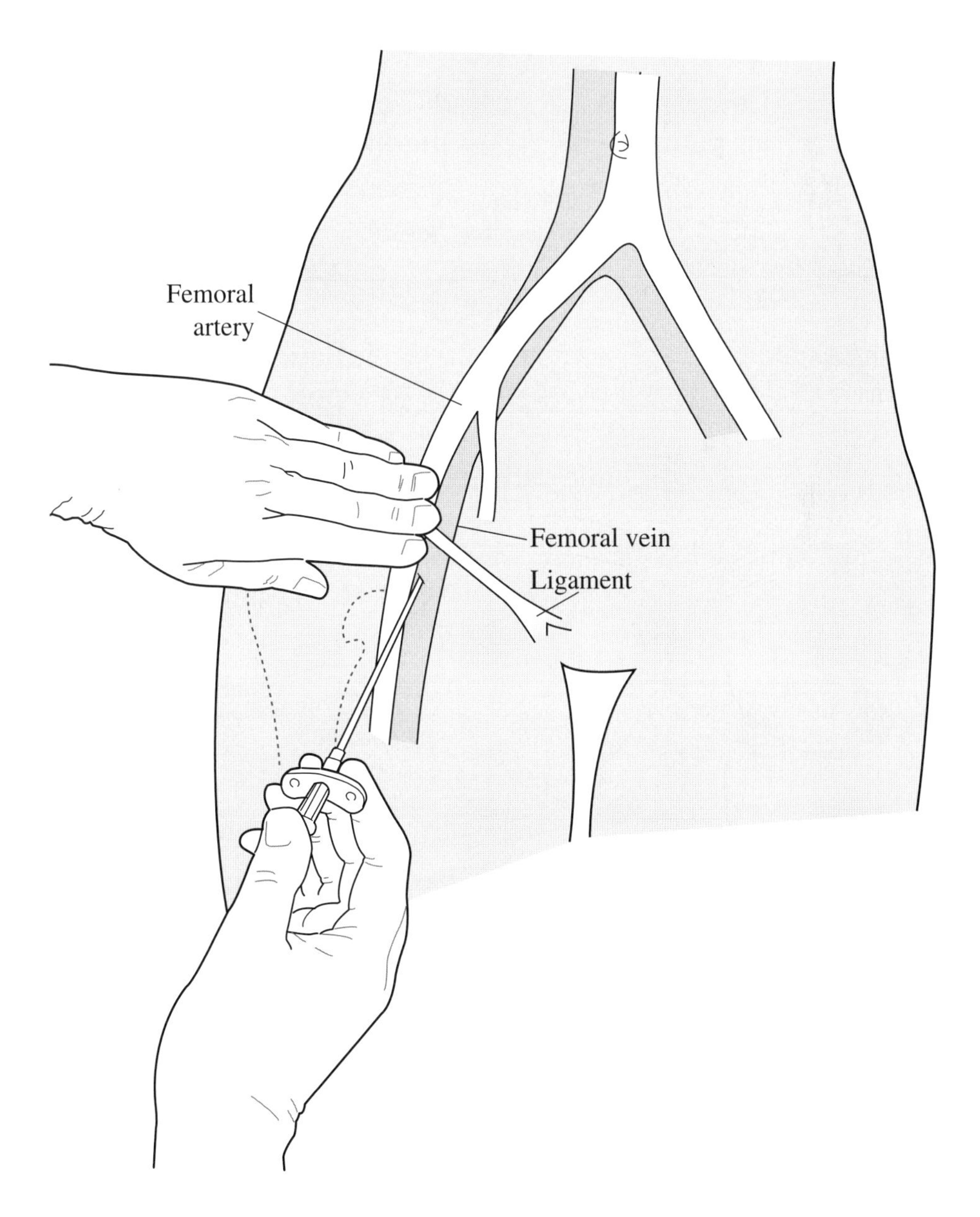

FIGURE 10-10a Catheterization.

is shown with the syringe and the compressed air pump ports. The most commonly used vascular clamps are shown in **Figure 10-10c.**

The use of a balloon is also shown in **Figure 10-11** in coronary angioplasty (to open a blocked coronary artery) with a stent placement. The stent is a metal or a plastic mesh-like material used to hold the structure open. When the balloon is positioned in the right coronary artery, the plaque is flattened against the arterial wall upon inflation and the obstructed artery is cleared. The prosthetic intravascular stent is then placed to maintain the opening of the artery.

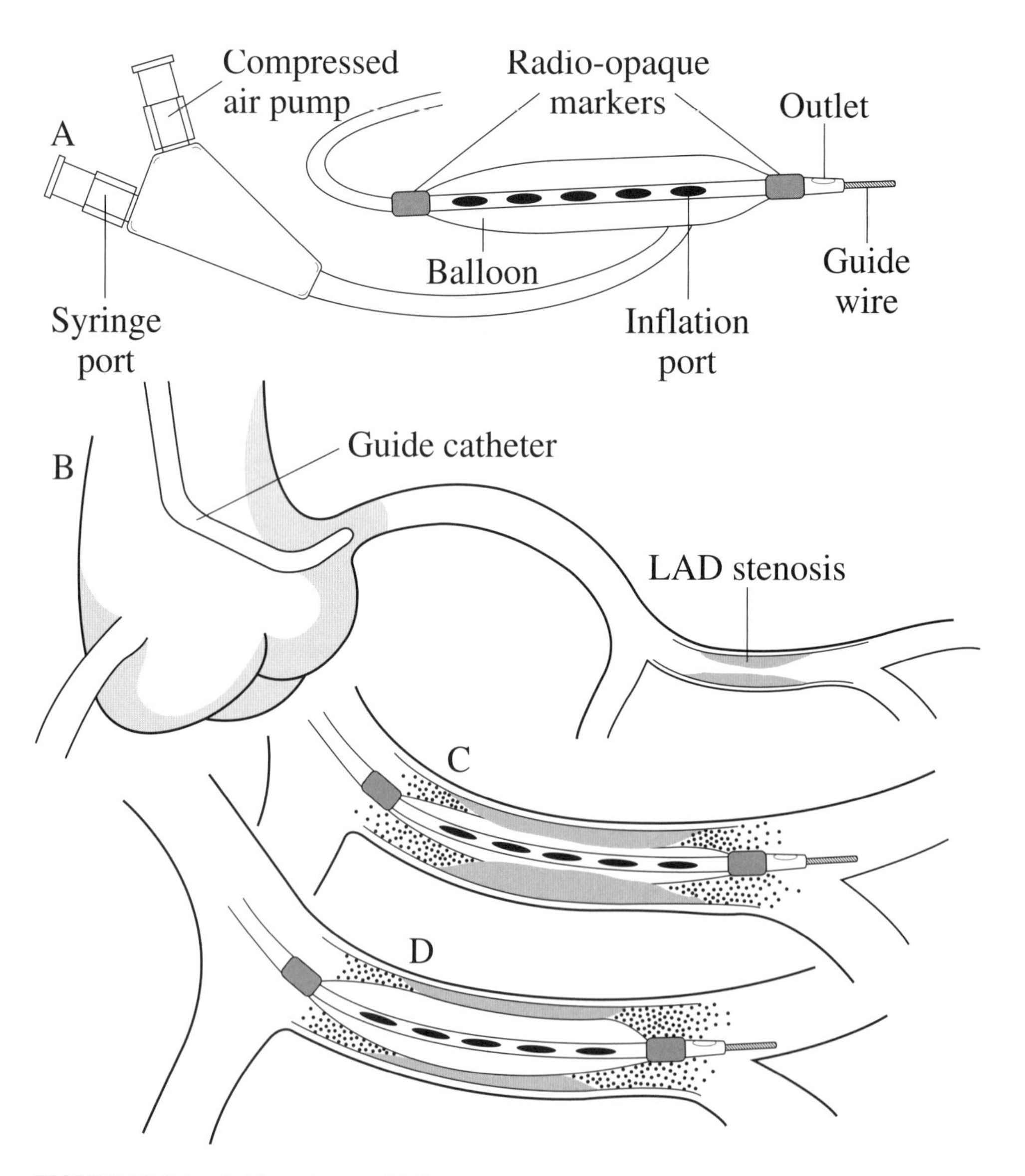

FIGURE 10-10b Guide catheter and balloon.

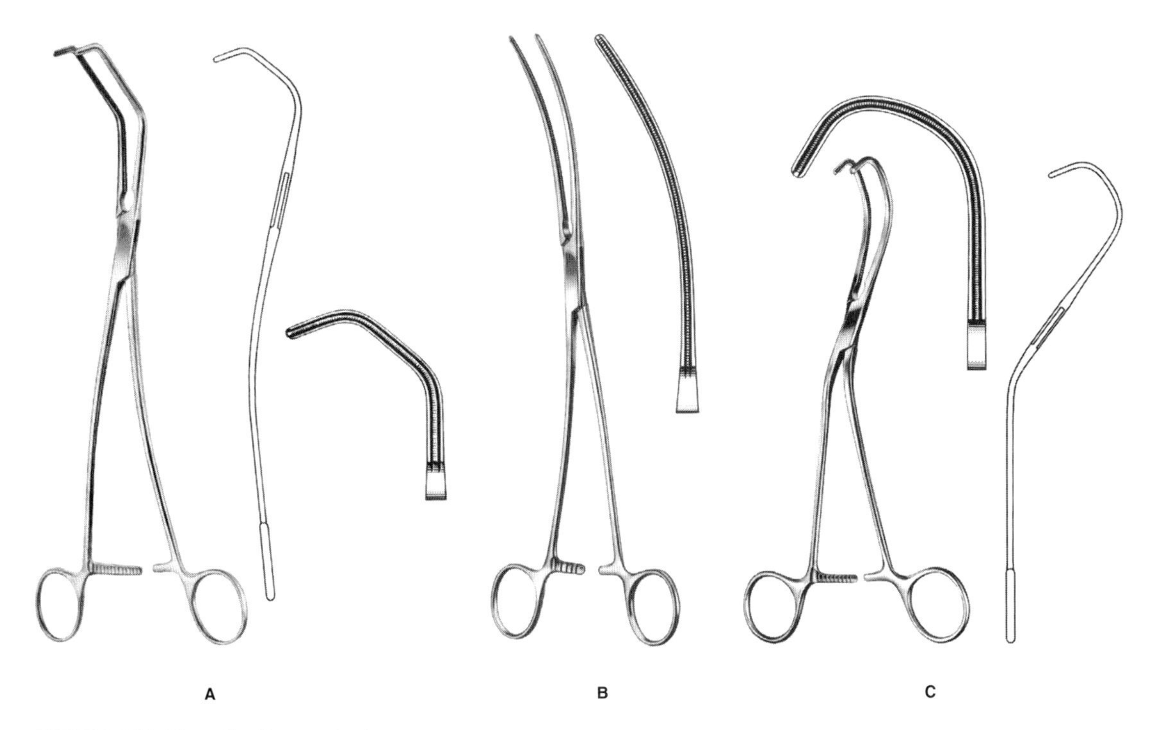

FIGURE 10-10c Cardiovascular instruments.

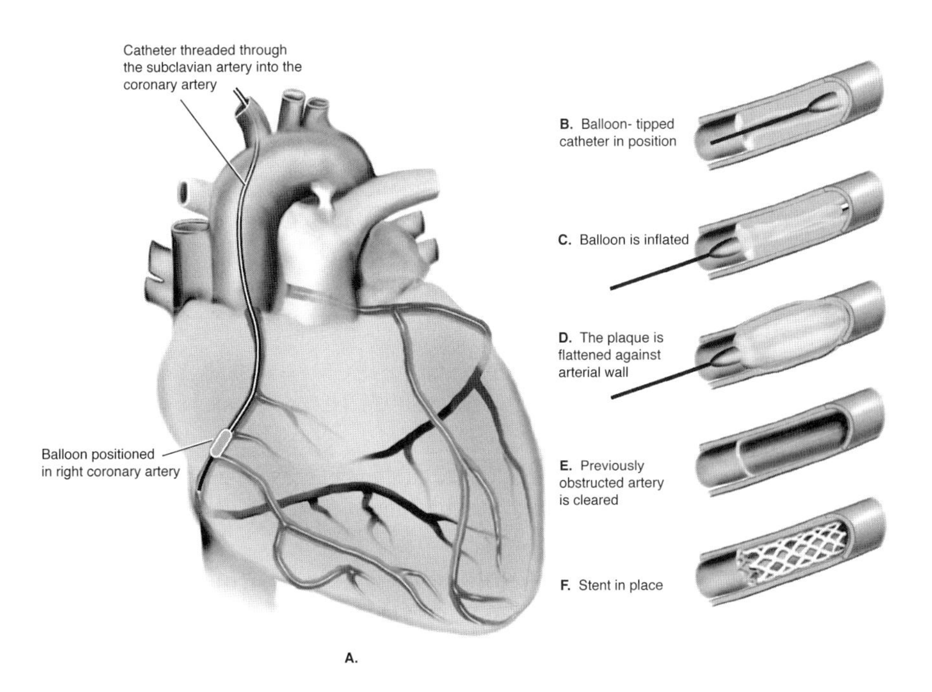

AU/ED: Figure 10.11 is missing. Please provide. —Comp.

FIGURE 10-11 Coronary angioplasty with stent placement.

SUMMARY

- Extracorporeal treatment is used to describe any sort of medical treatment that takes place outside the body. Most extracorporeal treatments are related to the circulatory system. Extracorporeal circuits, equipment, and systems are used to treat such organs as the heart, lungs, and kidneys.
- Dialysis is a treatment to replace kidney function in order to maintain the body's internal equilibrium of water and minerals. The treatment replaces the kidney functions through diffusion (waste removal) and ultrafiltration (fluid removal) across a semipermeable membrane. The blood flows on one side of the membrane, and a dialysate, or fluid, flows on the opposite side.
- In apheresis systems, the machine selects the blood's cellular components required while returning the remaining components back to the donor/patient.
- Extracorporeal membrane oxygenation (ECMO) is a technique that provides both cardiac and respiratory support oxygen to a patient whose heart and lungs are diseased or damaged and no longer have healthy function.
- A ventricular assist device (VAD) is a mechanical pump that assists the heart to pump blood through the body.
- An intra-aortic balloon pump (IABP) is a mechanical device used to decrease myocardial oxygen demand while increasing cardiac output (CO).

MEDICAL TERMINOLOGY

Apheresis: the removal of useless or pathological elements from a patient's blood by a constant flow separator. Hemodialysis is an example of this process.

Cannulas: a hollow tube or sheath utilized for the introduction or withdrawal of fluid from areas of the body.

Dialysate: a solution containing water and electrolytes that can pass through a human or artificial kidney to rid the blood of excess fluid and waste.

Dialyzer: device used to perform dialysis. The device usually contains two compartments composed of dialysate and blood that are separated by a semipermeable membrane.

Extracorporeal: situated or occurring outside and beyond the body.

Extracorporeal membrane oxygenation (ECMO): process that takes blood from a vein in a patient and pumps it through a mechanism that oxygenates it and removes carbon dioxide then returns the blood to the patient.

Hemodialysis: process to remove toxins and excessive fluid from the body by forcing the patient's blood through a dialysis machine for filtering and then returning the clean blood to the body.

Intra-aortic balloon pump (IABP): device inserted through an artery to the thoracic aorta. In the chest, a balloon inflates and deflates in harmony with the heartbeat to assist in blood pumping.

Left ventricular assist device (LVAD): automatic device positioned in a patient with end-stage heart disease when the heart cannot pump blood to an adequate level needed by the body to function properly. The device assists in pumping blood to the left ventricle.

Nephrologist: medical professional specializing in diagnosing and treating structural and functional diseases of the kidneys.

Oxygenerator: device that is capable of automatically oxygenating the blood. This mechanical device is used primarily for open-heart surgery.

Perfusion: the passing or flow of fluid or blood through vessels of an organ. For example, perfusion can be used as a chemotherapy technique to treat melanoma occurring on the arm or leg. The flow of blood in the limb is stopped and anticancer drugs are administered in the vessels of the limb.

Saline: solution of water and salt. The proper osmolarity of saline solution in the body is necessary for maintaining osmotic pressure, stimulation, and regulation of muscular activity.

Ultrafiltration: multiplicity of membrane filtration that can utilize hydrostatic pressure to force a liquid against a semipermeable membrane; filtration that is under pressure.

Ventricular access device (VAD): device to replace the functioning of a partially or completely failing heart; usually used to assist the patient awaiting a heart transplant. The mechanical device can be used on the right or left ventricle, or both at the same time, if required.

QUIZ

1. The mechanical circulatory assist device is ________________.
2. Blood is diverted to a machine for oxygenation that is called a(n):
   a) Dialysis machine. b) Intra-aortic balloon pump device.
   c) Heart-lung machine. d) Apheresis machine.
3. The intra-aortic balloon is ________________ and ________________ during diastole and systole, respectively.
4. In the hemodialysis machine, the extracorporeal circuit consists of a dialyzer, arterial blood line, venous blood line, and ________________ blood line.
5. The proper conductivity of a dialysis machine is in the range of:
   a) 5 mS to 8 mS. b) 12 mS to 16 mS. c) 1 mS to 5 mS. d) None of the above.
6. What are the two components of the dialysate in the dialysis machine?
7. Left ventricular assist devices (LVADs) are ________________.
8. An apheresis system involves two processes:
   1. ________________
   2. ________________
9. What is the main difference between venoarterial and venovenous procedures in ECMO?
10. Which meter is appropriate to measure the conductivity of the dialysate fluid?
    a) Voltmeter b) Ohmmeter c) Light meter d) Force meter

RESEARCH TOPICS

1. The current practices and techniques in extracorporeal circulation raise several issues of ethical and legal nature, including medical concerns. The operation of a life support system, appropriate therapies, blood conservation, and physiological interactions between patient and the machine are all important issues in cardiopulmonary bypass (CPB) and clinical perfusion. The research paper should discuss these issues including the psychological effects on the patient and family.
2. Remote monitoring of dialysis treatment has benefits and shortcomings. The research paper should discuss the conventional in-center dialysis and monitoring systems versus the home-based (nocturnal) dialysis and remote telemonitoring systems. The technology of telemonitoring should be discussed in some detail. With sufficient training and certification, home-based dialysis is considered a more gentle treatment.

CASE STUDIES

1. Transonic Systems' hemodialysis monitor can display measurements during hemodialysis. It can sense flow through dialysis tubing and provide computations of CO, access recirculation, and access flow on a laptop computer. The case study should compare this product with other products used in hospitals.

PROBLEMS

1. Describe the complication in ECMO procedures in general, then compare the specifics in neonatal and pediatric ECMOs.
2. List the hemodynamic parameters and the parameters that are affected by the IABP. Additionally, discuss the timing of the balloon inflation and deflation in the IABP procedure.
3. What are the indications for dialysis in chronic renal failure? Explain and provide numerical values of normal and abnormal circulations and their rates.
4. List the types of sensors in the hemodialysis machine and their placement in the dialysis circuit.
5. Define the following:

   a) Ultrafiltration
   b) Peritoneal
   c) Dialysis
   d) Left ventricular dysfunction
   e) Minimally invasive valve surgery
   f) Isolated limb perfusion

6. List the main components of a dialysis machine on the dialysate side and on the blood side (at least five on each side).
7. Explain the process of the transmembrane pressure (TMP), that is the pressure difference between the blood side and the dialysate side of the membrane in a dialysis machine.
8. Discuss the oxygenator in a heart-lung machine and compare various types of oxygenators used in heart-lung machines. You may use the Internet for your research.

9. Write equations relating pressure, volume, velocity, temperature, and flow in a heart-lung machine. Additionally, indicate normal values of these parameters used during cardiopulmonary bypass.
10. Discuss various types of sensors and transducers used in the heart-lung machine circuit. Indicate the range, resolution, and accuracy in the measurement by the sensors and the transducers.

CHAPTER 11

Instrumentation in Respiration

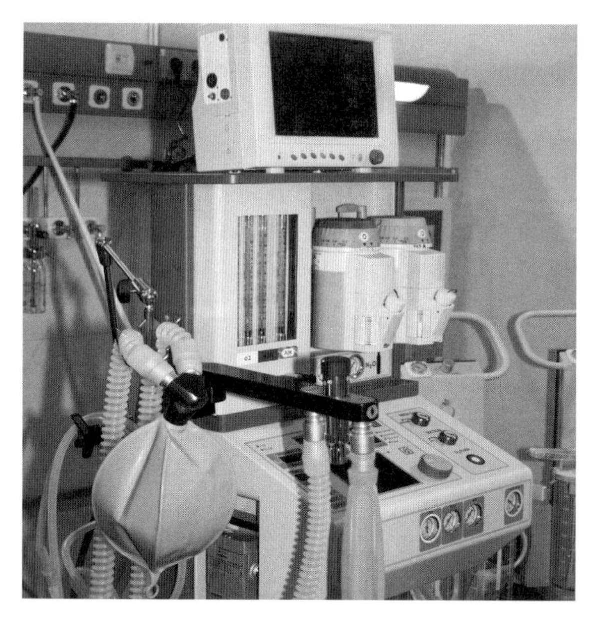

CHAPTER OUTLINE

OBJECTIVES

The objective of this chapter is to introduce the reader to biomedical devices used in respiration. Such instruments discussed include spirometers, respirators and ventilators, pulse oximeters, humidifiers, nebulizers, and aspirators.

Upon completion of this chapter, the reader will be able to:

- Compute pressure and respiration constants.
- Compare and contrast the characteristics of cardiopulmonary machines.
- Describe respirators and ventilators.
- Compare normal and abnormal data in respiratory care.
- Compare the various spirometers used in hospitals.
- Compare humidifiers, aspirators, and inhalers.
- Define oximetry.

INTERNET WEB SITES

http://www.aarc.org (American Association of Respiratory Care)
http://www.ajrccm.org (American Journal of Respiratory and Critical Care Medicine)
http://www.chestsurg.org (Division of Thoracic Surgery, Brigham and Women's Hospital)

http://www.cardinal.com (Cardinal Health)
http://www.lunglinks.com (Allegheny Center for Lung and Thoracic Disease)

■ INTRODUCTION

The human respiratory system functions to allow gas exchange. The anatomical features of this include airways, lungs, and the respiratory muscles. Molecules of oxygen and carbon dioxide are passively exchanged, by diffusion, between the gaseous external environment and the blood. Deprived of breath for even a few minutes, the human body can expire. Breathing disorders affect millions of Americans each year. Respiratory care is the medical field that works with patients with breathing disorders. These disorders can be malfunctioning lungs, lack of proper oxygen in the arterial blood, and, more seriously, cancers of the lungs or respiratory tract. This chapter discusses respiratory care and the gaseous transport process in blood circulation, the laws of gases, gas volumes, and respiration transducers and devices.

■

11.1 HUMAN RESPIRATORY SYSTEM AND PULMONARY CIRCULATION

Figure 11-1a shows the respiratory system and the major organs. The respiratory system of the human body consists of the upper and lower respiratory tracts, including the nasal cavity, nasopharynx, oropharynx, epiglottis, larynx, esophagus, trachea, right and left bronchus, the lungs, the alveolar sac, duct alveoli, and bronchioles.

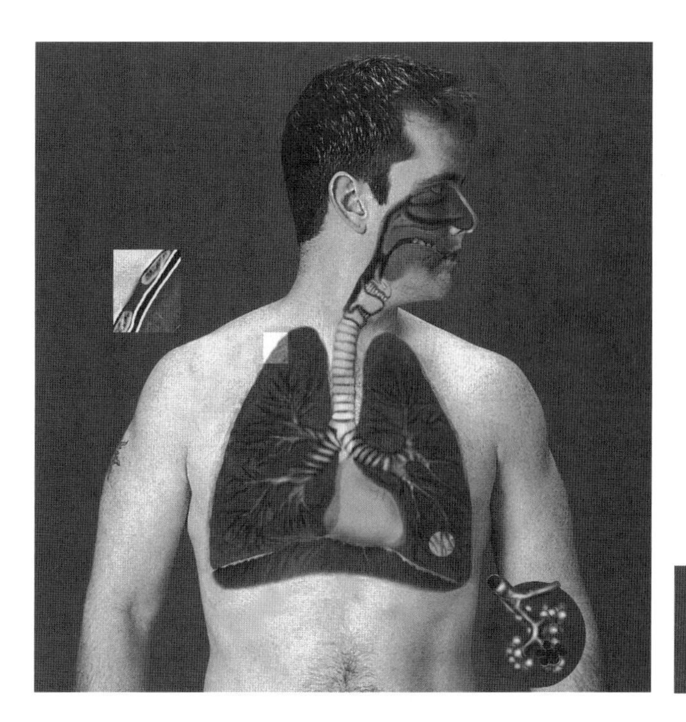

FIGURE 11-1a Structures of the respiratory system.

FIGURE 11-1b The trachea, bronchial, and alveoli.

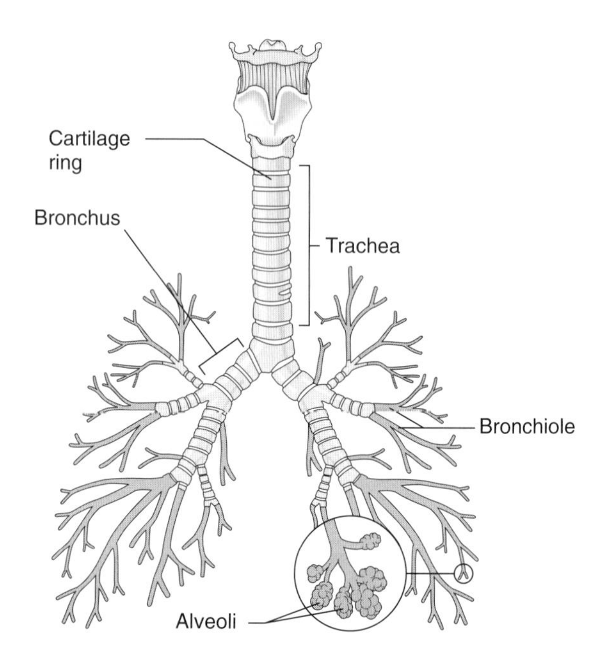

Figure 11-1b shows duct alveoli, also called the air sacs, which are tiny grape-like clusters located at the end of each bronchiole. Each lung has millions of alveoli filled with air from the bronchioles. **Figure 11-2** shows the function of the respiratory system and its interaction with the blood circulation in the pulmonary circuit.

Oxygen and carbon dioxide exchanges can be traced in the following steps:

1. External respiration (breathing) is the exchange of oxygen and carbon dioxide between air, alveoli, and blood in the pulmonary capillaries. The breathing process consists of inspiration (inhalation) and expiration (exhalation).
2. Internal respiration includes the exchange of oxygen and carbon dioxide between the cells.
3. Cellular respiration is the oxidation reaction occurring within the cells.

As the fluid dynamics of flow, volume, and pressure can explain the blood flow in arteries and veins, similarly, the gas flow and its dynamics can explain the process of respiration and medical gas therapy equipment. The following observations can be made in gas flow measurements:

1. Gas flows from an area of greater pressure to an area of lower pressure.
2. Some of the units of pressure are:

   a) 1 atm (unit of atmospheric pressure) = 760 mm Hg

   b) 1 mm Hg = 0.01934 lb/in^2
3. The rate of gas flow depends on the difference in pressure and the size of the opening between two areas. For large pressure differences, gas flow is faster. Similarly, for the large opening, the flow will be greater.

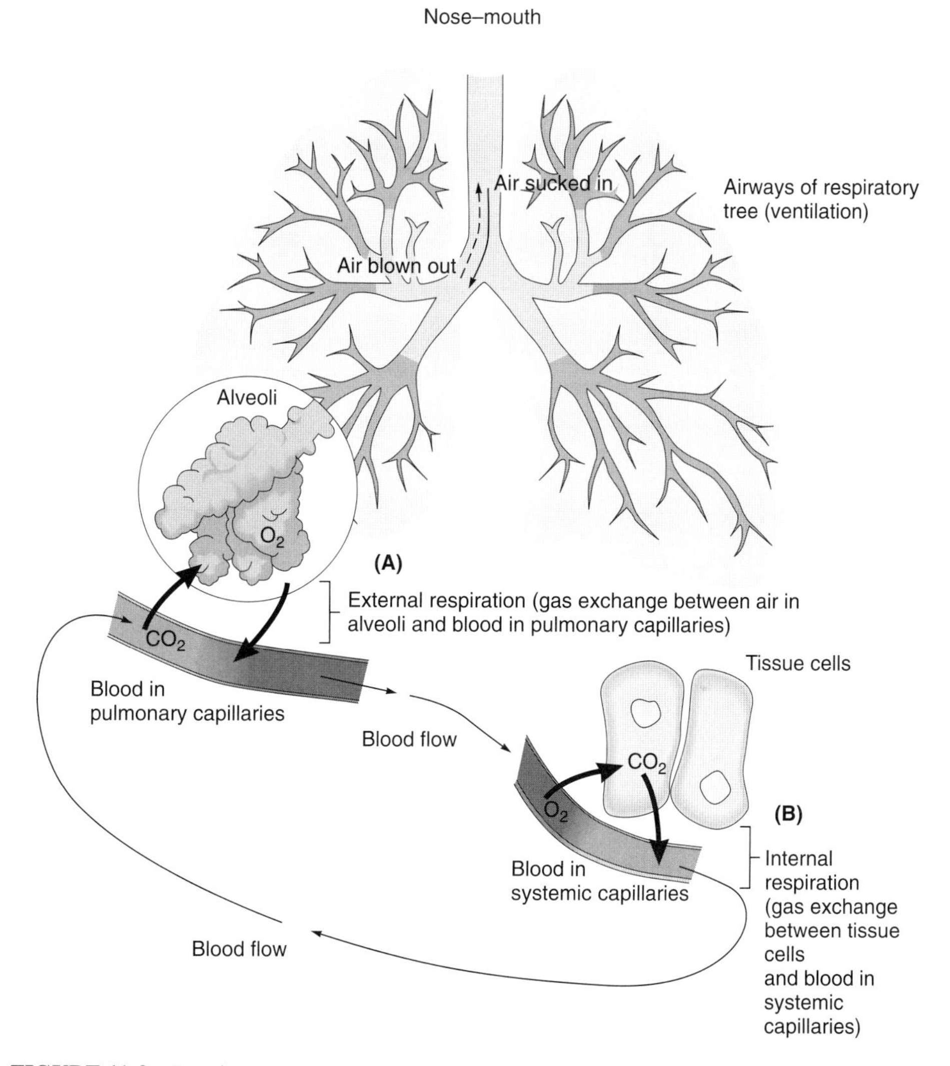

FIGURE 11-2 Respiratory system.

4. Bernoulli's principle states that as the rate of gas flow increases, the lateral pressure within the tube decreases. As the rate of gas flow increases, the pressure decreases such that the total energy of the gas remains constant.
5. The Venturi effect uses Bernoulli's principle to measure gas flow through a Venturi tube by measuring the pressure difference between the narrow center portion of the tube and the wider portion at the tube's exit, as shown in **Figure 11-3a**. If the diameter of the tube does not change, however, the pressure in the tube remains constant (see **Figure 11-3b**), even though the flow rate of gas at the jet remains very high.

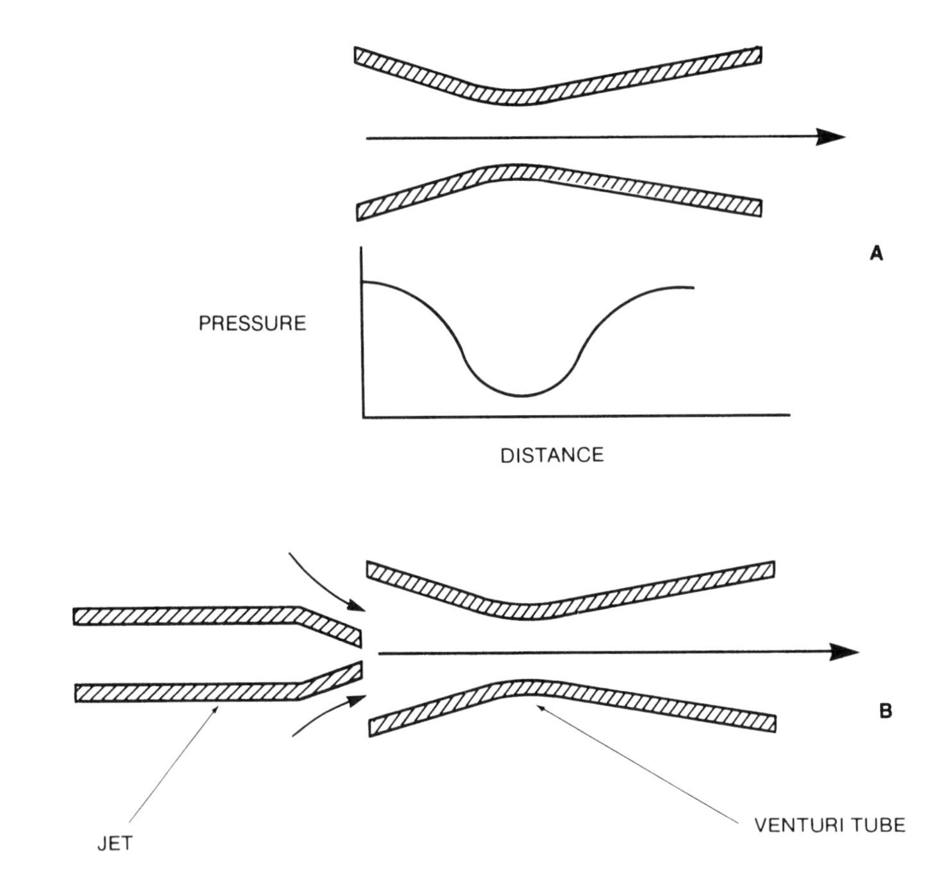

FIGURE 11-3a Venturi tube.

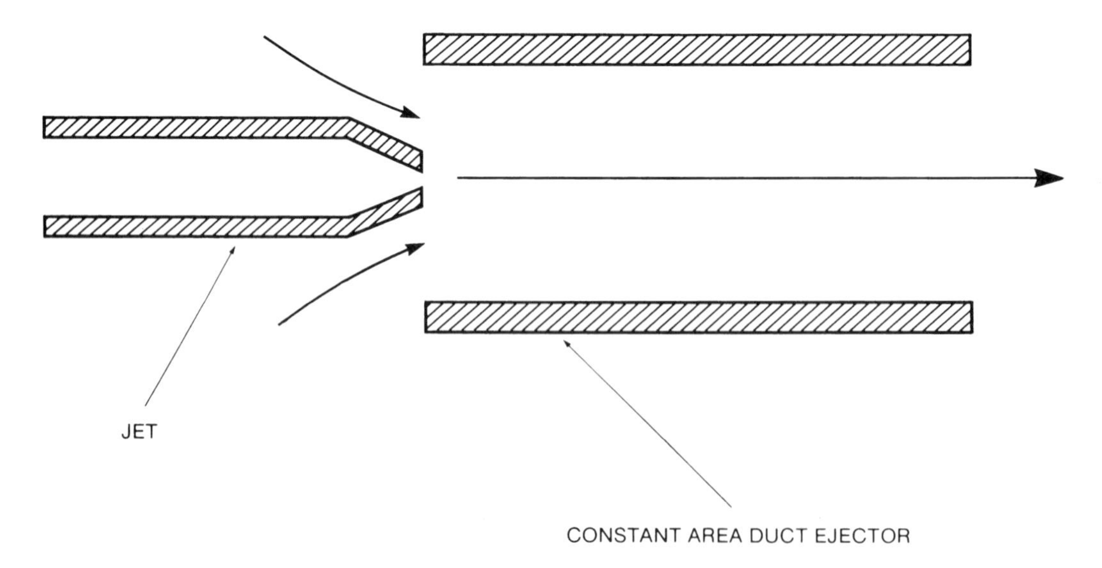

FIGURE 11-3b Constant area duct ejection.

The mechanics of breathing in the organs of the breathing circuit follow the same rules as discussed in the Bernoulli and Venturi principles. **Figure 11-4a** and **Figure 11-4b** show the graphs of lung volumes with respect to time. In a normal breathing cycle, the tidal volume is the amount of air (i.e., gas) inspired or expired with each normal breath. Normal inspiration is 3,000 ml and expiration volume is 2,500 ml. The forced maximum inspiration volume can go beyond the tidal volume up to 6,000 ml. Similarly, one can bring down the lung volume all the way to 1,000 ml by forced expiration.

The Relationship of Pressure and Volume in Respiration (Gas Laws)

There are three major laws that govern the relationship of gaseous pressure and volume in the respiration process. These laws are known as Boyle's law, Charles' law, and Dalton's law.

Gas molecules collide with one another inside the walls of the vessel and possess mass and velocity. These multiple collisions and the momentum (mass × velocity) of the gas molecules create a gas pressure inside the vessel. Gas pressure is calculated as force exerted per unit area of the vessel. There are several ways to measure gas pressure, such as by using an inspiratory force manometer.

The respiratory gases include oxygen, carbon dioxide, nitrogen, helium, and water molecules or a mixture of these.

As gas flows from one point to another due to pressure difference, the flow typically is steady, or laminar, but sudden pressure changes or changes in the geometry

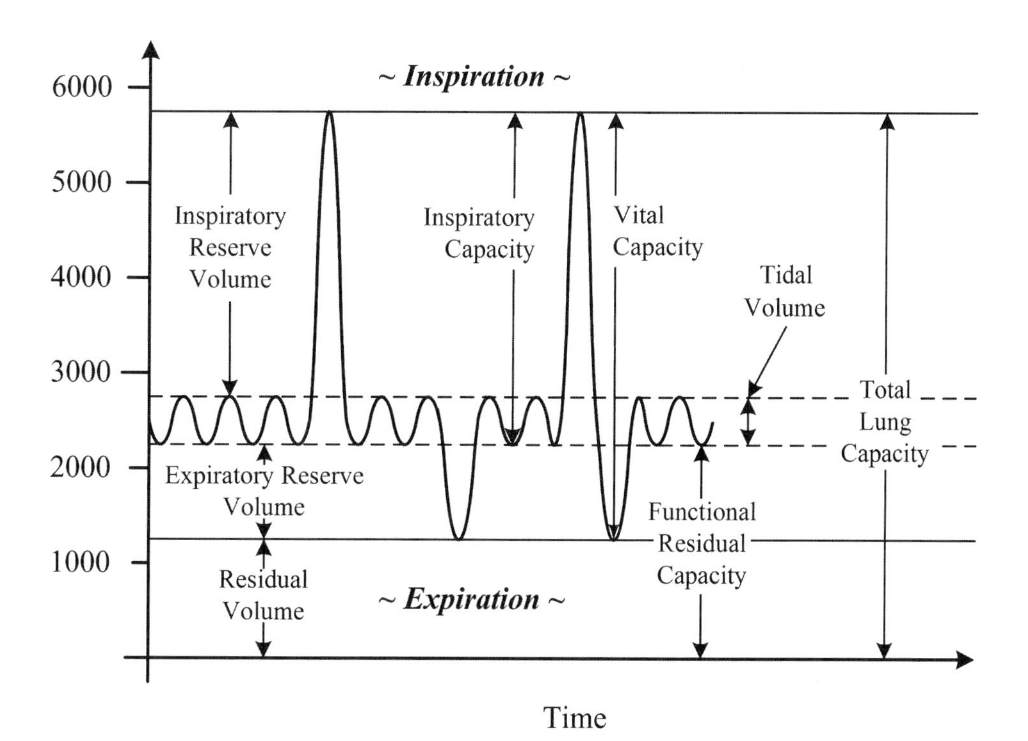

FIGURE 11-4a Respiration range.

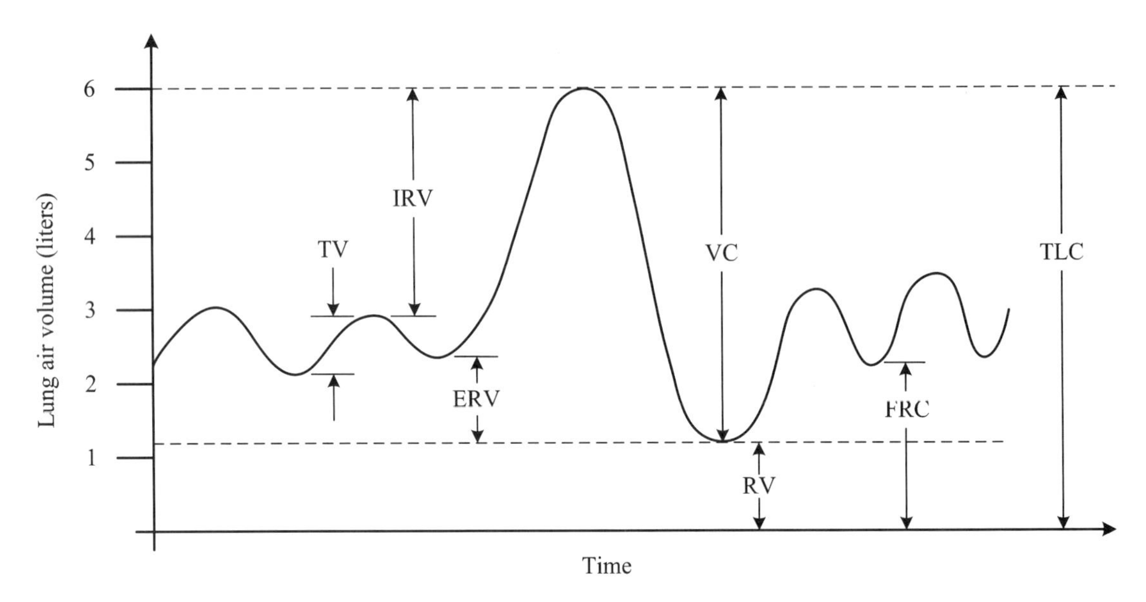

FIGURE 11-4b Respiration range abbreviated.

of the vessel can change this to a chaotic or turbulent flow. The laminar or turbulent flow is explained by the Reynolds number, just as in the fluid dynamics of blood flow circulation. The Reynolds number characterizes the flow when the viscosity and speed of flow are taken into account at the same time. The number is greater for faster flows and for more dense gas or fluid, and the number is smaller for more viscous gas or fluid.

Boyle's law states that the volume of a fixed amount of a gas varies inversely with the pressure when the temperature remains constant. This means that as the volume of the gas increases, its pressure decreases; the reverse also applies (i.e., a decrease in volume corresponds to an increase in pressure). The relationship is given as:

$$P_1 \times V_1 = P_2 \times V_2$$

Where P_1 and V_1 are the original pressure and volume of the gas respectively and P_2 and V_2 are the new values of pressure and volume.

The unit of the pressure is mm Hg and the volume is ml.

Charles' law states that the volume of the gas is directly proportional to the temperature when the pressure does not change. This is given as:

$$\frac{V_1}{T_1} = \frac{V_2}{T_2}$$

Where the unit of the volume is millimeters and the temperature is given in Kelvin.

Dalton's law states that the total pressure exerted in the vessel is equal to the sum of the partial pressures of the various gases in the mixture. Given as:

$$P\ (TOTAL) = P_1 + P_2 + P_3 + + +$$

Pulmonary Volumes and Capacities

Figure 11-4a and **Figure 11-4b** show the respiratory excursions during normal breathing and during maximum inspiration and expiration. The pulmonary volumes can be explained as:

Tidal volume (TV): the volume of air inspired or expired with each normal breath. This amount is about 500 ml averaged over 12 to 15 normal breaths per minute.

Inspiratory reserve volume (IRV): is the extra volume of air that can be inspired over the normal tidal volume. It amounts to about 3,000 to 3,500 ml.

Expiratory reserve volume (ERV): is the amount of air that can be expired after the end of the normal tidal volume and it amounts normally to about 1,000 to 1,200 ml with the forced expiration.

Residual volume (RV): is the volume of air still remaining in the lungs after the most forceful expiration. This volume amounts to about 1,200 ml. This amount is the amount that the person cannot breathe out. It is the functional dead space of the air remaining in the oxygen and carbon dioxide transfer mechanism.

Inspiratory capacity (IC): the amount equal to the sum of the tidal volume and the inspiratory reserve volume. The equation is written as:

$$\text{IC} = \text{TV} + \text{IRV}$$

This is when the person can breathe normally and then can force himself or herself to the maximum inspiration from the end of the normal expiratory level.

Vital capacity (VC): when the person can forcefully inspire to the maximum amount and then can expel the air to the maximum by forceful expiration. The equation is written as:

$$\text{VC} = \text{IRV} + \text{TV} + \text{ERV} \quad \text{or} \quad \text{VC} = \text{IC} + \text{ERV}$$

Total lung capacity (TLC): amounts to about 5,700 ml to 6,200 ml and is the maximum volume to which lungs can be expanded with the maximum inspiratory effort. The equation is written as:

$$\text{TLC} = \text{RV} + \text{VC}$$

Functional residual capacity (FRC): the amount of air remaining in the lungs from the end of the normal expiration level. This can be written as:

$$\text{FRC} = \text{RV} + \text{ERV}$$

Lung compliance: the elastic force of the lungs accepting a volume of inspired air. Lungs with high compliance (i.e., greater ease in filling) have low elastance, whereas lungs with low compliance (i.e., lower ease of filling) have high elastance. The formula for lung compliance is then:

$$\text{Compliance} = \frac{\text{Volume of the inspired air}}{\text{Intrapleural pressure}}$$

Elastance is the reciprocal of compliance and is the natural ability to respond to force and return to the original resting shape.

Peak inspiratory flow: the amount of inspiratory volume per second. It is given as:

$$\text{PIF} = \frac{\text{Inspiratory volume}}{\text{Inspiratory time}}$$

The airway resistance can then be calculated as the pressure difference between the mouth and the alveoli divided by the PIF. In respiratory disorders, any changes in the diameter or the length of the airway may alter the airway resistance, which in turn may alter the flow and the intrapleural pressures. The airway resistance can also be calculated in terms of the radius of the vessel, the length of the vessel, and the viscosity of air. It is given as:

$$R = \frac{8 \times \eta \times l}{\pi \times r^4}$$

where r and l are the radius and the length of the vessel respectively. η is the viscosity of the air.

Diffusion of Oxygen and Carbon Dioxide Through Respiratory Membrane

When the alveoli are ventilated with fresh air on inspiration, the process of diffusion begins as oxygen is transferred from the alveoli to the pulmonary blood, and carbon dioxide is simultaneously transferred from the pulmonary blood into the alveoli.

The process simply involves random motion of gas molecules as they make their way in both directions through the respiratory membrane.

Transport Mechanism of Oxygen and Carbon Dioxide in the Blood

For diffusion, a pressure gradient of the gas is required. A net diffusion of gas from a high-pressure area to a low-pressure area is equal to the number of molecules bouncing from the high-pressure direction minus the numbers bouncing from the low-pressure direction.

When oxygen is diffused from the alveoli into the pulmonary capillary blood, it combines with the hemoglobin and is transported throughout the body to the tissue capillaries, where it is released to the cells for processing. In the cells, the oxygen reacts with nutrients and forms large quantities of carbon dioxide, which in turn are diffused into the tissue capillaries and transported back to the lungs.

The presence of hemoglobin in the red blood cells allows the blood to transport 50 to 100 times more oxygen compared to the transport of dissolved oxygen in the water of the plasma. Similarly, transport of carbon dioxide increases 15- to 20-fold when carbon dioxide combines with the chemical substances of the blood.

The transport of oxygen and carbon dioxide by the blood depends on both the diffusion process and the movement of the blood. When the oxygen pressure (P_{O2}) in the alveoli is greater than the oxygen pressure in the pulmonary capillary blood, oxygen diffuses from the alveoli into the blood. Similarly, higher oxygen pressure in the capillary blood causes oxygen to diffuse to the cells.

We can say the same thing about the carbon dioxide diffusion. A higher carbon dioxide pressure (P_{CO2}) in the cells causes carbon dioxide to diffuse into the capillary blood, and it then diffuses out of the blood into the alveoli when the carbon dioxide pressure in the alveoli is lower than that in the pulmonary capillary blood.

Respiratory Abnormalities

Some diseases of the respiratory system result from inadequate ventilation or from abnormality of diffusion. Some of the more common respiratory abnormalities are:

- Eupnea (normal breathing).
- Tachypnea (rapid breathing).
- Bradypnea (slow breathing).
- Hyperpnea (over-respiration).
- Hypopnea (under-respiration).

The physical and chemical processes of respiration include external respiration, internal respiration, and cellular respiration. External respiration takes place in the lungs and internal respiration is between the cells of the body and the blood bathing the cells. Cellular respiration occurs within the cell structures. The respiration circuit (**Figure 11-2**) includes the external and internal respiration.

The alveolar air interacts with the blood flow from the heart through the lungs and back to the heart. Carbon dioxide and oxygen are transferred—carbon dioxide in the expired air and oxygen in the inspired air. The systemic arteries and veins then play important roles in the exchange of carbon dioxide and oxygen throughout the body's cells.

The sounds in the respiratory tract and the changes in respiration dictate the normal and abnormal respiratory conditions. The disorders mainly prevent the outside air from reaching the alveoli. The causes may include some type of infection in the upper or lower airway or an obstruction of the airway itself.

Common infectious diseases are:

Bronchitis: inflammation of the mucous membrane of the trachea and the bronchial tube.

Common cold: illness caused by a virus.

Influenza: inflammation of the mucous membrane of the respiratory system due to a virus.

Pneumonia: infection of the lungs caused by bacteria or a virus.

Tuberculosis: infectious disease of the lungs caused by the tubercle bacillus.

Laryngitis: inflammation of the larynx.

Pharyngitis: inflammation of the throat caused by bacteria or a virus.

EXERCISE A spirometer can measure lung capacity of 6,000 ml in a normal person without any respiratory disease. Determine the several factors that add up to the total lung capacity of 6,000 ml.

a) Normal tidal volume = ... 500 ml

b) Normal inspiratory reserve volume = ... 3,000 ml

c) Normal expiratory reserve volume = ... 1,000 ml

d) Normal residual air = ... 1,500 ml

Total = 6,000 ml

EXERCISE Calculate the vital lung capacity and the functional residual capacity from the previous question.

a) Vital lung capacity = Tidal volume + IRV + ERV

4,500 ml = 500 ml + 3,000 ml + 1,000 ml

b) Functional residual capacity = ERV + Residual air

2,500 ml = 1,000 ml + 1,500 ml

EXERCISE Which part of the brain affects the rate of breathing?

Medulla oblongata and pons monitor the level of carbon dioxide in the blood.

EXERCISE A volume of gas equaling 2 L at 20° C passes though a heater and heats up to 38° C before it is delivered to the patient. Does the volume of the gas change? If so, how much?

Charles' law states that the volume of the gas will increase or decrease as the temperature increases or decreases. This makes temperature and volume directly proportional. Thus:

$$\frac{V_1}{T_1} = \frac{V_2}{T_2}$$

Calculate V_2:

$$V_2 = \frac{T_2}{T_1} \times V_1$$

$$V_2 = \frac{38^\circ \text{ C}}{20^\circ \text{ C}} \times 2 \text{ L}$$

$$V_2 = 3.8 \text{ L}$$

EXERCISE Determine the partial pressure of Gas A in the mixture of other gasses, B and C. The gas mixture is made up of Gas A = 40 percent, Gas B = 30 percent, and Gas C = 30 percent. The total pressure is 500 mm Hg.

For this problem, we will use Dalton's law. Dalton's law states that the partial pressure of each gas is proportional to its volumetric percentage. Find the partial pressure of Gas A.

Gas A = Volumetric percentage × Total mixture pressure
= 40% × 500 mm Hg
= 0.4 × 500
= 200 mm Hg

11.2 TYPES OF RESPIRATORY EQUIPMENT

The lungs transfer oxygen from the ambient air to the blood on inspiration and exhaust carbon dioxide from the blood into the atmosphere on expiration. In turn, the blood carries oxygen to the cells of the body and brings back the carbon dioxide from them. This is a closed-loop system of gas transfer of the respiratory regulation. The following text describes the various types of equipment used for respiratory treatment and diagnosis in hospitals, as shown in **Figure 11-5**.

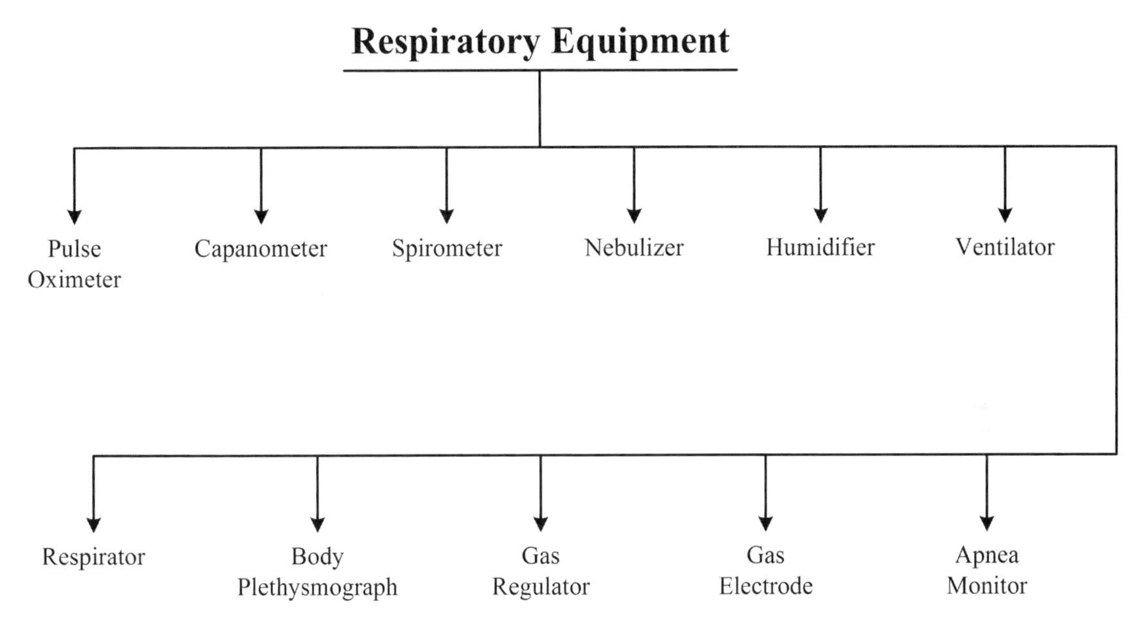

FIGURE 11-5 Table.

Pulse Oximeter

The use of light and optics in medical devices has increased in recent years. A pulse oximeter is a device that uses red and infrared light to measure oxygen saturation in the arterial blood; medical conditions can often be diagnosed by determining a patient's blood oxygen level. **Figure 11-6a** shows a finger probe. The sensor transmits infrared light through a capillary bed from one side and receives that light on the other side. Because highly oxygenated blood absorbs more infrared light than deoxygenated blood, less light is detected at the receiver.

Generally, when highly oxygenated or red blood (e.g., 100% saturated) is viewed in red light, less light is absorbed; when deoxygenated or blue blood (e.g., 0% saturated) is viewed

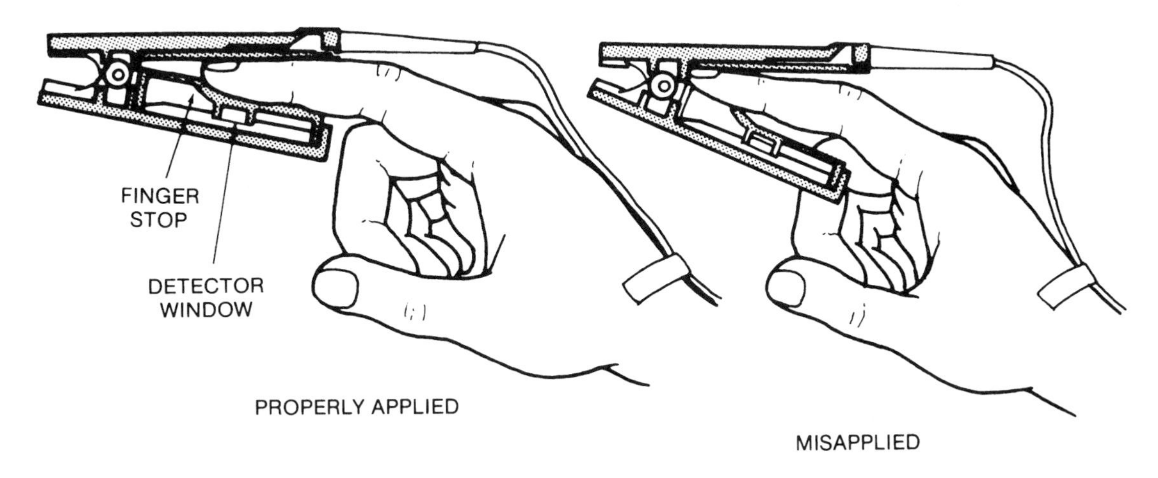

FIGURE 11-6a Finger probe shown with proper and misapplied usage.

in red light, more light is absorbed. In the case of infrared light, however, the opposite applies; red blood absorbs more and blue blood absorbs less. The composition and wavelengths of the red and infrared light determine how the light will be absorbed in the bloodstream. In general, the larger the wavelength, the greater the level of absorption (red light has a wavelength of 660 nm and infrared light has a wavelength of 940 nm). Therefore, arterial and venous blood each absorb red and infrared light differently. In addition, light absorption is affected by the volume of blood in the vessels during systole (a large volume of blood, resulting in greater absorption) and diastole (a small volume of blood, resulting in less absorption).

The pulse oximeter then uses this information to calculate the level of oxygen saturation as a percentage and displays the result as an oximetry signal, as shown in **Figure 11-6b**.

Oxygen saturation is determined by the ratio R of light absorption in the arteries and veins of the capillary bed and is given as:

$$R = \frac{(A_{660}) \div (V_{660})}{(A_{940}) \div (V_{940})}$$

where A_{660} and V_{660} are the 660 nm (red) light absorption by the arterial blood and the venous blood respectively. Similarly, A_{940} and V_{940} are the 940 nm (infrared) light absorption by the arterial and venous blood respectively.

In hospitals, various types of pulse oximeters are used. They provide continuous measurements of oxygen saturation, SpO_2, pulse strength measurements, and pulse rate. They are lightweight, transportable digital handheld devices, as shown in **Figure 11-6c.** Some patient monitors are capnograph/oximeters that provide respiration rate, heart rate, end-tidal carbon dioxide ($ETCO_2$), and inspired carbon dioxide levels in addition to the basic oxygen saturation readings. These devices reject spontaneous motions, artifacts, improper sensor positioning, and processed low perfusion signals.

A monitor block diagram of a pulse oximeter is shown in **Figure 11-7**. This oximeter contains a microcontroller chip. The microcontroller interfaces the analog sensor voltages and passes that information in the digital form to the microprocessor. The microprocessor

FIGURE 11-6b Oximetry signal.

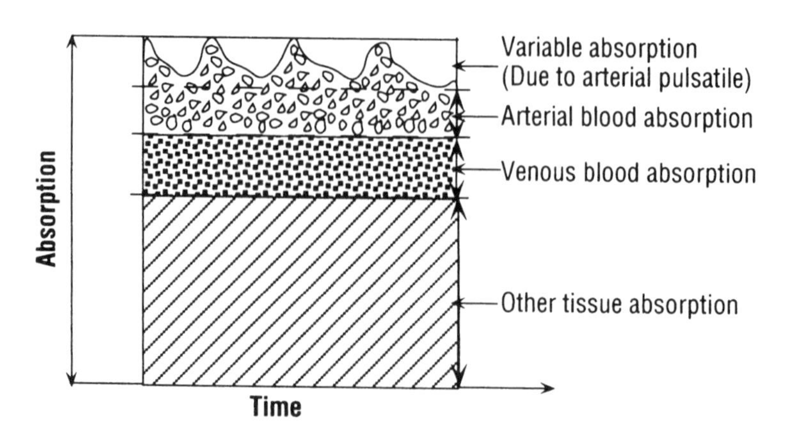

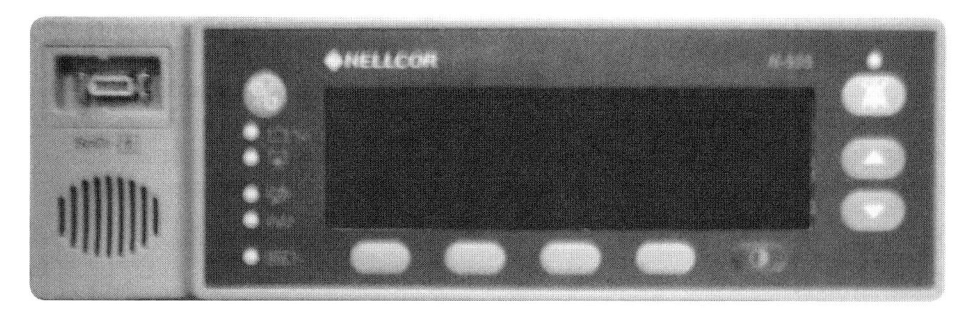

FIGURE 11-6c A photograph of a pulse oximeter.

acts as the master controller. It displays the oxygen saturation and pulse rate data on the membrane panel.

Capnometer/capnograph

The capnometer measures carbon dioxide in the respired gas and provides a single value called end-tidal partial pressure of carbon dioxide, or end-tidal carbon dioxide. The capnograph displays this single-valued capnometric data in the time domain as a continuous signal during the ventilatory cycle. See **Figure 11-8a** for the time-domain capnograph signal. The

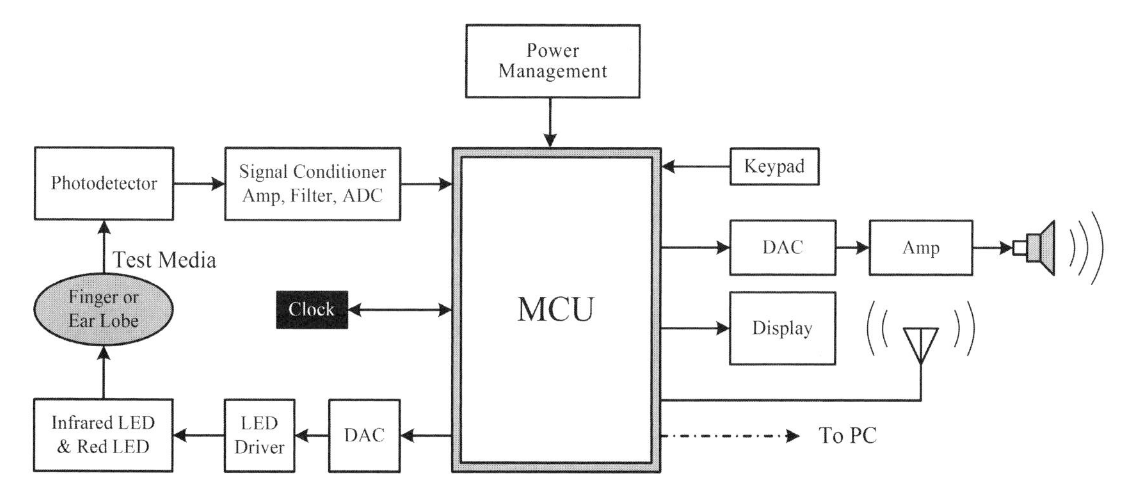

FIGURE 11-7 A capnograph/oximeter microprocessor control system.

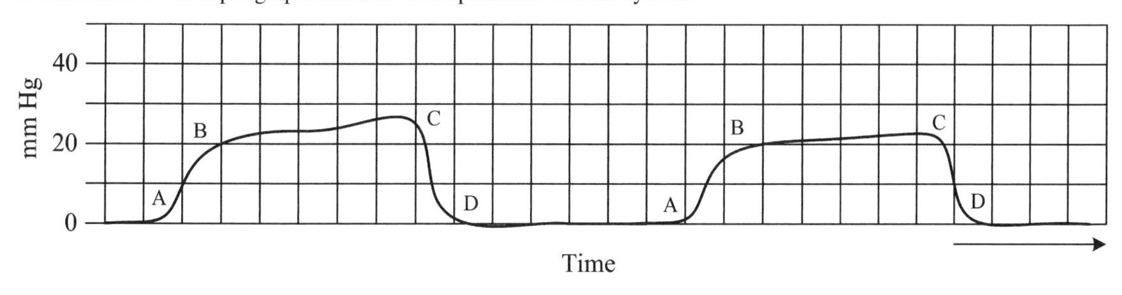

FIGURE 11-8a A capnograph.

vertical axis is the partial pressure of carbon dioxide in mm Hg, and the horizontal axis is the time axis.

The capnograph siphons gas from the patient circuit at variable rates, passes it through a water trap to remove patient secretions, and finally performs carbon dioxide analysis. The gas is sampled through nasal cannulas or a catheter is placed in the nasopharynx. As shown in **Figure 11-8b,** carbon dioxide is a unique gas with a characteristic infrared absorption band different than that of other gases of the respiratory circuit. The wavelength of the absorption band for carbon dioxide is right in the middle of the infrared absorption spectrum at around 4.25 μm. This analysis is called infrared spectrophotometry. The idea is that carbon dioxide absorbs maximum IR light at the wavelength of 4.26 μm.

When the IR light passes through the gas sample, the amount of IR light absorbed is proportional to the concentration of carbon dioxide in the sample. The more carbon dioxide there is in the gas, the more IR light will be absorbed. This is a sidestream technique because the gas is withdrawn from the patient's airway.

In the mainstream technique, a sensor is placed directly in the ventilator airway circuit. The sensor has an IR light source and a photodetector.

Pulse Oximetry Monitoring

This is a noninvasive method of assessing a patient's arterial oxygen level. These days pulse oximetry is one of the parameters in multiparameter patient monitors for measuring oxygen saturation.

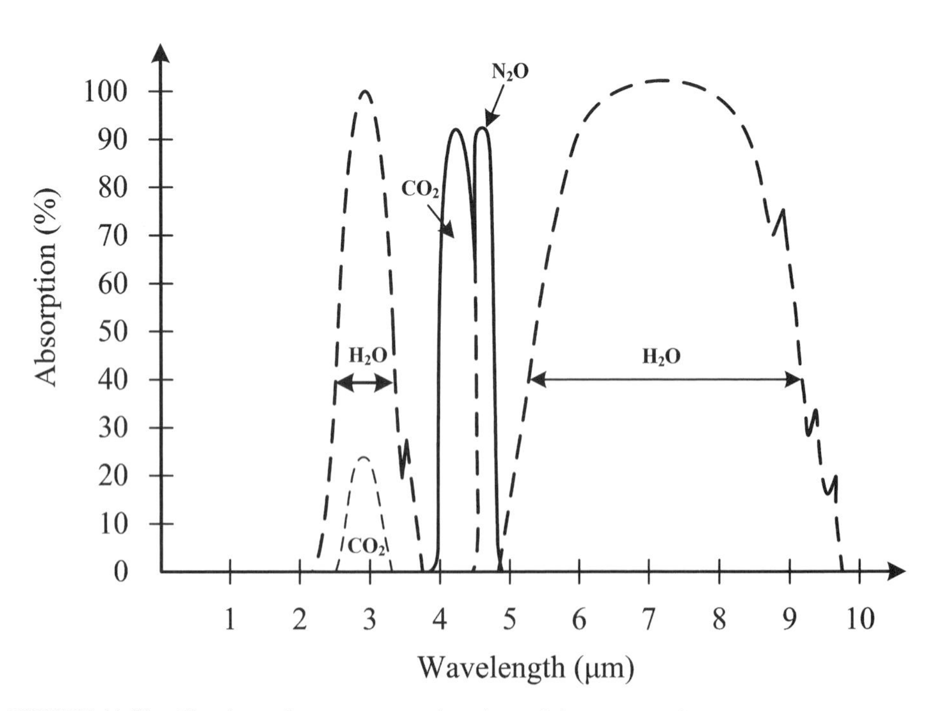

FIGURE 11-8b The absorption versus wavelength graph in capnography.

Capnography Monitoring

Also known as an end-tidal carbon dioxide monitor, it measures the concentration of carbon dioxide in the patient's inspired and expired air. By doing this, it determines whether the patient is properly ventilated. In the blood-air exchange, poor ventilation indicates pneumonia or excessive mucus in the lungs.

Spirometer

A spirometer is a device used to measure air volume when the patient inhales and exhales through a mouthpiece. **Figure 11-9a** is a photograph of the Stead-Wells spirometer. The functional diagram of a bellows-type incentive spirometer is shown in **Figure 11-9b.** The spirometer measures the inspired volume and the scale reading indicates that to the patient. The displacement in the bellows (as the air is removed) is shown when the patient inhales the air.

Spirometry is the measurement of a person's ability to inhale and exhale. This device then records the person's breathing capabilities and measures the amount of air expelled and the rate at which the air is expelled from the lungs. Spirometry indicates several parameters of breathing such as forced vital capacity (FVC) and forced expiratory volume (FEV). The physician then evaluates the patient's lung function with the data provided by the spirometer. The physician can diagnose asthma or other lung diseases and also measure the progression of respiratory diseases with the spirometry test. If the patient has abnormal spirometer measurements (values fall below 85% of the normal values), then other lung tests are recommended to diagnose lung disease or airflow obstruction. The recommendations of the spirometer tests with different patient populations (with respect to age, sex, and family history) are provided by the National Heart, Lung, and Blood Institute (NHLBI).

A satellite spirometer has the features of the desktop spirometer but can fit in the palm of your hand. Spirometers can be volume based or flow based, and all have their relative merits and minimum performance requirements.

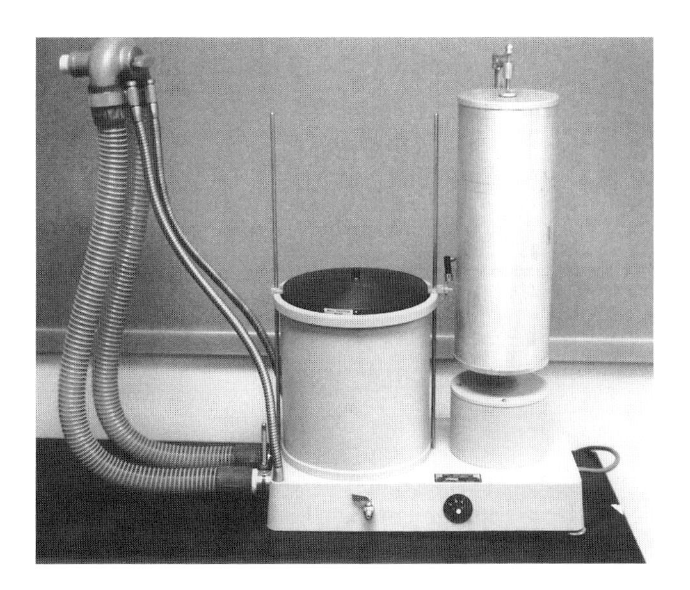

FIGURE 11-9a A Stead-Wells spirometer.

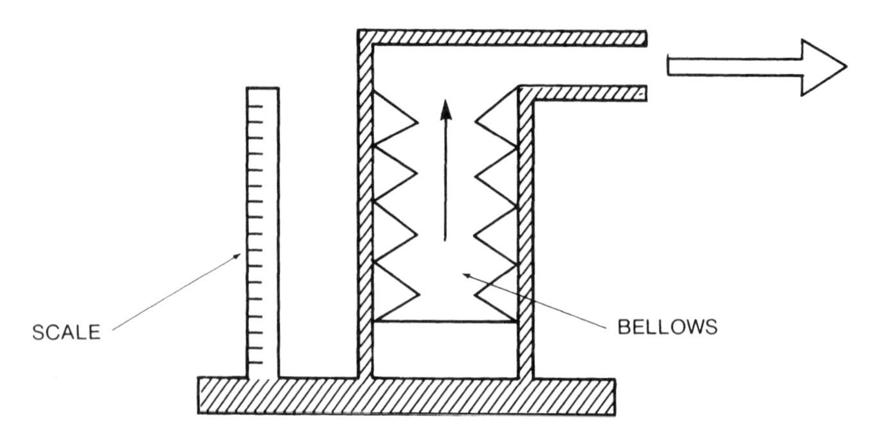

FIGURE 11-9b A functional diagram of a bellows-type incentive spirometer.

The spirometer consists of bellows and is linked to a potentiometer wiper such that the wiper moves when the patient breathes into the bellows. The output voltage of the potentiometer at the wiper is then given as:

$$V_{out} = V_{cc} \times \frac{\text{volume of the bellows at a wiper position}}{\text{maximum volume of the bellows}}$$

Where V_{cc} is the potentiometer battery voltage and

Maximum volume of the bellows = (area πr^2 of the bellows) $\times$ maximum height of the bellows

Nebulizer

This device is used for spraying liquid or medication into the patient's airway. **Figure 11-10a** and **Figure 11-10b** show a nebulizer and its functional diagram. The nebulizer delivers liquid or solid particles to a gas or air stream. In the mainstream nebulizer, the particles are in the main flow of the gas, but in the sidestream nebulizer, the particles need to change direction before they merge into the flow of the gas. The size of particles is small compared to the mainstream nebulizer. A handheld nebulizer is used at home by patients.

The gas is forced through the jet by squeezing the rubber bulb. The reservoir of the nebulizer is filled with medicine, and each time the patient squeezes the bulb a small amount of medication is delivered to the gas stream. This gas stream is then delivered orally to the patient by having one end of the nebulizer inserted into the mouth.

Humidifier

This device is used to combine water vapor with medical gases delivered to a patient. A room or central humidifier increases the humidity (moisture) of the air in the room or rooms. However, in respiratory oxygen therapy, the humidifier provides humidity to the oxygen flow. **Figure 11-11** is a bubble humidifier and its functional diagram. Oxygen enters at the inlet and flows down in a hollow tube to a diffuser. As the reservoir is filled with water, the

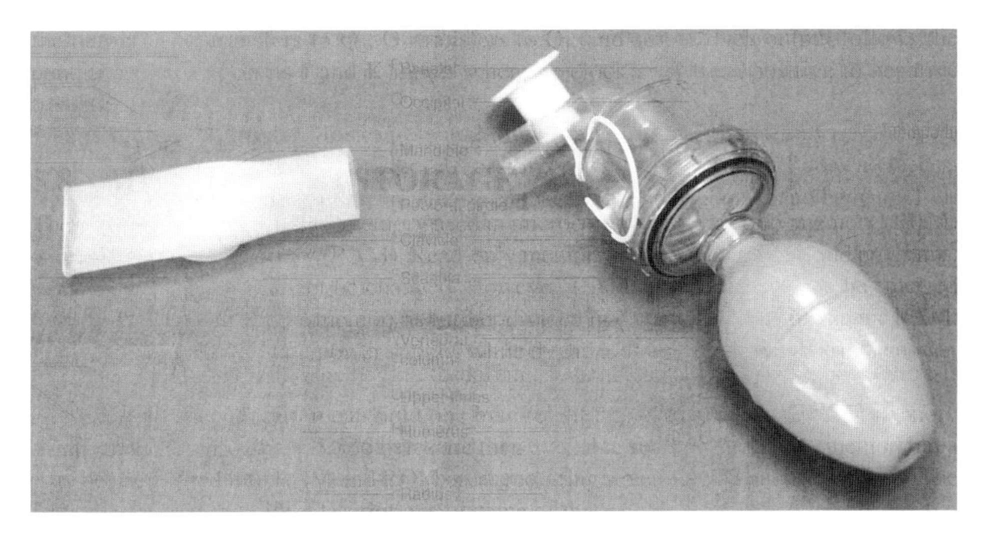

FIGURE 11-10a A bulb nebulizer for home use.

diffusing element bubbles the oxygen flow into the water and in turn, water evaporates into the air bubbles. The outlet is then connected to the patient ventilator circuit.

Because medical gases are free of water, they need to be humidified to prevent problems in the patient's pulmonary system. If these gases are not properly humidified, the patient can experience irritation, bacterial infection, retained secretions, and airway obstruction in the throat, trachea, and lungs.

Ventilator or Respirator

These are devices used to provide oxygen-enriched, medicated air to the patient for artificial respiration. Hospitals use a variety of mechanical ventilators that can fully or partially

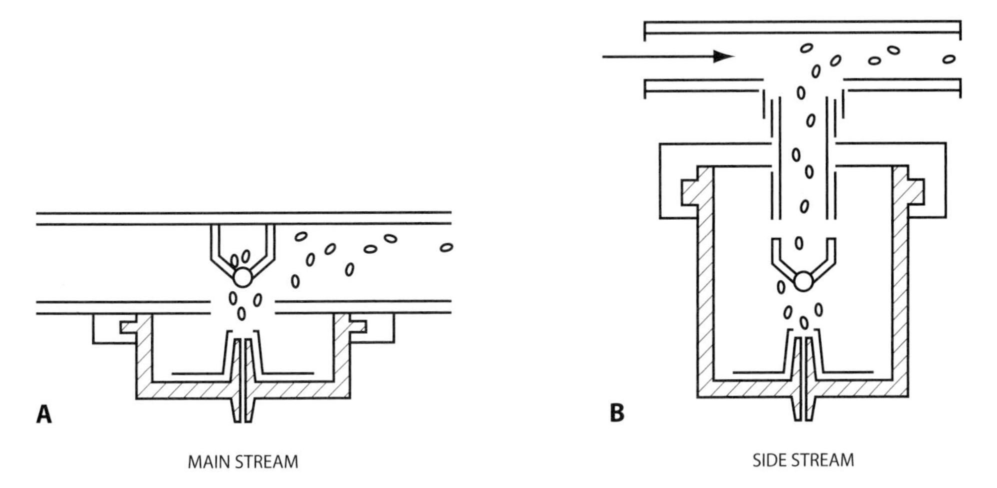

FIGURE 11-10b A diagram of a mainstream and sidestream small volume nebulizer.

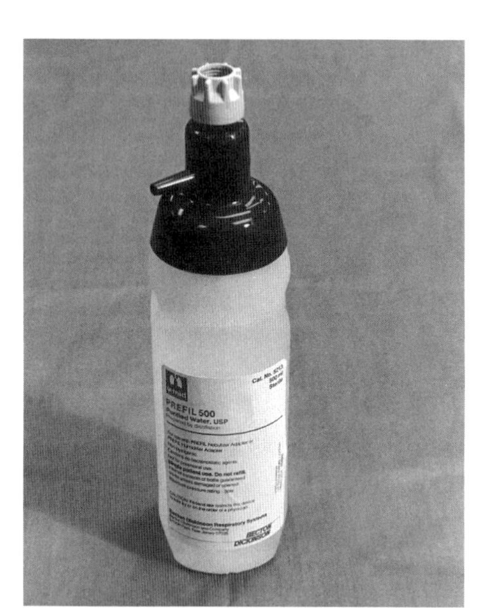

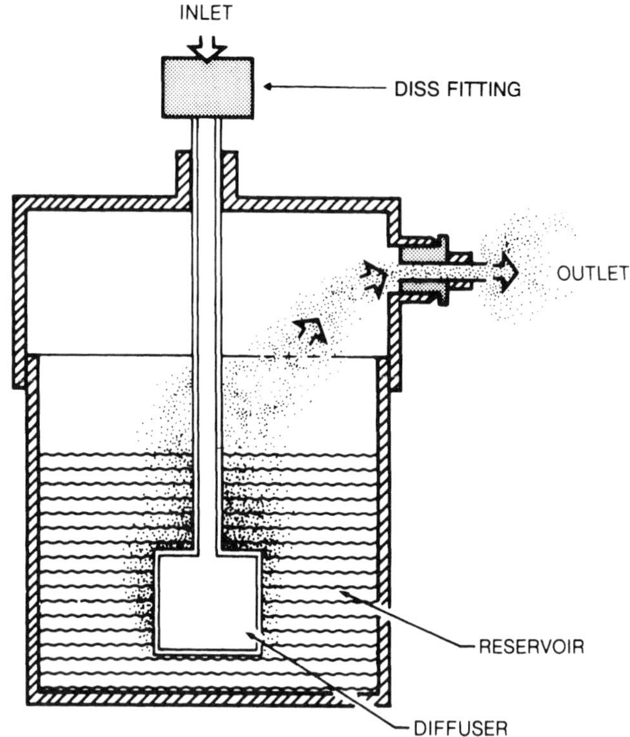

FIGURE 11-11 A bubble humidifier and its functional diagram.

substitute for the ventilator functions of the patient's muscles. When these muscles are paralyzed, the mechanical ventilator helps the patient to breathe. A simple ventilator is shown in **Figure 11-12**.

Ventilation is movement of air (gases) in and out of the lungs. Ventilation is pulmonary specific, but respiration refers to the wider context of breathing (inspiration and expiration) to include nose, pharynx, larynx, trachea, bronchi and the right and left lungs. The respiratory system combines with the cardiovascular system to deliver life-giving oxygen to the cells of the body.

Ventilators are devices or machines that provide artificial ventilation in respiratory care.

There is a wide spectrum of ventilators that differ in types and modes of operations. Ventilators can be classified as:

- Positive-pressure ventilators create pressure gradients by adding positive pressure to the airway.
- Negative-pressure ventilators support ventilation by exposing the surface of the chest wall to subatmospheric pressure during inspiration. The expiration occurs when the pressure around the chest wall increases and becomes atmospheric.
- Fluidic ventilators apply the Coanda effect to the movement of the flow of air or gases. The Coanda effect states that the surrounding air molecules not in the airstream acquire a higher pressure.
- Pediatric ventilators are specially designed for infants and newborns.

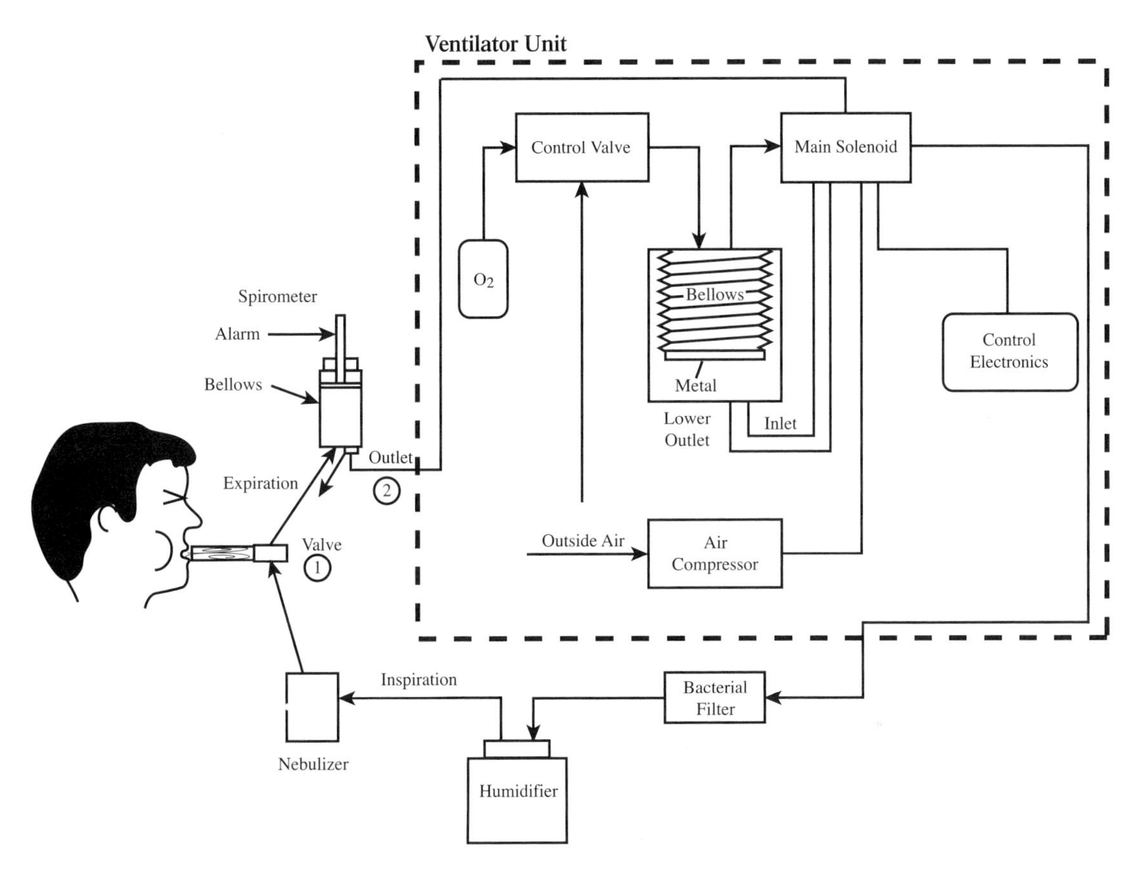

FIGURE 11-12 Block diagram of a ventilator.

There are also several ventilatory modes:

- Negative end-expiratory pressure (NEEP) is the subatmospheric pressure that develops at the airway at the end of expiration. An example is −5 cm H_2O pressure at the endotracheal tube during expiration.
- Positive end-expiratory pressure (PEEP) is the pressure applied at the end of expiration to maintain alveolar recruitment. The airway pressure is kept positive and is not allowed to return to the atmospheric pressure. When inspiration commences, the pressure is on top of the PEEP pressure.
- Continuous positive airway pressure (CPAP) is the positive pressure applied to the airway in inspiration and expiration.
- Continuous-flow ventilation (CFV) is the constant flow ventilation and maintains normal gas exchange.

High-frequency Oscillatory Ventilator

A high-frequency oscillatory ventilator such as those manufactured by SensorMedics or Hamilton Veolar is used for the ventilatory support and the treatment of respiratory failure and barotrauma in neonates who weigh less than 4.6 kilograms and are between 24 and 43 weeks of gestational age. It consists of eight subsystems:

1. External air/oxygen blender interfaced to the patient
2. External humidifier interfaced to the patient
3. Pneumatic logic and control
4. Patient circuit with patient interface
5. Oscillator subsystem
6. Airway pressure monitor
7. Electronic control and alarm system
8. Electrical power supply

The ties between electricity and the pressure generated by the ventilator are the solenoid valve and the movement of the oscillating piston. The mean airway pressure can be maintained and controlled by the ventilator control mechanism and the patient circuit.

An electronic square-wave driver (generator) in the oscillator subsystem drives a linear motor, which in turn drives a piston assembly. When the polarity of the square-wave driver is positive, it drives the electrical coil and the attached piston forward in the direction of the patient's inspiration. When the polarity is negative, the attached piston is driven in the opposite direction (expiration).

The distance the piston is driven in each direction is determined by the magnitude of the square-wave voltage, the patient circuit pressure encountered by the piston plate, the piston coil counterforce current, and the frequency of the square wave. The total transit time required for the displacement of the electrical coil and the piston is of the order of a few milliseconds. At lower oscillation frequencies, the piston will remain stationary at its full-travel position for the majority of that particular respiration phase (inspiratory or expiratory).

As the oscillation frequency increases, the transit time of the electrical coil and piston to its set full displacement will become a larger percentage of the total respiratory phase duration. The electrical coil and piston are unable to complete full displacement before the square wave driver switches polarity; thus, the displacement amplitude of the oscillator piston will decrease as the oscillation frequency is increased. **Figure 11-13** shows a photograph of the Hamilton Veolar volume ventilator. This is pneumatically powered and its microprocessor controls the flow and the various modes of ventilatory cycles. The control panel is shown in **Figure 11-14.** The schematic of the Hamilton Veolar ventilator is shown in detail in **Figure 11-15.** The inspiration and expiration lines are shown as directly connected to the patient's lungs. Also shown are the patient high-pressure valve, the nebulizer valve, the expiration valve, and the ambient valve. The mixture of oxygen and air is monitored at the front panel of the ventilator.

LTV-series Ventilator

The LTV-series ventilator is designed for use by adults and pediatrics weighing a minimum of 22 pounds and it needs positive pressure ventilation (delivered invasively or non-invasively). It uses turbine technology that allows the ventilator to operate without an external compressed gas source. It is designed for the oxygen blending from either a high-pressure oxygen source or a low-pressure oxygen bleed-in. A high-pressure source

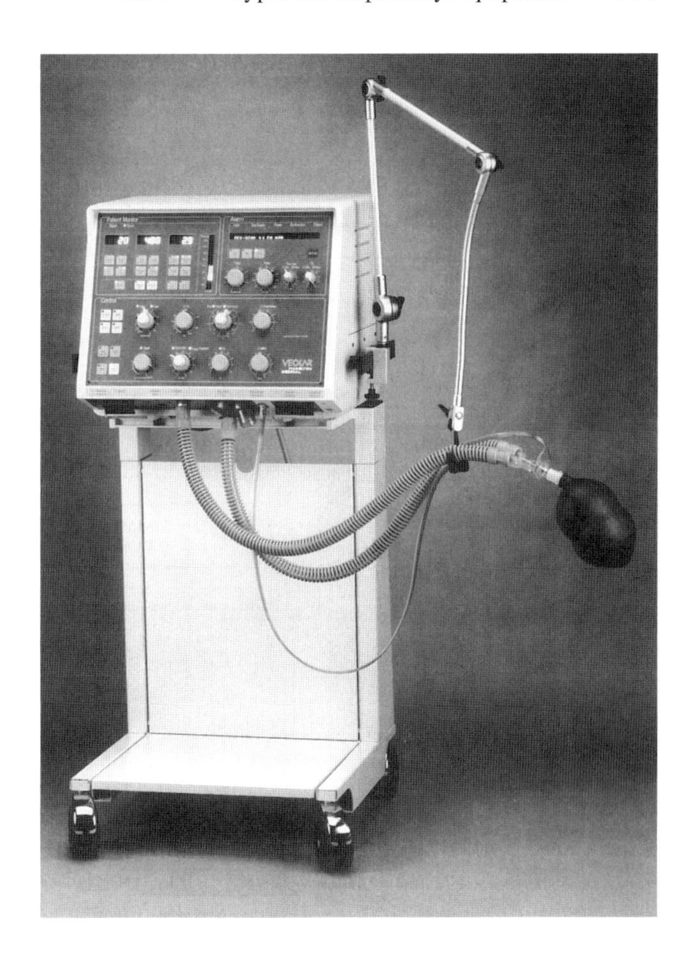

FIGURE 11-13 A Hamilton Veolar volume ventilator.

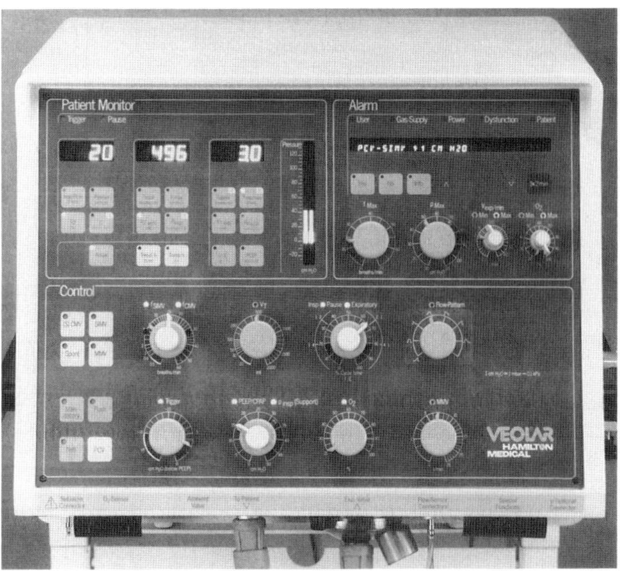

FIGURE 11-14 The control panel of the Hamilton Veolar ventilator.

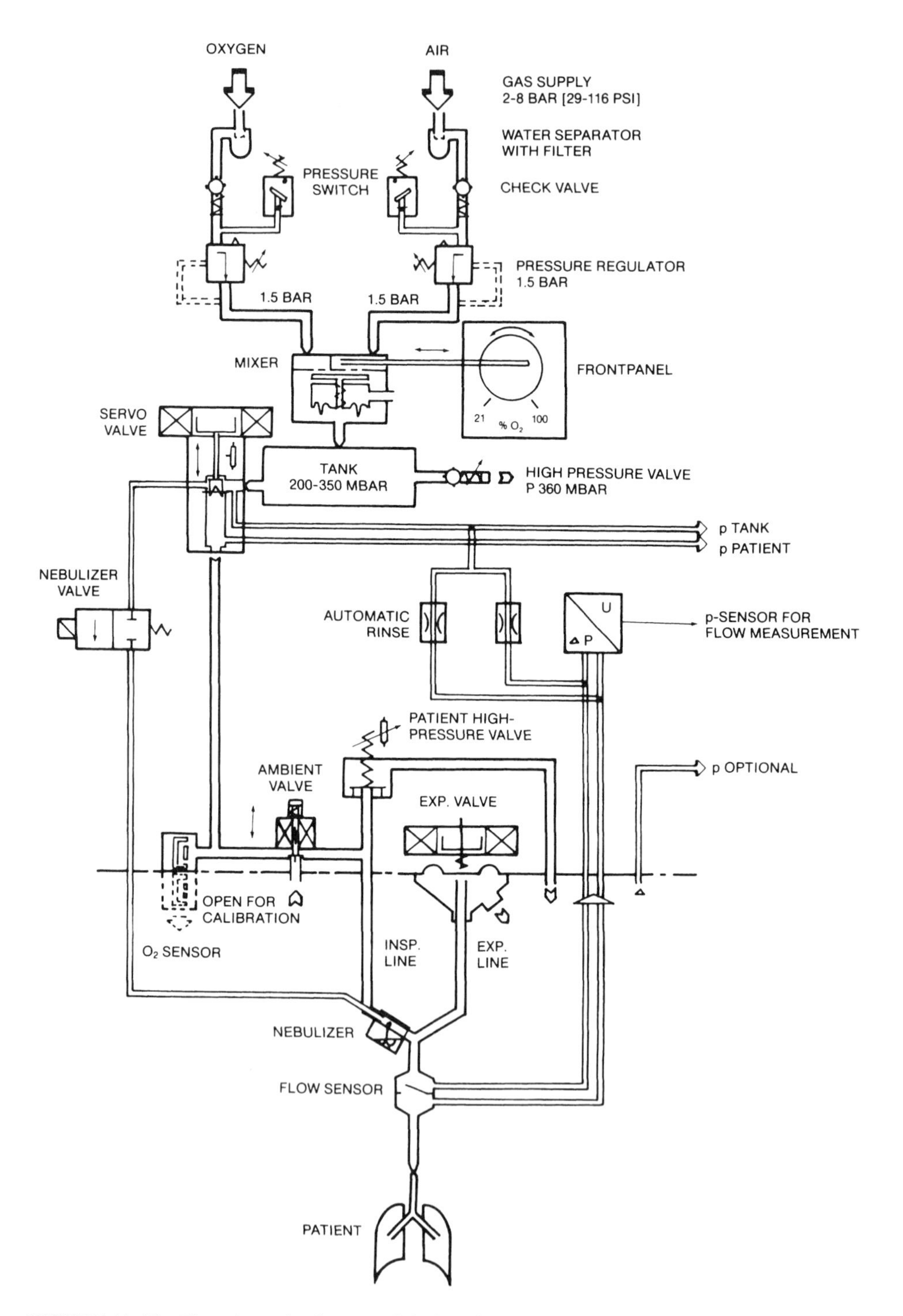

FIGURE 11-15 The schematic diagram of the Hamilton Veolar ventilator.

provides oxygen at 40 to 70 psig, while low-flow low pressure is less than 10 psig. The use of psig indicates that the unit of pressure is in pounds per square inch gauge (relative to the surrounding atmosphere); it indicates the pressure resulting from a force of one pound applied to an area of one square inch.

The electromechanical pneumatic system, under microprocessor controls, delivers ventilation to a patient. The process is as follows:

1. Room air enters the ventilator through INLET FILTER.
2. After exiting the filter, the air enters ACCUMULATOR/SILENCER where the air mixes with the oxygen delivered from the OXYGEN BLENDER.
3. Mixed gas then enters the ROTARY COMPRESSOR where energy is added to the mixed gas as required to meet the pressure and flow delivery requirements of the current ventilation settings.
4. Now the energized mixed gas enters another silencer after exiting the rotary compressor.
   a) Gas flow splits in two paths on exiting the silencing chamber. Gas flow for ventilation diverts to the flow valve, while excess flow is re-circulated through the bypass valve to the inlet accumulator/silencer.
   b) The flow valve now controls all inspiratory gas flow to the patient.
   c) Ventilation gas exiting the flow valve is connected to the exhalation valve by a patient circuit.

In this machine, the accumulator/silencer provides acoustic silencing to reduce the rotary compressor noise. The oxygen blender accepts pressurized oxygen from an external source and meters the oxygen flow to meet the requirements of the current oxygen percent setting and the ventilation flow demand.

The bypass valve maintains the flow valve inlet pressure high enough above the flow valve outlet pressure to ensure a positive pressure across the valve, yet low enough to ensure that excess energy is not wasted when operating from batteries.

The flow valve is driven by a rotary actuator, and translates circular motion to a poppet position, which in turn meters flow to the patient. The valve allows the gas flow as a function of the differential pressure across the valve and the actuator position. A differential pressure transducer is provided to measure the differential flow valve pressure.

The exhalation valve:

- Closes the exhalation port during inspiration (to divert gas to the patient).
- Opens the exhalation port during exhalation (to allow patient gases to be exhausted to the atmosphere).
- Provides variable positive end expiration pressure (PEEP) during the exhalation phase.
- Measures the exhaled flow using a fixed orifice type transducer. The transducer ports are located between the patient and ventilator connection ports.

The breath types available on machines such as the LTV-series ventilators are machine, assist, and patient. These types are either initiated or limited or cycled by the patient or the ventilator.

	Machine	Assist	Patient
Initiated by	Ventilator	Patient	Patient
Limited by	Ventilator	Ventilator	Ventilator
Cycled by	Ventilator	Ventilator	Patient

Breaths may be given in the following forms: volume control, pressure control, pressure support, and spontaneous. The breathing and ventilation controls for the patient can be graphed.

Body Plethysmograph

This device is used to measure airflow rate and lung capacity. The device follows Boyle's law and measures the thoracic volume changes. This is an airtight sealed chamber that completely encloses the patient chamber, as shown in **Figure 11-16**. As the patient's lungs expand and contract during breathing, the pressure changes in the chamber. By measuring this pressure change, the change in thoracic volume can be calculated.

The equation of total lung capacity can be given as

$$\text{TLC} = -\frac{(\text{volume of the chamber}) \times (\text{change in chamber pressure due to breathing})}{(\text{change in thorax pressure})}$$

Because every body plethysmograph has a given chamber volume, the changes in chamber pressure and thoracic volume are due to breathing motions.

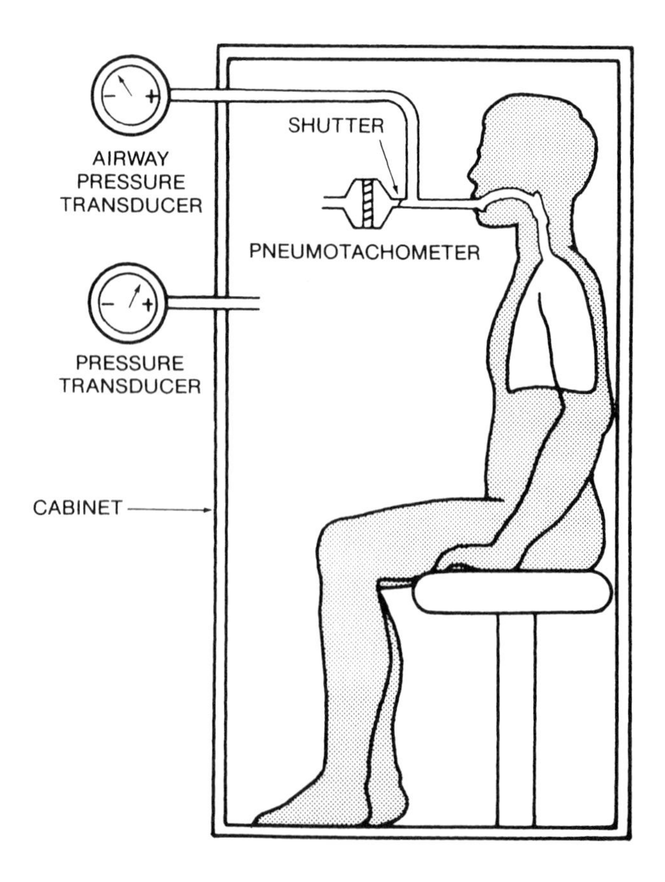

FIGURE 11-16 A functional diagram of a body plethysmograph.

Gas Regulators

Gas regulators are devices that regulate gas flow and control the rate of oxygen flow to the patient.

Gas Electrodes

Gas electrodes are devices that measure the percentage of a specific gas in a gas mixture.

Apnea Monitor

This is a device that measures the patient's respiratory rate when an irregular pause in the patient's breathing pattern is detected. A prolonged pause in breathing might indicate that the patient has actually stopped breathing for a short period, thus decreasing oxygen intake and possibly even interrupting sleep. In sleep apnea, the pauses in breathing during sleep are longer than 20 sec and are caused by an obstruction of the airway. **Figure 11-17** shows a diagram with the components of a four-channel sleep apnea monitor. The four channels are ECG, airflow, oxygen saturation or SpO_2, and the snoring microphone.

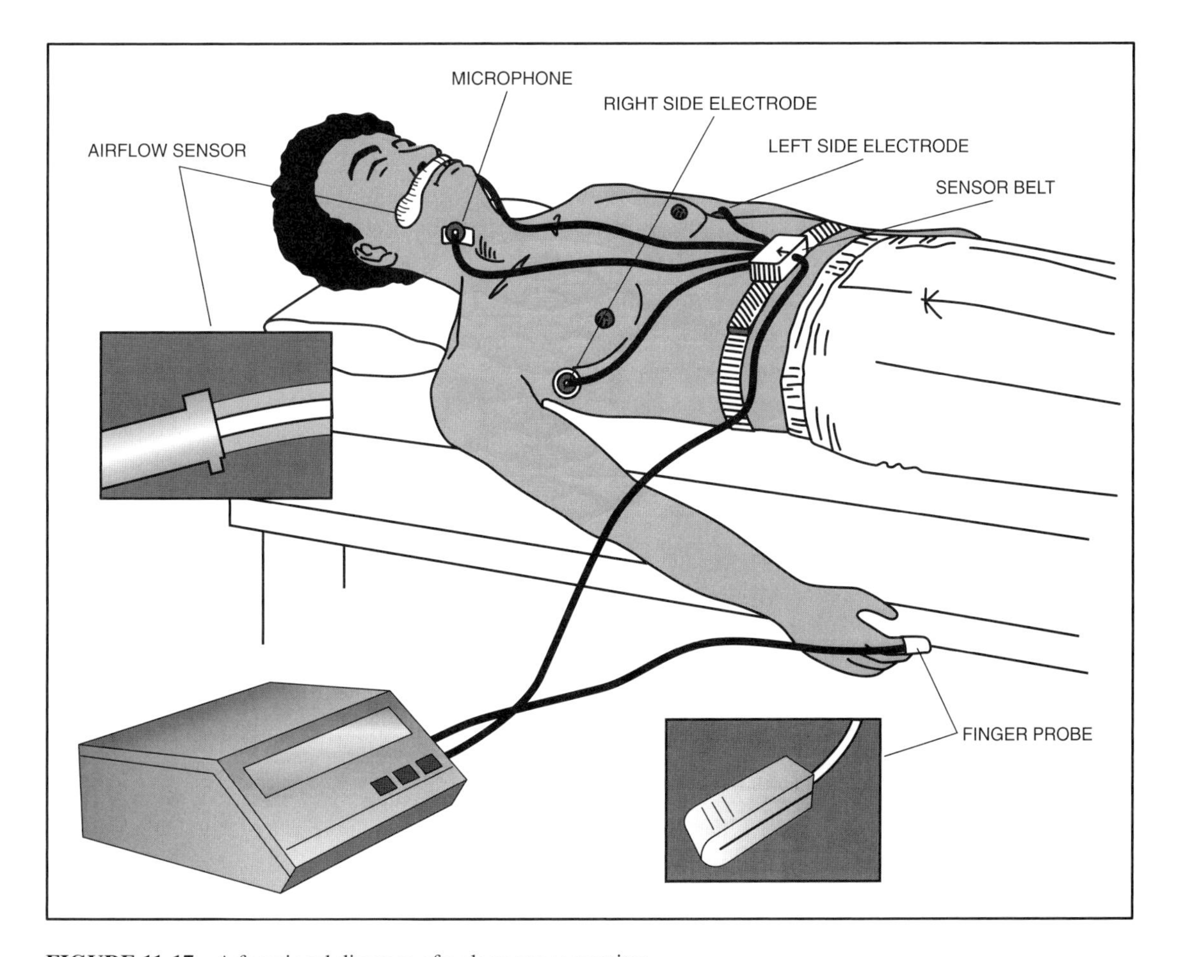

FIGURE 11-17 A functional diagram of a sleep apnea monitor.

11.3 PULMONARY FUNCTION TEST

Although physical examination and chest X-rays can provide a lot of information about the lungs, the pulmonary function test (PFT) provides additional information about the functions of lungs and the respiratory system. The test determines the amount of air the lungs can hold, the efficiency of the lungs in exchanging oxygen and carbon dioxide from the blood, and the effectiveness of the lungs in moving air into and out of the body. Patients may be tested while sleeping or sedated, or they may be on mechanical ventilation. These tests can be done in clinics, hospital laboratories, or in intensive care units. Some of the tests include:

Volume-time spirometry: the patient uses the spirometer and FEV_1 and FVC are determined.

Flow-volume spirometry: the patient uses the spirometer and the forced expiratory flow (FEF) at several FVCs is determined.

Arterial blood gases: arterial blood is the oxygenated blood flowing directly from the heart; analysis of arterial blood can determine the chemistry of the blood before it is used by tissues and cells. Apart from oxygen and carbon dioxide saturation, the pH of the blood is also determined.

Diffusion capacity measurement: the patient inhales a small amount of carbon dioxide and holds his breath for ten seconds before exhaling into a carbon dioxide detector. The amount of carbon dioxide remaining in the exhaled air determines how rapidly the patient exchanges gases from the lungs into the bloodstream.

Single-breath closing volume: this procedure determines the dilution of the residual nitrogen in the lungs after a single breath of 100% oxygen. On expiration, the dilution of the nitrogen gas predicts the patient's airway abnormalities.

Maximum mid-expiratory flow rate: this is a spirogram test that checks FEFs at 25 percent through 75 percent FVCs.

Lung volume measurement: the patient sits in the body plethysmograph and breathes in and out through the mouthpiece. The pressure change inside the box determines the volume of gas in the lungs.

SUMMARY

For a body to survive, oxygen must be in constant supply through respiration. The three processes of respiration are external respiration, internal respiration, and cellular respiration. The following topics are covered in this chapter on respiratory care and its instrumentation.

1. Human respiratory system and pulmonary circulation, including a diagram for further understanding are discussed in the first section. Respiration is achieved through the mouth, nose, trachea, right and left lungs, and diaphragm. The trachea splits into bronchi and bronchial tubes that lead directly into the lungs. Oxygen and carbon dioxide exchange occurs in the lung capillaries. The oxygen-rich blood then enters the pulmonary veins and returns to the heart.
2. Respiration laws are provided next, including: Boyle's Law, Charles's law and Dalton's law. Boyle's law states that the volume of a gas varies inversely with its pressure,

whereas Charles' law states that the volume of a gas varies directly with its temperature. Dalton's law states that the total pressure of a mixture of gases is the sum of the partial pressure of each gas in the mixture. Pulmonary volumes and capacities are explained with simple equations. Tidal volume is the volume of the air in normal inspiration or expiration, while total lung capacity is the maximum volume the lungs can hold with the maximum inspiratory effort.

3. Knowledge of diseases of the respiratory circuit can promote the understanding of other illnesses.
4. Respiratory equipment is discussed in depth covering a variety of devices to correct or minimize respiratory disorders. A list of such equipment is provided and discussed.
5. The pulmonary function test (PFT) is emphasized and explained in some detail.

MEDICAL TERMINOLOGY

The following is a list of medical terminology mentioned in this chapter.

Apnea: lack of spontaneous respiration. There is no movement of the muscles of respiration and the volume of the lungs at first remains unchanged.

Aspirator: device used for removing fluid from a body cavity. A hollow tubular instrument connected to a partial vacuum.

Autoclave: machine used to sterilize equipment by utilizing high pressure and heat, usually at 250° F (121° C) for a specified time period.

Body plethysmograph: airtight chamber surrounding the body that is used to measure lung volume and pressure for diagnosis of certain diseases.

Capnography: measurement of carbon dioxide in each breath of the respiratory cycle. The concentration of carbon dioxide at the end of exhalation is displayed.

Cardiopulmonary: pertaining to or involving both the heart and lungs. For example, cardiopulmonary resuscitation (CPR).

Continuous positive airway pressure (CPAP): technique to assist an individual's breathing by maintaining the air pressure in the lungs above atmospheric pressure throughout the respiratory cycle.

End-tidal carbon dioxide ($ETCO_2$): used to determine the partial pressure of carbon dioxide in the arterial blood to assess adequacy of ventilation.

Nebulizer: device used to deliver medication in the form of a mist that is inhaled through a mouthpiece or facemask. Air is pumped through a liquid medicine to produce a spray to be inhaled.

Oximeter: electronic instrument used to measure oxygen saturation of the arterial blood.

Pulmonary function test (PFT): a group of procedures that measure the functional capability of the lungs. The spirometry is the most common test used to measure how much and how fast air moves in and out of the lungs.

Respiratory care: field dedicated to assisting patients with cardiopulmonary disorders, such as asthma, cystic fibrosis, trauma, and so on. Respiratory care encompasses diagnostic evaluation, therapy, and education of patients.

Respiratory disorders: any disorder affecting the function of the respiratory system by inhibiting inspiration and expiration, such as common colds, flu, and coughs. Chronic problems may include cystic fibrosis or asthma.

Spirometer: device used for measuring the volume of air inspired and expired by the lungs to determine capacity.

Oxygen saturation (SpO_2): measurement of oxygen saturation of the arterial blood, often determined at the fingertip or earlobe with each pulse beat.

Ventilator: mechanical machine used for artificial ventilation of the lungs for the exchange of oxygen and carbon dioxide. It is used to replace or supplement the patient's natural breathing function.

QUIZ

1. The normal range of the respiratory rate for an infant is:

   a) 10 to 20 breaths per minute. b) 30 to 60 breaths per second.

   c) 30 to 60 breaths per minute. d) None of the above.

2. Pulse oximetry measures:

   a) Carbon dioxide saturation in the arterial blood.

   b) Oxidation reaction.

   c) Oxygen saturation in the arterial blood.

   d) Pulse rate.

3. Apnea is a (an):

   a) Sleep abnormality. b) Cessation of breathing.

   c) Nervous disorder. d) Infection.

4. CFV is an abbreviation of:

   ____

5. When a mechanical ventilator is switched to a mode enabling the patient to attempt to breathe by him- or herself, the mode is called:

   a) Controlled. b) Assist. c) Functional. d) Time-limited.

6. The difference between death due to carbon monoxide and death due to strangulation is:

   ____

7. Boyle's law states:

   a) Volume is proportional to the pressure in a tube.

   b) Volume is inversely proportional to the temperature in a tube.

   c) Pressure is inversely proportional to the volume in a tube.

   d) Temperature is proportional to the pressure in a tube.

8. Lung volume is measured by:

   a) Ohmmeter. b) Cardiometer. c) Oximeter. d) Spirometer.

9. Bernoulli's principle states:
   a) The relationship between pressure and volume of a gas.
   b) The energy balance between pressure and velocity.
   c) The relationship between pressure and temperature.
   d) None of the above.
10. If the Reynolds number is 912, the gas flow through a tube is:

    ____

RESEARCH TOPICS

1. Write a research paper on hazards and common faults in operating respiratory humidifiers. The paper should include the various safety and performance parameters and testing methodologies. The paper may concentrate on a few specific respiratory humidifiers used in hospitals.
2. Write a research paper describing the information you find regarding pulmonary hypertension.
3. Write a research paper on how the lung function test (PFT) may determine the impairment in patient's ability to blow air out of the lungs and why COPD (chronic obstructive pulmonary disease) is affecting a large population in the world. This research topic needs to cover not only emphysema and chronic bronchitis but also the various environmental factors in developing COPD.
4. Pulmonary artery catheters (PACs) are inserted by anesthesiologists and surgical technologists. These are used in patients with respiratory distress and in congestive heart failure cases. This research paper must include the guidelines of its utilization and the competency requirements.
5. Every year, there are ventilator-related deaths and injuries in hospitals. Investigate the reasons for such mishaps and then create a plan involving instrumentation to correct these problems. The researcher must acquire sufficient knowledge in various types of these ventilators and their functioning.
6. A research topic of "What are your daily air needs" can provide insight in measuring lung tidal volume, vital capacity and other parameters of a healthy person under resting and exercising conditions. The topic should also include patients with respiratory conditions and their air needs. The researcher is encouraged to make mathematical calculations of the respiration parameters.

CASE STUDIES

1. Apnea is a temporary stopping of the breathing movements. Neonatal apnea is more problematic and the breathing can be irregular. Caregivers must watch these children closely. A caregiver should rush to wake a child if the child stops breathing. A case study may be done on this subject and the following questions can be asked:
   a) What are the normal practices in watching and acting in apnea situations of infants?
   b) What kind of monitors and electronic systems are available to wake a child automatically without caregiver intervention?

PROBLEMS

1. Match the left column with the correct description in the right column:

1. Dyspnea is known as	a) volume of a gas to its pressure.
2. Influenza is characterized by	b) an aerosol therapy device.
3. Boyle's law relates the	c) painful breathing.
4. Maximum inspiratory volume is	d) total lung capacity.
5. A nebulizer is	e) partial sum of pressures to the total pressure in the mixture of gases
6. Normal expiratory volume is	
7. A spirometer is	f) tidal volume.
8. Dalton's law relates the	g) inflammation of the mucous membrane of the respiratory system.
	h) a device that measures lung capacity.

2. The body plethysmograph chamber has a volume of 25×10^4 cm^3. When the patient breathes in the extreme inspiration and expiration cycle, the chamber pressure changes from 15 psi to 15.5 psi and the patient's thorax pressure changes from 5 psi to 20 psi. Calculate the patient's total lung capacity.

3. A spirometer has a radius of 15 cm and the maximum height of 10 cm. Determine the maximum gas volume of the spirometer. Also, determine the output voltage of the potentiometer at the maximum height. Given: battery voltage 12 V.

4. The gas mixture is 20 percent Gas A, 30 percent Gas B, 35 percent Gas C, and 15 percent Gas D. Determine the partial pressure of Gas C when the total pressure of the gas mixture is 500 psi.

5. The volume of the gas exiting a delivery device is 1.5 liters at a temperature of 24° C. The gas then heats up to 35° C before it is delivered to the patient. Determine the volume of gas when patient receives it.

6. A valve separates two gas chambers, A and B. Chamber A contains one gas at 200 psi, while chamber B contains another gas at 300 psi. What will happen when the valve is opened? Can the gas pressures in chambers A and B be predicted?

7. Using proper medical terminology, discuss the process of respiration, tracing the taking of a breath of air through the mouth to the use of the oxygenated blood in the muscle tissue.

8. Determine vital capacity, given the following data:

TLC = 6 L. Volume of air left in two lungs at the end of maximum expiration = 2 L.

9. The volume of air expired and inspired in the lungs during exercise varies from 0.2 L to 4.1 L during each respiratory cycle; discuss the meaning of these values.

10. Write the average normal numerical values (or range) for the pulmonary function tests for an adult in the following table. When the values are not provided in the chapter, you may use Internet or other resources.

a) Volumes and capacities:

Tidal volume (TV) = ______________________________

Total lung capacity (TLC) = ______________________________

Vital capacity (VC) = ______________________________

Residual volume (RV) = ______________________

Inspiratory reserve volume = ______________________

Expiratory reserve volume = ______________________

b) Gas exchange and diffusion:

Oxygen consumption = ______________________

Carbon dioxide output = ______________________

Diffusing capacity of lung oxygen = ______________________

Diffusion capacity of lung carbon dioxide = ______________________

c) Arterial blood:

Oxygen partial pressure = ______________________

Carbon dioxide partial pressure = ______________________

pH = ______________________

Oxygen percent saturation of hemoglobin = ______________________

d) Mechanics of breathing:

Compliance of lung and thorax = ______________________

Compliance of lungs = ______________________

Airway resistance = ______________________

e) Ventilatory function tests:

Forced expiratory volume = ______________________

Forced expiratory flow = ______________________

Forced vital capacity = ______________________

f) Alveolar gas:

Oxygen partial pressure = ______________________

Carbon dioxide partial pressure = ______________________

11. Determine a patient's inspiratory reserve volume given the following information:

Total lung capacity = 5 L. Vital capacity = 4.1 L.

Tidal volume = 700 ml. Expiratory reserve volume = 1.1L.

12. The radius of the bronchial tube is reduced by one-half due to mucosal swelling. Determine the flow rate in milliliters per second through the swollen bronchial tube when the gas flow through the tube prior to swelling was 15 ml/sec.

13. The radius of the bronchi is reduced by one-half due to swelling. Determine the gas pressure in the swollen bronchi when the gas pressure in the tube prior to swelling was 1.2 cm H_2O.

14. Determine lung compliance when the intrapleural pressure is -5 cm H_2O during inspiration and the lungs accept a new volume of 200 ml of air. Also, if the pressure changes to -10 cm H_2O, what is the new compliance with the new volume of 400 ml?

15. Determine the inspiratory time when the patient is receiving continuous mandatory ventilation (CMV) in the control mode at a rate of 15 breaths/min and the expiratory time is 4 sec.

16. Determine the frequency of breathing when the patient is receiving continuous mandatory ventilation in the control mode and has an inspiratory time of 2.2 sec and an expiratory time of 4.3 sec.

CHAPTER 12

Electroencephalography and EMG Instrumentation

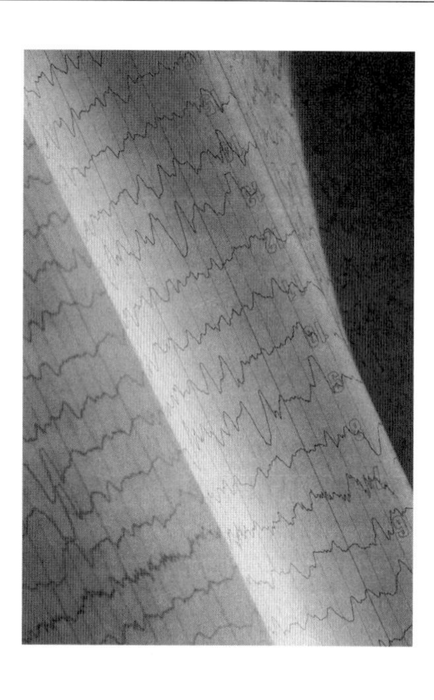

CHAPTER OUTLINE

OBJECTIVES

The objective of this chapter is to introduce the reader to the bioelectric function of the brain, and the contracting skeletal muscles using EEG and EMG instrumentation respectively.

Upon completion of this chapter, the reader will be able to:

- Describe the differences in the frequencies of various EEG waves.
- Explain the patient's physiological environment in acquiring various EEG waves.
- Define evoked potentials in EEG and EMG.
- Describe EEG leads placed on the scalp.
- Describe EEG and EMG electrodes.

■ INTERNET WEB SITES

http://www.aanem.net (American Association of Neuromuscular and Electrodiagnostic Medicine [AANEM])

http://www.eeginfo.com (Woodland Hills, California)

■ INTRODUCTION

Neuroimaging techniques such as electroencephalography (EEG) and electromyography (EMG) provide real-time temporal resolution tools for measuring brain function and electrical activity of muscles respectively. This measurement of the brain functions can predict the patient's abilities in areas of memory, spatial perception, attention to details, and information processing. Early signs of conditions such as Parkinson's disease and Alzheimer's disease, neuromuscular disease, or brain injury can be diagnosed using EEG neuroimaging techniques. An EMG can be used to detect abnormal electrical activity of muscle tissue that can occur in diseases such as muscular dystrophy, amyotrophic lateral sclerosis (ALS), and myasthenia gravis.

Electroencephalographic technicians are trained to use machines that record electrical activity of the brain. The EEG technician records the patient's brain activity by placing electrodes on the patient's scalp and connecting them to the EEG machine. The resulting data is then analyzed by neurologists to diagnose head injuries and brain diseases.

12.1 THE ORGANIZATION OF THE BRAIN AND ITS MEASUREMENTS

The nervous system is the most complex of all the systems in the body. It is composed of the brain, several sensors, and a high-speed communication link to all parts of the body. It determines a person's comprehension, memory, ability to interact with others, and his or her personality. The brain is a collection of neurons and is protected from light and heat by the skull. **Figure 12-1** shows the basic unit of neurons in the nervous system.

A neuron is a single cell with a cell body, called soma, and has one or more input fibers called dendrites. The neuron has a long transmitting fiber called an axon. Both axons and dendrites are called nerve fibers and a bundle of these nerve fibers is called a nerve. The brain, as the center of the nervous system, controls neural communication throughout the entire body. Before we explain neural communication, however, we will discuss the functions of the various parts of the brain.

Functions of the Brain

Certain parts of the brain play a dominant role in some functions; however, the parts of the brain interact to perform multiple roles as well. **Figure 12-2a** shows the brain components and **Figure 12-2b** indicates the brain functions. Each area of the brain controls different types of functions. The following section describes each area and its functions.

Medulla

This segment of the brain, located in the brainstem, controls the heart rate, breathing, and kidney functions.

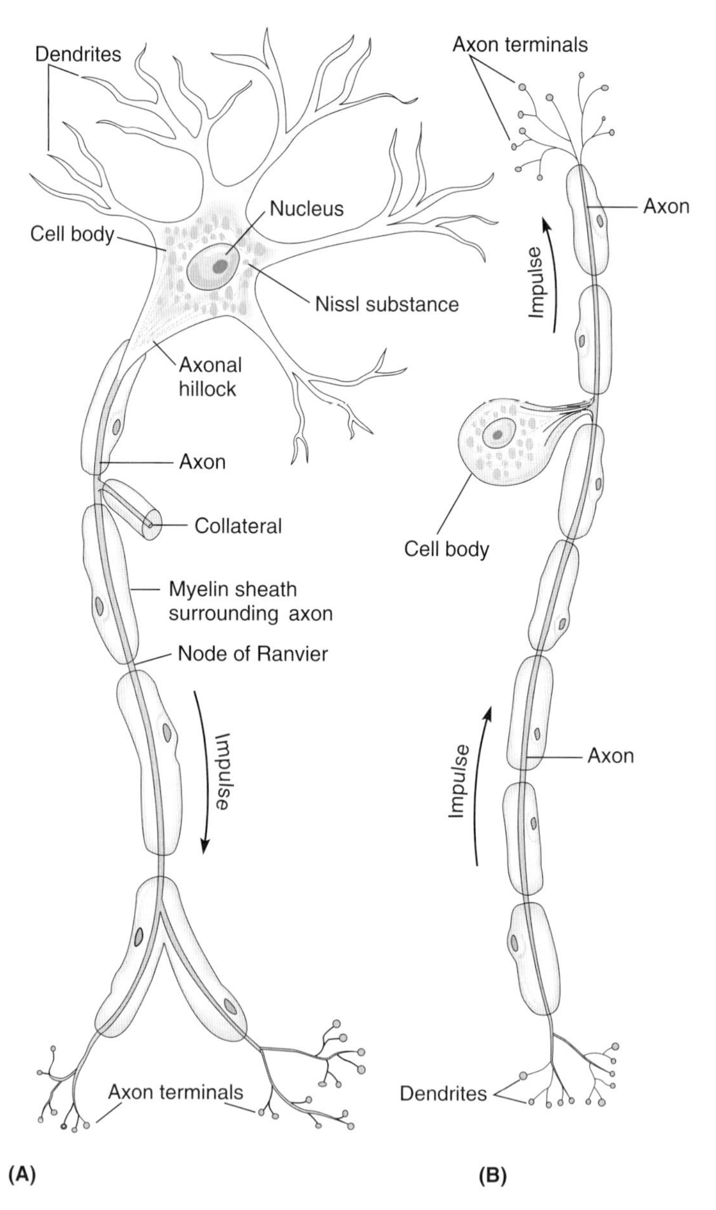

FIGURE 12-1 Multipolar and unipolar types of structural neurons.

Pons

This segment of the brain controls salivation, facial expression, respiration, and auditory function.

Cerebellum

This segment of the brain controls the motions of the muscles and maintains proper balance of the body.

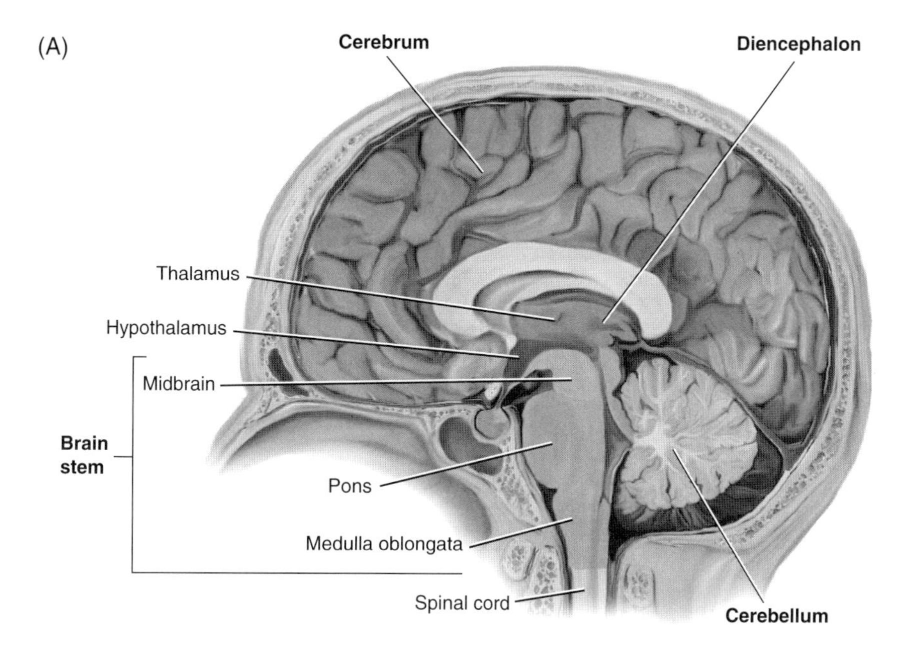

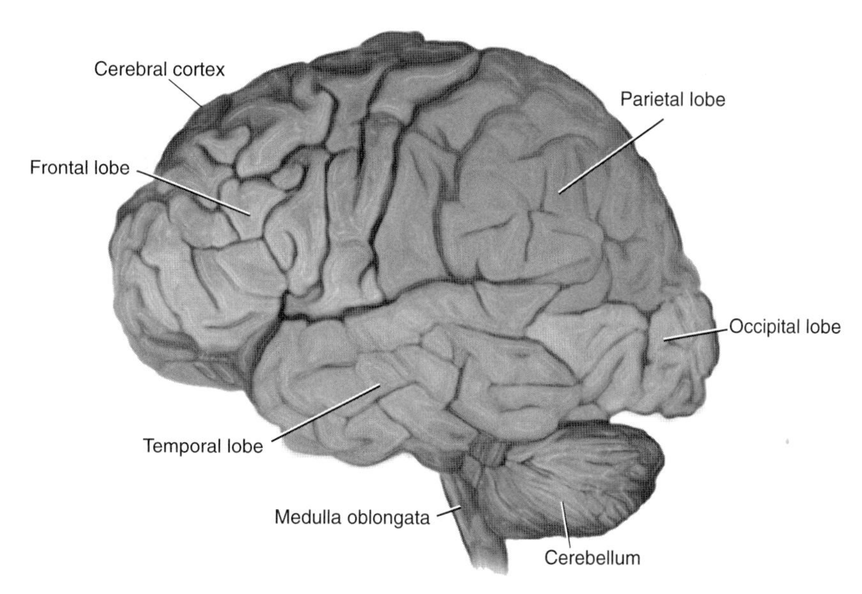

FIGURE 12-2a Cross-section of the brain.

Thalamus

This segment of the brain controls the visual and auditory sensory systems.

Hypothalamus

This segment of the brain is the center of emotions. It controls the sympathetic nervous system.

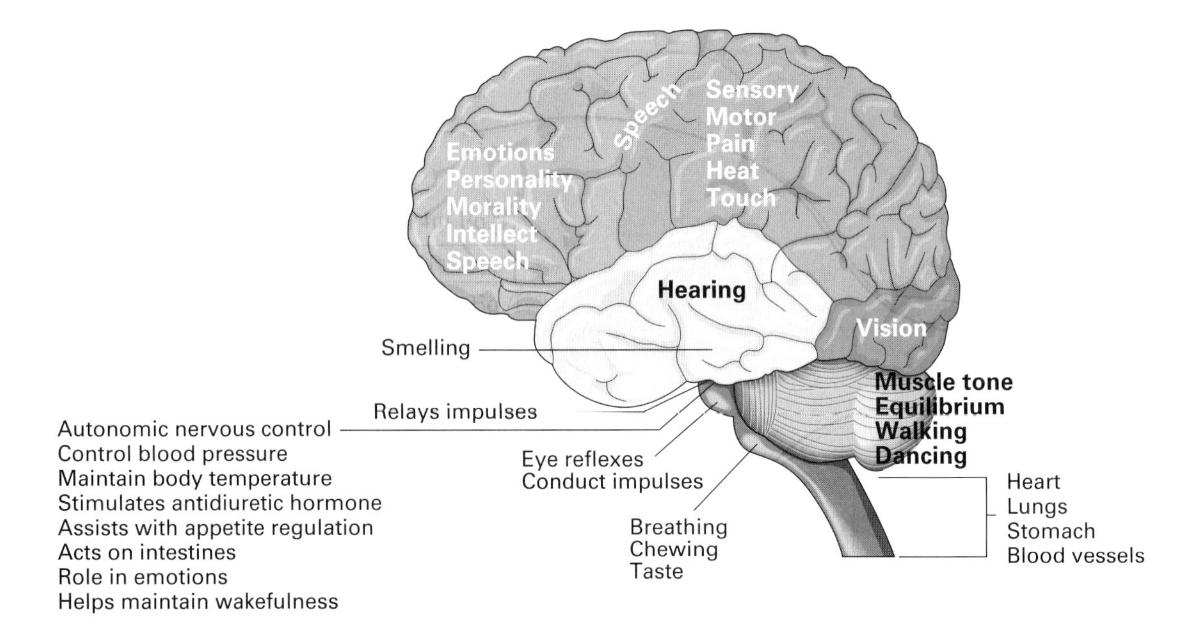

FIGURE 12-2b Cerebral functions.

Basal Ganglia

This segment of the brain is associated with a variety of functions such as motor control, cognition, emotions, and learning.

12.2 NEURAL COMMUNICATION

When excited, neurons generate brief action potentials called spike discharges. The sequence of these spikes are transmitted down a neural path. The neurons communicate with each other through synapses, or the spaces between two nerve cells. The speed of synapses can be as fast as 65 meters per second!

Sodium and potassium ion transfers cause the rapid and reversible potential changes across nerve and muscle cell membranes. At rest, the action potential is approximately −70 mV. When stimulated, however, it can change from a negative to a positive potential of approximately 20 mV. This is the depolarization phase. During depolarization, the extracellular fluid contains more sodium ions than does the intracellular fluid. It returns to the resting potential during the re-polarization phase as the inflow of sodium into the intracellular fluid increases.

The EEG potentials recorded at the surface of the scalp are caused by the combined effect of spike discharges, or the action potentials, over a wide region of the cortex and from various surrounding points. EEG recording is more complex than ECG recording because the action potentials vary greatly with the location of the electrodes attached to the surface of the scalp.

Another form of EEG measurement is called evoked potential response. This is a measurement of the disturbance in the EEG pattern due to external stimuli, such as a flash of light or the click of a sound. The evoked responses are distinguishable from the normal EEG activity and the noise in the EEG recordings. They tend to be low amplitudes—less than a microvolt to several microvolts—compared to tens of microvolts for EEG.

12.3 ELECTROENCEPHALOGRAM

The electroencephalogram (EEG) is a graphic record of the electrical activity of the brain as produced by a machine called an electroencephalograph. The delivery of any information through stimuli in the human body is received by the brain, which then interprets and responds to the information by carrying out an activity.

The brain is encased inside the cranium (the bony part of the skull minus the mandible (jawbone)) for protection. The cranium, in turn, is covered by skin (the scalp). Because the cerebral cortex is just under the cranium and is the largest part of the brain, EEG electrodes are placed on the scalp to detect electrical activity from the millions of neurons in the brain. One square millimeter of cortex contains more than 100,000 neurons!

The recordings from the brain, once any artifacts have been suppressed, are called brain waves. These brain waves are acquired when the patient is in different states of physiological activities, such as sleeping, or in an emotional state. **Figure 12-3** shows the brain wave through a differential circuit. **Figure 12-4** shows the brain wave patterns called alpha, beta, theta, and delta waves. A set of EEG-evoked potential graphs is also shown in **Figure 12-5.** These are averaged from several responses from a patient. The top graph is an average of ten responses, the middle graph is an average of fifteen responses, and the bottom graph is an average of twenty responses. The frequencies and amplitudes (rhythms) of alpha, beta, delta, and theta patterns in the brain waves are recorded by the electrodes on the scalp. They can range from 10 to 200 μV and have a frequency range of 1 to 30 Hz.

12.4 BIOELECTRIC POTENTIALS AND BRAIN WAVES

The characteristic of the brain waves depends on the degree of the activity of the cerebral cortex. Brain waves change significantly between the states of wakefulness and sleep and can show distinct and not-so-distinct patterns. The electrical potential is recorded when a large number of nerve fibers in the brain discharge simultaneously. The waves can be classified as follows.

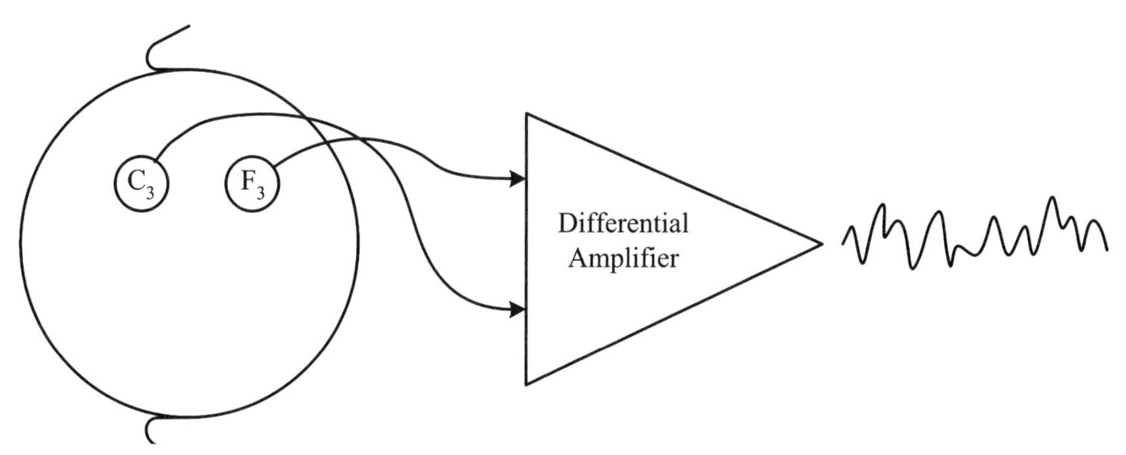

FIGURE 12-3 A differential amplifier circuit for the brain wave.

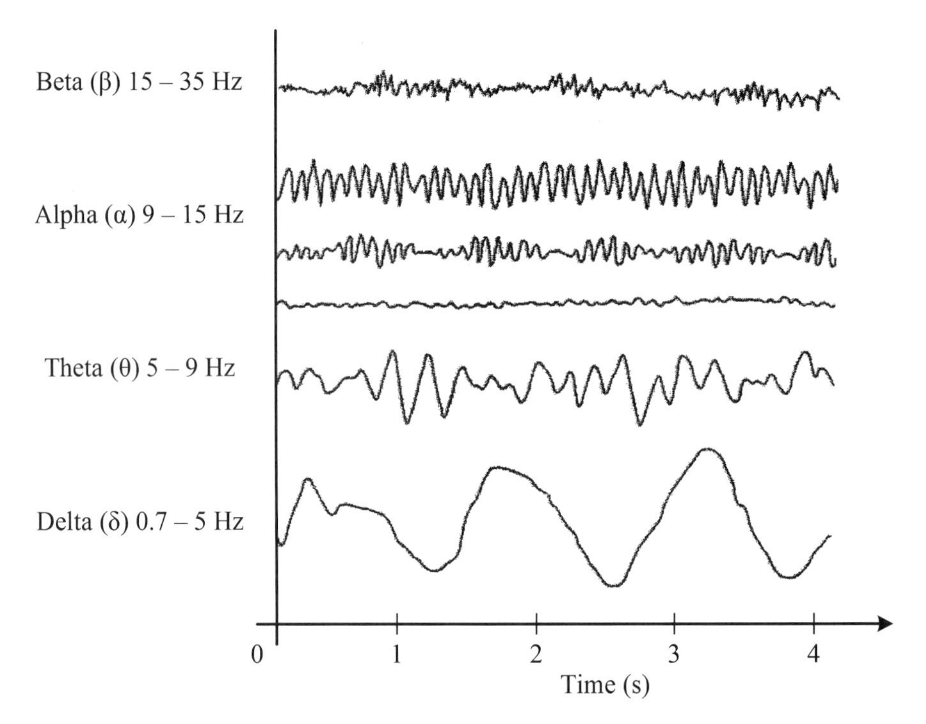

FIGURE 12-4 Brain waves.

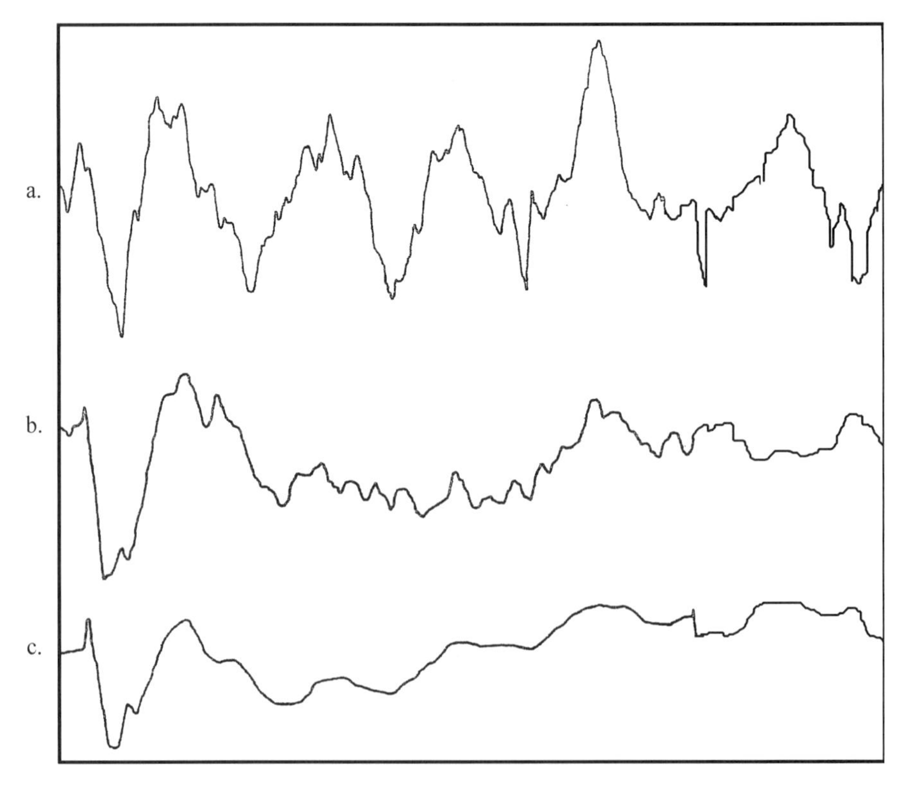

FIGURE 12-5 Averaging of the brain waves.

Alpha Waves

When healthy adults are awake, quiet, and in resting state, alpha waves are the rhythmic brain waves, with amplitudes of approximately 50 μV and a frequency range of 8 to 13 cycles per second. They are generated by synchronous activity of the cortical neurons in the thalmo-cortical region; during sleep, the alpha waves disappear.

Alpha waves are usually recorded in the occipital region; however, they can also be recorded from the frontal and parietal regions of the brain. **Figure 12-6** shows recorded alpha brain waves.

Beta Waves

Beta waves are asynchronous and have lower amplitudes than the alpha waves, but they range in higher frequency (25 to 50 Hz). These waves are recorded from the frontal and parietal regions. **Figure 12-7** shows recorded beta brain waves. Beta waves are often associated with active, busy or anxious thinking, wakefulness and active concentration.

Theta Waves

Theta waves have lower frequencies than alpha waves and the frequency range is four to seven cycles per second. They are recorded from the parietal region and occur when a person in some emotional stress. **Figure 12-8** shows recorded theta brain waves.

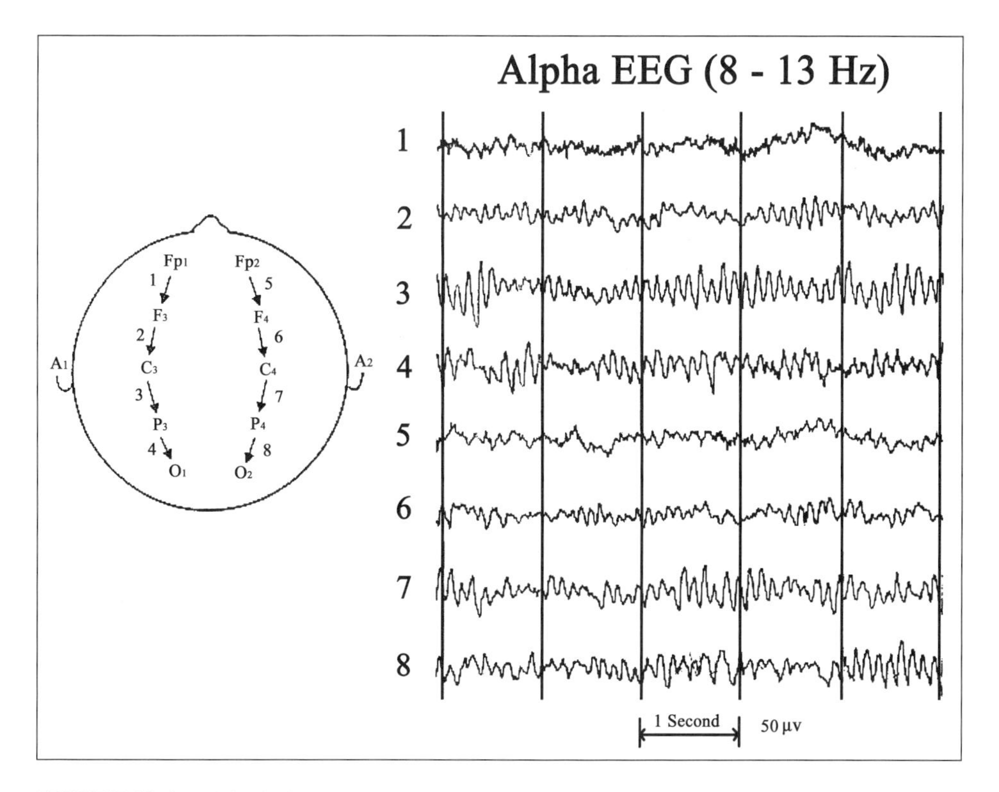

FIGURE 12-6 Alpha brain waves.

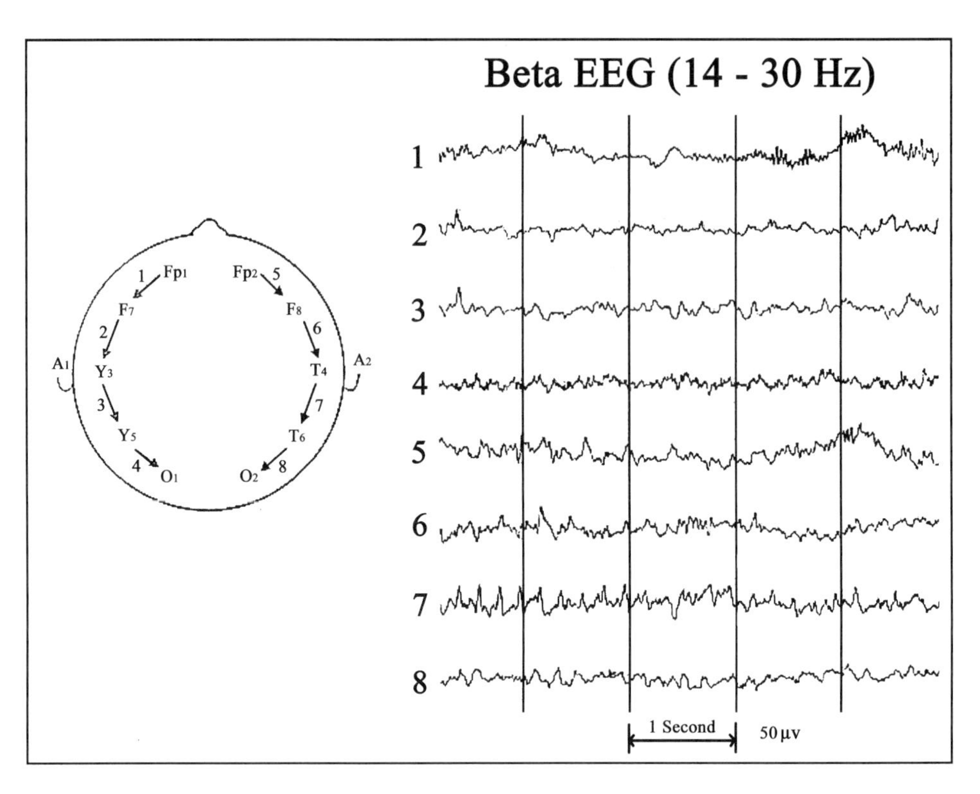

FIGURE 12-7 Beta brain waves.

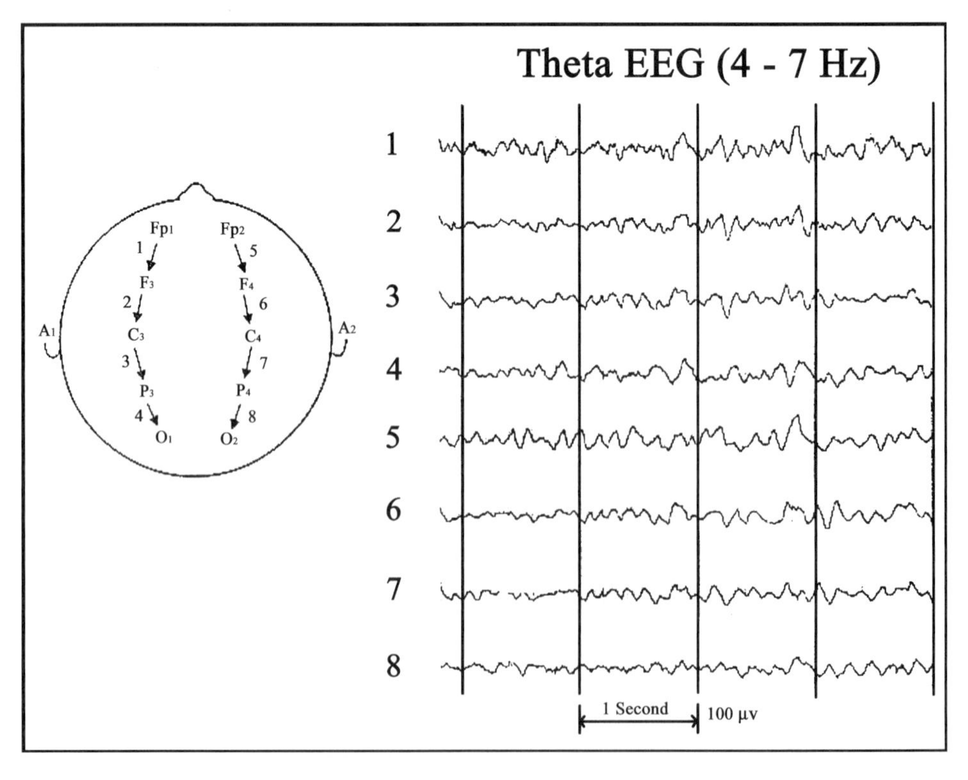

FIGURE 12-8 Theta brain waves.

Delta Waves

These are the lowest frequency signals (less than 3.5 Hz) from the cortex of the brain and occur when the person is in deep sleep. **Figure 12-9** shows recorded delta waves.

EXAMPLE Design an EEG filter that has cutoff frequencies of 25 Hz (high-pass) and 50 Hz (low-pass) with sharp roll-offs.

Consider including a combination of a high-pass filter (with low-frequency cutoff) and a low-pass filter (with high-frequency cutoff). A buffer circuit is needed between these two filters to avoid a loading problem. A sharp roll-off filter such as a Chebyshev filter can be considered for the roll-off requirement.

Also, there are band-pass filters that can provide a flat bandwidth between two frequencies and the low and high cut-offs can then be designed at the 3-dB gain.

■

EXAMPLE Design an EEG system that amplifies the raw EEG signal and detects the alpha wave if present in the raw EEG signal. The alpha activity is displayed in real time.

The differential amplifier gain can be adjusted to 1:10000 by selecting proper feedback and input resistances. Also, a band-pass filter is designed for 8 to 13 Hz bandwidth to detect the alpha activity.

■

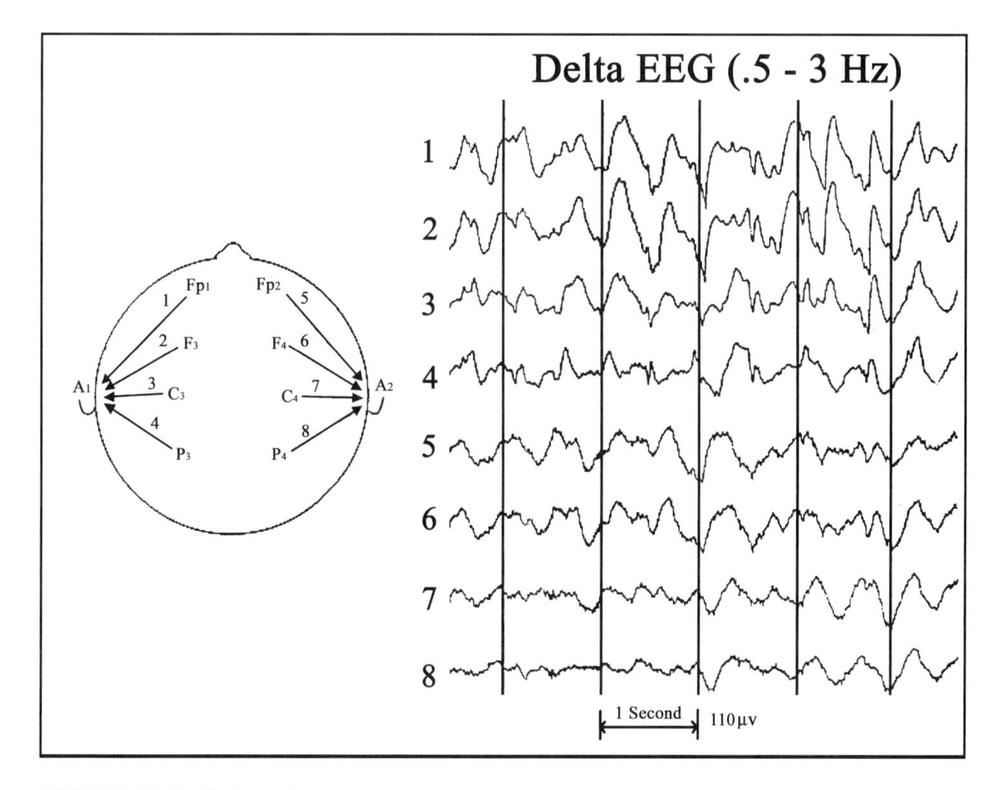

FIGURE 12-9 Delta brain waves.

EXAMPLE Generally, when is the amplitude of the EEG highest?

Amplitude denotes the intensity of synchronous neural activities in cortex, such as in deep sleep.

■

12.5 EEG LEADS

The standard spontaneous EEG is recorded by a 10–20 electrode system, and this system is an international standard. **Figure 12-10** shows these electrodes on the surface of the scalp. The reference points of the positions of these electrodes are called nasion and inion. Nasion is the top of the nose at the level with the eyes. Inion is the base of the skull on the back of the head. The skull perimeters are measured from these reference points in the transverse plane (across the scalp in the vertical axis) and the median plane (around the scalp in the horizontal axis), as shown in **Figure 12-11.**

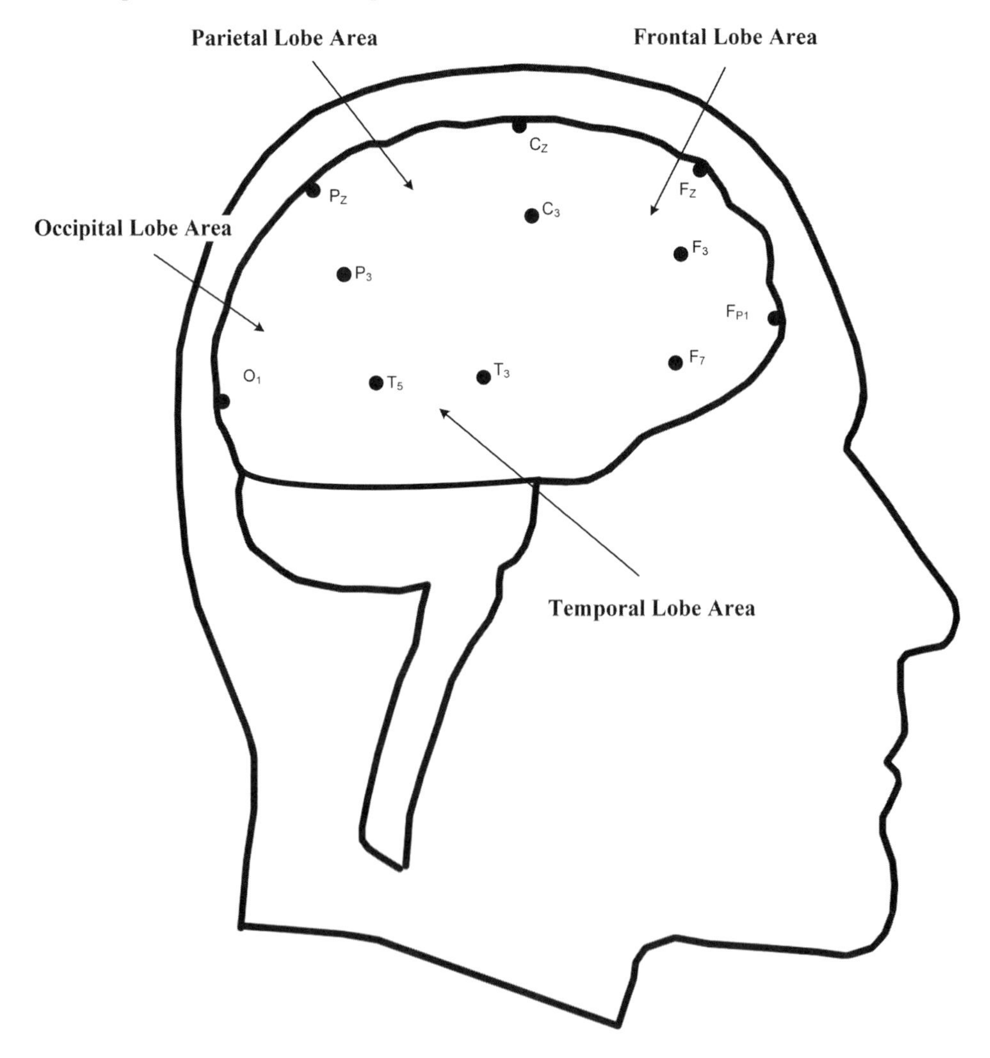

FIGURE 12-10 10- to 20-EEG electrode system.

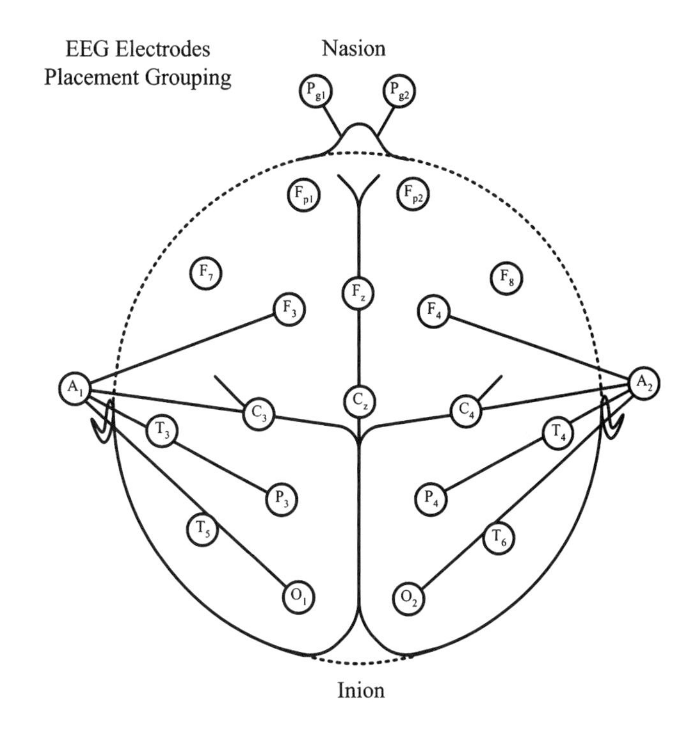

FIGURE 12-11 Grouping of the EEG electrode system.

Notice the symbols used in this electrode positioning: C = central, F = frontal, P = parietal, O = occipital, A = ear lobe, F_p = frontal polar, P_g = nasopharyngeal, and T = transverse.

The perimeters are then divided in 10 percent and 20 percent distances and electrodes are placed on those points. These electrodes can also be used to detect EEG signals based on unipolar or bipolar referencing. In the unipolar method, potential of each electrode is compared with respect to a reference neutral electrode. However, in the bipolar method, the potential difference is detected between two electrodes.

12.6 EEG ELECTRODES AND ACCESSORIES

Surface electrodes can be used to detect EEG signal, but they are smaller in size than the surface electrode for ECG. A cup electrode can be attached to the scalp by a conducting gel or paste. These are noninvasive electrodes, but EEG signals are also recorded using invasive electrodes to detect signals from inferior frontal regions. **Figure 12-12a** shows types of invasive electrodes and **Figure 12-12b** shows noninvasive cup electrodes.

EEG recordings may show the variability of frequency and amplitude depending on the mental state of an individual. The prominent alpha rhythm in an EEG signal is influenced by certain conditions, such as relaxation, eyes closed or open, abnormal breathing, visual attention, or even personality. **Figure 12-13** provides the Fourier spectrum of an EEG signal with frequency and amplitude changes. Due to the alpha rhythms, the maximum amplitude is approximately 10 Hz.

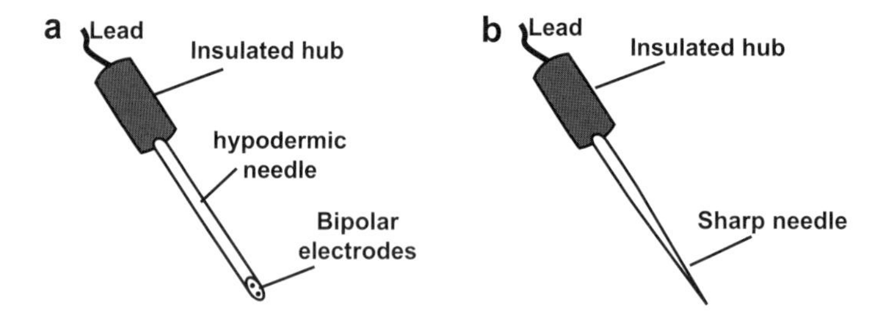

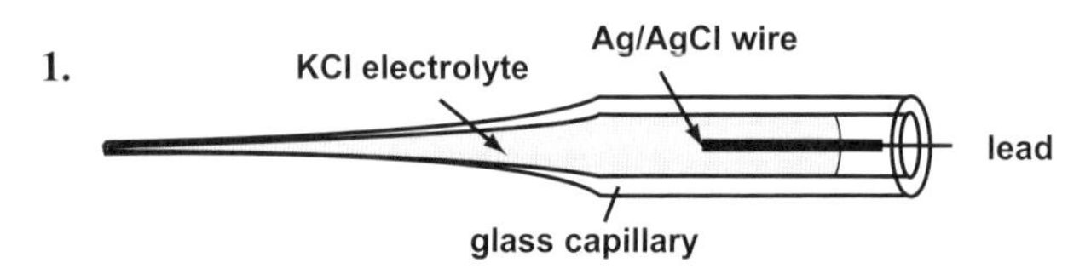

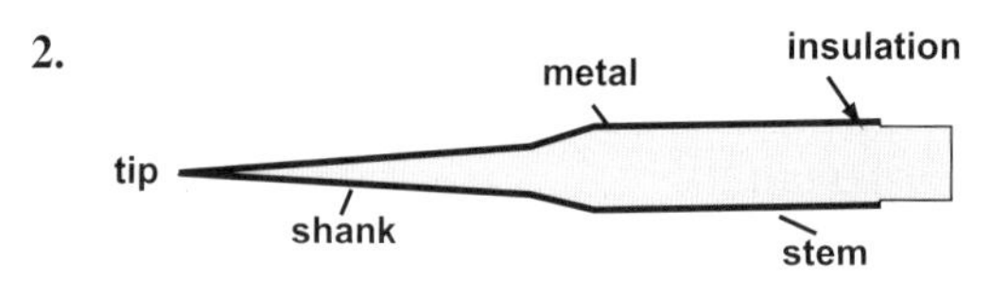

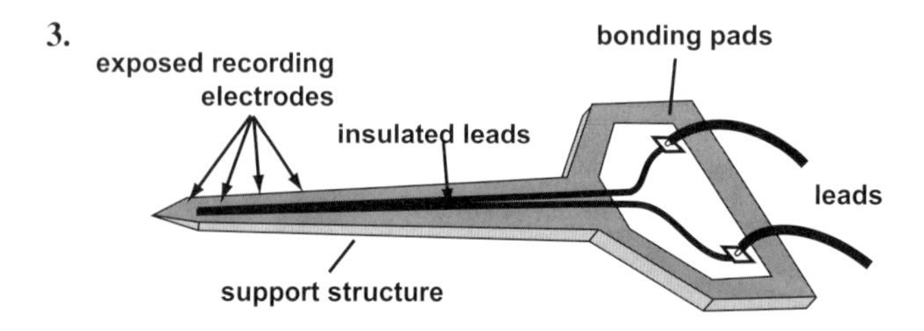

FIGURE 12-12a Illustrations of various EEG electrodes.

FIGURE 12-12b A photograph of EEG electrodes.

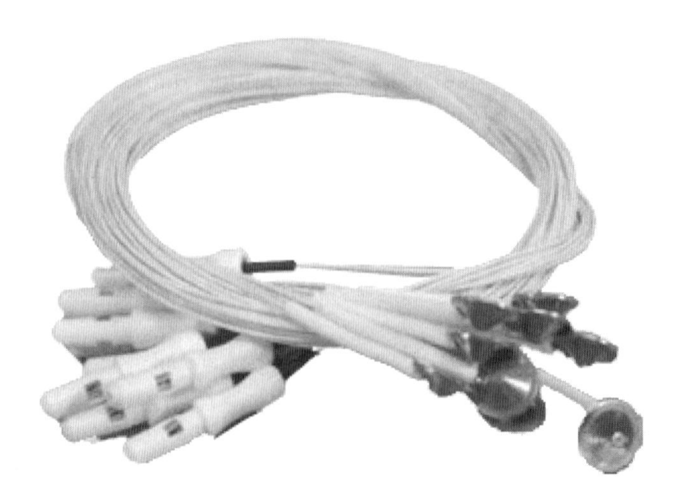

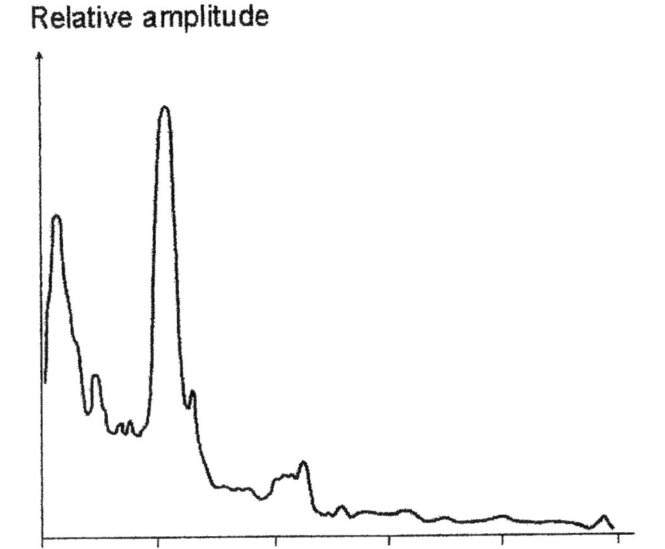

FIGURE 12-13 Fourier spectrum of an EEG wave.

12.7 EEG MACHINES

The Nicolet Corporation's EEG computer system is shown in **Figure 12-14a.** The main component in this system is the 32CTE amplifier, which collects analog EEG signals from up to 32 electrodes. The 32CTE amplifies and multiplexes them and sends them to the ISO coder.

All inputs are capacitive coupled and diode clamped for patient safety and hardwired to 32 differential amplifiers. This is also a 32-to-1 analog multiplexer. One 32CTE unit can combine other 32CTE units for recording from 128 electrodes.

The 32CTE modular unit is shown in **Figure 12-14b.** The pin-out for the 32CTE input connector is listed in **Figure 12-14c** for the 32PJA jack adapter. Apart from the 32 electrode connections, there are two ground leads and two connections for the reference electrodes.

The international 12 20-label set allows the standard 10–20-electrode positions plus ground and reference on the 32PJA adapter. The conversion table can show the pins to the proper montages.

Additionally, the nonscalp EEG electrodes are of either the referential type or the bipolar type. Referential-type electrodes are placed on the ear, mastoid, mandible, chin, or nose; bipolar-type electrodes are placed front to back, side to side, around the circumference of the hat band.

In the computer system, ISO code digitizes the 32 EEG analog channels, inserts checksum, time, date, and calibration information. The video camera input is combined with the 32 EEG waveform channels and is shown on the video monitor. The 32-channel computed output in analog form can be sent to the EEG machine.

Figure 12-15 shows the Nicolet EEG Machine front panel. The preamplifier arm connects to several channels. Each channel is connected to an EEG electrode. The ISO

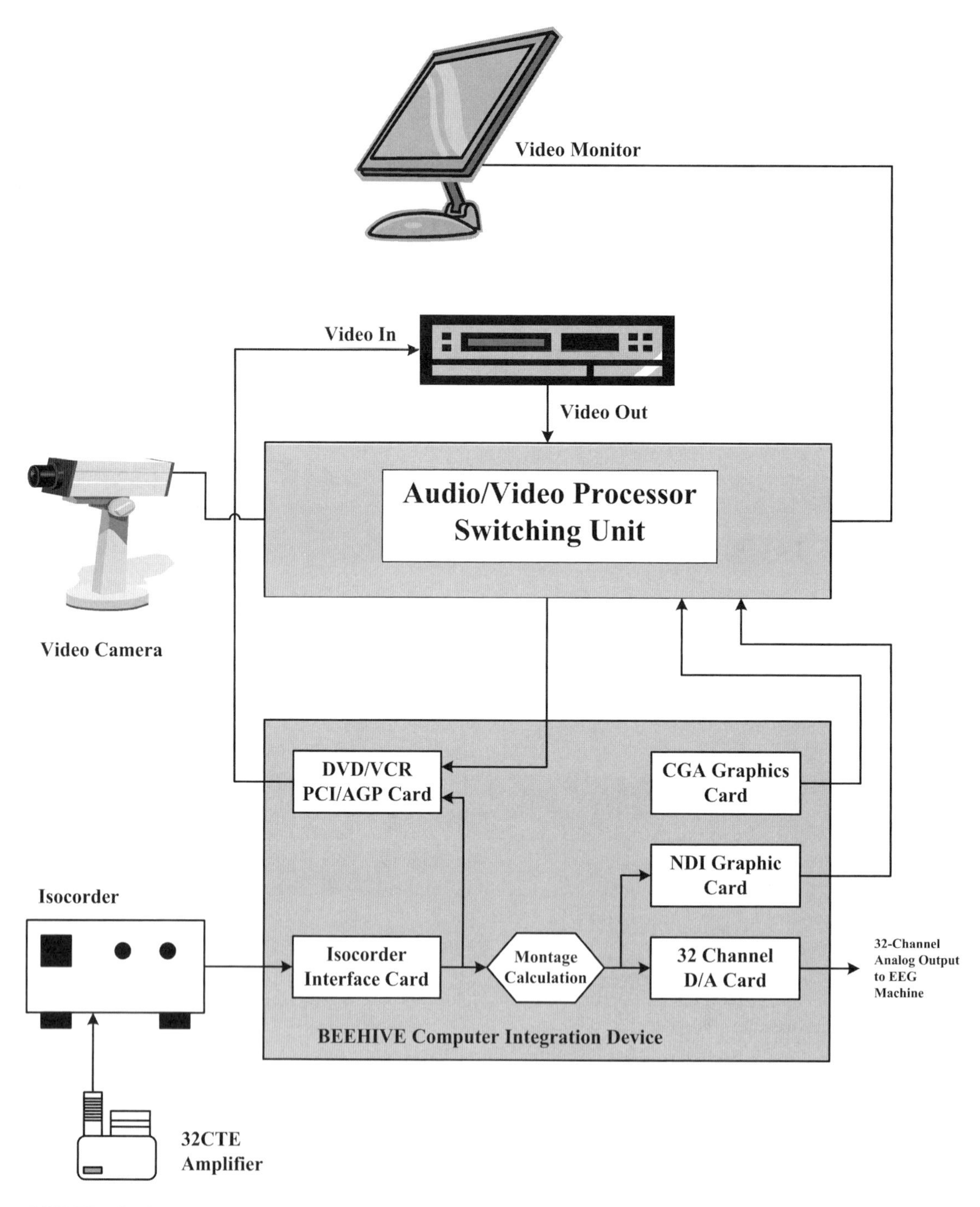

FIGURE 12-14a A block diagram of the EEG system.

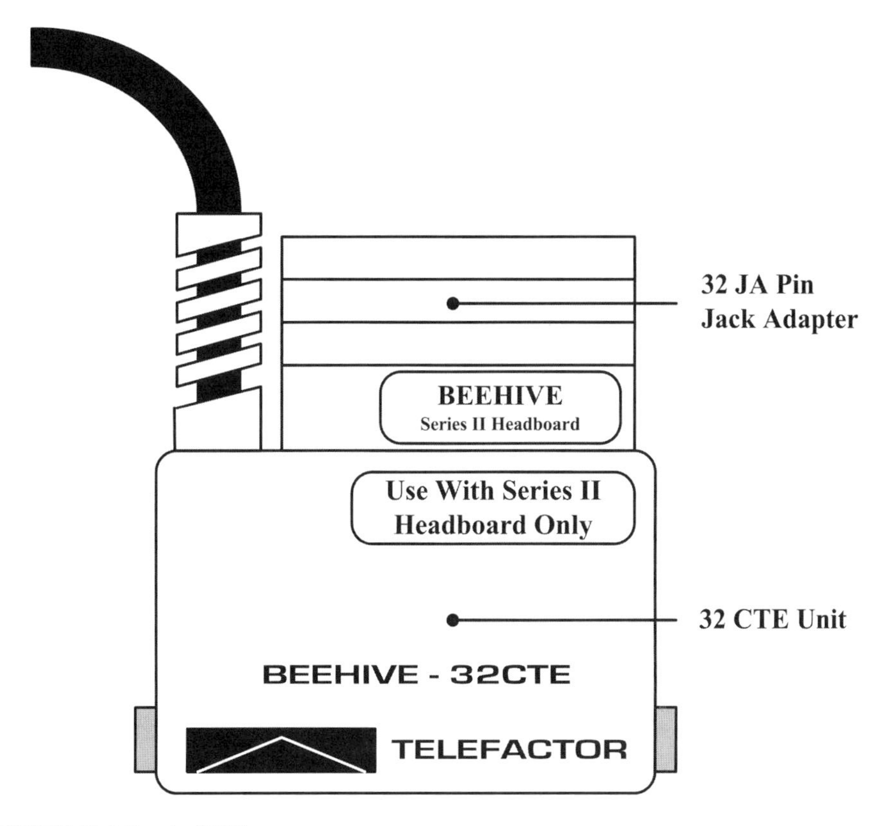

FIGURE 12-14b An EEG connector.

Input Channel	10-20 Electrode	Input Channel	10-20 Electrode
Input Ch 1:	Fp1	Input Ch 14:	T6
Input Ch 2:	F3	Input Ch 15:	P4
Input Ch 3:	F7	Input Ch 16:	O2
Input Ch 4:	C3	Input Ch 17:	Fz
Input Ch 5:	T3	Input Ch 18:	Cz
Input Ch 6:	T5	Input Ch 19:	Pz
Input Ch 7:	P3	Input Ch 20:	A1
Input Ch 8:	O1	Input Ch 21:	A2
Input Ch 9:	Fp2	Input Ch 22:	Pg1
Input Ch 10:	4	Input Ch 23:	Pg2
Input Ch 11:	F8	Input Ch 24:	Sp1
Input Ch 12:	C4	Input Ch 25:	Sp2
Input Ch 13:	T4	Input Ch 26:	T1
		Input Ch 27:	T2

FIGURE 12-14c EEG pins.

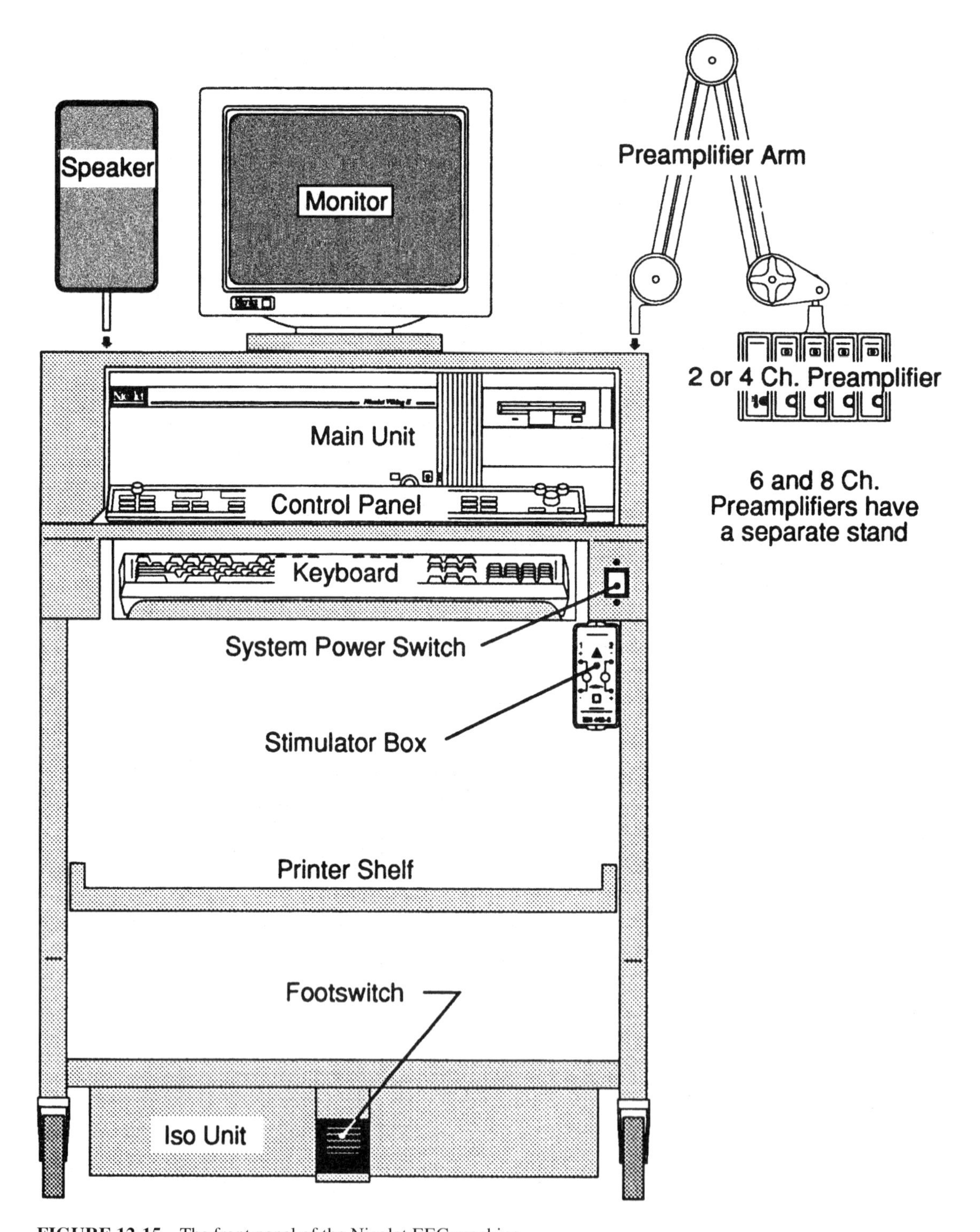

FIGURE 12-15 The front panel of the Nicolet EEG machine.

unit is the isolation transformer unit that connects to the wall outlet. **Figure 12-16** shows the master menu of the Nicolet EEG machine. By pressing any soft key, a variety of operations can be activated. There are several levels of relevant functions under each operation.

The EEG signal is also detected after the application of several types of stimulations such as visual, electrical, or auditory stimulations. **Figure 12-17** shows several stimulator and I/O boards. In a visual stimulator, either single or continuous strobe flash activation can be selected. Duration of the flash is at least 100 msec and the background illumination intensity is controllable from 2 fL to 30 fL. For the electrical stimulator, 0 to 100 mA or 0 to 400 V continuously adjustable intensity is provided into a 4 kΩ load. The auditory stimulator deals with tone frequencies ranging from 250 Hz to 8,000 Hz.

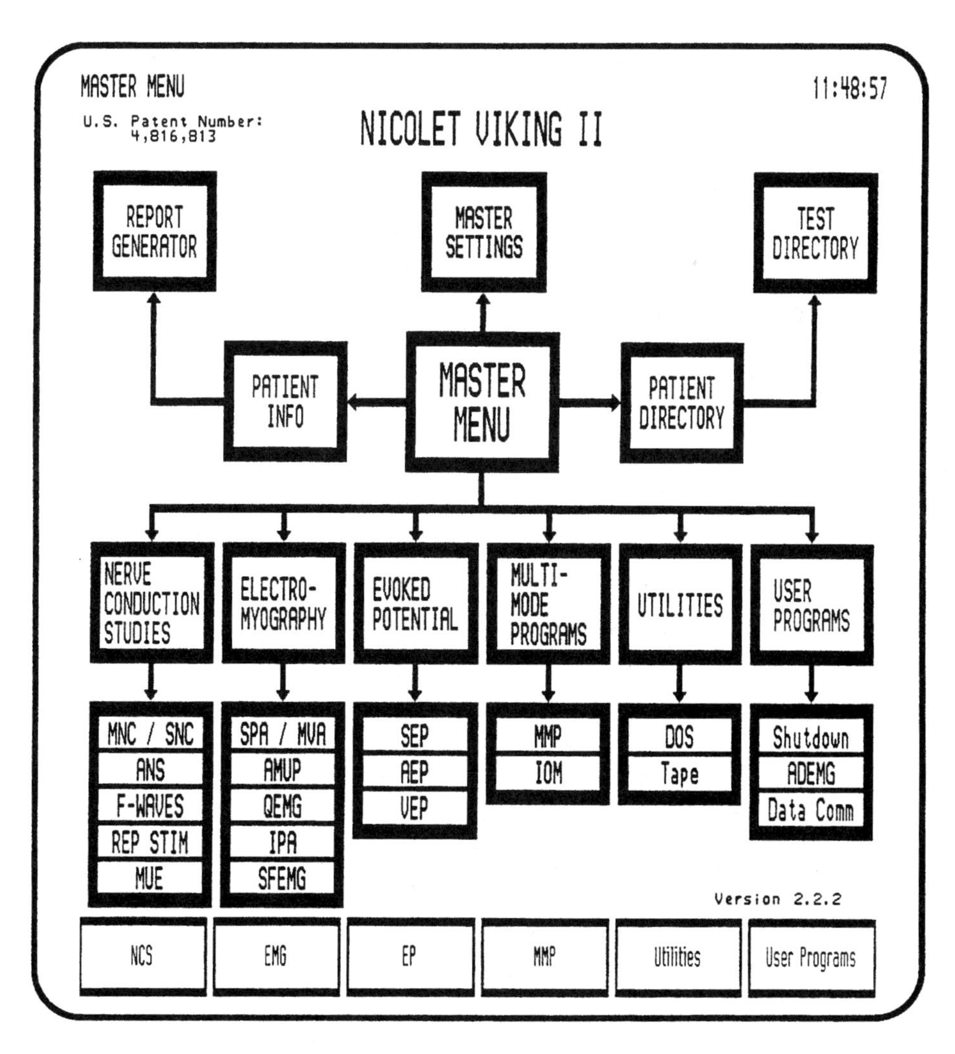

FIGURE 12-16 Master menu of the Nicolet EEG machine.

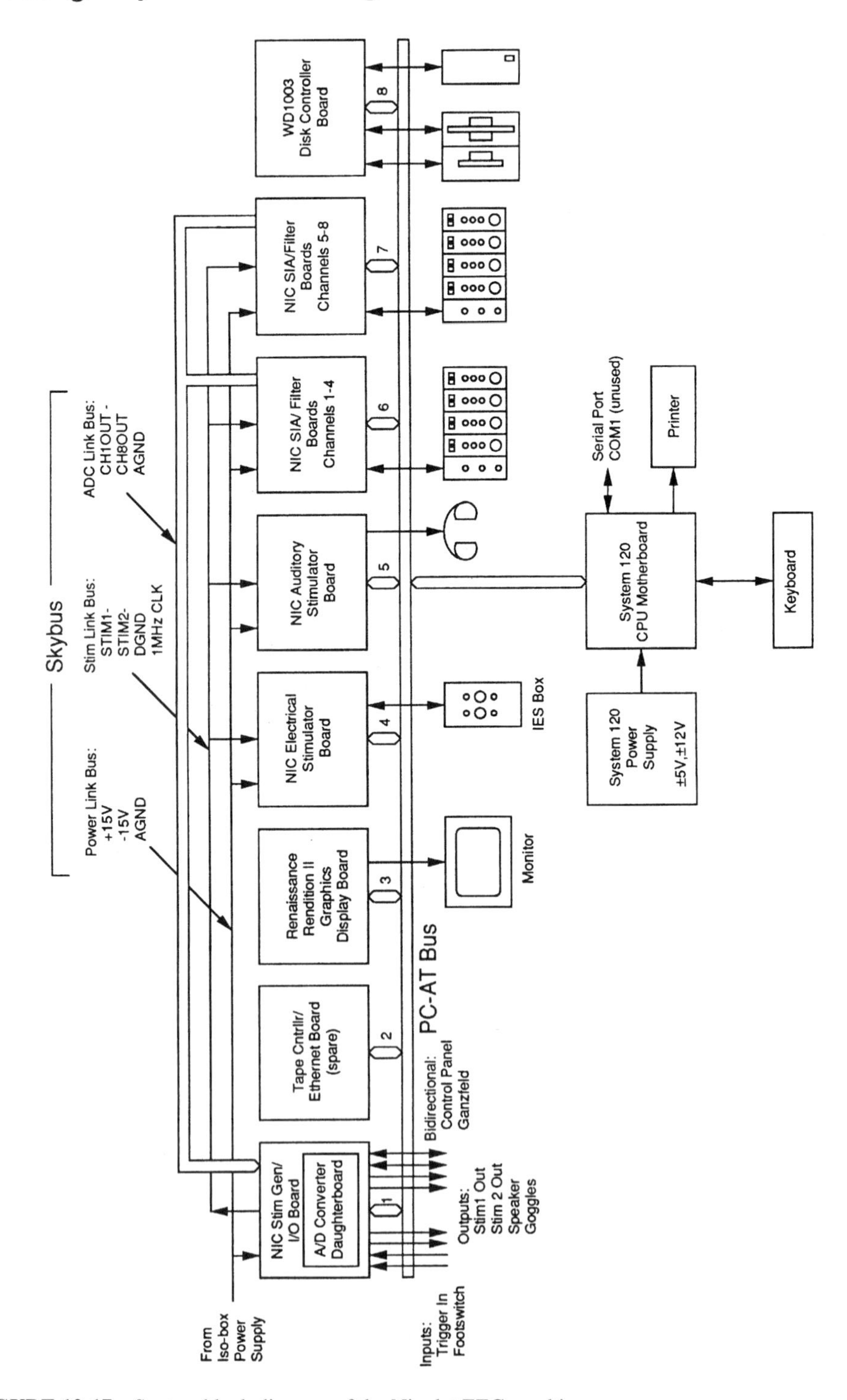

FIGURE 12-17 System block diagram of the Nicolet EEG machine.

12.8 EEG PROCEDURE

For a **regular EEG,** the EEG technician attaches 16 to 20 electrodes to the patient's scalp. For improved electrical conduction, gel is used on the electrodes and then glue is used to attach these electrodes to the skin of the scalp. This is a noninvasive procedure and no medical stimulation is transmitted to the brain. The procedure for proper measurement of the electrical activity in multiple parts of the brain can take approximately one hour. The patient may be asked to breathe slowly or quickly or a flash of light may be used for to visually stimulate the brain activity.

For the **sleep EEG,** the same procedure as the regular (awake) EEG is used; however, the patient is in a quiet room and asleep for up to three hours.

Similar to the Holter monitor for recording an ECG signal, the **ambulatory EEG** uses a portable recording device to record EEG activity. Electrodes are placed on the scalp. The electrode cables are attached to the recording device, which is belted to the patient. The patient conducts regular activity for 24 hours while the device records the EEG signals.

In studies of seizure disorders, the patient is asked to not take any anti-seizure medication for two days prior to the EEG test. Then, during the EEG test, the patient is exposed to flashing lights or other stimuli to induce a seizure. There is no pain involved in the EEG test and the patient can go home immediately afterwards.

A neurologist interprets the recordings. If abnormalities are found in the brain wave patterns, the patient's doctor is alerted for further evaluation, such as a CT or MRI.

EEG Patient Data

The EEG is an important neurological test used to diagnose brain disorders. The patient submits in-depth evaluation forms explaining his or her medical history. This information is stored in databases used to collect important data on patients suffering from epilepsy, brain damage, degenerative diseases, mental disorders, sleep disorders, and brain death.

12.9 NEUROMUSCULAR MEASUREMENTS

An EEG is a measurement of the bioelectric potentials at the scalp and represents the combined effect of action potentials over a wide region of the cortex. Electromyography (EMG), however, is a measurement of the bioelectric potentials at the surface of the body near a particular muscle or muscles and measures the combined effect of action potentials from the fibers of those muscles.

Electromyography (EMG) and electrodiagnostic medicine involve the testing of nerves and muscles for conditions such as pinched or damaged nerves or back or neck pain. The EMG is the measurement of the electrical activity in muscle tissue in response to nerve stimulation. An EMG is performed when patients complain of muscle weakness. The EMG can then distinguish between muscle conditions in which the problem begins in the muscle and muscle weakness that is due to nerve disorders.

12.10 EMG MACHINES

Most EMG laboratories use computers in addition to EMG electrodes, amplifiers, and audio speakers. In EMG testing, there are three types of electrodes placed on the patient: a recording electrode, a reference electrode, and a ground electrode. The most commonly used electrode is a needle electrode, which is a small (0.1 mm) metallic wire that is encased in an external cannula. The amplifier is a differential amplifier with a high CMRR, large gain, and very high input impedance.

Electrodes are also used to stimulate peripheral nerves using square waves. The peak amplitudes of the square waves are in the order of hundreds of volts, and the pulse widths also vary in the range of hundreds of microseconds.

The EMG machine, such as Nicolet's Viking, has preamplifiers for eight EMG channels, apart from stimulator channels (electrical, auditory, and visual). The control panel is used for all user interface functions except entering data. It contains the hard keys, soft keys, adjustment dials, and cursor wheel.

Data from nerve conduction studies, EMG, and evoked potential tests are collected in the Viking master menu. The spontaneous activity, maximum voluntary activity, automatic motor unit potential, interference pattern analysis, and single fiber EMG can be performed on the patients in the EMG section.

Filter boards are connected to the EMG channels. The CPU is a 25 MHz, 32-bit Intel 80386, 8-megabyte memory system. Each A/D converter is a 12-bit converter for each EMG channel. The resulting parallel processing capability allows simultaneous waveform acquisition, display, and real-time signal analysis.

The sensitivity of an amplifier is 1 μV/div to 10 mV/div in 13 steps with 2 V(p-p) max full scale output. The input impedance is greater than 1,000 MΩ, and the CMRR is greater than 110 dB at 60 Hz. The amplifier/filter board has optical isolation circuits with several notch, low-, and high-pass filters. The electrode impedance is DC to 500 kΩ at 20 or 500 Hz.

When acquiring EMG waveforms, two surface electrodes (red and black) and a ground plate electrode are applied to the patient using conductive gel.

A patient diagnosed with muscle or nerve abnormalities, such as muscle pain or cramping or numbness, weakness, or tingling sensations in the body, should be tested in an EMG lab. The lab will generally perform one of the following tests: a nerve conduction study (NCS), a needle EMG, or an evoked potential test.

Nerve Conduction Study

A nerve conduction study is performed on several nerves, as shown in **Figure 12-18** through **Figure 12-20.** In this test, a small shock is delivered to the nerve to determine how well electrical signal reaches the nerve or how well the nerve responds. The electrical stimulation signal (shock) can travel extremely fast on some nerves (100 miles an hour!).

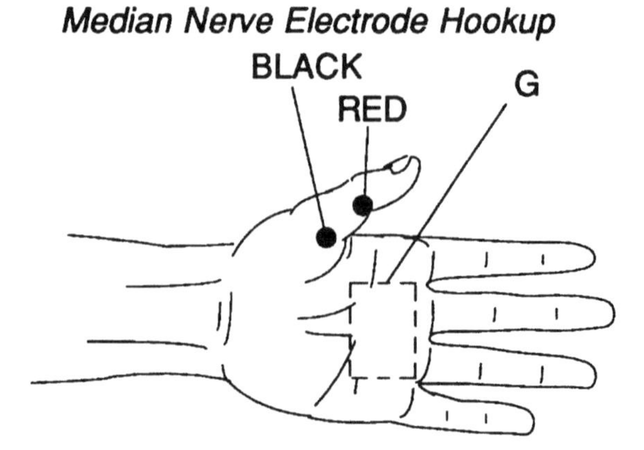

FIGURE 12-18 EMG electrode hook-up on the hand.

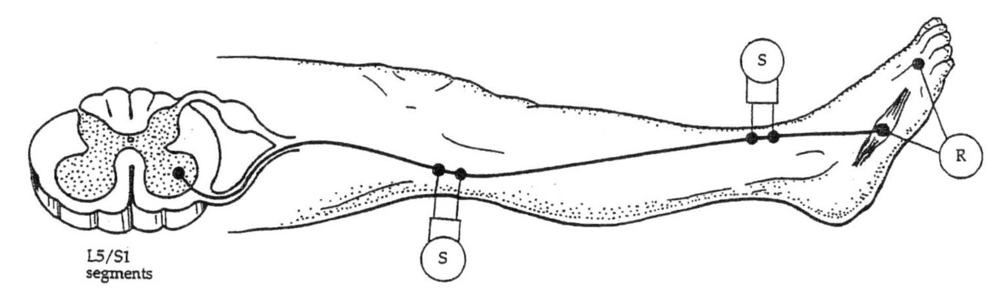

FIGURE 12-19 EMG electrode hook-up on the leg. S = stimulator electrode, R = recording electrode.

Needle EMG

In a needle EMG, a disposable needle is inserted into the patient's muscle. The EMG machine records the electrical signal from the needle to the machine. These signals can also be audible using headphones. This test is performed a specialist such as a neurologist or a rehabilitation doctor, and there can be minor pain involved when the needle is inserted.

Evoked Potentials

This test allows a specialist to check nerve pathways through the spinal cord, eyes, or ears. Similar to the EEG recording, often the patient is subjected to an external stimulation, such as an electrical stimulation or a flashing light or sound.

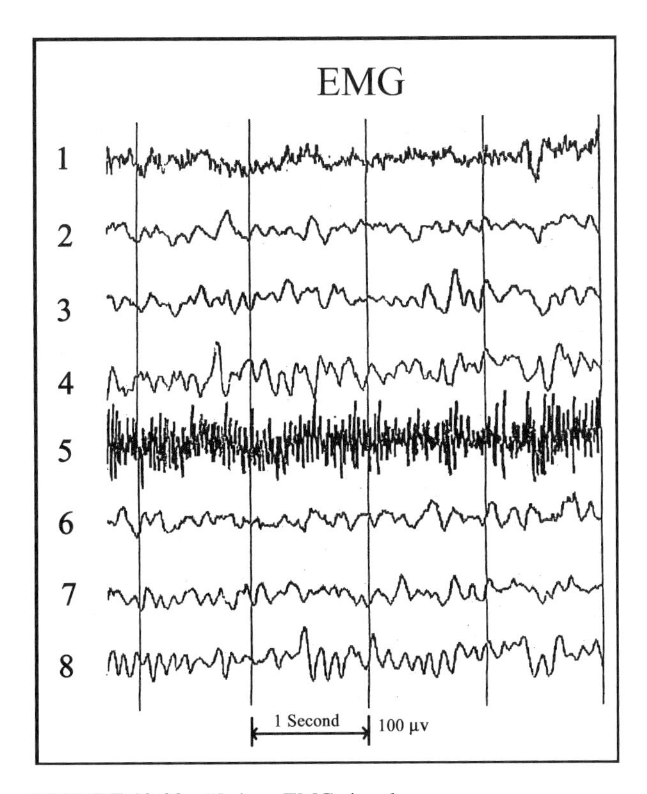

FIGURE 12-20 Various EMG signals.

SUMMARY

The brain is the seat of intellect and its association with the central nervous system coordinates the communication with the body functions.

1. The organization of the brain and its neural communication is carried out by two complementary processes: electrical conduction and chemical transmission. Electrical conduction allows the nerve impulses to travel rapidly within a neuron, whereas the chemical transmission takes place in the synapses between neurons and allows nerve impulses to be transmitted from one neuron to the next.
2. EEG is the recording of electrical activity along the scalp produced by the firing of neurons within the brain. The recording is of the brain's spontaneous electrical activity over a short period of time, usually about 30 minutes, as recorded by multiple electrodes placed on the scalp. The association of bioelectric potentials and brain waves is discussed next in the chapter.
3. EEG is described as a composite wave of different frequencies. The frequency bands are delta (less than 4 Hz), theta (4–8 Hz), alpha (8–12 Hz), and beta (13–30 Hz).
4. The EEG machine is discussed in detail. It consists of EEG electrodes, amplifiers, filters, ADC, EEG computer, and the monitor for display.
5. EMG measures muscle response or electrical activity in response to a nerve's stimulation of the muscle. It is used along with nerve conduction study to differentiate a muscle disorder from a nerve disorder.

MEDICAL TERMINOLOGY

The following is a list of medical terminology mentioned in this chapter.

Alzheimer's disease: progressive and debilitating disease caused by degenerative changes in the brain, beginning with memory loss and progressing to complete loss of mental, emotional, and physical functioning.

Ambulatory EEG: electroencephalography is a sample of the brain's electrical activity recorded over a prolonged period of time when a patient can move and walk around or even when the patient is in a sleep state.

Brain seizure: abnormal electrical disturbance in the brain resulting in irregular synchronization of electrical neuronal activity.

Brain waves: rhythmic oscillations of electric potential between the parts of the brain. An electroencephalogram is used to view brain waves.

Cerebral cortex: outer portion of the brain composed of gray matter and arranged in deep folds called fissures.

Cerebro-vascular: pertains to the blood vessels that supply blood to the brain.

Cortical: pertains to or consists of the cortex. It refers to the outer layer of an organ beneath its membrane. For example, the outer portion of the cerebrum is the cerebral cortical area.

Dendrites: root-like processes that accept impulses and conduct them to cell bodies. Dendrites comprise most of the receiving surface of neurons.

Electroencephalography: process of measuring electrical activity produced by the brain and recorded through the use of electrodes attached to the scalp.

Electromyography: a diagnostic procedure that records the strength of a contraction of a muscle in response to nerve stimulation by an electric current.

Epilepsy: group of neurological disorders with recurring episodes of irregular electrical activity (seizures) of the nervous system.

Evoked potentials: measurement of the electrical activity of the brain in response to stimulation of nerve pathways by sensory input.

Intracranial: refers to within the cranium or skull. For example, intracranial pressure is the amount of pressure inside the skull.

Magnetoencephalography: noninvasive imaging technique used to detect and measure the magnetic fields produced by electrical activity in the brain.

Needle EMG: recording and study of electrical activity of muscle using a needle electrode. It assesses the upper motor neurons, lower motor neurons, and neuromuscular junction.

Neuromuscular: refers to the functional relationship between a nerve and muscle or is in reference to the whole unit of a nerve and all muscle fibers that innervate it.

Neurons: basic cell of the nervous system used to carry neurological impulses throughout the body via electrochemical processes. A neuron consists of three basic parts: a cell body, one axon, and one or more dendrites.

Occipital: pertaining to or relating to the back part of the head. For example, the occipital bone is distinguished by a large hole through which the spinal cord passes.

Parietal: pertaining to or forming the walls of a body part, organ, or cavity. For example, the parietal bones form the top and upper sides of the cranium.

Parkinson's disease: chronic and degenerative central nervous system disorder with a slow deterioration of nerves in the brain stem's motor system. The condition results in progressive loss of control over movement with tremors and a shuffling gait.

Sleep EEG: a sample of the brain's electrical activity recorded over a two- to three-hour sleep period.

Stimuli: agent, action, or factor that elicits or influences a physiological or psychological response.

Synapse: space between the end of one nerve and the beginning of another nerve where nerve impulses are transmitted for communication to a target cell.

QUIZ

1. Maximum peak amplitudes of the EEG waveforms typically are:

a) 120 mV. b) 100 mV. c) 100 μV. d) 10 μV.

2. The difference between afferent and efferent nerves is ______________.

3. The thalamus and hypothalamus are part of the ______________.

4. EEG electrode positions are named according to the brain regions: Frontal, parietal, occipital, and ______________.

5. There are two basic methods of electrode placements when recording the EEG:

1. ______________. 2. ______________.

6. There are three kinds of muscle tissue:

1. ______________. 2. ______________.

3. ______________.

7. Why is a larger area of the motor cortex of the cerebrum required to control the muscles of the fingers than the muscles of the thorax (chest)?
8. Plotting integrated EMG data (as the raw EMG data is being received) facilitates the:
   a) Detection of the slopes of the raw EMG data.
   b) Running summation of the raw EMG data.
   c) Positive and negative deflections of the raw EMG data.
   d) None of the above.
9. When attaching a surface electrode, you may squeeze a drop of electrode gel onto the surface of the skin or onto the electrode for:
   a) Removing hair form the skin. b) Amplifying the EMG signal.
   c) Making good electrical contact. d) None of the above.
10. The lowest frequency signal in an EEG waveform occurs in the:
   a) Alpha wave. b) Beta wave. c) Delta wave. d) Theta wave.

RESEARCH TOPICS

1. The number of electrodes and their placements on the scalp in EEG studies follow international standards. However, these standards are not always followed by some doctors. Investigate the reasons why some doctors do not use the standards and critique the protocols used by these doctors.
2. Discuss the amplification and frequency response of amplifiers in EEG, EMG, and ECG machines or circuits.
3. In neurofeedback, a patient can change the characteristics of his or her brain waves as measured by sensors on the scalp in the form of a video display, sound or vibration. The neurofeedback is a therapy technique and presents the patient with real-time feedback on brainwave activity. Discuss the possible instrumentation needed in recording this kind of activity.

CASE STUDIES

1. An unmarried, 30-year-old female patient complains of nervousness and low self-esteem whenever she attends parties. She is also preoccupied with her weight and appearance. There is a history of nervous problems in the family, but the patient has no physiological problems. Is the patient a candidate for EEG studies? What kind of EEG data would need to be collected, if any?
2. EEG neurofeedback is a clinical tool in the treatment of behavioral disorders such as Attention deficit disorder (ADD), depression, anxiety, panic attacks, and several other conditions. In neurofeedback, the patient can experience how his or her brain is reacting to different situations and then can learn to change the abnormal brain waves into normal brain waves. The researcher performing the case study on the EEG neurofeedback can assess the software and hardware techniques and must collect data from the Internet or public surveys in the treatment of various brain-related disorders.

PROBLEMS

1. Name the organs that make up the central nervous and peripheral nervous systems.

2. Match a term in left column with its correct description in the right column.

1. Spinal cord	a) where the messages go from one cell to the next cell
2. Thalamus	b) comprises of the sensory area
3. Cerebellum	c) neuron has extensions of cytoplasm from the cell body
4. Hypothalamus	d) acts as a relay station for the incoming and outgoing nerve impulses
5. Parietal lobe	
6. Dendrites	e) a conduction pathway to and from the brain
7. Synapse	f) a bulb-shaped structure between the pons and the spinal cord
8. Medulla oblongata	g) maintains the normal body temperature
	h) located behind the pons and below the cerebrum

3. Show the models of ECG and EEG electrodes and differentiate their electronic circuits in terms of resistance and capacitance. What kinds of voltages are expected from these two groupings of electrodes before any amplifiers are connected to them?
4. Design a complete signal conditioning circuit for the alpha brain waves using proper EEG electrodes and their placement on the scalp.
5. Design an electronic circuit including electrodes to deliver electric shock to the brain for psychiatric patients. This will require research on the patients and the type of shock therapy conducted, including the placement of the electrodes.
6. Compare amplifiers (in terms of amplification, bandwidth, and noise requirements) in ECG, EEG, and EMG measurements.
7. Design a first-order band-pass filter for beta waves in the frequency range of 13 to 22 Hz. Also, plot the gain curve for this band-pass filter using MATLAB in the frequency range from 1 to 40 Hz.
8. Design a differential amplifier circuit to process an EEG waveform with an input impedance that exceeds 10 MΩ, a gain of 10^6, and a CMRR of more than 80 dB. You may use the Internet to search for a suitable differential amplifier chip or a specialized op-amp.
9. Design an electrical stimulation circuit to stimulate the forearm to move right and left when the elbow is resting on a table.
10. Four EEG-evoked potential responses (caused by a flash of light stimuli) are shown in **Figure 12-21**. These responses are recorded from one patient and are timed from the same flash of light. Create a plan to determine the average of these four responses.

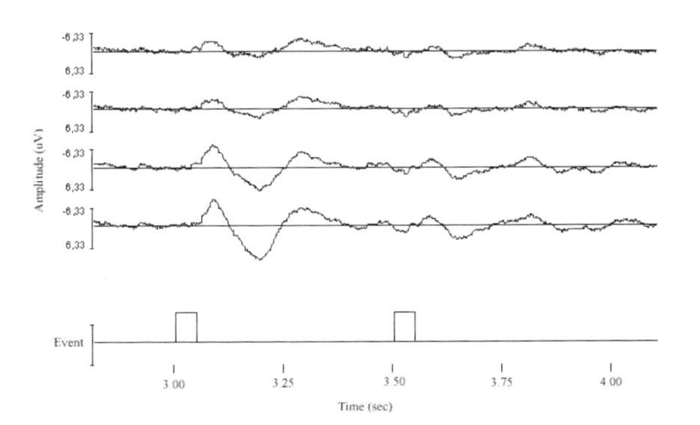

FIGURE 12-21 Averaging of brain waves.

CHAPTER 13

Artifacts and Noise in Medical Instrumentation

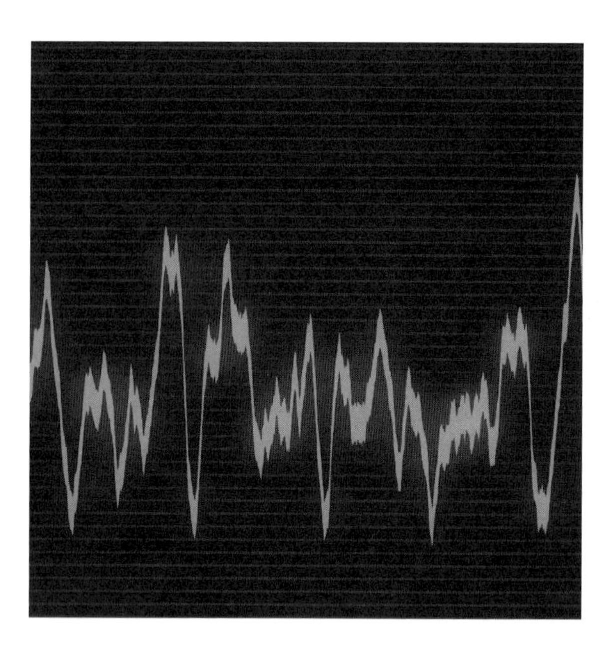

CHAPTER OUTLINE

OBJECTIVES

In this chapter, the reader will learn the various types and sources of noises that affect the biomedical signals. The chapter also provides simple noise reduction techniques used in hardware circuits and in software processing in computers.

Upon completion of this chapter, the reader will be able to:

- Describe noise sources in biomedical instrumentation.
- Name the types of noises in biomedical instrumentation.
- Name the filters used in noise reduction.
- Discuss mathematical tools in noise reduction.
- Name the steps taken in reducing motion artifacts in hospitals.

INTERNET WEB SITES

http://www.ti.com Texas Instruments
http://www.nationalinstruments.com National Instruments

http://tc-biomedsignal-processing.embs.org Technical committee Biomedical Signal Processing, IEEE Engineering in Medicine and Biology Society
www.physionet.org PhysioNet sponsored by National Institute of Biomedical Imaging and Bioengineering

INTRODUCTION

In biomedical instrumentation, "noise" is considered a disturbance that affects a signal and may distort the information carried by that signal. Some sources of noise can be operator error, machine malfunction, or other influences. Noise is characterized as external or internal. Examples of external sources of noise are 60 Hz electric line frequency or magnetic field interference. An internal source of noise may be patient motion, such as eye blinking or muscle movement while the signal is being recorded. This chapter discusses various types of noise and the suppression of noise by digital signal processing techniques.

13.1 EXAMPLES OF NOISE IN MEDICAL INSTRUMENTATION

Artifact is a term used to describe a wave on an ECG or an EEG that arises from sources other than the heart or brain. **Figure 13-1a** is an example of a recording of muscle artifact, **Figure 13-1b** shows a recording of a wandering baseline artifact, and **Figure 13-1c** shows a recording of electromagnetic interference. Patient movement or the respiration at frequencies between 0.15 Hz to 0.30 Hz can affect how the signal is recorded. Power line interference can also occur with a narrow-band noise centered at approximately 60 Hz or 50 Hz radiated with a bandwidth less than 1 Hz.

Arterial blood pressure waveforms are also affected by noise. **Figure 13-2** is a list of various graphs showing normal, flattened, erratic, rounded, and slow uptake waveforms that a healthcare provider may need to interpret.

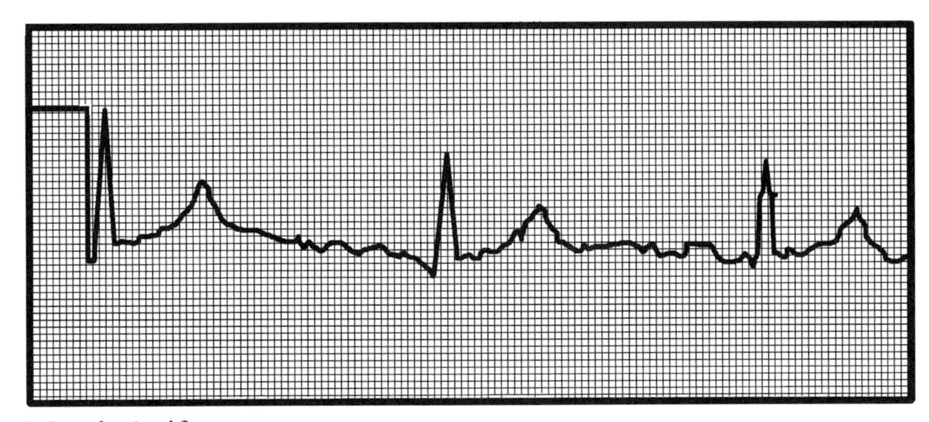

FIGURE 13-1a Muscle artifact.

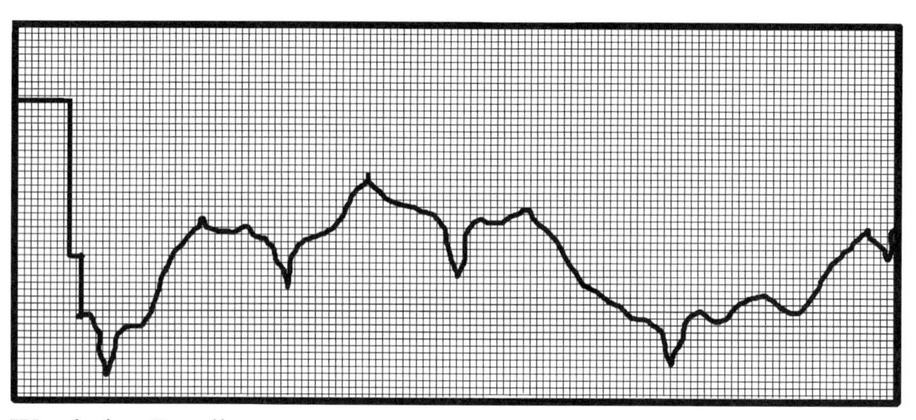

FIGURE 13-1b Wandering baseline artifact.

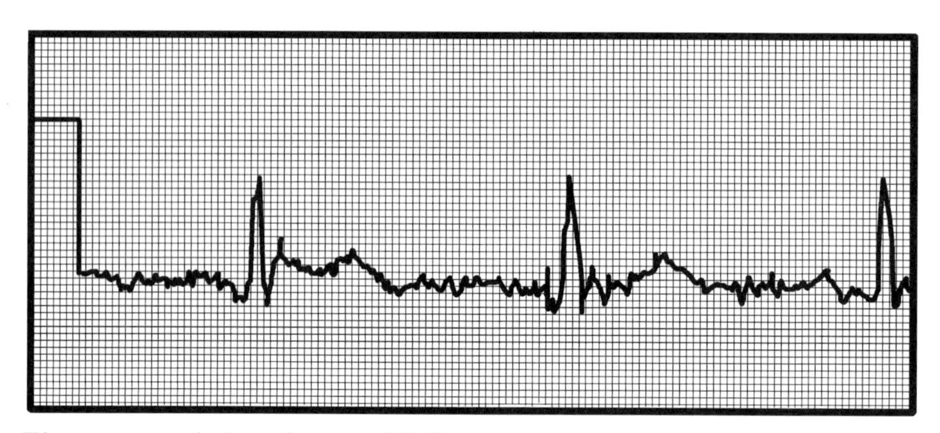

FIGURE 13-1c Electromagnetic interference (EMI).

An otherwise good signal can be corrupted by noise and often can be indecipherable unless signal processing is done. **Figure 13-3** gives a few examples of how noise impositions on good signals can appear.

Figure 13-4 shows an example of the susceptibility of the medical devices at the operating frequencies of cell phones, two-way radios, and very high frequency (VHF), and ultra high frequency (UHF) communication devices. The susceptibility is given in terms of electric field strength received at the site of medical devices. Pulse oximeters are most susceptible to all the high-frequency communication devices.

FIGURE 13-2 Noisy blood pressure signals.

Normal waveform

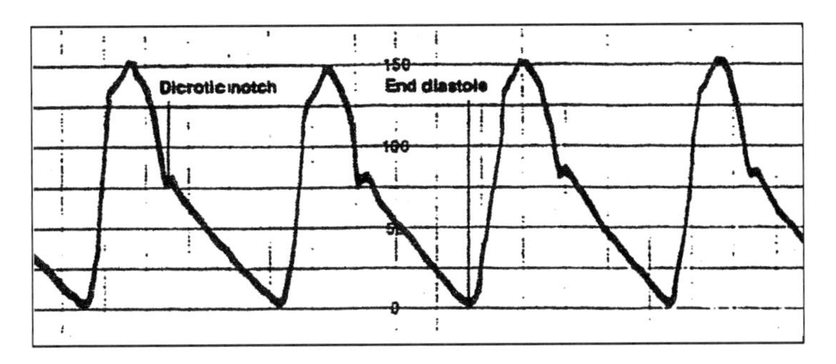

Alteration of high and low waves in a regular pattern

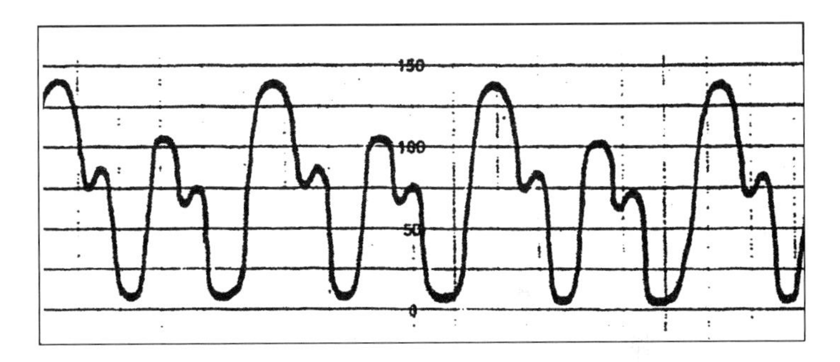

Flattened waveform

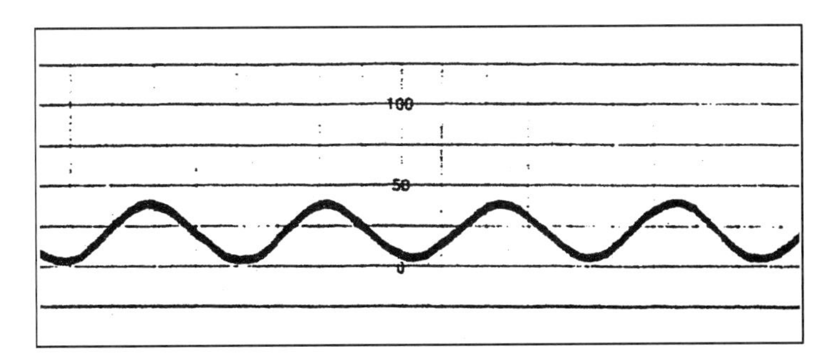

Erratic ragged waveform

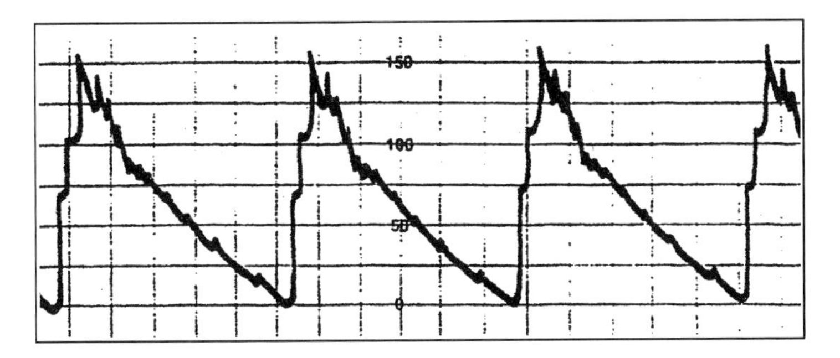

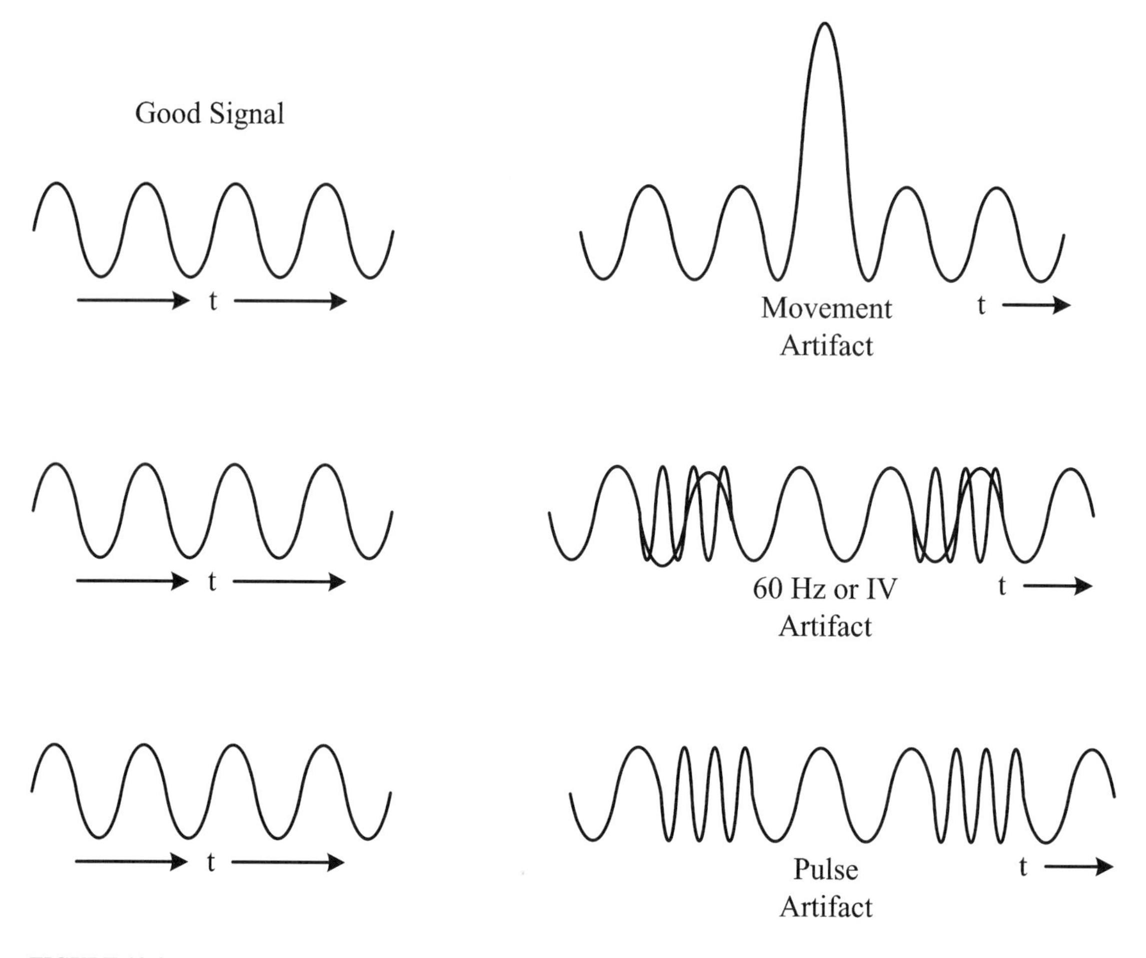

FIGURE 13-3 Various artifacts that affect a good signal.

Computer software processing or filtering with computer hardware can be used to correct respiration artifacts or the effects of wandering baseline in an ECG signal. The results of this processing can be seen in **Figure 13-5** and **Figure 13-6**.

13.2 NOISE AND BIOMEDICAL SIGNALS

Following is a categorization of the noise that can superimpose on such biomedical devices as an ECG, EEG, or blood pressure monitor.

Power Line Interference

The 60 Hz line frequency and its harmonics from a power line can interfere with biomedical signals either from the 60 Hz radiation in the room or through leakage in the wires.

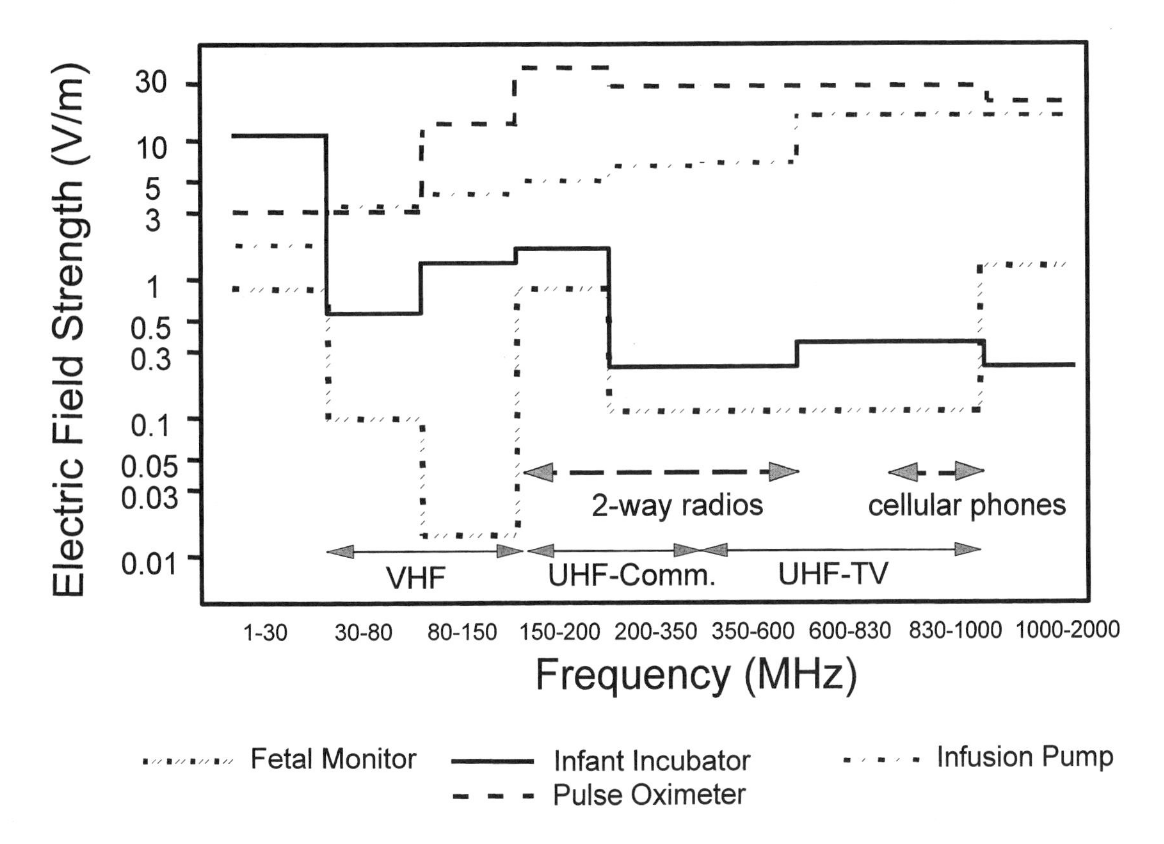

FIGURE 13-4 Susceptibility of medical devices to RF signals.

FIGURE 13-5 Respiration artifacts.

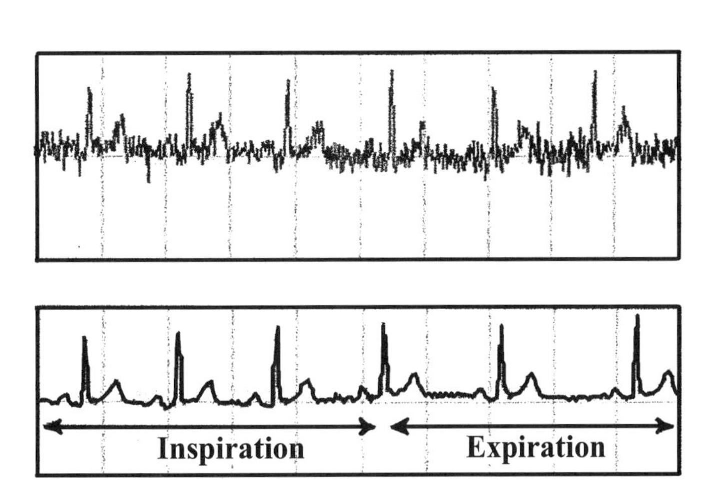

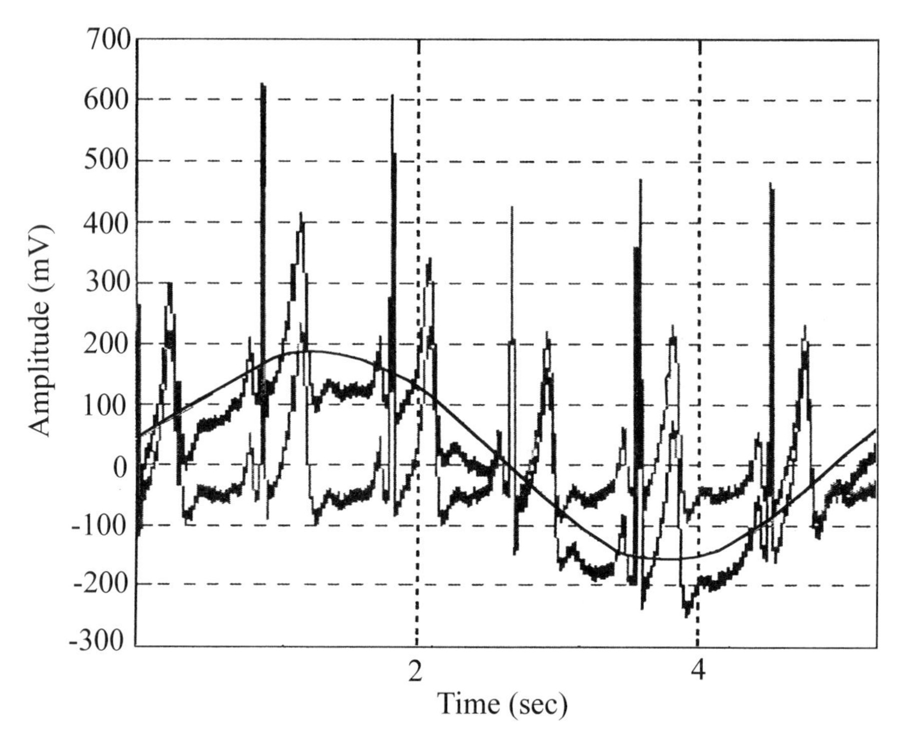

FIGURE 13-6 Wandering artifacts on ECG.

Sometimes this 60 Hz noise is at least 50 percent peak to peak of the amplitude of the bio-signal. Additionally, this noise may result in periodic interference.

Electrode Contact Noise

If the electrode is not properly in contact with the skin, there are rapid and random baseline transitions of the bio-signal. The transitions decay back to the baseline.

Respiration Noise

Respiration can also damage the real signal by moving the baseline with the waveform of the respiration. The amplitude and frequency of respiration can vary. This is called the breathing artifact.

Motion Artifacts

A shift in the baseline of the bio-signal can be caused by patient vibration or movement. This baseline shift is similar to a DC offset of the signal and the change can be abrupt. These transient baseline changes are due to electrode motion resulting in changes in electrode-skin impedance. The electrode-skin impedance is similar to a source impedance of the bio-signal source and if there are abrupt changes to its integrity, the resulting input voltage to the amplifier will also change.

Motion artifacts are the noise caused by movement of the electrode. This movement results in skin deformation, which changes the impedance and capacitance of the skin around the electrode site. For example, a patient walking on a treadmill during an ECG procedure may generate motion artifacts in his or her ECG traces. These motion artifacts may lead to misdiagnosis or inappropriate decisions.

Muscle Contraction Noise

Muscle contractions can generate EMG noise in ECG signals. This is because this type of EMG signal has smaller amplitudes but has a larger bandwidth than the ECG signal. There are more than one type of EMG signals with varying amplitudes and frequency ranges.

Electronic Devices Noise

If the input amplifier gain is such that the bio-signal sends the amplifier into saturation or cut-off mode, then the output amplified signal is not a true representation of the bio-signal. All electronic devices are temperature-sensitive and the circuit should never be allowed to operate in the saturation or cut-off mode.

Electro-Surgical Noise

An electro-surgical machine operates at frequencies over 100 kHz, and high-frequency noise from the machine can radiate or leak into the ECG signals. As a result, the ECG signal will be noisy and this noise will appear in the trace.

Image Artifact Noise

Images can have distortions due to patient movement, metallic artifacts, or operator errors. In MRI imaging, three types of noise can appear in the actual images: 1) patient motion and the resulting blood flow; 2) electromagnetic spikes due to MRI electromagnets and abrupt or intense changes in the object discontinuities (such as brain/skull interface); and 3) chemical shift and the sensitivity to any metal around.

An image artifact is a structure not normally present in the image as a result of changes in patient position, electromagnetic spikes or even malfunction in the software. The image distortions may appear and the quality of the image can be affected due to these artifacts. These are possible in CT, MRI, or any other types of image modalities. Several techniques using computer software or hardware have been developed to identify and reduce these artifacts.

Operator Errors

Operator errors can result in bad signals. For example, the operator may unintentionally fail to follow the correct procedure in collecting patient data.

Machine Malfunctions

If the noise cannot be recognized as one of the preceding types, it could be the result of a machine malfunction.

Electro-Magnetic Interference (EMI) from Wireless Communication

If unwanted RF signals are transmitting at the same carrier frequency as a medical radio signal in the hospital environment, it can cause the medical signal to be corrupted or interrupted.

Now that we have an understanding of the different types of noise, let's look into the theories of noise reduction or suppression by digital signal processing (DSP) techniques. Processing techniques either can be performed in the DSP chip or computer software can apply it on the noisy signals once interfaced to the computer.

13.3 NOISE REDUCTION WITH DIGITAL SIGNAL PROCESSING

In digital signal processing, the sampled amplitudes are mathematically manipulated and modified to extract information using simple mathematical operations, such as addition, subtraction, multiplication, and division. The sampling rate and the number of bits play important roles too. The DSP algorithms for processing are stored in the embedded DSP chips. The high-resolution chips or systems use a large number of bits. An 8-bit system allows only 256 quantized values, but a 24-bit system will allow over 16 million values. The quantized noise is then greatly reduced.

In biomedical applications, the purpose of digital signal processing is to extract low-amplitude actual bio-signals out of a detected noisy signals. This process is apart from the signal conditioning of amplification, filtering, and even the digitizing process itself.

Correlation and convolution are two methods of DSP. Each method must follow three operations: 1) shifting, 2) multiplication, and 3) addition.

Correlation

Correlation is a relationship between signals, and DSP measures the similarities between two or more signals. The process is called autocorrelation if the two signals are exactly the same and cross-correlation if the two signals are different. Correlation measures the similarity between two signals, and it is useful in identifying a signal by comparison with a set of known reference signals. The following steps are used in cross-correlation of two sampled signals:

1. Determine the amplitudes of two signals at finite samples in time.
2. Determine cross-correlation values between these samples of the signals by multiplying and then by adding.
3. Shift one of the signal samples to the right or left and again calculate the cross-correlation value.
4. Continue right or left shifts and calculate the cross-correlation value at discrete intervals.

Autocorrelation uses the same process and the same calculations as cross-correlation; the only difference is that in autocorrelation, both signals are identical. **Figure 13-7** shows an example of the cross-correlation process between two signals.

With no shifts:

$$
\begin{aligned}
&C = \text{cross-correlation value}\\
&C = x[-3] \times y[-3] + x[-2] \times y[-2]\\
&\quad + x[-1] \times y[-1] + x[0] \times y[0]\\
&\quad + x[1] \times y[1] + x[2] \times y[2]\\
&\quad + x[3] \times y[3] + x[4] \times y[4]\\
&\quad + x[5] \times y[5]\\
&C = 0 + 0 + 0 + 0 + 0.5 + 1 + 0 + 0 + 0\\
&C = 1.5
\end{aligned}
$$

With one right shift of the triangular signal, the cross-correlation value is then:

$$
\begin{aligned}
C &= 0 + 0 + 0 + 0 + .5 + 0 + 0 + 0\\
&= 0.5
\end{aligned}
$$

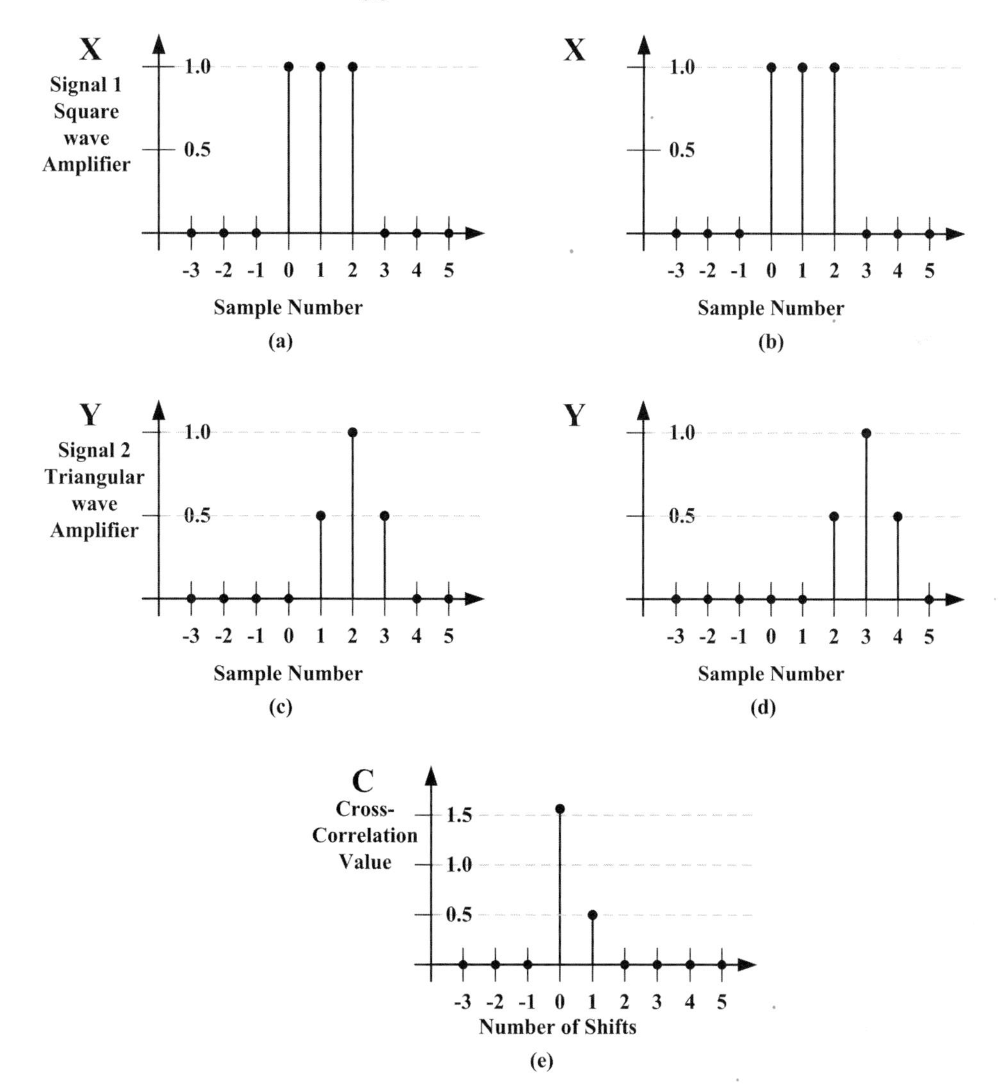

FIGURE 13-7 Cross-correlation.

FIGURE 13-8 Convolution.

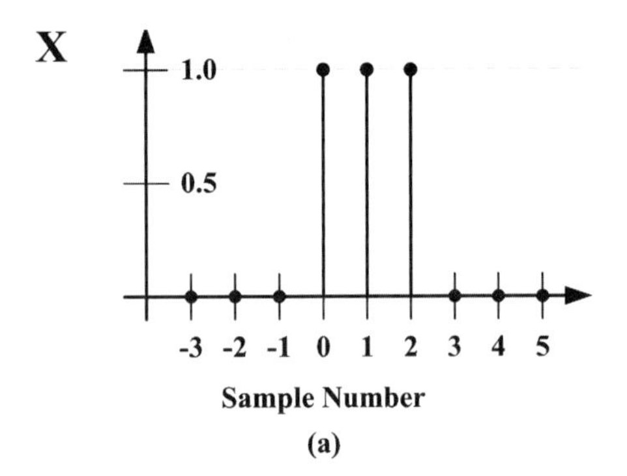

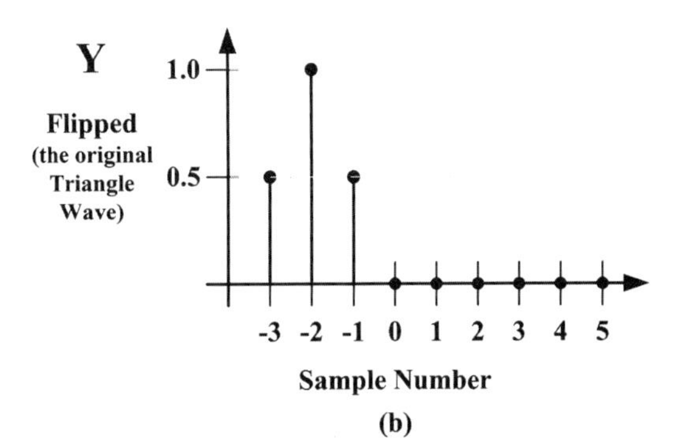

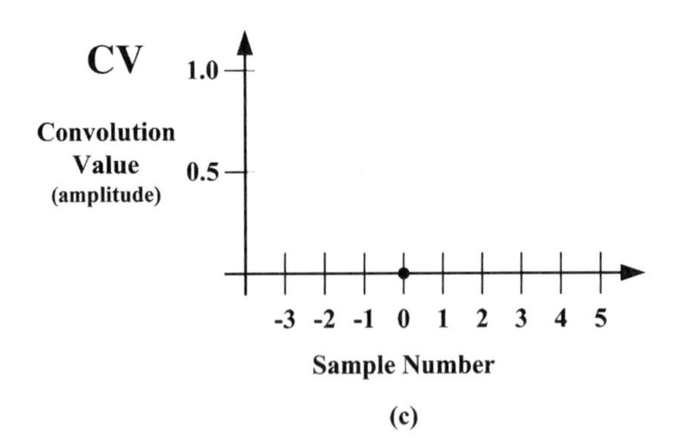

Convolution

Convolution uses the same steps as in cross-correlation except that one of the signals is first flipped (that is, it is the mirror image), and then the same steps of shifting, multiplication, and adding are applied between the flipped and the non-flipped signals.

We will take the example of the previous two signals to determine the convolution amplitude. This is shown in **Figure 13-8.**

With no shift of the flipped signal:

$$\text{Convolution value (CV)} = 0 + 0 + 0 + 0 + 0 + 0 + 0 = 0$$

Other convolution values can be achieved with the shifts (right or left) of the flipped signal and by keeping the square-wave signal not flipped and not shifted.

Application of Cross-Correlation, Autocorrelation, and Convolution on Medical Signals

Figure 13-9 shows the upper trace with so much noise that the periodicity of the actual signal is not visible. However, the lower trace is the result of autocorrelation of the upper trace. The actual signal can be seen in the lower trace. In general, correlation measures the degree of similarity between two signals, that is, how the two signals are related.

FIGURE 13-9 An example of autocorrelation.

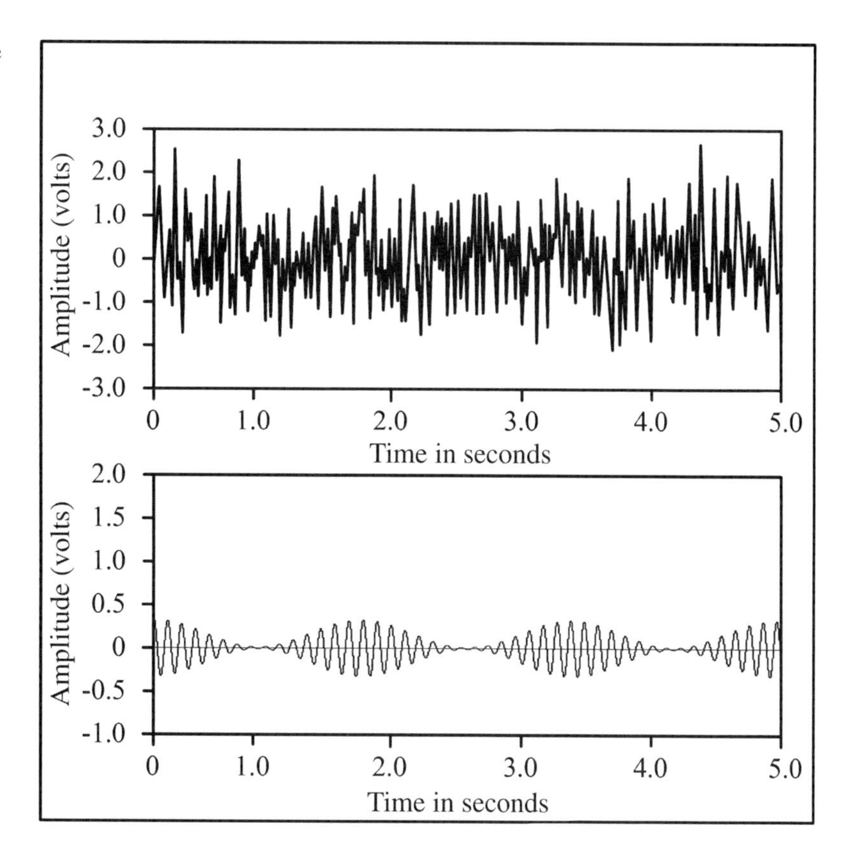

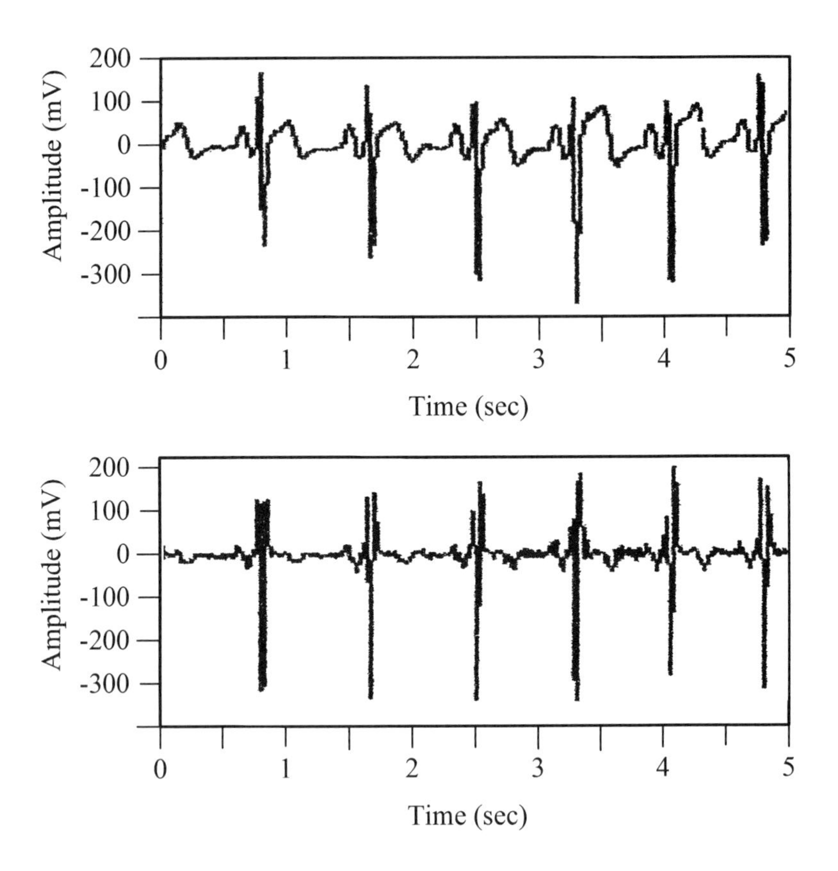

FIGURE 13-10 An example of convolution.

Another example of the convolution process is shown in **Figure 13-10,** when the upper trace has P and T waves of an ECG signal, but the lower trace filters them out. Here, the convolution results in the lower trace when the upper trace is convolved with [1,-1] signal and the high-pass filtering is achieved with P and T (slow frequency) waves are eliminated.

13.4 MOVING AVERAGE DIGITAL FILTER

In DSP, a digital technique of moving average digital filter or multiply and accumulate (MAC) out process can be used to filter undesirable frequencies. Filtering can be done by electronic digital circuits or by the software implementations. The expensive DSP techniques will not need active filter components and the temperature variations will not affect the performance. The steps of a low-pass digital filter using the moving average process are as follows:

1. Sample the analog signal into discrete sampled amplitudes.
2. Add the first 3, 5, or more discrete values.
3. Calculate their average value.
4. Convert the average value to an analog value.
5. Add the next three, five, or more discrete values, but follow the same number as in step 2. If first three values were used earlier, then go to second, third, and fourth values.

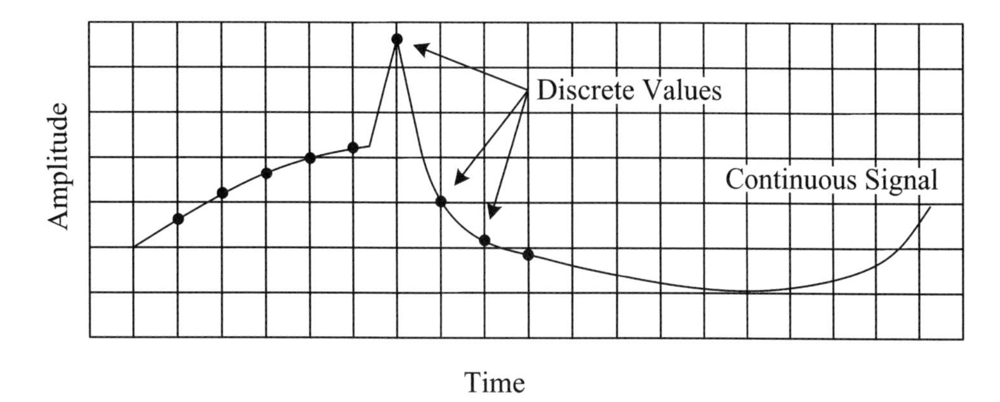

FIGURE 13-11a Discrete values in sampling.

6. Calculate the average.
7. Convert to analog value.
8. Continue next the adding of third, fourth, and fifth values.
9. Continue the process.

Figure 13-11a and **Figure 13-11b** show examples of this type of low-pass digital filtering. **Figure 13-11a** has the discrete sampled values shown. **Figure 13-11b,** shows the averaged discrete values that are computed and plotted after conversion to analog. Each dot represents binary (discrete) value. In **Figure 13-11b,** the noise spike is reduced in amplitude.

The process smoothes out high-frequency fluctuations into a low-pass signal.

As in the above process, divisions are used in calculating averages; it is time-consuming in microprocessors. Instead of division, MAC implementation used multiplications that are faster to implement. The moving average digital filter is now a MAC implementation in **Figure 13-12.**

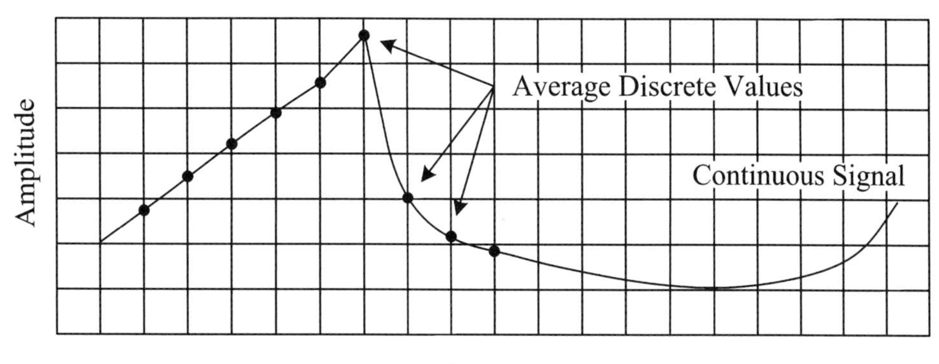

FIGURE 13-11b Averaging of the discrete values of Figure 13-11a signal.

The clock starts the A/D of the analog signal, the first quantized value is multiplied by 0.333, and the result goes to an accumulator (adder). After a delay of one clock period, the first quantized value is multiplied by the coefficient 0.333 and summed in the accumulator with the second quantized value after it has been multiplied by the first coefficient 0.333. The process then continues in the second delay circuit. The end result is a smoothed out signal at the output of the D/A converter. The clock period is the reciprocal of the clock frequency. The coefficient of 0.333 is used, because the average of the three discrete values

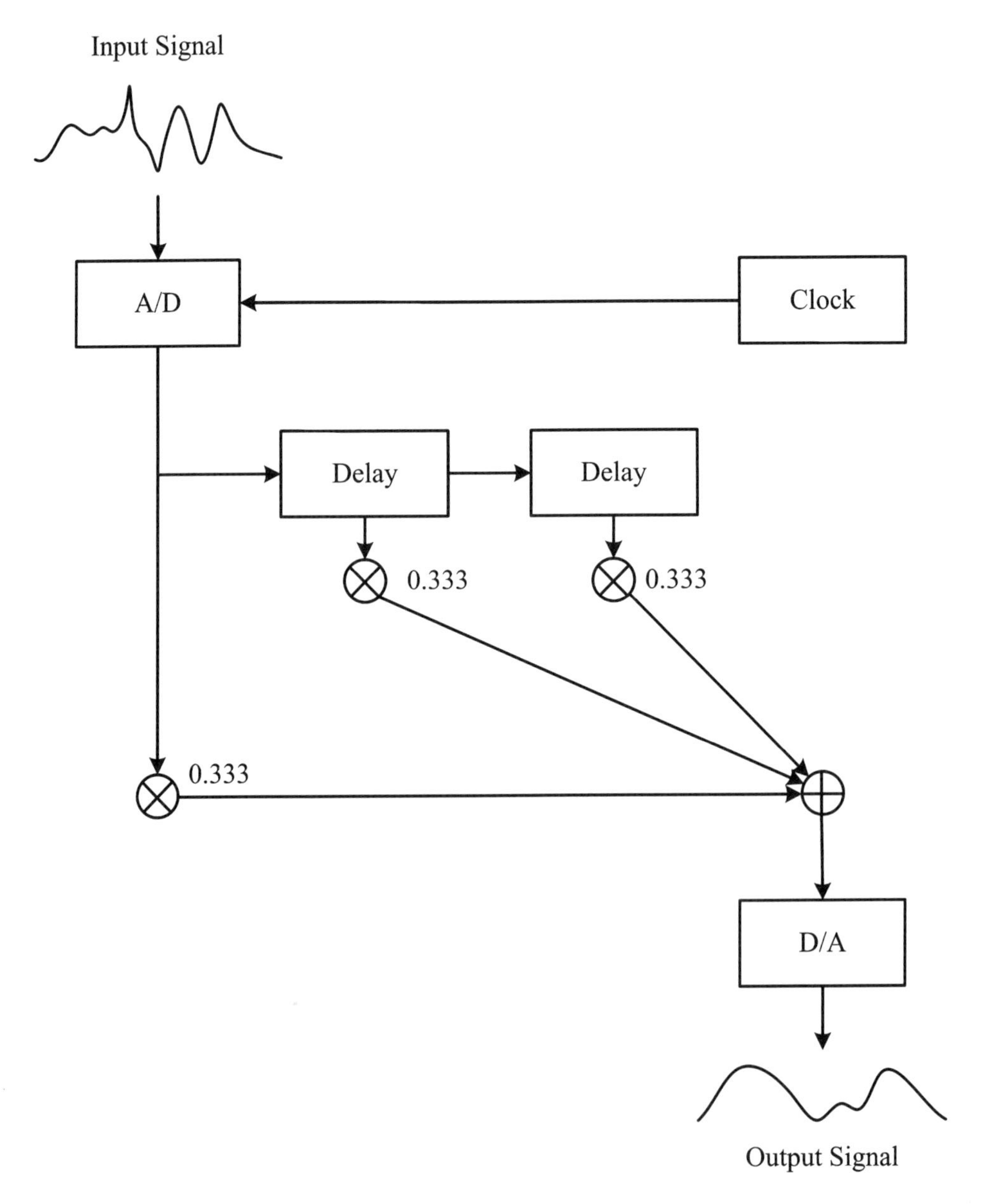

FIGURE 13-12 Process in a digital filter.

was computed by dividing by three in the moving average filter method. We are using (1/3) = 0.333 for multiplication in the MAC implementation.

SUMMARY

This chapter provides information on various types of noise that can corrupt the recording of bio-signals. The chapter also provides information on digital signal processing techniques used in DSP chips in suppressing the noise. The processes of autocorrelation, cross-correlation, convolution, and moving average digital filter are introduced in this chapter.

1. Autocorrelation is the correlation of a signal with itself and is unlike cross-correlation, which is the correlation of two different signals. Autocorrelation is useful for finding repeating patterns in a signal when the signal has been buried under noise.
2. Cross-correlation measures the similarity of two signals. It is commonly used in pattern recognition and signal detection. It can be used to detect the presence of known signals as components of a more complicated signal.
3. Convolution relates the input signal, the output signal, and the impulse response. It combines two signals to form a third signal.
4. The moving average digital filter reduces random noise while retaining a sharp step response.

TECHNICAL TERMINOLOGY

The following is a list of technical terminology mentioned in this chapter.

Artifact: noise from a source other than the actual signal source. When added to an actual signal, noise may change the signal's amplitude, frequency, or phase. Examples include audio or video defects that occur due to digital conversion and/or compression, data errors, and even analog noise.

Baseline wandering: a destructive effect that occurs when the baseline (i.e., zero voltage reference line) of an analog or digital signal changes. This change may saturate the dynamic ranges of A/D converters. One example of this effect is that it can mislead ECG annotators into inaccurate identification of the ECG features.

Digital signal processing (DSP): the study of digital signals and the methods of processing these signals. Digital signal processing includes audio signal processing, digital image processing, and speech processing.

Electromagnetic interference: unwanted electromagnetic noise produced by electrical or electronic equipment. This noise can induce itself on signal wires and can obscure the instrument signal.

Filtering: a process designed to remove undesirable signal components and/or to enhance desirable ones. Used in electronic circuits that perform signal processing functions.

Motion artifact: smearing, blurring or ghosting resulting from involuntary movements (e.g., respiration, cardiac motion and blood flow, eye movements, and swallowing).

Radio frequency (RF) noise: frequencies generated by something other than the transmitter. Usually sounds like hiss or static. RF noise may be AM or FM, but the effect is that it either alters the audio signal, or adds background noise to the audio signal.

Surge: over-voltage or over-amplified condition. Surges can damage electronics and corrupt or destroy data.

QUIZ

1. Motion artifacts are caused by the patient moving his or her body. However, wandering artifacts are caused by ______________________________.
2. In hospitals, a cell phone most affects:
   a) an infusion pump.
   b) an incubator.
   c) a pulse oximeter.
3. A DC offset is similar to:
   a) a 60 Hz noise.
   b) a wandering signal.
   c) a moving artifact.
4. List three types of digital signal processing techniques.
   ____
   ____
   ____
5. True or False: Autocorrelation involves the shifting of the signals.
   a) True
   b) False
6. The RF interference in a hospital comes from a/an:
   a) 60 Hz noise to the patient's ECG signal.
   b) Activation of the false alarm circuit of the hospital security system.
   c) A disruption in the operation of a pacemaker.
   d) None of the above.
7. Convolution in a DSP chip means:
   a) Combining two signals to form a third signal.
   b) Combining a signal twice.
   c) Detecting similarity between two signals.
   d) None of the above.

8. In a noisy ECG signal, a band-pass filter with a range of 0.5 to 40 Hz can suppress the noise:

   a) Somewhat.

   b) Completely.

   c) Not at all.

9. Explain your answer selection in quiz question 8.

   ____

10. Cross-correlation:

    a) Finds the repeating patterns, such as the presence of a periodic signal, buried under noise.

    b) Combines two signals into a third signal.

    c) Is a method to estimate the correlations between signals in time.

    d) None of the above.

PROBLEMS

1. Identify and explain the noise in the following ECG graphs in **Figure 13-13.**

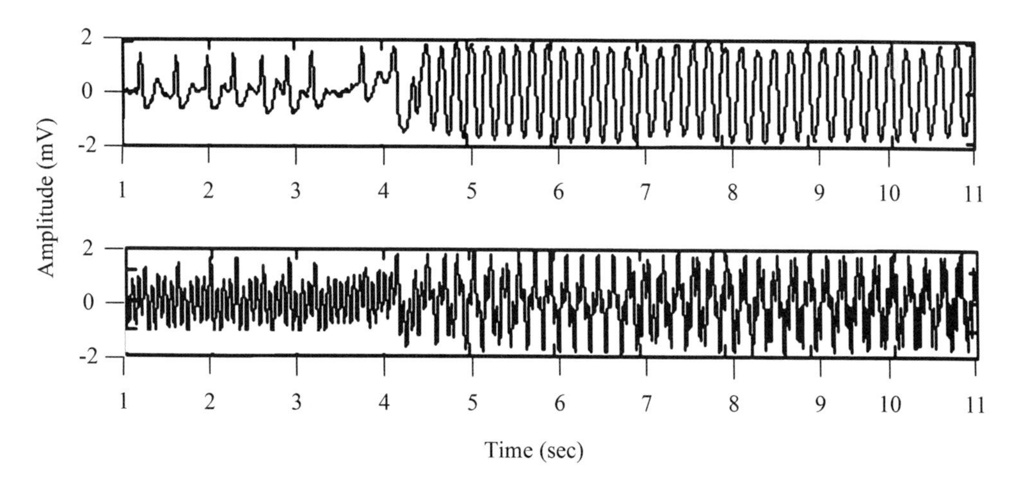

FIGURE 13-13 Noisy ECG signals.

2. Design analog electronic circuits in suppressing the noise for the applicable noisy ECG graphs of problem 1.
3. Design digital electronic circuits for problem 2 instead of analog types.

4. Determine cross-correlation values for the given two signals with the given discrete values shown in **Figure 13-14.**

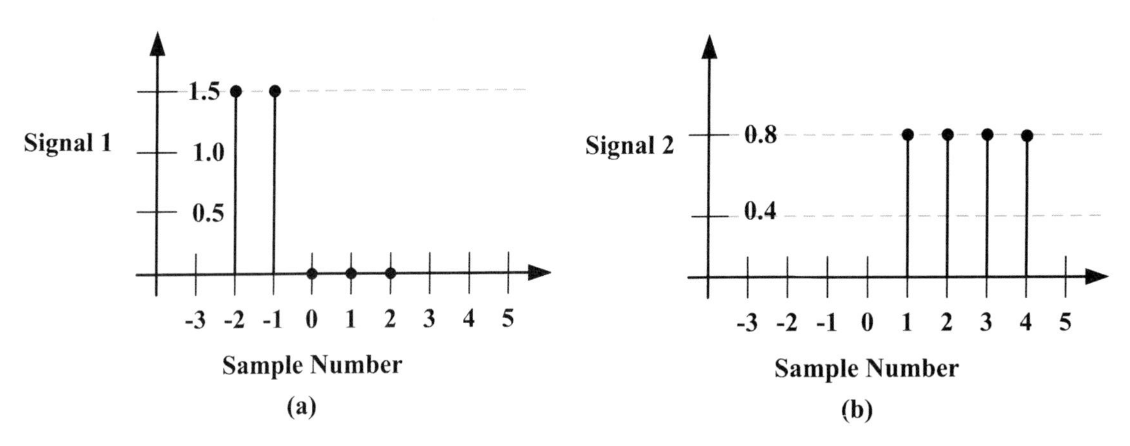

FIGURE 13-14 Cross-correlation of two signals.

5. Determine the convolution values between the two signals of problem 4.
6. Determine the averaged discrete values for the given signal in **Figure 13-15** using the moving average digital filter technique. Also plot the values to see whether the given signal is smoothed.
7. The dots in **Figure 13-15** represent binary (discrete) values such as in a four-bit A/D and D/A system. The values are as follows: 1010, 0010, 0101.

FIGURE 13-15 Moving average filter values.

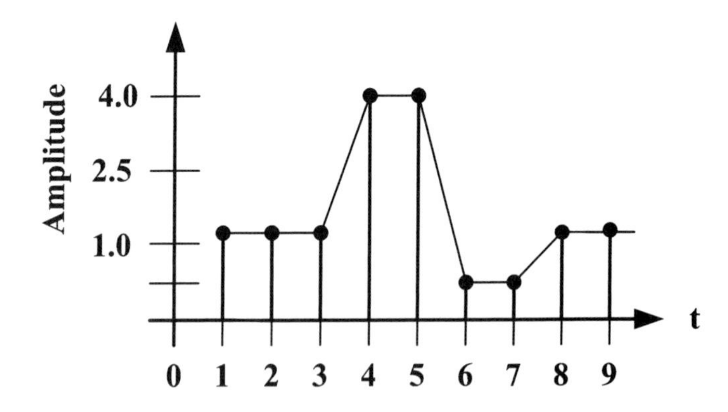

Determine the summation of digits for 1010, 0010, and 0101. Does this represent the summation of discrete values? Provide proof for your answer. (Suggestion: add digits separately than adding discrete values.)

8. Identify the types of noise that generally occur in EEG and EMG signals, and discuss the ways noise can be suppressed.

9. Discuss typical bandwidths of the following signals: ECG, EEG, EMG, arterial blood pressure, respiration, pulse oximetry, and capnogram.
10. Differentiate digital signal processing from digital image processing in terms of technology, resolution, and bandwidth requirements.

RESEARCH TOPICS

1. Simple to complex DSP algorithms are now used not only to extract real signals in the noisy situations, but also in developing new applications in medical areas. DSP is a mathematical application tool. The input and the output could be different discrete values depending on the DSP application. The research topic may include explanations of the algorithms, design of electronic circuits, and discussion on vendor-specific DSP chips.
2. FIR (finite impulse response) and IIR (infinite impulse response) digital filters are widely used in medical applications. Discuss their characteristics and explain the algorithms in simple terms. You can use block diagrams to explain.
3. Write a research paper about the effects of two-way radios, PDAs, and cell phones on medical equipment and devices. Discuss frequency ranges, carrier strengths, types of effects on medical devices, and possible changes made to the device circuits.

CASE STUDIES

1. The American Heart Association has database of ECG recordings and you can download an ECG trace. Discuss the following for each trace:

   a) Can it be considered an appropriate signal? If not, what are the reasons?

   b) How can the problem, if any, be solved?

   c) Can you design an electronic circuit to detect the problem? Can a low-pass or band-pass filter be used?

   d) What role does application of gel play at the skin-electrode interface?
2. The MAC5000 ECG monitor lists calibration steps in acquiring good quality ECG traces. Write a case study emphasizing calibration of modules and electrodes. Include patient preparation for the ECG study.

CHAPTER 14

Instrumentation in Diagnostic Ultrasound

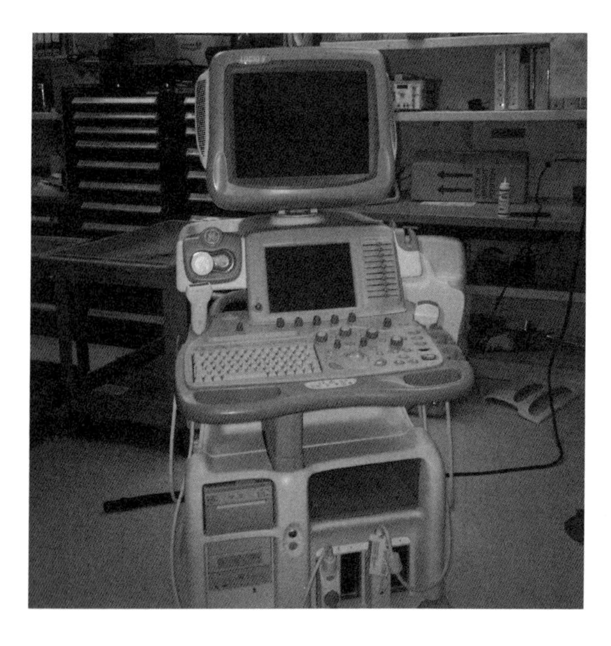

CHAPTER OUTLINE

OBJECTIVES

This objective of this chapter is to familiarize the reader with the physics of ultrasound and the various types of ultrasound equipment in hospitals.

Upon completion of this chapter, the reader will be able to:

- Compute ultrasound attenuation, reflection coefficient, and other parameters.
- Compare ultrasound imaging of A-mode, B-mode, and M-mode.
- Describe the components of an ultrasound machine.
- Name various ultrasound transducers.
- Discuss ultrasound applications in medicine.
- Describe safety issues of medical ultrasound.

INTERNET WEB SITES

http://www.ehealthmd.com   Health Information Publications
http://www.diagnosticimaging.com   Direct Medical Data, Des Plaines, IL
http://www.echoincontext.com   Duke University Center for Echo
http://www.medlineplus.gov   U.S. National Library of Medicine & National Institute of Health

INTRODUCTION

Ultrasound is a safe and painless technique used in biomedicine for examining the internal organs using high-frequency sound waves. Ultrasound is cyclic sound pressure with a frequency greater than the upper limit of human hearing. The production of ultrasound is used in many different fields, typically to penetrate a medium, such as soft tissue and internal organs, and measure the reflection signature or supply focused energy. The reflection signature can reveal details about the inner structure of the medium. The most well known application of this technique is its use in obstetric sonography to produce pictures of fetuses in the human womb, but ultrasound is used in many other areas of patient care, such as gynecology, cardiology, neurology, and orthopedics. Ultrasounds are most frequently performed in outpatient clinics or in the imaging departments of hospitals. This chapter will discuss the physics of ultrasound, types of ultrasound transducers, Doppler ultrasound, ultrasound imaging techniques, and patient preparation.

14.1 ULTRASOUND PHYSICS

Ultrasound is a frequency greater than the upper limit of human hearing. Although it varies from person to person, the frequency range for human hearing is between approximately 20 Hz and 20 kHz in healthy, young adults. Thus, 20 kHz serves as a useful lower limit in describing ultrasound.

As ultrasound travels through different media of solid, liquid, or gas, its speed is affected by the density and the stiffness of the media. This is called the propagation velocity. **Figure 14-1** provides a list of the propagation speed of the ultrasound through soft tissues, bones, and several organs. Notice that the speed of ultrasound through bone is twice that through muscle.

The characteristics of an ultrasound can be summarized as follows:

1. The speed of ultrasound through dry air is 330 m/sec. It cannot travel through a vacuum.
2. Ultrasound is a mechanical wave rather than an electromagnetic wave.
3. The denser the media, the faster the propagation of the ultrasound through that media.
4. Ultrasound intensity is the concentration of the energy in the beam.
5. Acoustical impedance changes the propagation of the ultrasound wave.
6. Ultrasound can be transmitted, reflected, refracted, scattered, or absorbed as it travels through different media.
7. Attenuation occurs as the ultrasound wave reflects and refracts as it passes through the body.

Material	Speed (m/s)	Speed (mm/μs)
Air	330 m/s	33 mm/μs
Lung	500 m/s	0.50 mm/μs
Fat	1450 m/s	1.45 mm/μs
Brain	1520 m/s	1.52 mm/μs
Muscle	1580 m/s	1.58 mm/μs
Liver	1550 m/s	1.55 mm/μs
Kidney	1560 m/s	1.56 mm/μs
Soft Tissue	1540 m/s	1.54 mm/μs
Bone	4000 m/s	4.00 mm/μs

FIGURE 14-1 Propagation velocity of ultrasound in tissues, bones, and various organs.

Mechanical Wave

A mechanical wave is a longitudinal pressure wave composed of periodic compressions and rarefactions in the material carrying the wave. **Figure 14-2** shows the wave direction of a moving mechanical wave (a string attached to the wall). Similarly, the molecules in the material vibrate back and forth in the same direction as the ultrasound travels. This is shown in **Figure 14-3a** when a piezoelectric crystal as a source generates the ultrasound wave. One complete cycle consists of the compression and rarefaction (relaxation) phase of the wave. How well ultrasound can be transmitted through the material depends on the

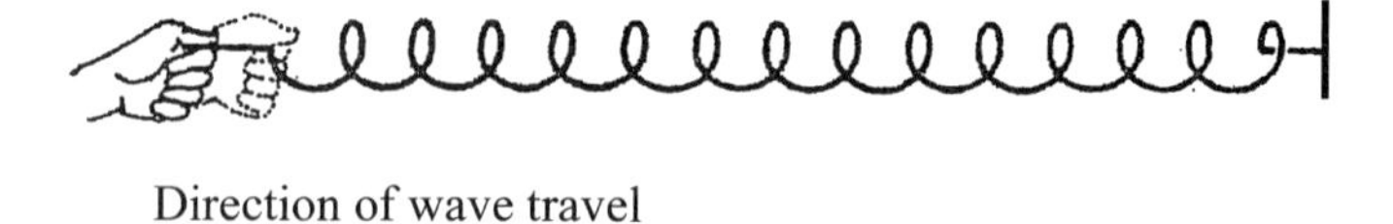

FIGURE 14-2 Mechanical wave in a string attached to a wall.

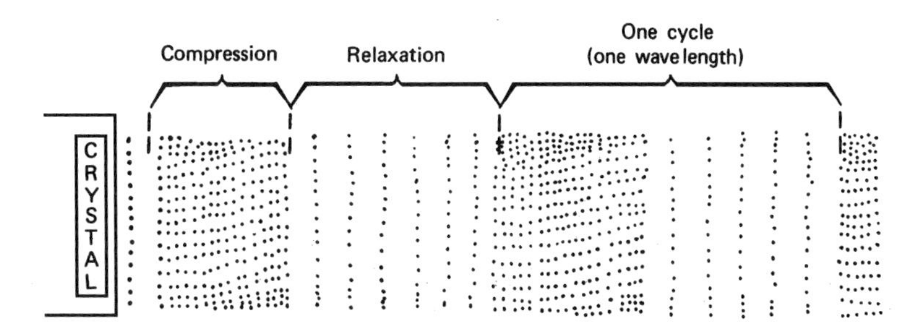

FIGURE 14-3a Wave generated by a piezoelectric crystal.

density and the elasticity of the material. If the molecules in the material are close as in the dense material, the propagation of the ultrasound is fast because the ability to couple the movement of molecules from one part of the material to the next has increased. In that case, more compressions and rarefactions will form.

Figure 14-3b shows an interface between a low impedance and a high impedance for the ultrasound to propagate (that is, a more dense material has a high acoustic impedance). An ultrasound wave coming to the interface with an angle can either reflect or refract. Reflection sends the wave back to the same media from which it came, while refraction causes the wave to bend and move into the next media.

Propagation

As a wave travels, propagation is the movement of that wave through a medium. The denser a media is, the faster the propagation of the ultrasound through that media. In a solid, ultrasound takes 0.3 sec to cover a distance of 1 km, whereas it takes 3 sec to cover the same

FIGURE 14-3b Ultrasound travel through a low impedance and a high impedance interface.

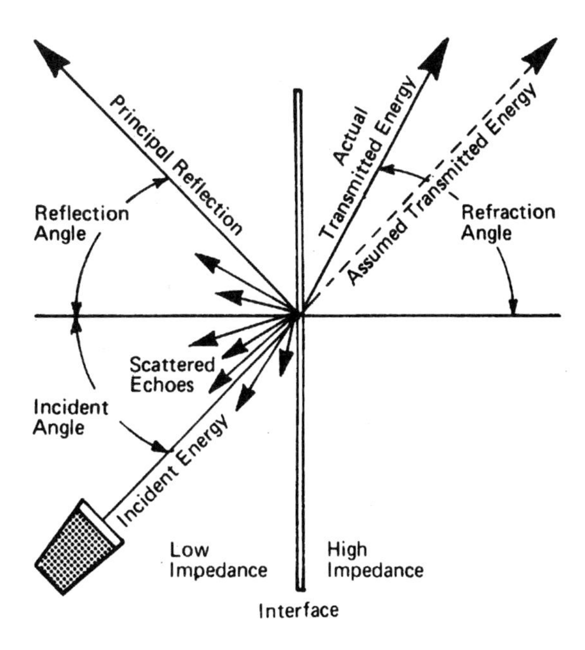

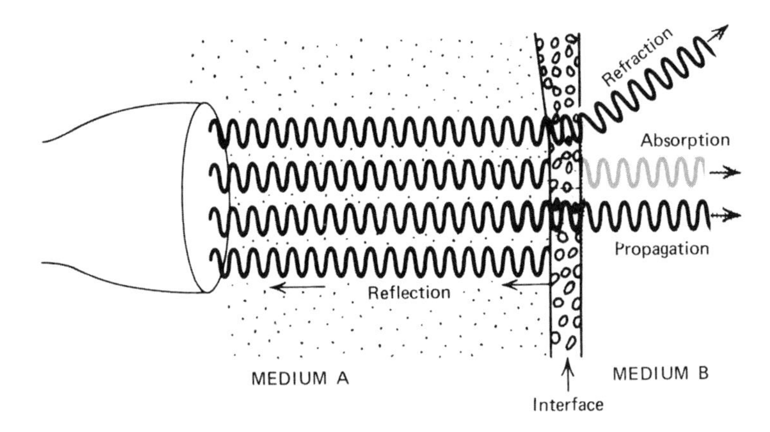

FIGURE 14-4a Ultrasound refraction at an interface.

distance through a gas medium. In **Figure 14-4a,** medium A and medium B are shown and the traveling wave can reflect or refract at the interface. Additionally, part of the wave can propagate or be absorbed. Each of these possibilities depends on the angle made at the interface and the medium density. **Figure 14-4b** shows the ultrasound velocities through media of gas, liquid, and solid.

The velocity in most biological material is close to 1,550 m/sec. This can be related as:

$$C = f \times \lambda$$

Where C is the ultrasound velocity in the material, f is the frequency of the ultrasound wave, and λ is the wavelength of the ultrasound wave and is the distance covered in one cycle of the compression and rarefaction phase.

Intensity

The amplitude and the intensity of the ultrasound are directly related. Amplitude is the size of the signal, small or large, but the intensity is the concentration of the energy in the beam

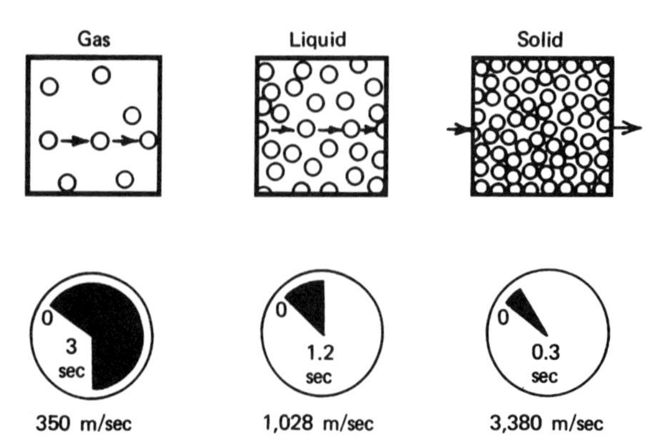

FIGURE 14-4b Length of time an ultrasound wave takes through gas, liquid, and a solid material.

and varies in space and time. Intensity is proportional to the square of the amplitude. The intensity decreases as the ultrasound travels through muscles and bones in the body.

Acoustic Impedance

As the media becomes more dense, the acoustical impedance increases. This changes the propagation of the ultrasound wave. The acoustical impedance is related to the compressibility of the material. In a dense material, the molecules are not easily compressible, and this affects the formation of compressions and rarefactions in the ultrasound wave.

The acoustical impedance of some of the materials is given in the table shown in **Figure 14-5.** Notice that bone is a dense material and its impedance is larger compared to the less dense water material. Interestingly, the ultrasound can propagate faster through this dense material as discussed in the previous section. The formula for the acoustical impedance can be given as:

$$Z = \rho \times C$$

Where Z is the acoustical impedance, ρ is the density of the material, and C is the velocity of ultrasound in the material. The unit of the acoustical impedance is gm/cm^2-sec.

Ultrasound Reflections

Similar to light propagation, ultrasound can be transmitted, reflected, refracted, scattered, or absorbed as it travels through the different media. Ultrasound propagation also follows the Snell's law as in optics. Snell's law states that the propagation depends on the various densities of materials and the geometry of their interfaces as ultrasound passes through them. The Snell's law for sound though states that a ray of sound coming onto a denser medium will bend away from the normal. This is different in optics as a light ray bends towards the normal when it enters onto a denser medium. The velocity of sound increases in a denser medium whereas the velocity of light decreases in a denser medium.

As the ultrasound beam encounters an interface where the acoustical impedance changes, reflections and/or refractions take place. The angle of incidence of the wave to the interface plays an important role in whether there will be a reflection or refraction.

Material	Acoustical Impedance (Z) (x 10^5 gm/cm^2s)
Air	0.0001
Fat	1.4
Water	1.5
Kidney	1.6
Muscle	1.7
Lens of Eye	1.8
Bone	8.0

FIGURE 14-5 A table of acoustical impedances to ultrasound in tissues.

Interface	Percent Reflection (%)
Blood-brain	0.3
Blood-kidney	0.7
Water-brain	3.2
Blood-fat	7.9
Muscle-fat	10.0
Muscle-bone	64.6
Brain-skull bone	66.1
Water-skull bone	68.4
Air-any soft tissue	100.0

FIGURE 14-6 A table of percent reflections of ultrasound at tissue interfaces.

In **Figure 14-6,** a table is provided for the percent reflection between two interfaces such as a muscle and a bone interface in the body. Approximately 64.6 percent of wave energy will be reflected from the muscle-bone interface.

The incident energy of the ultrasound wave is partially reflected to the low impedance material and the remaining energy will then be transmitted in the high impedance material. As the transmission path has changed in the high impedance material, the beam is called a refracted or bent beam. The incident energy consists of waves that will interact with the interface at different angles.

Figure 14-7 and **Figure 14-8** illustrate the various possibilities of whether an incident wave will be reflected or refracted.

If the incident wave is nearly perpendicular to the interface, or if the incident angle is larger than the critical angle, the wave will be reflected back to the same medium. In ultrasound imaging, the reflections are collected by the ultrasound detector. Snell's law relates the angles and the densities by the following equation:

$$\eta_1 \times \sin(\theta i) = \eta_2 \times \sin(\theta_r)$$

Where η_1 and η_2 are refractive indexes of the two mediums and θi and θr are the angles with the normal. Refractive index is defined as a ratio of the velocity of ultrasound in the material to the velocity of ultrasound in the air.

When we substitute η_1 and η_2 in the Snell's equation, the modified equation relates the velocities to the opposite angles. That is,

$$C_2 \times \sin(\theta i) = C_1 \times \sin(\theta r)$$

$$\frac{C_1}{C_2} = \frac{\sin(\theta i)}{\sin(\theta r)}$$

As with the difference in the acoustical impedances at an interface, the reflection coefficient Γ will indicate the percent of reflection and can be given as:

$$\Gamma = \frac{(Z_1 - Z_2)}{(Z_1 + Z_2)}$$

where

Z_1 and Z_2 = acoustical impedances.

Air has an impedance of 0.0001×10^5 gm/cm^2-sec and the muscle (like a soft tissue) has an impedance of 1.7×10^5 gm/cm^2-sec. The percent reflection is approximately 100 percent. However, the muscle-bone interface has comparatively less (approximately 65 percent) reflection.

The effect of the refraction is negligible when the ultrasound beam is perpendicular to the interface (the surface between two impedances). This is important because the idea is to collect the reflections, but not the refractions, from the interfaces in ultrasound diagnostics. The transducer is kept as perpendicular as possible at the surfaces and the organs of interest.

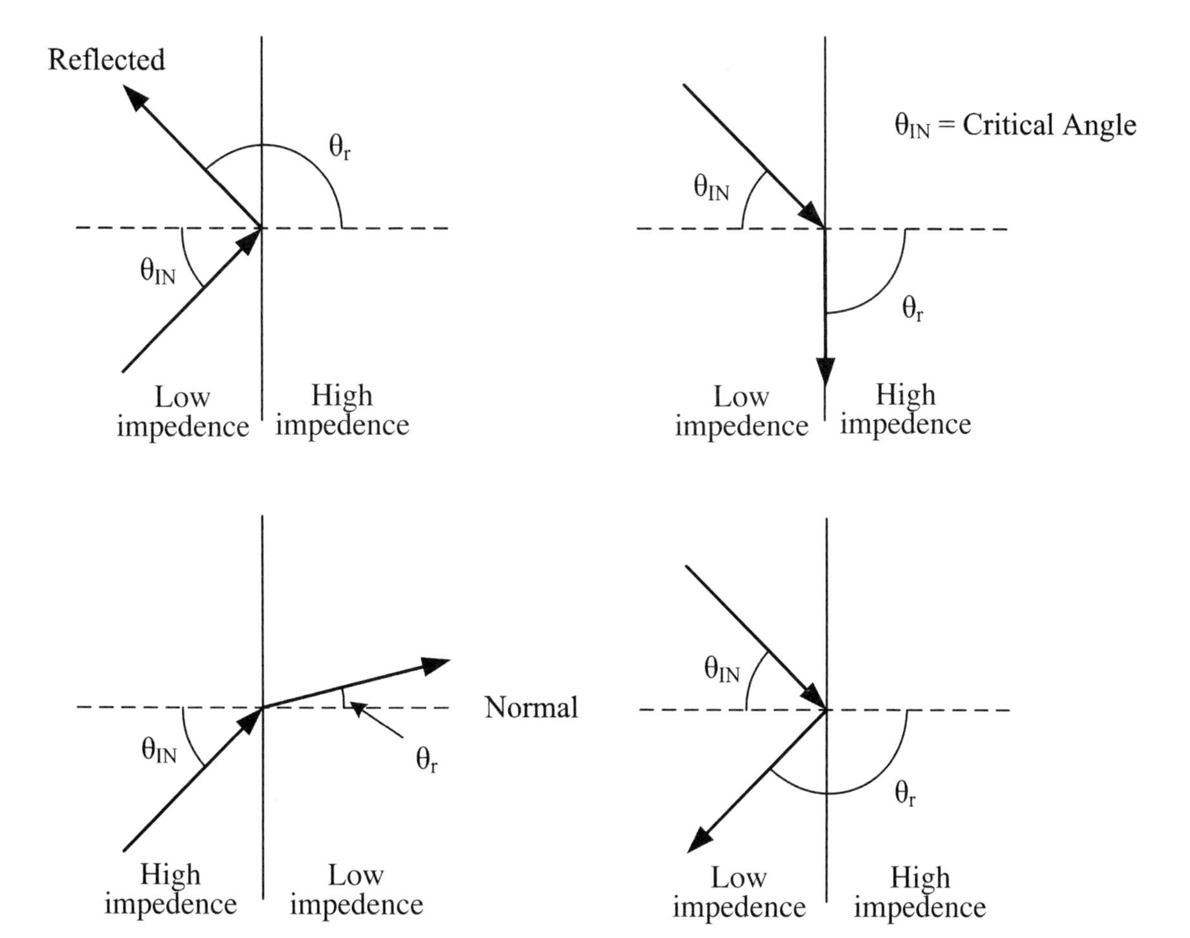

FIGURE 14-7 Refraction angles at interfaces.

FIGURE 14-8 Refraction angles at interfaces.

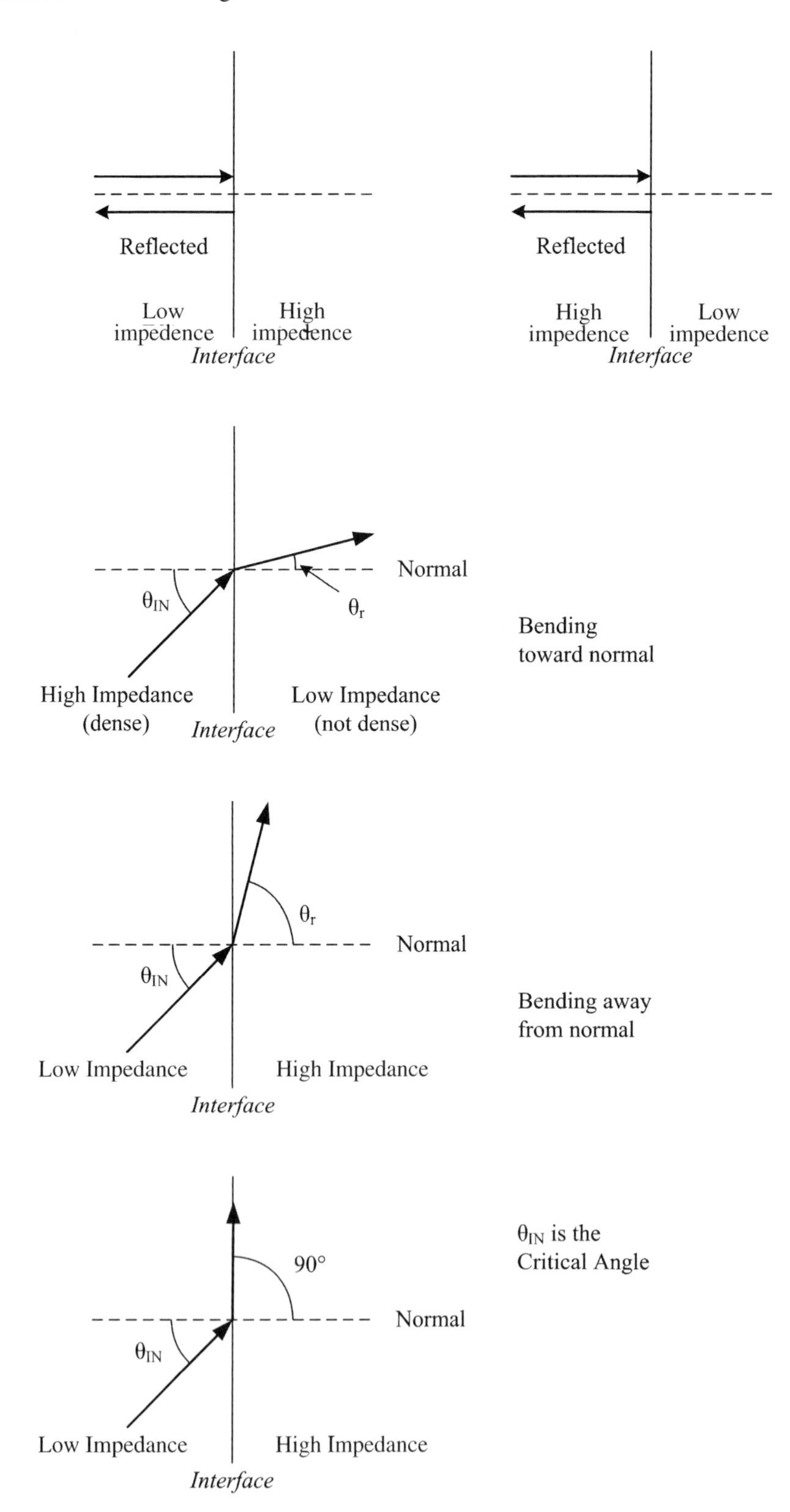

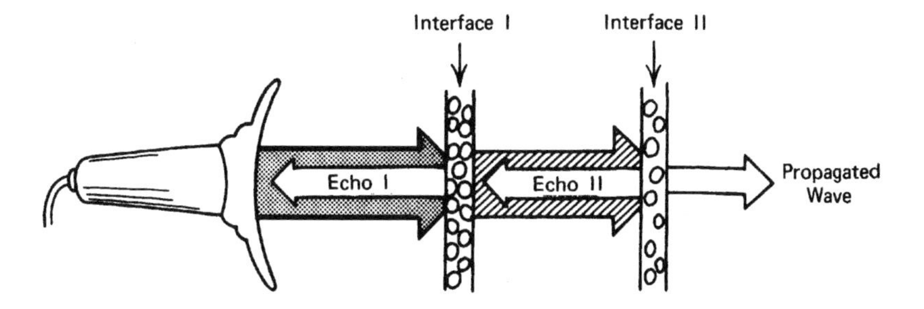

FIGURE 14-9a Ultrasound transducer at the soft tissue interface.

When the beam (which consists of rays of different incident angles) is nearly perpendicular to the interface, most of the ultrasound energy is reflected and is collected by the transducer, but the remaining energy is transmitted to the next medium as refractions. However, the next interface will reflect more, but with some time delay, and the remaining energy will then be transmitted to the next medium. This process is shown in **Figure 14-9a.** Echo 1 and echo 2 are produced at interface 1 and interface 2, respectively, due to the differences in density of the two materials. In **Figure 14-9b,** the ultrasonic gel is placed between the soft tissue and the lead zirconate titanate (PZT) transducer.

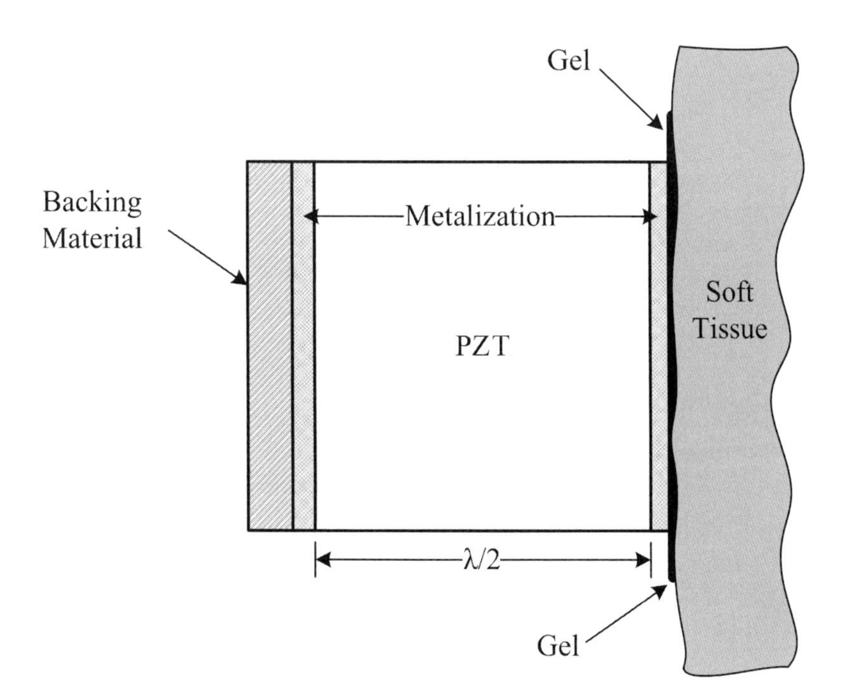

FIGURE 14-9b Reflections from interfaces in sequence.

Attenuation

When the ultrasound wave propagates through the body, undergoing reflections and refractions at several interfaces, it starts losing energy. This energy loss is caused by the transformation of some of the wave energy into heat energy, a process referred to as attenuation. Ultrasound energy causes the particles of the medium at which it is directed to vibrate, which allows further propagation of the wave. The amount of heat created depends on the frequency and intensity of the ultrasound energy, as well as the ability of the medium to permit propagation. The formula for calculating attenuation is as follows:

$$\text{Attenuation (in dB)} = 10 \log (I_1 / I_2)$$

Where

I_1 and I_2 are the ultrasound intensities in two mediums.

EXAMPLE An ultrasound signal passes through bone tissue with a frequency of 4 MHz. Compute the wavelength, period, and the phase constant.

$$\text{Wavelength } \lambda = \frac{C}{F} = \frac{\text{Velocity in the bone tissue}}{\text{Frequency}}$$

$$\text{Wavelength } \lambda = \frac{3{,}360 \text{ m/sec}}{4 \times 10^6 \text{ cycles/sec}} = 0.00084 \text{ m}$$

$$T = \text{Time period} = \frac{1}{F} = \frac{1}{4 \text{ MHz}} = 0.25\mu\text{s}$$

$$\text{Phase Constant} = \beta = \frac{2\pi}{\lambda} = \frac{6.28}{\lambda} = \frac{6.28}{0.00084} = 7476.19$$

■

EXAMPLE Compute the reflection coefficient of the ultrasound at the boundary of fat and bone. Given: Bone density = 1.85 gm/cm³ and speed of ultrasound 3,360 m/sec; Fat density = 0.93 gm/cm³ and speed of ultrasound 1,480 m/sec.

$$\Gamma = \text{Reflection coefficient}$$

$$\Gamma = \frac{Z_2 - Z_1}{Z_2 + Z_1}$$

$$\Gamma = \frac{\rho_2 C_2 - \rho_1 C_1}{\rho_2 C_2 + \rho_1 C_1}$$

$$Z_2 = (1.85 \text{ gm/cm}^3) \times (3{,}360 \text{ m/sec}) \times (100 \text{ cm/m})$$

$$Z_1 = (0.93 \text{ gm/cm}^3) \times (1{,}480 \text{ m/sec}) \times (100 \text{ cm/m})$$

■

EXAMPLE At the fat-bone interface, the direct incident power of the ultrasound wave is 2 W/cm²; how much power is reflected back toward the ultrasound receiver transducer?

$$\text{Reflected power} = \Gamma^2 \times \text{Incident power}$$

■

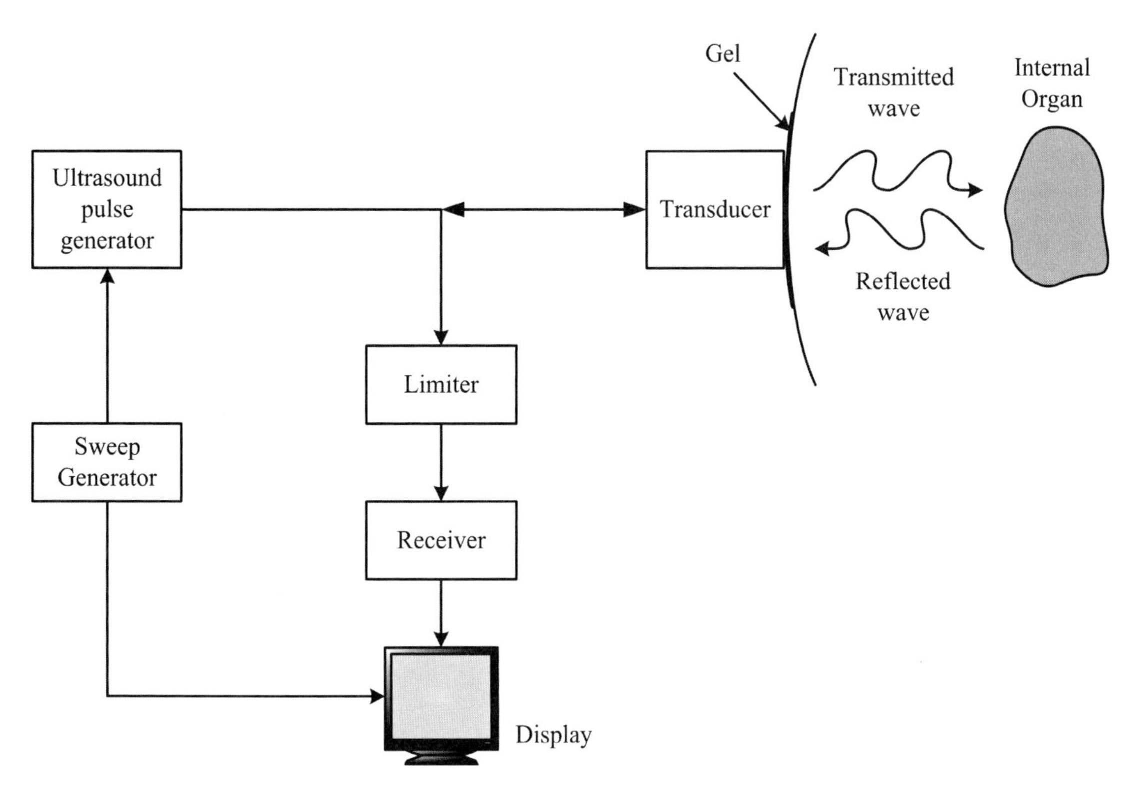

FIGURE 14-10 A simple block diagram of a ultrasound system.

14.2 ULTRASOUND SYSTEM

Figure 14-10 shows a block diagram of the ultrasound imaging system. The ultrasound signal generator activates the piezoelectric transducer with short-duration RF electric pulses that then generate ultrasound RF pulses traveling into the muscles and tissues. The ultrasound RF pulses are then reflected from the tissue-muscle boundaries and received at the machine and displayed after signal processing. The RF pulse generator is ON when sending the ultrasound signal and then it is OFF at the time of echo reception.

Note that the feedback signal is a series of echoes from the interface. These echoes are collected by the same transducer, amplified, and displayed based on various modes of imaging.

14.3 ULTRASOUND DOPPLER AND FLOW DETECTOR

The Doppler effect is a change in the observed frequency of the ultrasound wave when the source and the observer are in motion with respect to one another. The frequency increases when the source and the observer approach each other; in contrast, it decreases when they move apart from each other. The effect is used in monitoring blood flow. The ultrasound transducer or the blood molecules can be considered either the source or the observer.

The Doppler ultrasound instrument detects the motion of blood flow through a vessel and creates an audible trace. It is commonly used to detect vessel stenosis, or the narrowing of a blood vessel. The ultrasound transducer is placed on an area of the body where blood flow can be detected. The technician can then listen for changes in the pitch of the sound over the area. The pitch of the sound created increases due to higher flow velocity when the transducer lies directly over a stenotic segment of a blood vessel.

The Doppler effect is shown in **Figure 14-11a** through **Figure 14-11d.** The ultrasound transducer transmits pulses toward the target. In this case, the target is the blood molecules in the vessels. The reflections will also be detected by the same transducer. The reflections will always be about same if the blood molecules are stationary for any pulse transmitted. However, the reflections from the moving molecules will be different depending on the angle of interaction and the velocity of the blood molecules.

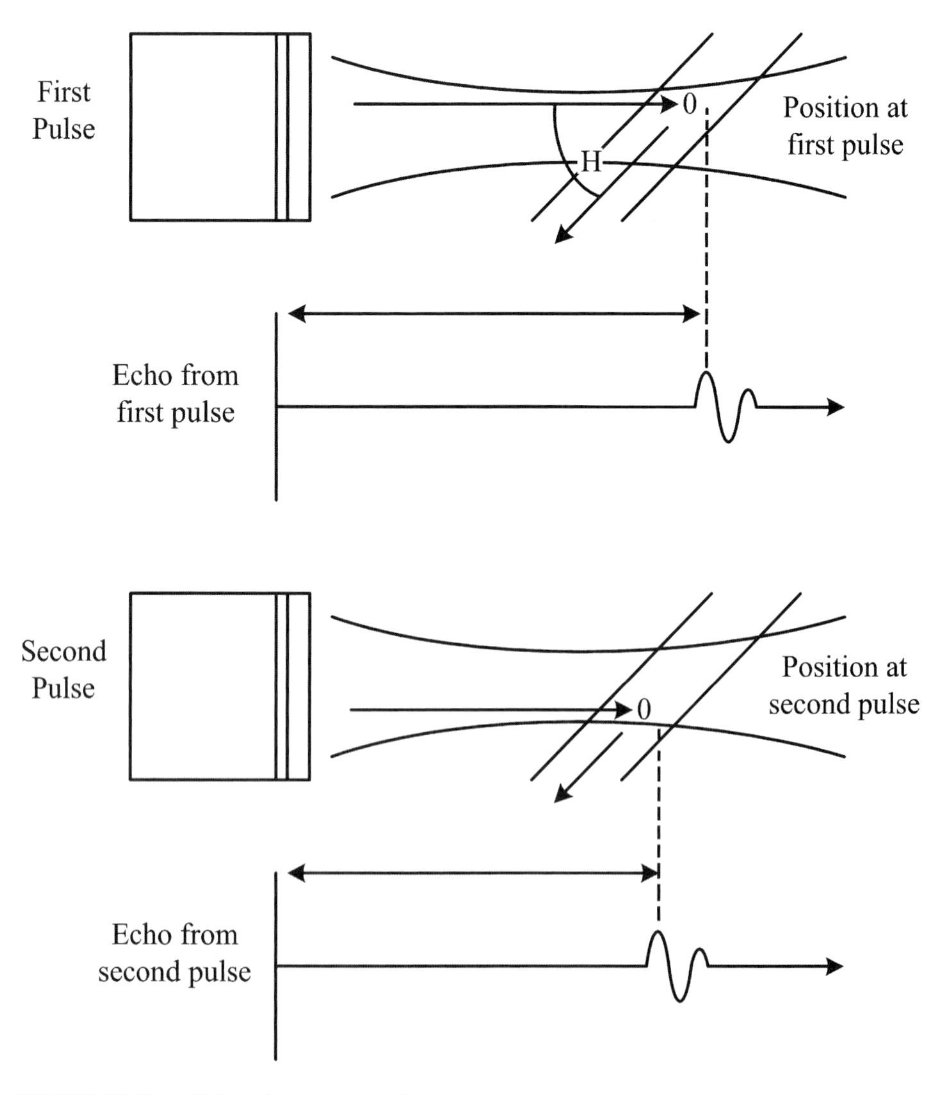

FIGURE 14-11a Echoes from moving blood stream.

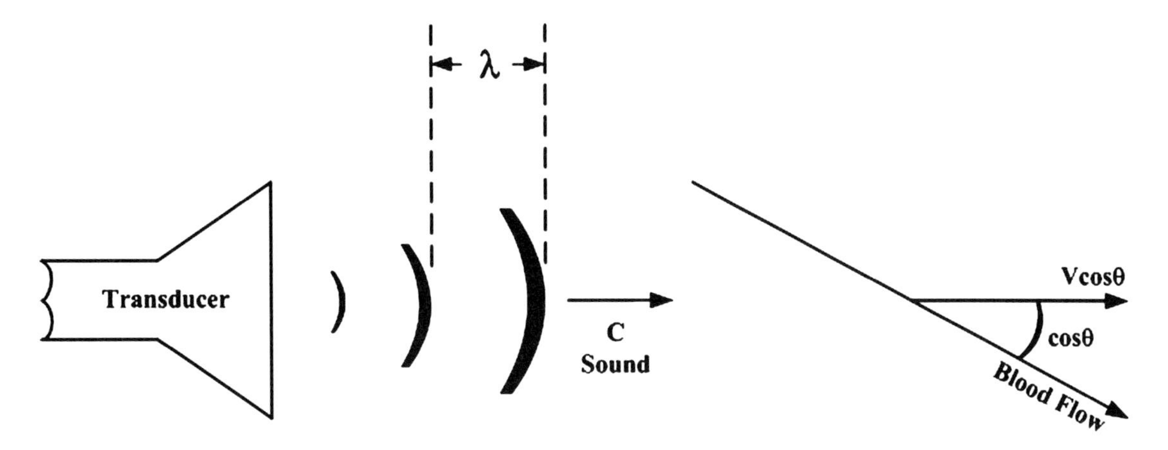

FIGURE 14-11b Ultrasound angles at the moving blood stream.

Analysis of the Doppler Effect

In **Figure 14-11d,** an ultrasound transducer is generating the sound waves. Ultrasound waves then produce compressions in the air with a wavelength of λ. The frequency then can be given as:

$$f = \frac{C}{\lambda}$$

where C is the velocity of ultrasound

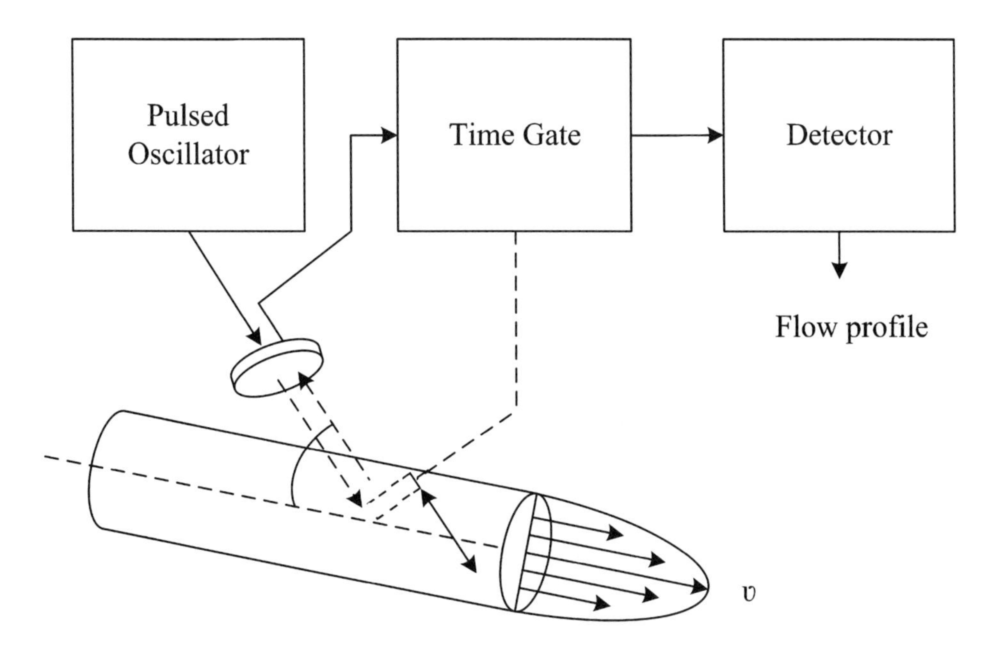

FIGURE 14-11c Detection of ultrasound echoes by the same transducer that transmits.

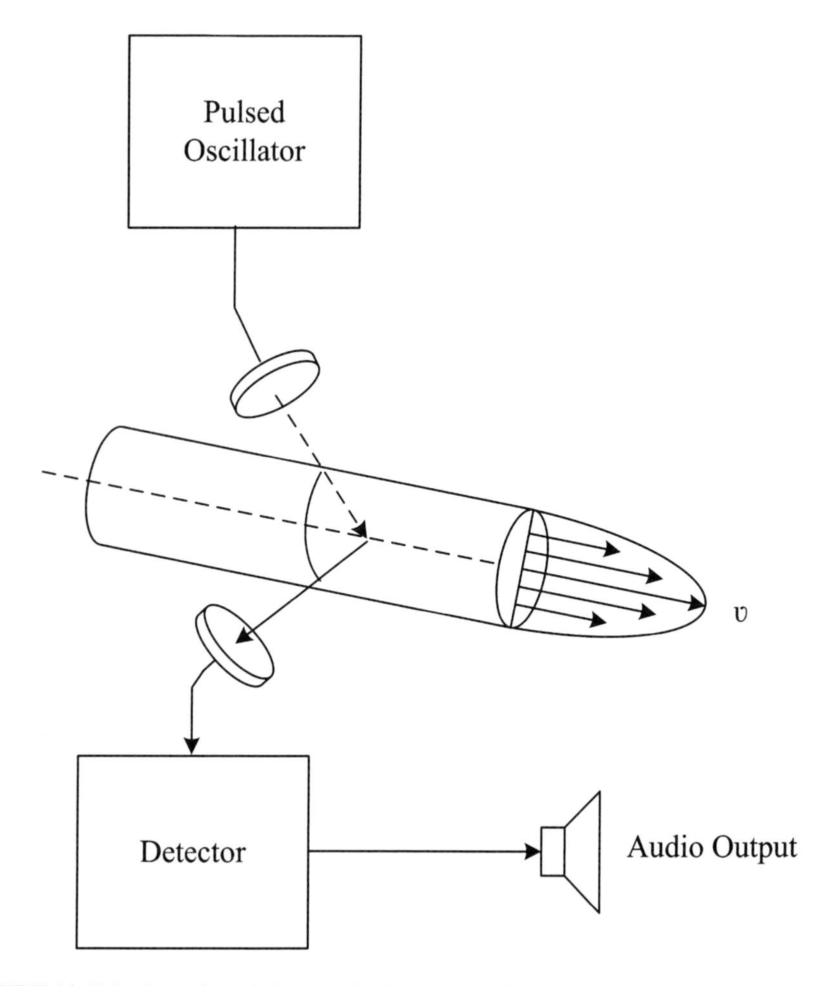

FIGURE 14-11d Detection of ultrasound echoes by a different transducer.

The wave interacts with the blood flow having a velocity of V and its component Vcosθ (which is in the same direction as the wave). This interaction is now affecting the frequency of the ultrasound and the changed frequency $\mathbf{f_p}$ (based on the difference of two velocities in the same direction) is given as

$$\mathbf{f_p} = \frac{(C - V \times \cos\theta)}{\lambda}$$

This is the frequency for the ultrasound still traveling in the same direction; however, this intersection also generates a reflected ultrasound wave that will travel back to the transducer. The frequency of the reflected wave can now be stated as if the intersection interface were a new source. That results in the returning frequency of $\mathbf{f_S}$ such that:

$$f_S = \frac{(C - V \times \cos\theta - V \times \cos\theta)}{\lambda}$$

$$f_S = \frac{C - 2 \times V \times \cos\theta}{\lambda}$$

$$f_S = \frac{C}{\lambda} - \frac{2 \times V \times \cos\theta}{\lambda}$$

$$f_S = \frac{C}{\lambda} - \frac{2 \times V \times \cos\theta}{C \times f}$$

$$f_S = f - \frac{2 \times V \times \cos\theta}{C} \times f$$

$$f_S = f\left(1 - \frac{2 \times V \times \cos\theta}{C}\right)$$

The term f_S is the echo frequency and the transducer can detect the difference between its initial traveling frequency and the echo frequency being received, thus:

$$\Delta f = f - f_S$$

$$\Delta f = f - f\left(1 - \frac{2 \times V \times \cos\theta}{C}\right)$$

$$\Delta f = \frac{2 \times V \times \cos\theta}{C} \times f$$

This change in frequency (Δf) is measured in the circuit and the flow velocity is computed by manipulating the Δf equation.

$$V = \frac{\Delta f \times C}{2 \times f \times \cos\theta}$$

The velocity of the blood flow is then computed when the difference frequency is measured by the electronic circuit. The other parameters in the equation are easily derived.

14.4 MODES OF ULTRASOUND SCANS

Ultrasound images are displayed in three major modes: A-mode, B-mode, and M-mode.

A-Mode

A-mode (amplitude mode) displays echoes by representing the amplitude of the echo as the height of a signal peak (vertical deflection) from the horizontal baseline. The distance of each signal peak deflection along the horizontal baseline represents the depth of the tissue from which that echo was received. In a way, the display relates the distance between tissue boundaries and can measure organ thickness. This mode is quite useful in the measurements of the brain (echo-encephalography) to find the distances of bones and muscles in the complex brain structure. This is shown in **Figures 14-12a.** The echo pulses are smaller than the original transmitted pulse. The distance can be determined with the half of the sound travel time and the velocity of ultrasound in tissue. This mode is not much used in imaging, but

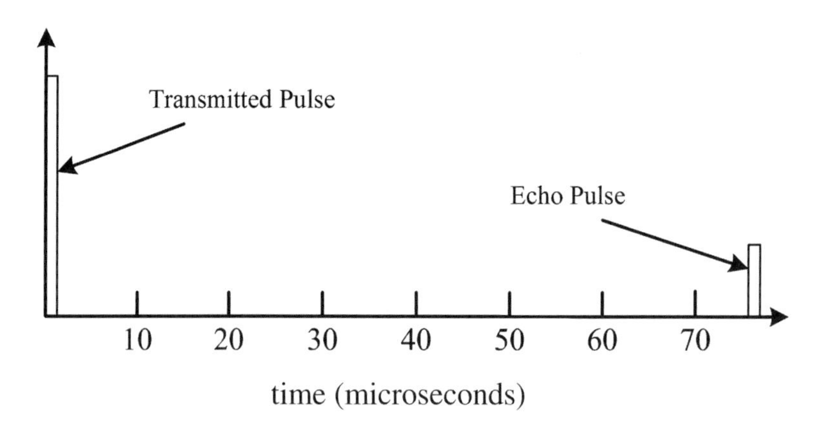

FIGURE 14-12a A-mode ultrasound reflections.

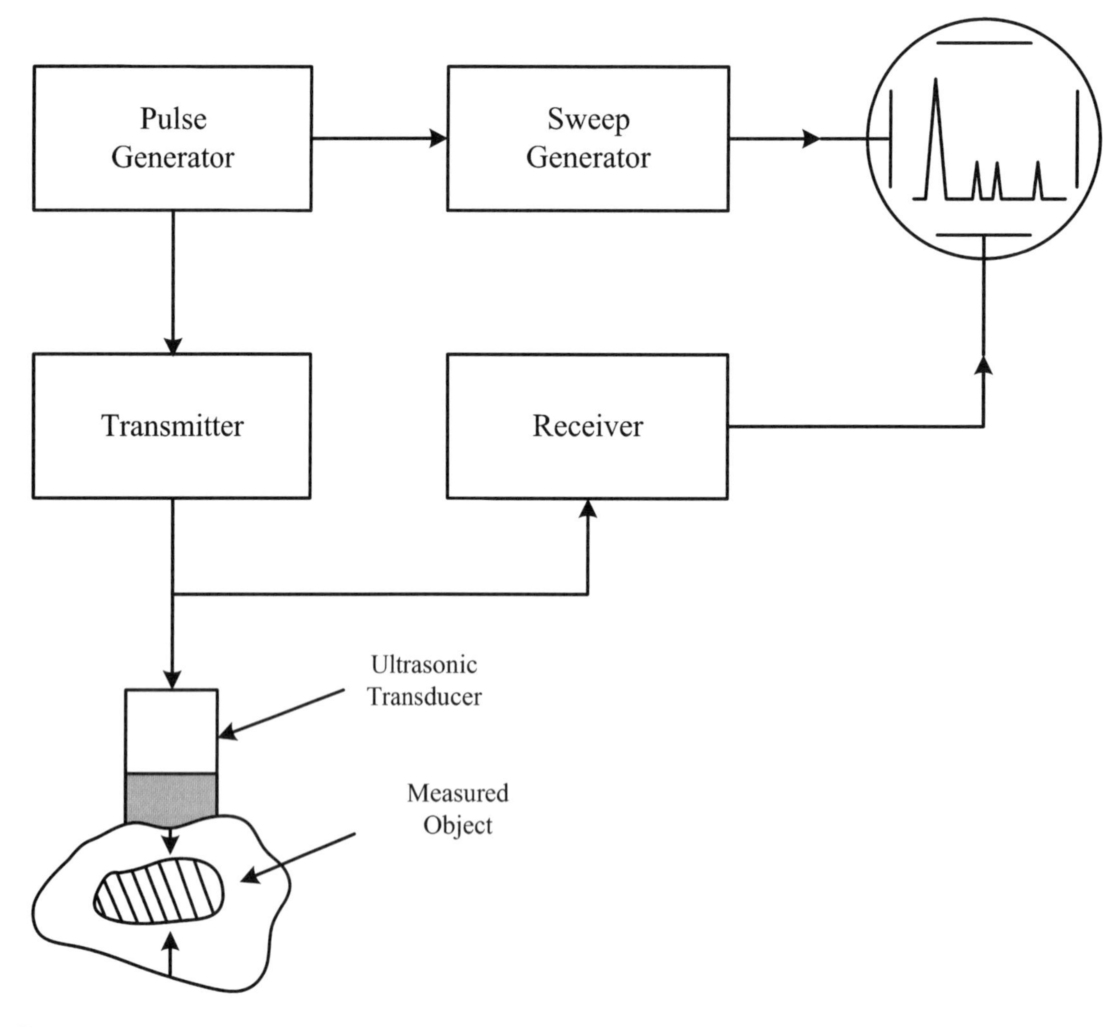

FIGURE 14-12b Block diagram of the A-mode ultrasound system.

the idea of echoes coming back to the receiver one after another from several reflectors at different times as spikes with smaller amplitudes really provide insight to understand other modes. A block diagram of the A-mode is shown in **Figure 14-12b.** The transmitter and the receiver are two separate units in the diagram and the sweep generator synchronizes the first pulse being transmitted and the reflected pulses being received.

B-Mode

B-mode (brightness mode) represents echoes as dots rather than vertical deflections and the brightness represents the strength of the reflected echo. The brightness increases with the echo amplitude. A scan of the B-mode is constructed by passing the ultrasound transducer over the body and then displaying the returning echoes on a monitor as more data points are acquired. A composite of these dots produces a two-dimensional picture of the area examined. A series of these B-mode scans can be made in various directions providing longitudinal and transverse views of the body. The advantage of the B-mode scan is that it can display a two-dimensional cross-sectional view of the anatomy and is often referred to as ultrasonic tomography.

There are at least two ways to generate B-mode scans. One way is to use a rotating transducer from side to side displaying the bright dots in their geometrically correct direction and distance. The second method is to use a phased array transducer. This transducer has several piezoelectric transducers positioned in a line and each one of them transmits and receives pulsed ultrasound successively in time. This type of scanning is faster than the rotating scan. **Figure 14-13a** shows the image outline with the dots representing the reflected pulses on a line in a specific direction. **Figure 14-13b** is a block diagram for the

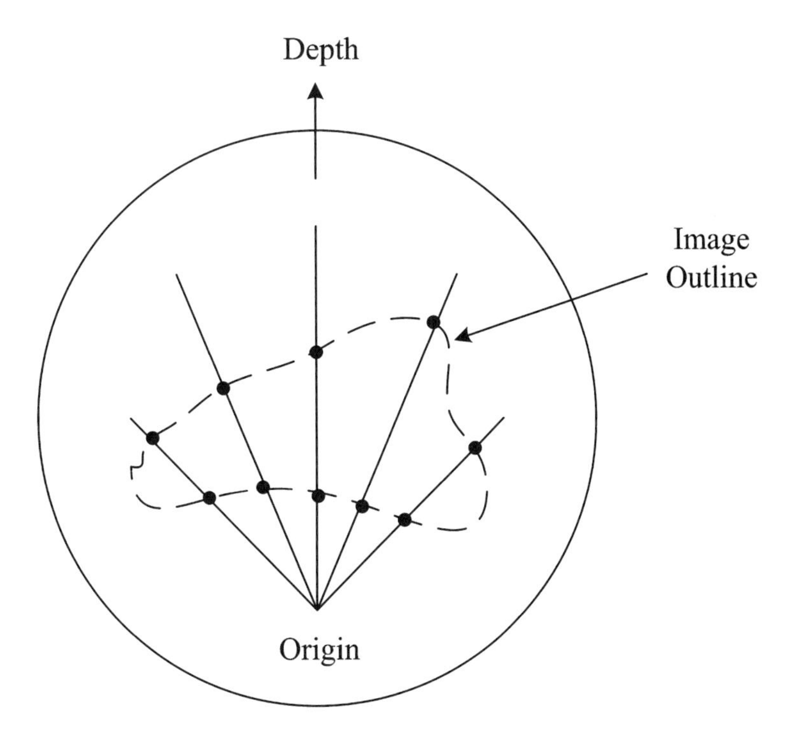

FIGURE 14-13a B-mode ultrasound reflections.

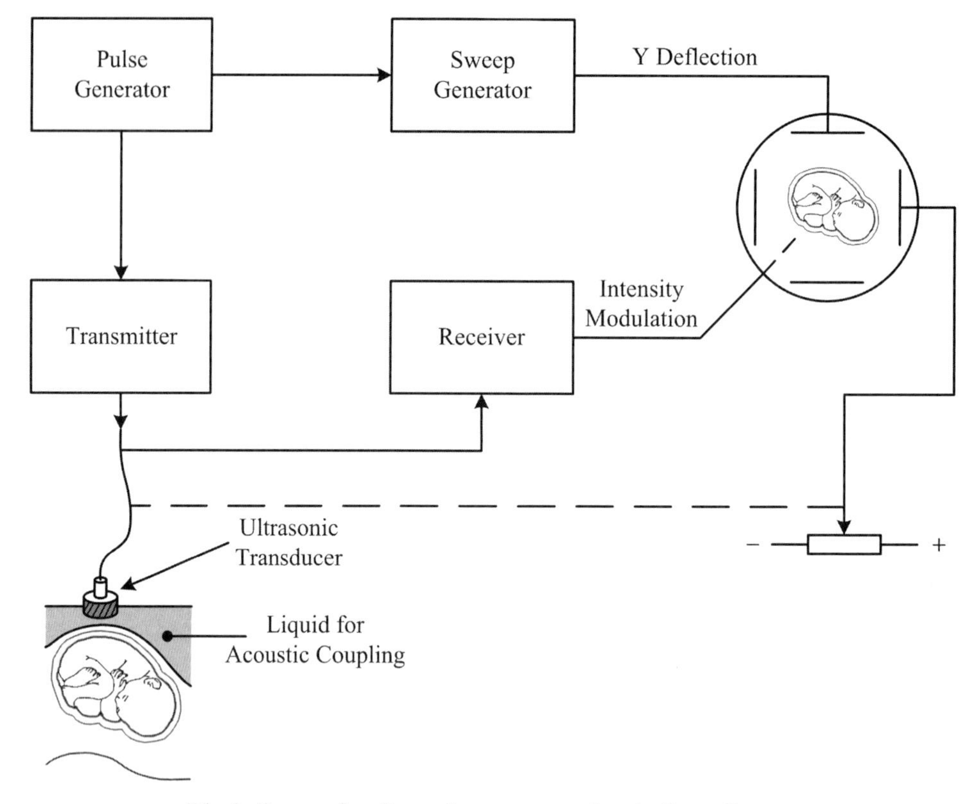

FIGURE 14-13b A block diagram of B-mode ultrasound system.

B-mode. Notice the block diagram of the B-mode is more complex than that of the A-mode. The transducer is moving in the horizontal direction and continuously collecting data from the depth of the tissue structure. The spikes of the A-mode are now intensity modulation.

M-Mode

Neither the A-mode nor the B-mode is capable of providing a graphical record of motion. M-mode (motion mode) is a time-motion display mode; it displays motion of the echo sources toward, and away from, the transducer with respect to time. M-mode is commonly used in echocardiography. In this display, a B-mode scan is moved as a function of time and the successive patterns of dots are swept electronically across the display monitor in a vertical direction. The motion of any structure in the horizontal direction along the beam path can be recorded by the time-exposure photography.

It is also possible to determine the rate of motion of the tissue or an organ by receiving the echo dots (B-mode) on a moving light-sensitive paper. As the speed of the moving paper and the number of dots per scan become known, the motion can be calculated. **Figure 14-14a** shows an M-mode waveform in time. The display shows the distances, or the depths, from where the reflected pulses are being received in time. **Figure 14-14b** shows a comparison between the A-mode pulses

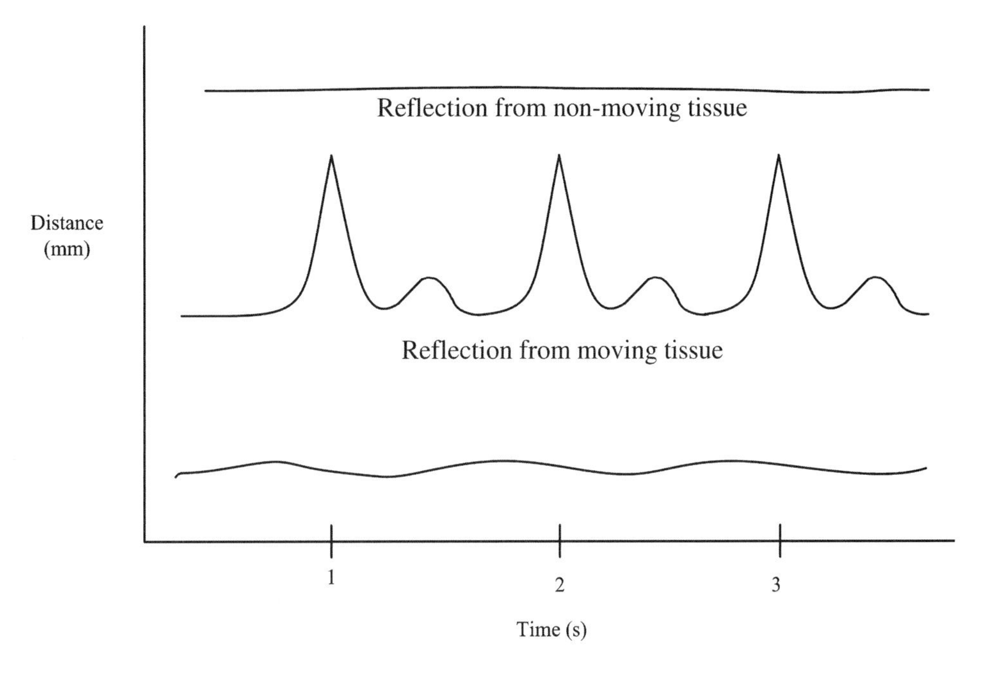

FIGURE 14-14a M-mode ultrasound reflections.

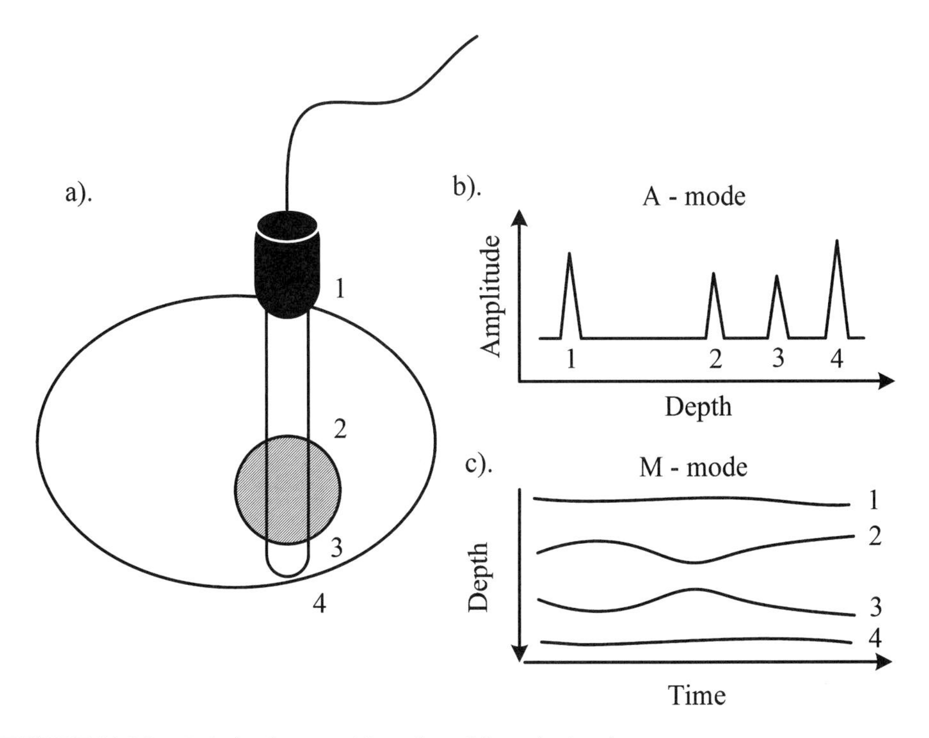

FIGURE 14-14b Relation between M-mode and A-mode signals.

and the M-mode display in time. When the transducer is placed over a muscle, for example, the A-mode displays the received echoes from various depths, whereas the M-mode displays the received echoes in time. The electronic circuit for the M-mode is more complex compared to the B-mode. This allows for more data to be collected in moving tissue, such as a heart valve.

14.5 ECHOCARDIOGRAM

Cardiologists, anesthesiologists, and thoracic surgeons rely on ultrasound to give them a minute-to-minute evaluation of cardiac function. An echocardiogram is also known as an ultrasound examination or a sound wave picture of the heart. It uses the same technology used to take pictures of the fetus in a pregnant woman. These pictures of the heart are taken by a highly trained ultrasound technician who places a hand-held plastic ultrasound probe against the patient's chest. **Figure 14-15a** shows an ultrasound machine.

The probe is connected to the computer with a video screen in the ultrasound machine. The computer reconstructs the reflected signals received through the probe into a picture

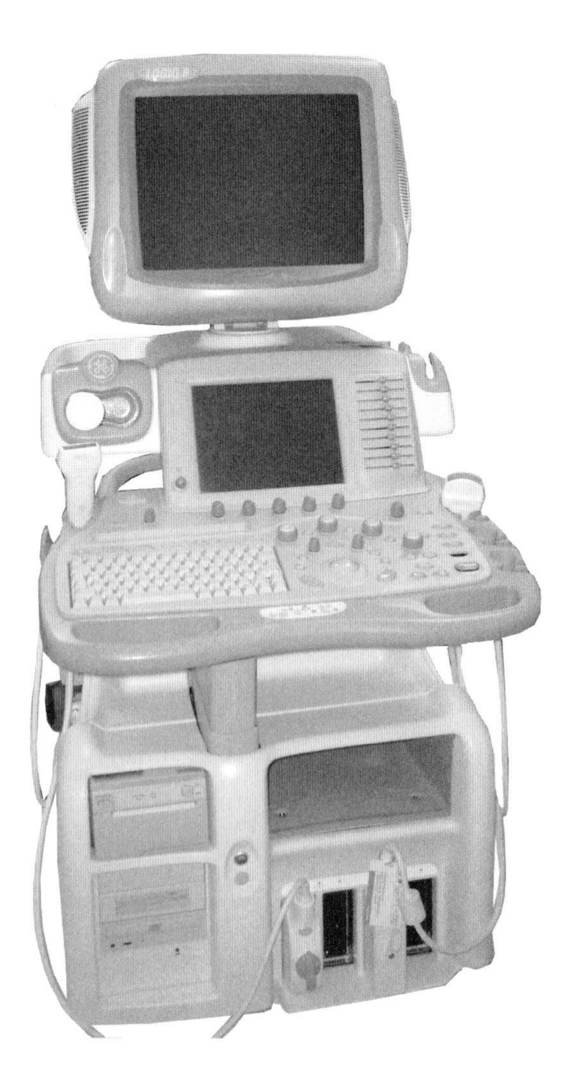

FIGURE 14-15a Ultrasound machine.

of the heart; this picture is then displayed on the screen and records on a digital storage medium. The echocardiogram shows:

1. The sizes of the four chambers of the heart.
2. The strength of the heart muscle. This is invaluable to the doctors in assessing the damage done to the heart after heart attack or heart failure conditions.
3. Any problems with the valves of the heart. The four valves of the heart must open or close properly in order for the heart to function properly. There are serious problems associated with the abnormal valve function such as heart murmurs, swelling, chest discomfort, and the difficulty in breathing.
4. Presence of fluid around the heart. It is a life threatening condition.
5. Congenital heart disease can be detected by the echocardiogram. The holes and abnormal connections between the heart chambers can be diagnosed.
6. Abnormal pressures within the chambers of the heart if the echocardiogram uses Doppler technique.
7. To determine the erratic heart beat due to tumors or calcification.

In **Figure 14-15b,** the M-mode imaging demonstrates the motion from cardiac structures. A series of lines now represent the position and also motion of a reflector in time.

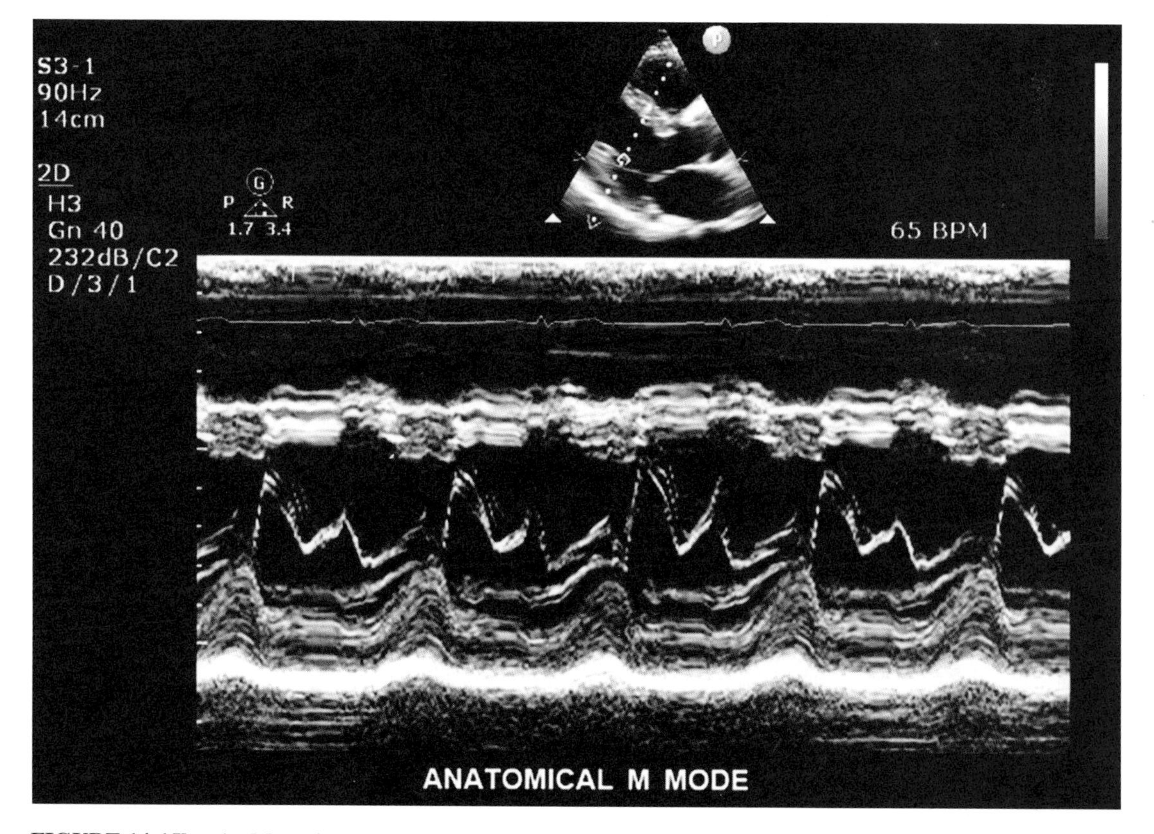

FIGURE 14-15b An M-mode ultrasound image.

14.6 VASCULAR DOPPLER ULTRASOUND

Doppler ultrasound is performed to evaluate blood flow and pressure in blood vessels. It can achieve several results, such as:

1. Detect blood clots or narrowed and blocked blood vessels in any part of the body, particularly in the legs, arms, and neck.
2. Determine the amount of blood flow to the transplanted kidney or liver.
3. Evaluate the blood flow after a stroke.
4. Determine the arterial plaque.
5. Determine leg pain due to atherosclerosis.

An example of the vascular Doppler is shown in **Figure 14–16.** The test can identify the specific arteries that are blocked in the neck.

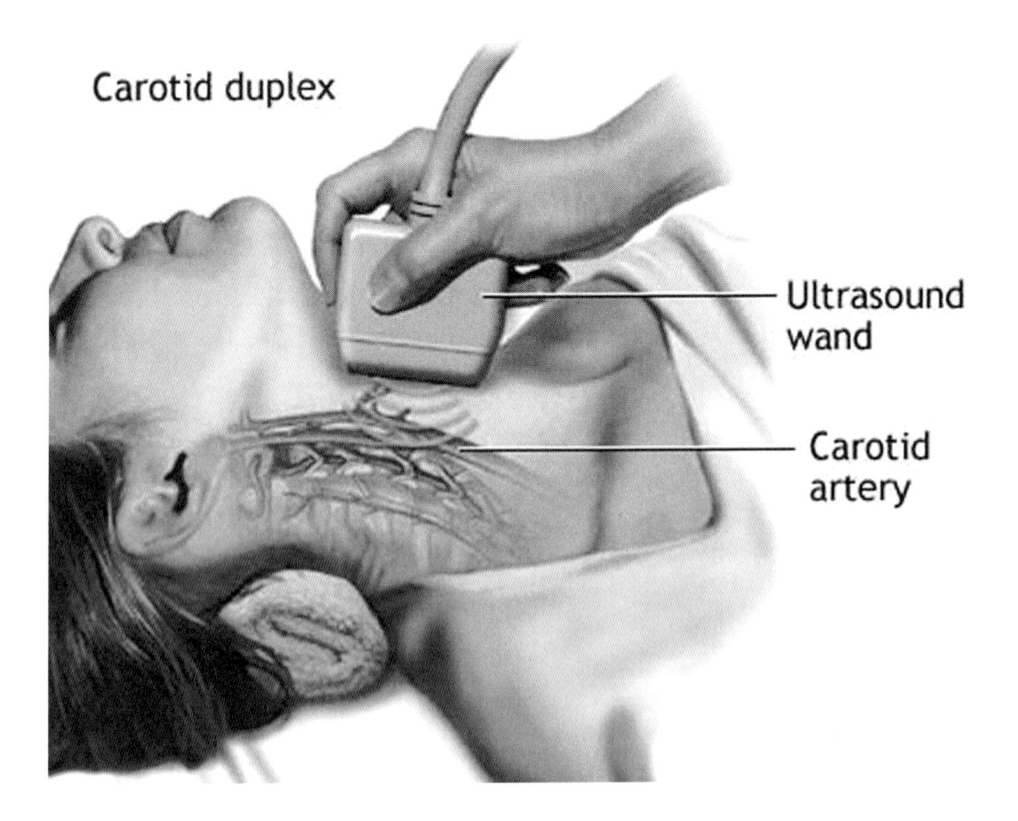

FIGURE 14-16 Vascular Doppler ultrasound procedure.

14.7 ULTRASOUND SYSTEM BLOCK DIAGRAM

A Texas Instruments block diagram for the transmission and reception of the ultrasound signal is shown in **Figure 14-17.** The ultrasound pulse is generated and transmitted from each of the 8 to 512 transducer elements. The timing and magnitude of the pulse is scaled and just after transmission of these pulses, these transducer elements switch to the receive mode. The frequencies range from 1 mHz to 15 mHz.

The strong amplitude echoes reflect surface body area (near fields) while the weak amplitude echoes reflect deeper areas (far fields) within the body. Stronger echoes need little amplification while the echoes received from the far fields must be amplified by 1,000 times or more. In the block diagram of **Figure 14-17,** the low noise amplifier (LNA) is a special gallium-arsenide circuit used in the amplification process. The analog-to-digital converter (ADC) is a 10- to 12-bit converter and the digital signal processing (DSP) chip is interfaced to the user.

Ultrasound Transducers

Commonly used ultrasound transducers, also called scanheads or ultrasound probes, are mechanical, annular, or vector transducers, and each type has a specific use in the imaging and Doppler techniques. **Figure 14-18** shows a few examples of transducers. These are linear, phased, and curved linear types of transducers.

The quartz piezoelectric crystal is used most commonly in ultrasound transducers. Other types of crystals used are ammonium dihydrogen phosphate (ADP) and lead zirconate titanate (PZT). For maximum power output, the crystal is cut to half the wavelength ($\lambda/2$)

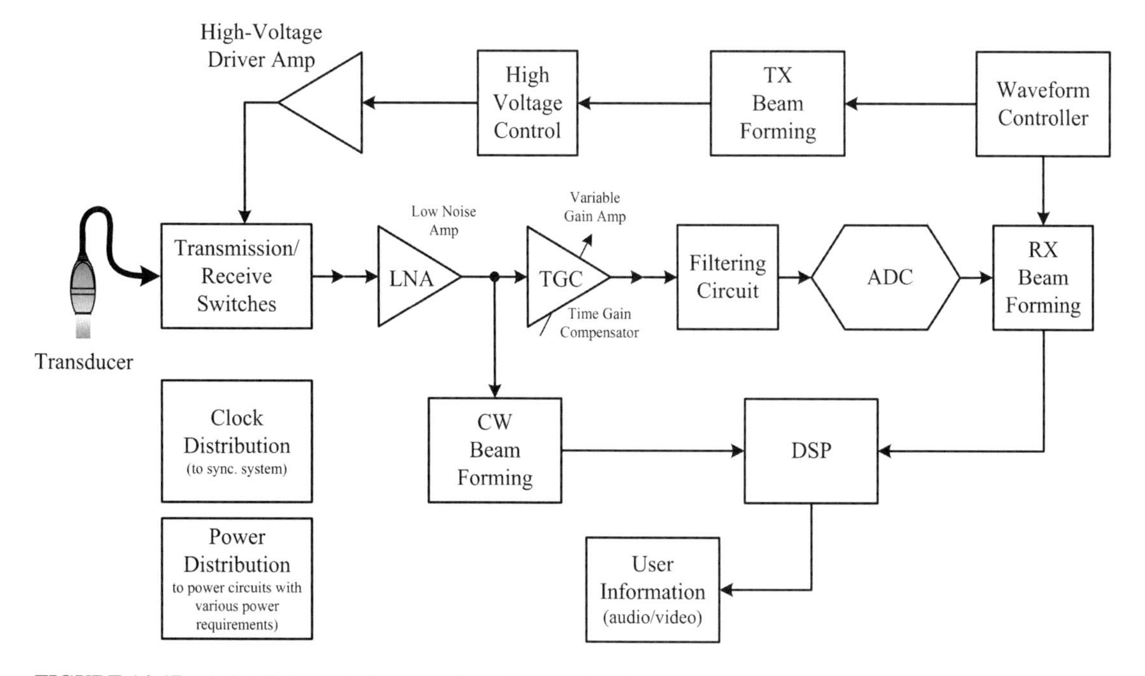

FIGURE 14-17 A detailed block diagram of an ultrasound system.

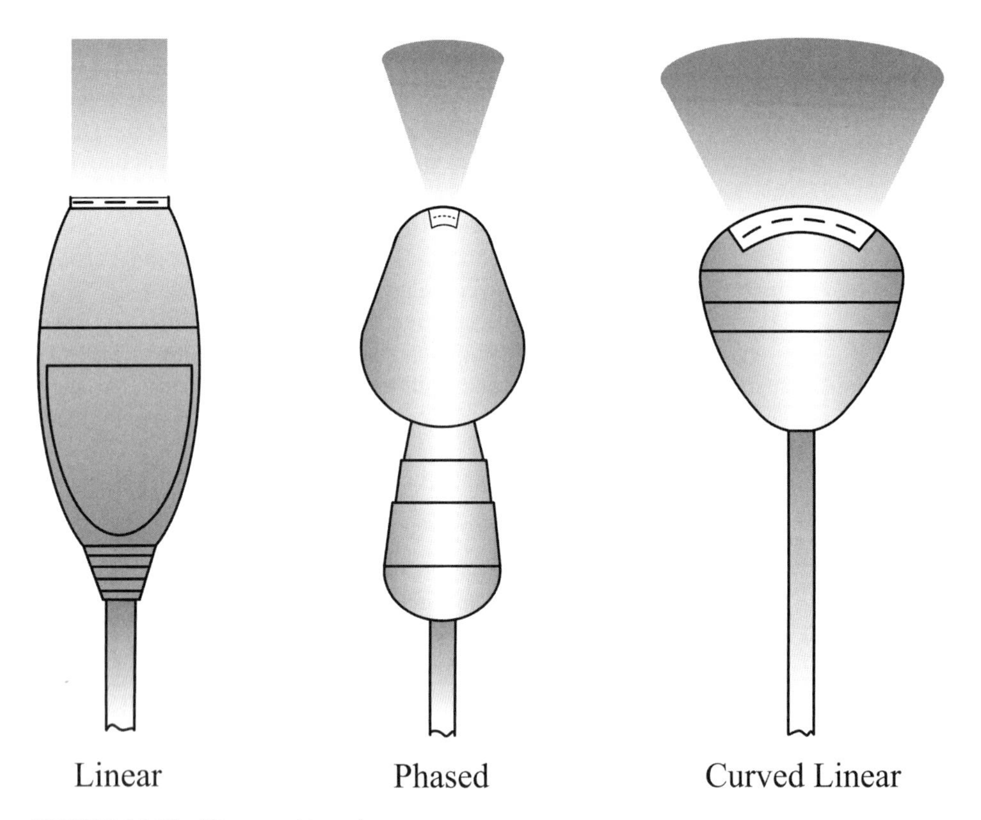

FIGURE 14-18 Ultrasound transducers.

of the ultrasound signal, and for impedance matching between the transducer and the skin surface, gel is placed between the two. The acoustic impedance of the gel is then adjusted by changing its viscosity (diluting with additional oil), thereby matching the overall impedance with the skin.

The piezoelectric effect for the human-made or natural crystals allows materials to vibrate when voltage is applied. It also creates a voltage when deformed due to pressure changes. This property is the basis of imaging transducers.

There are different methods in naming transducers. Some manufacturers include the various arrangements of crystals and the frequency range in the name. For example, P12-5 means a phased array transducer in the frequency range of 12 MHz to 5 MHz.

Similarly,

- L6-4 means linear with range of 6 MHz to 4 MHz.
- C8-5 means curved with range of 8 MHz to 5 MHz.
- S12 means sector transducer with the highest operating frequency of 12 MHz.

14.8 ACUSON SEQUOIA 512 ULTRASOUND SYSTEM

Figure 14-19a shows a full view of the Acuson Sequoia 512 Ultrasound System. Various modes of imaging are possible with this machine: two-dimensional, M-mode, color Doppler, pulsed wave spectral Doppler, and continuous wave spectral Doppler. **Figure 14-19b** shows the keyboard of the Acuson system.

The scans in **Figure 14-20a** and **Figure 14-20b** show the two-dimensional display of an image of the tissues that lie within the scan plane. Note the data fields in each image providing specific information about the transducer and the time and date.

M-mode: Displays a graphic representation of a line of interest (within the two-dimensional image) and displays a graph that shows how that line changes over time. In the image shown in **Figure 14-20b,** it documents the cardiac functions and precisely measures the chamber dimensions.

Spectral Doppler: Allows the monitoring of the blood flow through vessels or within the heart.

Color Doppler: Real-time spatial visualization of blood flow patterns in the heart and discrete vessels.

Figure 14-21a provides the information on array transducers and **Figure 14-21b** shows the Acuson transducer formats in imaging.

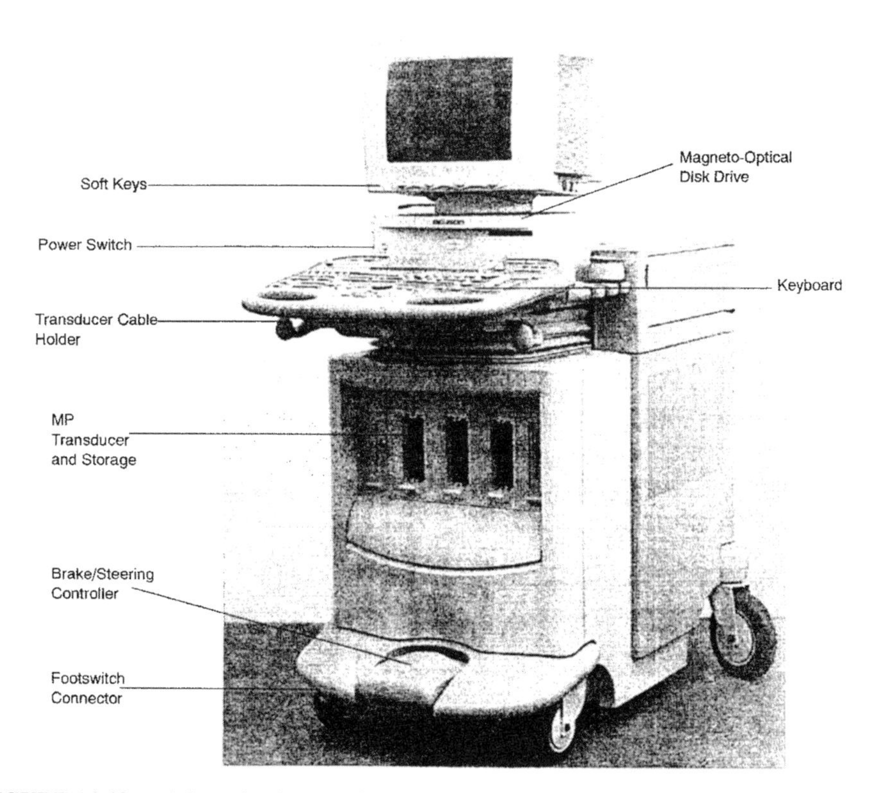

FIGURE 14-19a A Sequoia ultrasound machine.

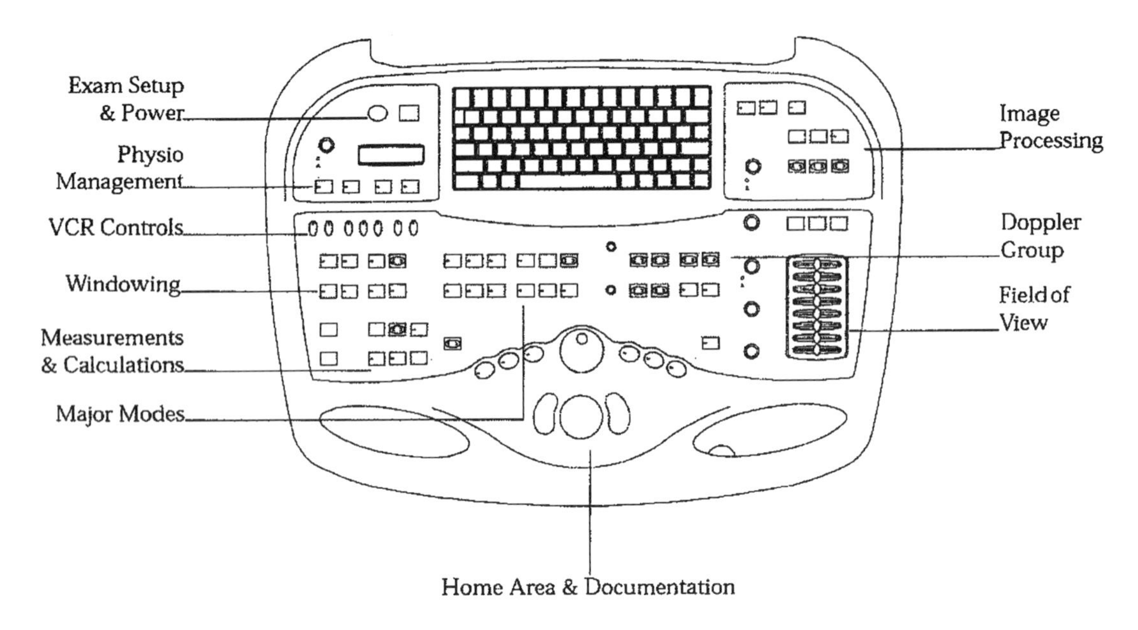

FIGURE 14-19b The keyboard of the Sequoia ultrasound machine.

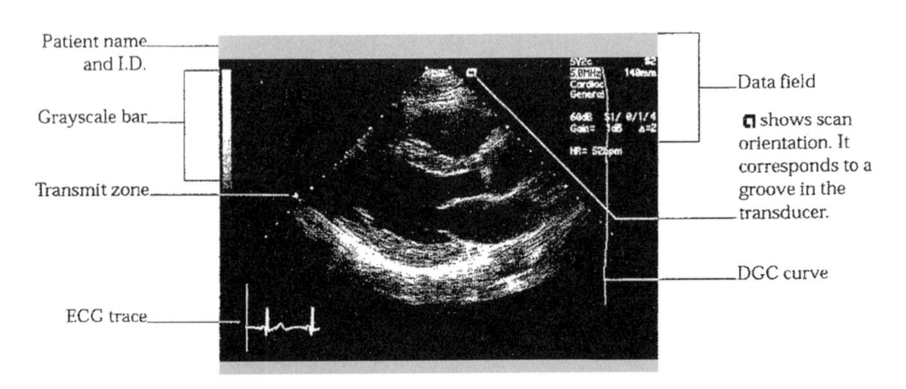

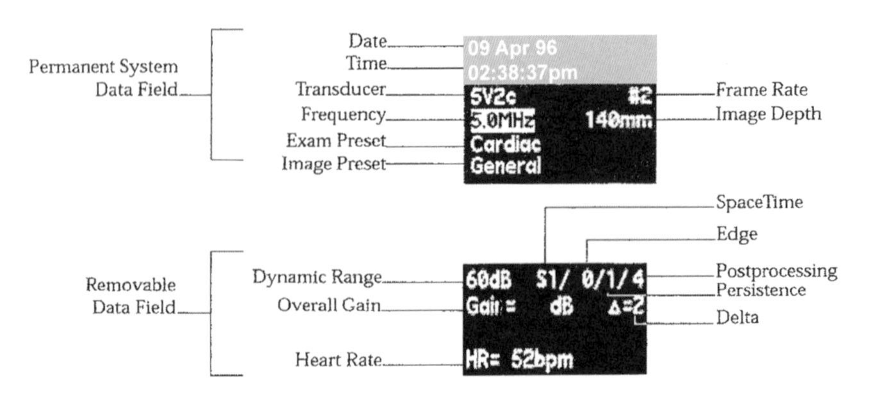

FIGURE 14-20a The data field display of the Sequoia ultrasound machine.

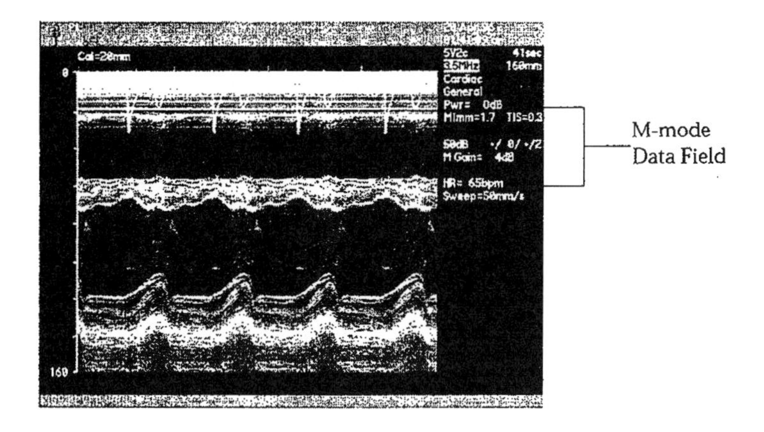

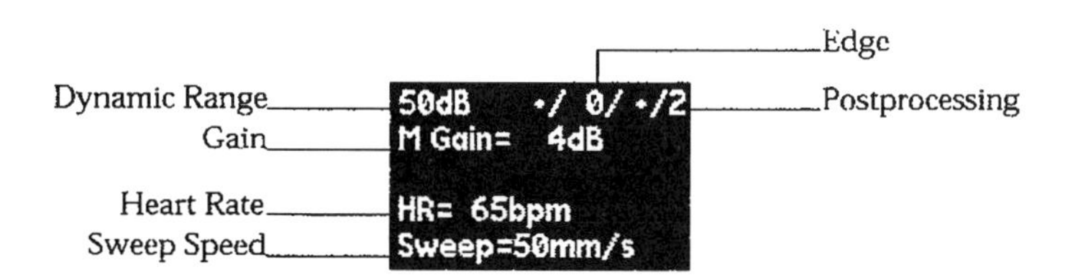

FIGURE 14-20b A display of an ultrasound image on the Sequoia ultrasound machine.

Format	Description
Linear Array	A linear transducer has a medium to large footprint that uses parallel ultrasound scan lines that are perpendicular to the face of the transducer to produce a rectangular image. Linear transducers usually have a large footprint, thus they typically produce a wide near field of view.
Vector Wide View Array	Vector is Acuson's trademark for its proprietary omni-steerable, omni-originating image formation technology. A Vector wide view array transducer forms ultrasound scan lines that can originate from any point on the transducer face and can be steered in any direction. A Vector wide view array transducer has a small footprint for imaging when access is difficult, however the near field image width is almost as wide as the transducer footprint. Vector wide view array transducers allow access in areas where underlying structures may create an obstruction, such as in intercostal scans.
Curved Array	A high-performance curved array transducer forms ultrasound scan lines that are perpendicular to the face of the transducer. Because the face of the transducer is curved, it produces an image with a wider far field than near field.

FIGURE 14-21a M-mode display on the Sequoia ultrasound machine.

General Applications Transducer Specifications

Transducer Format	Imaging Format	Footprint Size	Use	Frequency (MHz)				
				2D	PW	CW	CD	M-mode
5C2	Curved linear array	66 mm	Abdomen, Fetal, Ob/Gyn	5.0 3.5 2.5	2.5	—	5.0 3.5 2.5	5.0 3.5 2.5
8L5	Linear array	38 mm	Small parts, Vascular, Intraoperative	8.0 7.0 6.0 5.0	4.0	—	7.0 5.0 4.0	8.0 7.0 6.0 5.0
EV-8C4	Curved linear array	29 mm	Endovaginal	8.0 7.0 5.0 4.0	5.0	—	7.0 6.0 5.0 4.0	8.0 7.0 5.0 4.0
4V2	Vector array	28 mm	Abdomen, Ob/Gyn	4.0 3.5 2.5	3.5	—	4.0 3.5 2.5	4.0 3.5 2.5
8C4	Curved linear array	44 mm	OB, Neonate, Abdomen, Pediatrics	8.0 6.5 5.0	4.0	—	7.0 6.0 5.0 4.0	8.0 6.5 5.0

FIGURE 14–21b A table of ultrasound transducers for the Sequoia ultrasound machine.

SUMMARY

Medical ultrasound is based on two principles: 1) Reflections from interfaces and 2) Doppler effects due to motions within the body. This chapter presents these principles through physics and the imaging techniques of ultrasound.

1. Ultrasound physics is explained in terms of mechanical wave theory, acoustic impedance, reflection, and refraction. Attenuation and absorption in muscles and bones are also explained in this section. The acoustic impedance of a material is defined as the product of its density and ultrasound velocity. The impedance determines the transmission and reflection of ultrasound at the boundary of two materials. Attenuation is the reduction in amplitude and intensity of the ultrasound beam as a function of distance through the imaging medium.
2. Next, the theory of the Doppler ultrasound is given in some detail. The emphasis is on the detection of the blood flow by bouncing ultrasound off red blood cells. Doppler ultrasound can estimate how fast blood flows by measuring the rate of change in its pitch (frequency).

3. A block diagram of an ultrasound system is provided explaining the components of transmission and reception.
4. Various modes of ultrasound scans are provided. However, a greater concentration on two-dimensional scans extending into M-mode scans is the main focus in this section.
5. The application of ultrasound in an echocardiogram and in vascular Doppler is also covered in this chapter.
6. Ultrasound machines, particularly Acuson Sequoia ultrasound systems, are described in some detail in this chapter.

MEDICAL TERMINOLOGY

The following is a list of medical terminology mentioned in this chapter.

Attenuation: the reduction in amplitude and intensity of a signal. Usually, it is measured in decibels as a signal strength that varies with distances.

Doppler ultrasound: a technique that uses reflected high-frequency sound waves to measure the blood flow in a vessel to identify narrowing (stenosis) or clots. A transducer is passed over blood vessels, and the movement of blood cells in the vessels causes a change in the frequency of the sound waves that can be used to generate a picture.

Duplex ultrasound: a technique that uses Doppler and conventional ultrasound to observe blood flow in vessels and organs. A computer converts the sound waves into a two-dimensional image to produce information on the speed and direction of blood flow.

Echo: effect that occurs when sound waves reflect back to a source. For example, echocardiography is an ultrasonic diagnostic procedure used to assess the structure and motion of the heart.

Echocardiogram: the record that is produced by echocardiography. An image of the heart and surrounding tissues is produced by using high frequency sound waves.

Echocardiography: the use of ultrasound imaging to analyze the structures and motion of the heart; sometimes referred to as ECHO. The resulting test is used as a diagnostic tool to detect abnormalities and infections of the heart.

Echoencephalography: the use of ultrasound imaging to analyze midline structures of the brain. The procedure can detect abscesses, blood clots, injury, or tumors.

Reflection: the return of beams, rays, or sound from a surface; a mirror image.

Refraction: the ability of a lens to bend light rays to help focus on a particular point. Used in eye examinations to evaluate an eye's refractive error to determine the best corrective lenses needed.

Resolution: level of detail in a system to distinguish, detect, and/or record details to discern an image or object.

Ultrasonic tomography: technique in which acoustic pulses are released from an acoustoelectric transducer to produce an image used in mapping and identifying information about the structures and functions of organs and tissues.

Ultrasound: high frequency range of sound waves (over 20,000 kHz) that is inaudible to humans. Ultrasound has different velocities in different types of tissue, which allows for uses in imaging processes and physical therapy for musculoskeletal injuries.

Wavelength: the distance between replicating units in a wave pattern. A wavelength is measured from the crest of one wave to the crest of the next wave.

QUIZ

1. The range of ultrasound frequencies is called:
   a) Resolution.
   b) Sampling rate.
   c) Characteristic.
   d) Bandwidth.
2. Which of the following statements is not true in ultrasound transmission?
   a) Ultrasound is a sound wave greater than 20 kHz.
   b) Ultrasound cannot travel in a vacuum.
   c) Ultrasound travels with the same speed in tissues, muscles, and bones.
   d) Ultrasound energy decreases as it travels through the body.
3. A better resolution is detected when the ultrasound transducer is placed:
   a) At an angle over the muscle.
   b) Directly over the muscle.
   c) Over the bone-muscle interface.
   d) None of the above.
4. Ultrasound absorption is directly proportional to:
   a) The ultrasound frequency.
   b) The density of the structure.
   c) The characteristic impedance of the structure.
   d) All of the above.
5. Ultrasound transducers use:
   a) Silica material. b) In-organic material.
   c) Piezoelectric crystals. d) Bi-metal layers.
6. Ultrasound velocity in air is approximately:
   a) 1,540 m/sec. b) 1,450 m/sec.
   c) 330 m/sec. d) 4,020 m/sec.
7. True or False: Ultrasound velocity in bone is less than in the brain.
   a) True b) False
8. True or False: As far as acoustics are concerned, soft tissue behaves as a liquid.
   a) True b) False

9. Gel is used to provide an air-free contact for an ultrasound transducer because:

a) Moving it over the skin is easier.

b) Air absorbs ultrasound.

c) Air reflects ultrasound back to the transducer.

d) It keeps the transducer warm.

10. A certain phenomenon occurs at ultrasound intensities that do not occur at intensities below this threshold:

a) 3 W/cm^2 b) 0.3 W/cm^2

c) 1 W/cm^2 d) 30 W/cm^2

PROBLEMS

1. If 4 W/cm^2 of ultrasound power is incident on the fat-bone interface, how much of the power is reflected back to the transducer?

2. If 2 W/cm^2 ultrasound wave is incident on the muscle-bone interface, determine the reflected power in watts and the pressure of the reflected wave in N/m^2.

3. What is the wavelength of an ultrasound signal having a velocity of 1,500 m/sec. at 2.5 MHz?

4. Compute the reflection coefficient of the ultrasound wave at the interface of muscle and bone, given:

a) Muscle density = 1.07 g/cm^3. b) Speed in muscle = 1,580 m/sec.

c) Bone density = 1.82 g/cm^3. d) Speed in bone = 4,000 m/sec.

5. Find the refractive angle, θr, for the ultrasound beam at the muscle-bone interface, shown in Figure 14-22.

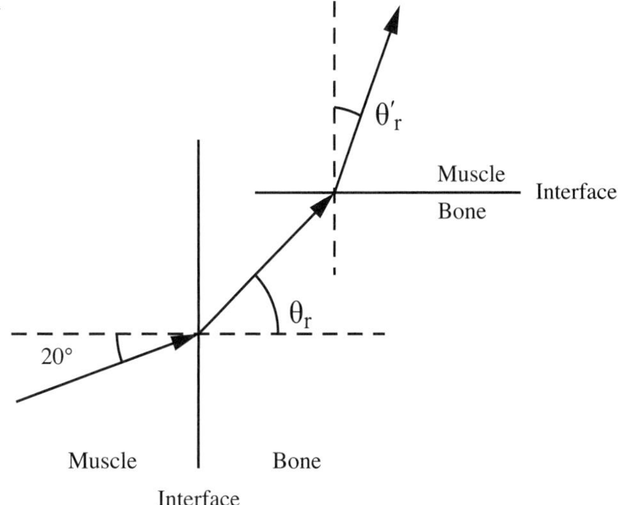

Figure 14-22 Refractions of an ultrasound wave.

Velocity of the ultrasound in muscle = 1,500 m/sec.

Velocity of the ultrasound in bone = 4,000 m/sec.

$\theta in = 20°$.

6. In a Doppler ultrasound system, the blood velocity is indicated as 2 m/sec. Find the transducer angle θ, given:

$$\text{Transducer transmit frequency} = 2\ \text{MHz.}$$
$$\text{Receiver transmit frequency} = 2.1\ \text{MHz.}$$
$$\text{Velocity of the ultrasound in blood} = 1{,}500\ \text{m/sec.}$$

7. Find the attenuation in decibels, when an ultrasound propagates with 7 W/cm^2 in one medium and with 0.5 W/cm^2 in another medium.

8. Compare the effect of bone and air on ultrasonic imaging. Show the changes in reflection and absorption when ultrasound passes through bone and air.

9. Discuss the advantages and disadvantages, such as resolution, cost, and efficiency, of two-dimensional and three-dimensional ultrasound imaging techniques. You may visit a hospital or use the Internet to gather information to answer the problem.

10. Discuss the advantages and disadvantages of B-mode and M-mode ultrasound imaging techniques.

CASE STUDIES

1. A 60-year-old woman was experiencing pelvic pain. Her gynecologist did a pelvic exam and looked for any sign of infection. The doctor then placed a small ultrasound probe inside the vagina and generated ultrasound images. The ultrasound exam confirmed the doctor's suspicion of infection. In this case:

a) What type of ultrasound was used?

b) Many times this type of ultrasound exam will show fibroids or cysts. How can an infection be differentiated from fibroids or cysts?

c) What is laparoscopy?

d) Is ultrasound used in the treatment of pelvic pain? Explain.

2. Roger, age 55, was having difficulty breathing during exercise, and sometimes, experiencing chest discomfort with any type of increased physical activity. He also noticed he was tiring easily. Roger was hospitalized and batteries of tests were performed. An ECG and chest X-ray proved inconclusive, but an echocardiogram confirmed that Roger had mitral stenosis. He did not need any surgery but he was put on medications immediately.

a) What is mitral stenosis and what are the other symptoms, not including the symptoms Roger was presenting?

b) For what reasons did Roger's ECG and x-ray exam results come out inconclusive for mitral stenosis?

c) Why was an MRI not done?

d) Could Doppler ultrasound have detected this disease?

RESEARCH TOPICS

1. How is ultrasound used in detecting aortoiliac occlusive disease?
   a) Present a research area that engages the reader in the research data on the subject. This is a peripheral arterial disease (PAD) and Doppler ultrasound is widely used for diagnosis.
   b) The paper may include a comparison study of other devices or instruments in detecting aortoiliac occlusive disease.
   c) Discuss the various types of transducers used in the medical devices used for detecting this disease.
2. With high-resolution transducers, the transesophageal echocardiogram (TEE) can assess the results of the transthoracic surgery by obtaining good images when the patient still has a fresh thoracotomy scar and is ventilated artificially.
   a) The research topic must include the vast uses of TEE in surgery, particularly in cardiac surgery.
   b) Discuss M-mode, color M-mode, and color Doppler imaging modes.

CHAPTER 15

Instrumentation in Medical Imaging

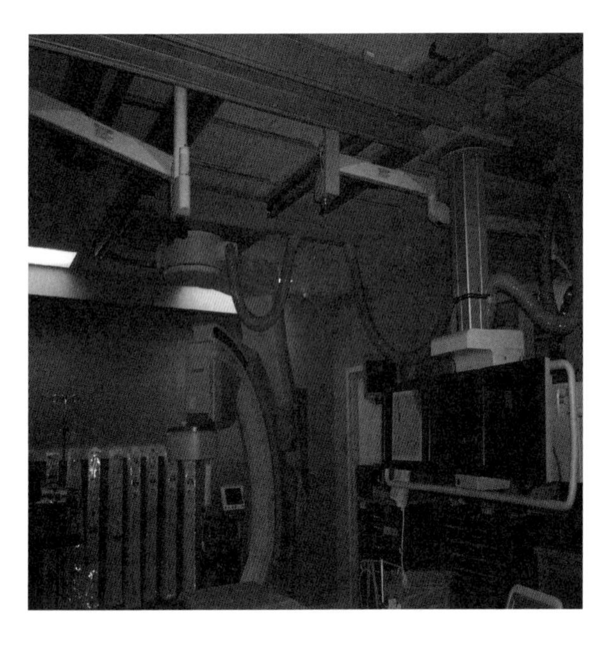

■ CHAPTER OUTLINE

Introduction

15.1 The X-ray Machine

15.2 Physics of X-rays

15.3 Characteristics of X-rays

15.4 X-ray Equations

15.5 Safety Issues with X-ray Radiation: Regulations in Hospitals

15.6 X-ray Images and Data

15.7 Vertical Bucky Stand

15.8 Computer Tomography: Principles and Scans

15.9 Fluoroscopy

15.10 Nuclear Medicine

15.11 Positron Emission Tomography

15.12 Magnetic Resonance Imaging

■ OBJECTIVES

The objective of this chapter is to familiarize the reader with the theory and instrumentation in radiological systems and machines such as X-ray, CT, MRI, and nuclear medicine machines.

Upon completion of this chapter, the reader will be able to:

- Compute X-ray intensity and power.
- Describe the components of an X-ray machine.
- Explain the process of X-ray generation.
- Compare X-ray and computer tomography machines.

- Compare X-ray and fluoroscopic machines.
- Discuss components of a magnetic resonance imaging machine.
- Describe the process of nuclear medicine in positron emission tomography scanners.

INTERNET WEB SITES

http://www.doh.wa.gov Department of Health, Washington State
http://www.mrisafety.com Institute for Magnetic Resonance Safety, Education & Research

INTRODUCTION

The history of medical imaging can be traced back to 1895, when Wilhelm Konrad Roentgen discovered the X-ray. Since then, medical imaging has become an important branch of medical science concerned with radiation devices for the purpose of obtaining visual information of organs, body fractures, the structure of the intestines, tumors, and much more. Traditionally, the technology of radiology included X-rays, computer tomography (CT), and nuclear medicine for medical diagnoses and treatment; however, today radiology includes such technology as ultrasound and magnetic resonance imaging (MRI) and the technology is growing quickly.

This chapter discusses the physics of the X-ray, its application in biomedicine, as well as other important imaging technologies, such as CT, MRI, and nuclear medicine.

15.1 THE X-RAY MACHINE

An x-ray machine is a device used by radiographers to acquire an x-ray image. Wilhelm Konrad Roentgen began observing and documenting X-rays in 1895 while experimenting with vacuum tubes. One of the first x-ray photographs was made of his wife's hand. The image displayed both her wedding ring and bones. A block diagram of an x-ray machine is shown in **Figure 15-1a**. The x-ray tube consists of a cathode and an anode. The cathode is connected to the filament transformer and receives proper filament current to so that it can

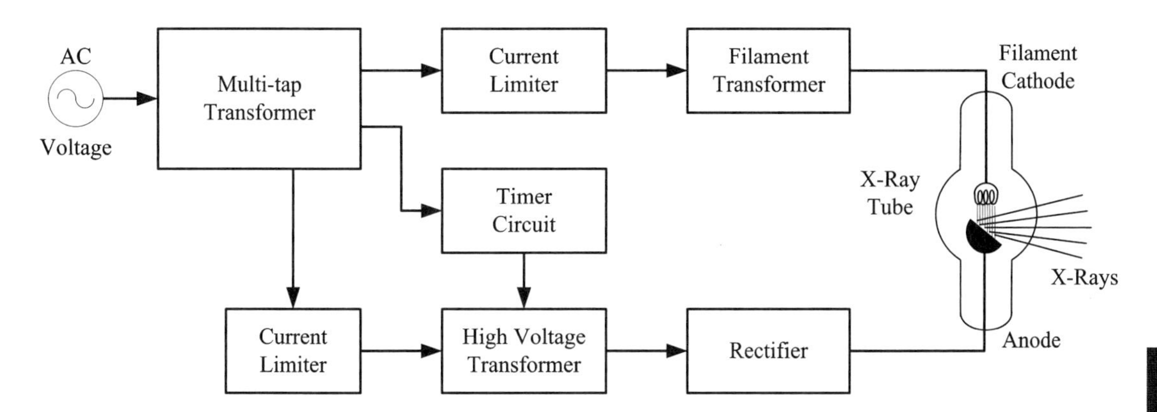

FIGURE 15-1a Block diagram of an x-ray machine.

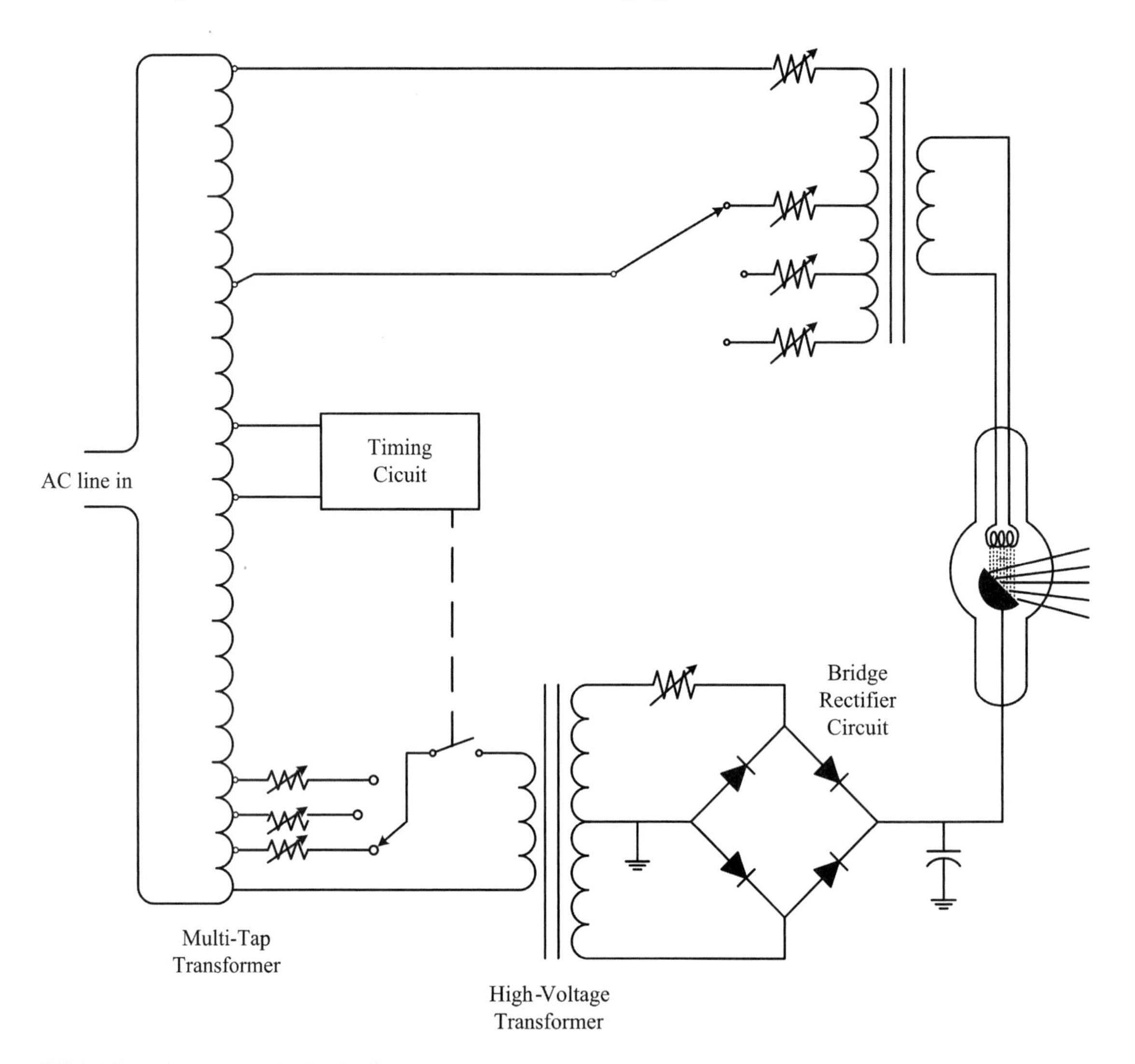

FIGURE 15-1b A simple circuit of an x-ray machine.

emit electrons in the x-ray tube. The anode is on the other side of the tube connected to a bridge rectifier and the high-voltage transformer. The tube current in milliamperes (mA) is then adjusted for the anode to receive the emitted electrons from the cathode. The cathode is negatively charged and the anode is positively charged. In the process of receiving of these electrons at the anode target, X-rays are generated.

In **Figure 15-1b,** a multi-tap transformer is shown. The x-ray equipment is operated from an incoming line of 210 volts (V) to 220 V (rms) and the voltage is then modified to a very high range to produce X-rays. The proper electrical and electronic circuits control the amperage, voltage, exposure, and the efficiency of the x-ray production.

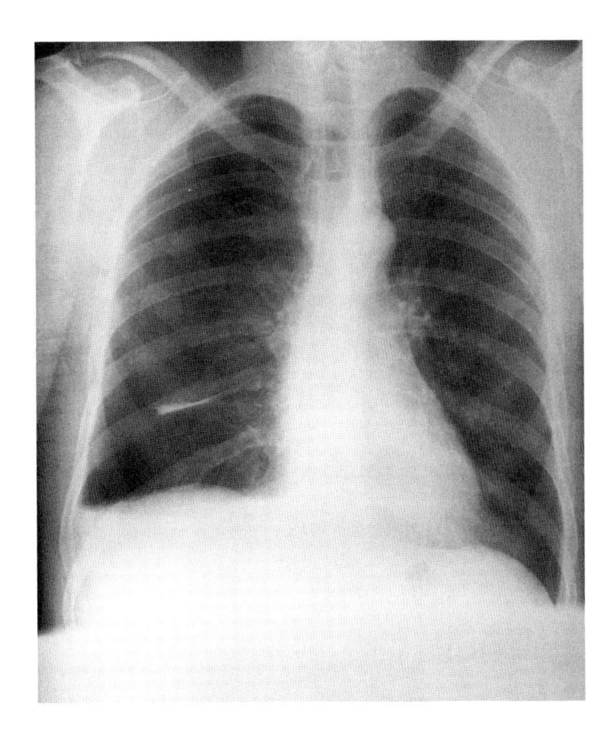

FIGURE 15-2 An x-ray image.

These X-rays can then pass through the human body and strike a photographic film or a screen on the other side of the body to generate an image of bones, muscles, and organs. This image is called an x-ray picture as shown in **Figure 15-2.** When X-rays pass through dense tissues such as bones, the resulting image appears white on the x-ray picture. This is because many of these rays are blocked, or absorbed, by dense tissues. An image in shades of gray is generated when X-rays pass through less dense tissues such as muscles and organs. X-rays that pass through air, such as X-rays of the lungs, will appear black.

15.2 PHYSICS OF X-RAYS

The negatively charged cathode is the source of electrons (e^-) and these electrons are then accelerated toward the anode by the electrical potential difference established between these electrodes (i.e., the cathode and the anode). In **Figure 15-3a,** this is all done in an evacuated glass tube. The accelerated electrons attain kinetic energy and about 1 percent of this kinetic energy is converted into X-rays when electrons impact on the nucleus of the anode target. The law of the conservation of energy is achieved when the kinetic energy of these electrons is lost but converted into x-ray photon radiation.

Figure 15-3b shows the path of the incident electrons to the anode target atom and the release of X-rays. This process is called the bremsstrahlung process. This is a German word meaning "braking radiation." The closest is the approach to the nucleus of the atom, the result is the loss of all of the electron's kinetic energy and the production of the maximum-energy X-rays. The radiation depends on the "applied brake" to the electron speed. With the high speed, electrons reach closer to the target and more brake is applied to convert into

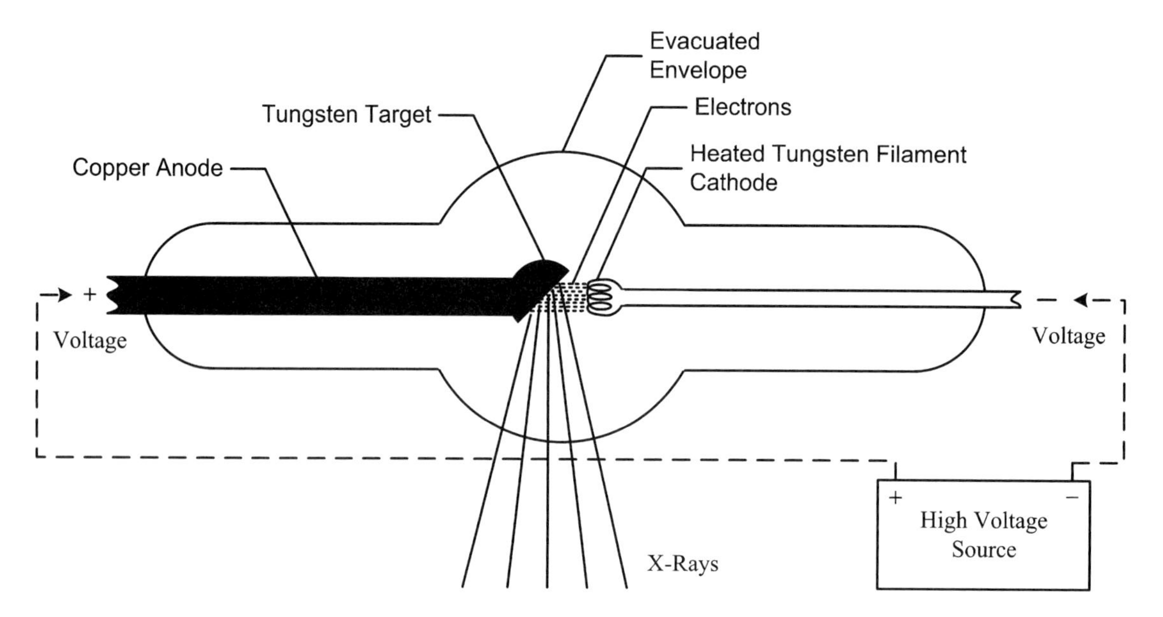

FIGURE 15-3a An x-ray tube.

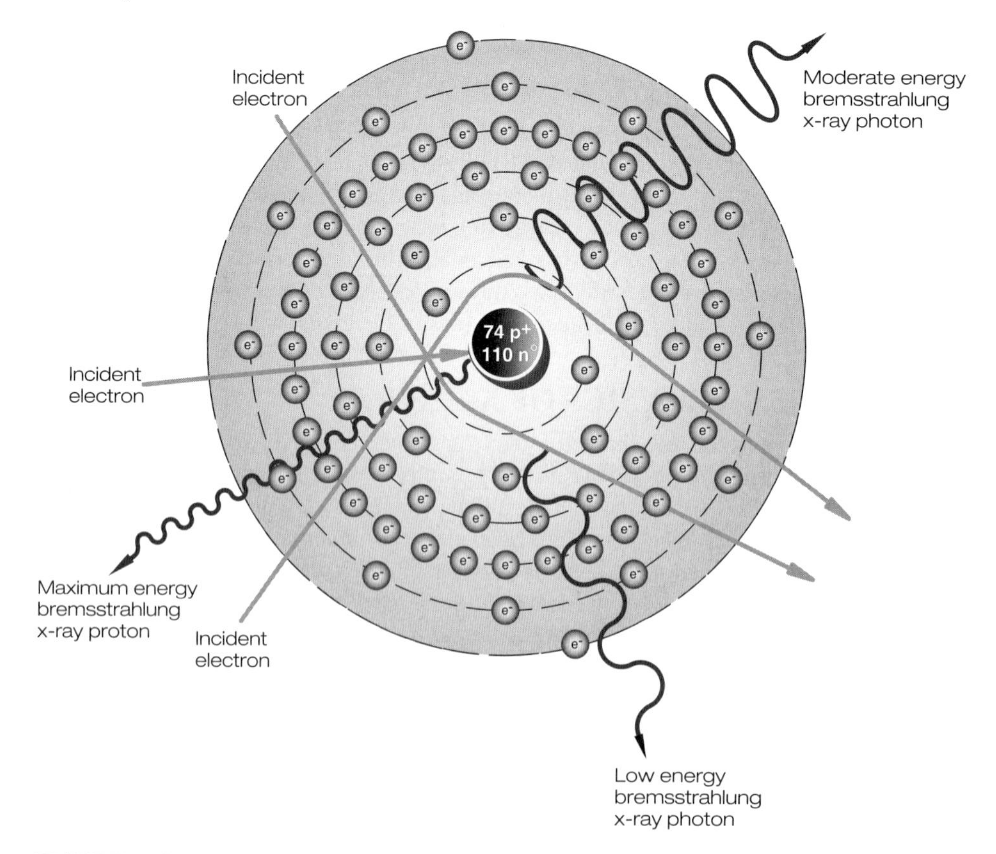

FIGURE 15-3b An x-ray interaction in a tungsten atom.

higher x-ray energy. About 99% of the kinetic energy converts into heat on the collisions of the incoming electrons with the anode target.

15.3 CHARACTERISTICS OF X-RAYS

The electromagnetic spectrum is shown in **Figure 15-4** with the values of energy, frequency, and wavelength given for the various waves. Notice X-rays start at 1 kilo-electronvolt (keV) of energy with a frequency of 10^{17} Hertz (Hz) and a wavelength of 10^{-9} meter (m). The photons of various radiations such as microwaves, visible light, or X-rays, all have sinusoidal electric and magnetic fields and they all travel with the velocity of light.

In an x-ray machine, X-rays contain energies based on the machine's set-up peak voltages (V_p), between cathode and anode. A machine operated on 80 kilovolt peak (kV_p), will generate X-rays with energies from 0 to 80 keV. An eV is the amount of kinetic energy acquired by an electron when it is accelerated through a potential difference of 1 V.

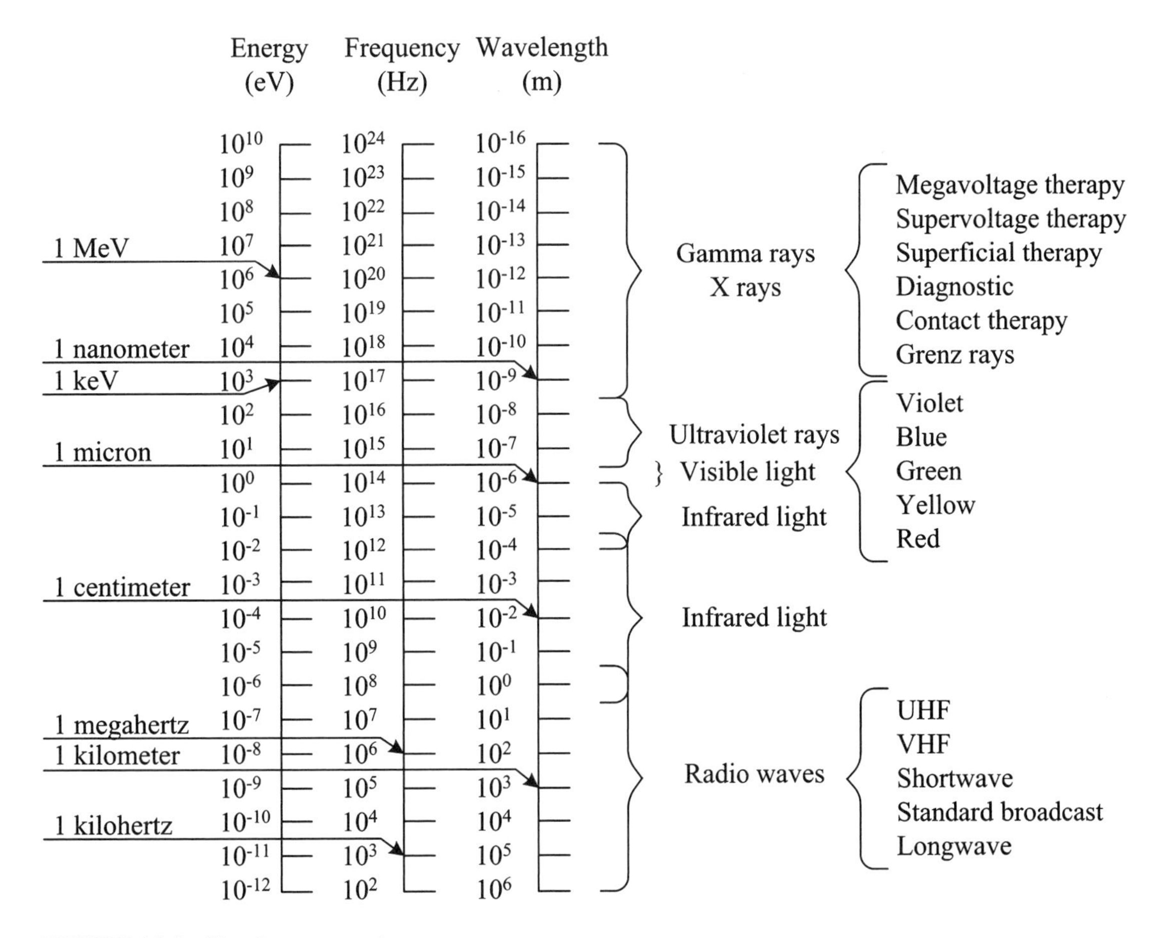

FIGURE 15-4 The electromagnetic spectrum.

The following list contains some of the primary factors in determining x-ray emission and the image quality at the receiving end.

1. The filament circuit has a variable resistor between the incoming line and the step-down transformer. The variable resistance then sets up the mA current for the filament.
2. The kV_P voltage selection is done at the autotransformer and it is meant to deliver high voltage to the anode circuit.
3. The x-ray emission (i.e., number of x-ray photons) depends on the milliamperage (mA) of the tube circuit, milliamperage time in seconds (mAs), and the kV_P. The milliampere seconds is the milliamperage multiplied by a set time measured in seconds. It indicates how many X-rays will be produced and for how long. An example is 100 mA × 0.2 sec = 20 mAs.
4. Although the kV_P is the primary controller of the differences in radiographic image densities, the mAs and the distance between the x-ray tube and the (film/screen) image receptor greatly affect the image quality.
5. In addition to the main switch and the circuit breakers, the exposure switch is a remote control switch that begins the exposure and the timer switch that ends the exposure. The exposure switch is depressed halfway to activate the rotating anode, and then depressed completely to initiate the x-ray exposure. To prevent the exposure from continuing, releasing the switch terminates the exposure.
6. The timer switch is capable of short exposure with a small delay. The timer circuit has a silicon-controlled rectifier (SCR) that triggers the exposure and the programmed microprocessor circuit to calculate the length of time the current can flow through the x-ray circuit.
7. The filament circuit gets its power from the main circuit power supply, and its current control device, then regulates the mA_S supplied to the filament of the x-ray tube. The mA ratings are in proper steps between 50 mA to over 1 ampere (A).

15.4 X-RAY EQUATIONS

Several equations follow to relate the x-ray intensity and exposure in milli-roentgen (mR) for imaging purposes.

X-ray Exposure mA and kV_P

The x-ray exposure changes based on the inverse square law given as:

$$\frac{I_1}{I_2} = \frac{D_2^2}{D_1^2}$$

or

$$I_1 \times D_1^2 = I_2 \times D_2^2$$

where I_1 = original intensity of radiation at a distance of D_1
and

I_2 = a new intensity at a new distance of D_2.

The inverse square law states that the intensity of radiation in mR at a given distance (from the point of the source) is inversely proportional to the square of the distance. Hence, if a distance increases by a factor of three, the intensity would decrease by nine times.

Let's determine the following: If an x-ray exposure of 200 mR is recorded at a distance of 15 inches, what is the exposure in mR at a distance of 30 inches?

In the following example,

$$I_1 = 200 \text{ mR}$$
$$D_1 = 30 \text{ inches}$$

thus,

$$I_2 = I_1 \times \frac{D_1^2}{D_2^2}$$

$$I_2 = 200 \times \frac{15^2}{30^2} = 50 \text{ mR}$$

One of the primary controlling factors of the x-ray intensity and the radiographic film density is mAs, the direct square law is applied to adjust mAs to maintain film density. As the distance increases, the intensity decreases which causes a decrease in exposure to the image receptor. This causes the image to appear less dense. The film density can be controlled by adjusting the mAs as shown in the following formula:

$$\frac{mAs_1}{mAs_2} = \frac{D_1^2}{D_2^2}$$

If the radiograph is taken at a distance of 15 inches and the x-ray tube is operating at 20 mAs and 80 kV_P, then the x-ray tube's amperage will increase to 80 mAs at a distance of 30 inches, provided the radiographic film is of the same density.

Similarly, changing the kV_P affects radiation intensity by the square of the ratios of the kilovoltage peaks. The formula for kV_P and the radiation intensity is given as:

$$\frac{(kV_{P1})^2}{(kV_{P2})^2} = \frac{I_1}{I_2}$$

If kV_P produces an intensity of 200 mR, then 200 kV_P will increase intensity to 800 mR (four times more) if no other factors have changed.

Electromagnetic Radiation

Electromagnetic radiation at high frequencies acts like a small bundle of energy, called photon or quantum energy. This is X-ray energy radiated when electrons collide at the annode. The photon energy and the frequency of the radiation are then directly proportional, given as:

$$E_p = h\nu$$

E_p = photon energy in eV

h = Planck's constant $(4.15 \times 10^{-15}$ eV-sec$) = 6.625 \times 10^{-34}$ joules-sec

ν = Photon frequency in hertz

The frequency of an X-ray can be calculated using the above formula when photon energy is given. The frequency of 80 keV x-ray photon is given as:

$$\nu = \frac{E_P}{h}$$

$$\nu = \frac{80 \text{ keV}}{4.15 \times 10^{-15} \text{ eV-sec}}$$

$$\nu = 1.92 \times 10^{19} \text{ Hz}$$

Cooling Time for an X-Ray Tube

In an x-ray tube, the anode must take time to cool sufficiently before the next exposure is made. An anode cooling chart is provided in terms of radiographic heat units. The heat unit (HU) is calculated as $kV_P \times mA \times$ time of exposure $\times$ heat unit constant. The analog cooling curve is an exponentially decaying curve with respect to time.

EXAMPLE How many heat units are generated by an exposure of 100 kV_P, 100 mA for a 0.1 second exposure in a single-phase and three-phase x-ray machine? Given the HU constant is 1.00 and 1.35 in a single-phase and three-phase unit, respectively.

Answer:

In the single-phase unit

$$100 \text{ kV}_P \times 100 \text{ mA} \times 0.1 \text{ second} \times 1.00 = 1{,}000 \text{ HU}$$

In the three-phase unit

$$100 \text{ kV}_P \times 100 \text{ mA} \times 0.1 \text{ second} \times 1.35 = 1{,}350 \text{ HU}$$

■

Radiation Intensity

Radiation intensity varies in direct relationship with the mAs and the square of KV_P, and inversely with the square of the distance. The formula is given as:

$$I = \frac{(mA) \times (kV_P)^2}{d^2}$$

X-Ray Exposure

A typical mR/mA reading is recorded for each kV_P and it estimates the entrance exposure to the skin or to the organ of interest. A measurement of mR/mA is recorded typically for an image receptor distance (SID) of 40 inches (100 cm). The inverse square law is then applied to determine the exposure for the source to entrance skin distance. The following formula explains the relationships:

$$\frac{mR_1}{mR_2} = \frac{SOD^2}{SID^2}$$

Where,

$$\begin{aligned} SID &= SOD + OID \\ SID &= \text{Source to image receptor distance} \\ SOD &= \text{Source to object distance} \\ OID &= \text{Object to image receptor distance} \end{aligned}$$

mR_1 and mR_2 are exposures at different distances. If $kV_P = 100$, mR/mA = 6, mA = 30 at a SID of 100 cm, then:
Exposure at 100 cm is

$$\text{Exposure at 100 cm} = 6\frac{mR}{mA} \times 30\ mA$$

$$\text{i.e. Exposure at 100 cm} = 180\ mR$$

SOD is calculated as

$$SOD = SID - OID = 100\ cm - 40\ cm = 60\ cm$$

$$\frac{mR_1}{mR_2} = \frac{SOD^2}{SID^2} = \frac{60^2\ cm^2}{100^2\ cm^2}$$

$$\frac{180\ mR}{mR_2} = \frac{60 \times 60}{100 \times 100}$$

thus,

$$mR_2 = 180 \times \frac{10{,}000}{3{,}600}$$

$$mR_2 = 500\ mR$$

In **Figure 15-5,** the (SID = SOD + OID) distances are shown. The computation of mR_2 is done based on the given value of mR_1.

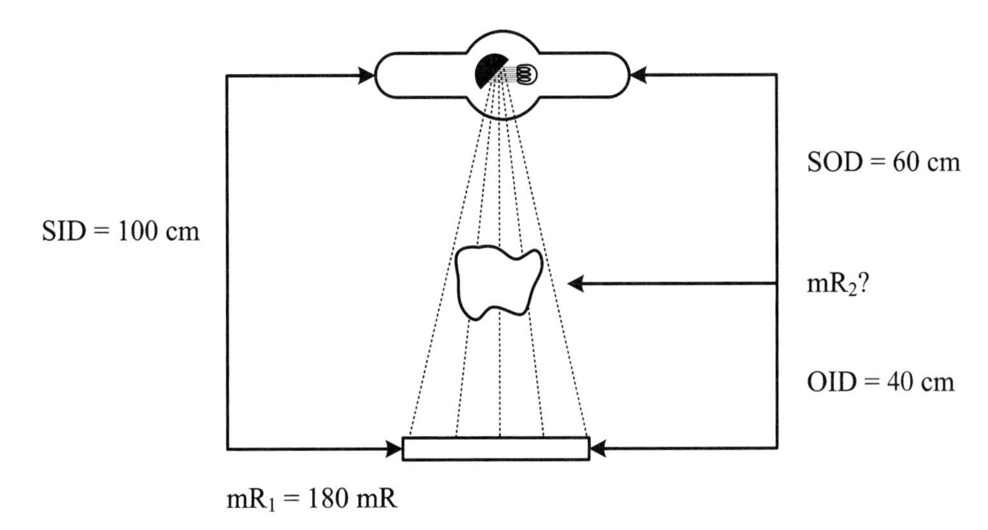

FIGURE 15-5 Image distances.

Half-Value Layer

Half-value layer (HVL) is defined as the thickness required for a material to reduce the power of an x-ray beam to one half its original value. In general, there is an exponential relationship between the number of incident photons (N_O) and those that transmitted (N) through thickness x without interaction, given as:

$$N = N_O e^{-\mu x}$$

Where,

μ = mass (density of the material included) attenuation coefficient of the material in cm^{-1}

when,

$$N = \frac{N_O}{2}, \; x = HVL$$

resulting in,

$$\frac{N_O}{2} = N_O \times e^{-\mu \times (HVL)}$$

simplifying to

$$HVL = \frac{0.693}{\mu}$$

If a material of 5 mm thickness allows only 30% of photons in an x-ray beam, first the μ is calculated and then the HVL of the beam. Assume $N_O = 1$, $N = \frac{30}{100}$, so:

$$\frac{30}{100} = 1 \times e^{-\mu(0.5\text{ cm})}$$
$$\ell n(0.3) = -\mu(0.5\text{ cm})$$
$$\frac{-(\ell n(0.3))}{0.5\text{ cm}} = \mu$$
$$2.40\text{ cm}^{-1} = \mu$$

thus,

$$HVL = \frac{0.693}{\mu}$$
$$HVL = \frac{0.693}{2.40}$$
$$HVL = 0.288875\text{ cm}$$

This suggests that the material thickness of 0.28 cm will reduce the number of photons by 50%.

Energy of the Electron

The energy of the electron when it strikes the anode is given in electronvolts (eV) and the formula is given as:

$E_E = e \times$ anode voltage
$e =$ the negative charge of an electron given as 1.602×10^{-19} coulombs

So for the 100 kV anode voltage, the energy of the electron, (i.e., photon energy of the X-ray radiated) is given as:

$$E_E = 1.602 \times 10^{-19} \text{ coulombs} \times 100 \times 10^3 \text{ V} = 1.602 \times 10^{-19} \text{ joules/volt} \times 100 \times 10^3 \text{ V}$$

$$E_E = 1.602 \times 10^{-14} \text{ joules} = 100 \text{ keV}$$

Given 1 eV is 1.6×10^{-19} joules.

Equivalent Energy of a Proton and an Electron

The equivalent energy of 1 atomic mass unit (amu) is computed as:

$$E = m \times c^2 = (\text{mass of a proton})(\text{speed of light})^2$$

$$E = (1.66 \times 10^{-24} \text{ gram}) \times (3 \times 10^{10} \text{ cm/sec})^2$$

$$E = 1.49 \times 10^{-3} \text{ g} - \text{cm}^2/\text{sec}^2$$

$\text{g} - \text{cm}^2/\text{sec}^2$ is also called ergs, so

$$E = 1.49 \times 10^{-3} \text{ ergs} = 1 \text{ amu}$$

$$1 \text{ eV} = 1.6 \times 10^{-12} \text{ ergs}$$

ergs can be converted in eV

$$1.49 \times 10^{-3} \text{ ergs} = 931 \text{ MeV}$$

One amu is then converted into another unit of energy in 931 MeV. As the mass of an electron is 1/1838 of the mass of a proton, the equivalent energy of an electron is 0.52 MeV.

EXAMPLE Calculate the amount of scatter from a source at four feet if the intensity at six feet is 50 mR/hour.

If

$$\frac{I_1}{I_2} = \frac{D_2^2}{D_1^2}$$

then,

$$I_2 = \frac{D_1^2}{D_2^2} \times I_1$$

$$I_2 = \frac{6^2}{4^2} \times 50$$

$$I_2 = 112.5 \text{ mR/hr}$$

■

EXAMPLE Discuss the range of the following parameters for a typical x-ray system.

a. kV

b. mA

c. Exposure time

▪

EXAMPLE Draw a graph of the x-ray intensity with respect to the distance through a muscle. Given: Anode voltage as 100 kV, and the intensity of the X-ray is 15 W/m^2 at the muscle surface, distance ranges from zero to 3 cm, mass attenuation coefficient = $\mu = 0.523\ cm^2/g$

$$\text{Muscle density} = \rho = 1.06\ g/cm^3$$

Use the formula:

$$I = I_0 \times e^{-\mu\rho d}$$

where d = distance

▪

EXAMPLE Use the same instructions as in the previous example, but, for this example the X-ray is incident on the bone surface. Given: μ (bone) = 2.5 cm^2/g, ρ = 1.85 g/cm^3

▪

15.5 SAFETY ISSUES WITH X-RAY RADIATION: REGULATIONS IN HOSPITALS

Alpha, beta, gamma, and X-rays are types of electromagnetic radiation that can penetrate through various materials as shown in **Figure 15-6.** This is a kind of shield around a radiation source. Alpha particles can be stopped even by a sheet of paper; beta particles can pass through paper and can travel a farther distance but they can be stopped by plastic or aluminum sheets. Medical X-rays can be stopped by a relatively thin layer of lead (a few inches) or by a thick layer (several feet) of concrete.

X-ray shielding is an important regulatory safety issue in hospitals. Radiation is absorbed by the body tissues. The unit of this absorbed dose is called a Rad. When a Rad is multiplied by a quality factor (Q) (also known as a radiation weighting factor) to account for the type of radiation, the new unit is then called Rem. The quality factor is 1 for beta rays, gamma rays, and X-rays, but it is 20 for alpha particles. 20 Rem of X-rays (20 Rads $\times$ a Q of 1 = 20 Rem) will have the same biological effect as 20 Rem of alpha particles (1 Rad $\times$ a Q of 20 = 20 Rem), even though the absorbed dose (in Rads) is different. The following list compares some of the absorbed doses:

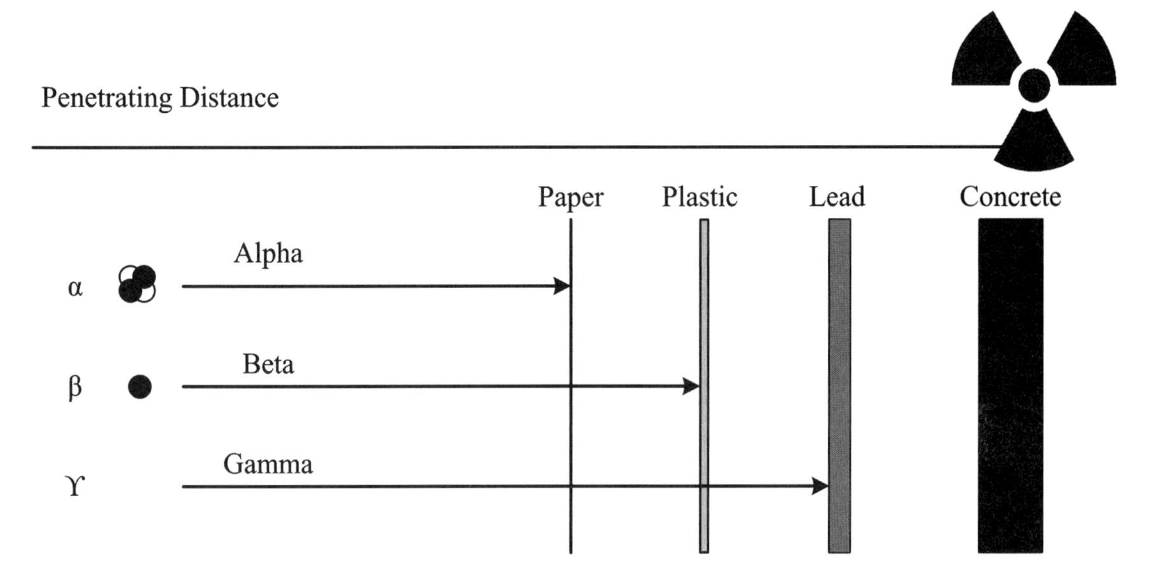

FIGURE 15-6 X-ray penetration through various materials.

Chest X-ray	10 millirem per scan
Dental X-ray	12 millirem per scan
Smoking	300 millirem per year
Drinking water	5 millirem per year

The human body can absorb only a certain recommended dosage of X-ray radiation before it starts to suffer tissue damage. To limit patient exposure to radiation, therefore, a lead cover is used to channel the X-rays to the target area; X-rays cannot penetrate lead, so the cover protects both the patient and the technician.

The NFPA99 describes codes dealing with the wiring and installation requirements on X-ray equipment, the nature of hazards, grounding reliability, receptacles, isolated power systems, and many more types of circuitry. Some of the codes are discussed below:

1. Double-insulated appliances shall have two conductor cords, however, there are other appliances used in patient care that are provided with a three-wire cord and three-pin grounding-type plug.
2. The resistance between the appliance chassis and the ground pin of the attachment plug should be less than 0.5 ohms (Ω).
3. The leakage current from frame to ground should not exceed 5 mA in patient care areas for fixed equipment. For portable equipment the tolerance is much lower. The chassis leakage current for portable equipment is not to exceed 300 μA.
4. Beyond 1 kHz, the leakage current limits are multiplied by the frequency (in kHz) up to a maximum of 10 mA.

5. The patient leads connected to the intra-cardiac catheters or electrodes should be isolated from the appliance's power (120 V) source.
6. Electrical appliances should be tested at least annually in the general care areas, although the interval between testing periods for appliances for critical care in wet areas (e.g., bathrooms, the shower) should not exceed six months.
7. The primary winding of an isolated transformer is not to exceed 600 V input power and its neutral must be grounded.
8. Each isolated power system is provided with a continually operating line isolation monitor. The monitor indicates possible leakage current or fault current from an isolated conductor to ground.
9. The voltage and impedance measurements must be done with respect to a reference point. This point is either a grounding point or a grounding contact of a receptacle that is powered from a different circuit.
10. The voltage and impedance measurements should be made with an accuracy of ±20 percent.
11. The NFPA diamond shaped labeling system indicates the radiation hazard (0: no hazard, 4: severe hazard) and is posted on exterior walls of a facility.

15.6 X-RAY IMAGES AND DATA

The types of x-ray machines used in hospitals can be classified as:

- Radiographic systems (for visualizing bone structures and other dense tissues)
  - □ Chest x-ray radiography
  - □ Portable or mobile units
  - □ Dental radiography
  - □ Chiropractic systems
- Fluoroscopic radiologic systems (moving X-rays to assess an organ or object in real time)
  - □ Heart catheterization
  - □ Barium studies
  - □ Surgical systems
  - □ Mammographic radiology
  - □ Bone densitometers
  - □ Computer tomography (CT)

The chest X-ray is the most common type of diagnostic procedure in hospitals and clinics. These black and white x-ray pictures can detect problems with the organs and structures inside the chest. Heart, lungs, blood vessels, bones of the chest including ribs and collarbone, and the upper portion of the spine, all will appear in a chest X-ray. For abnormal chest X-rays, the physician may suggest additional tests such as CT, MRI, or ultrasound. An example of an x-ray picture is shown in **Figure 15-7.**

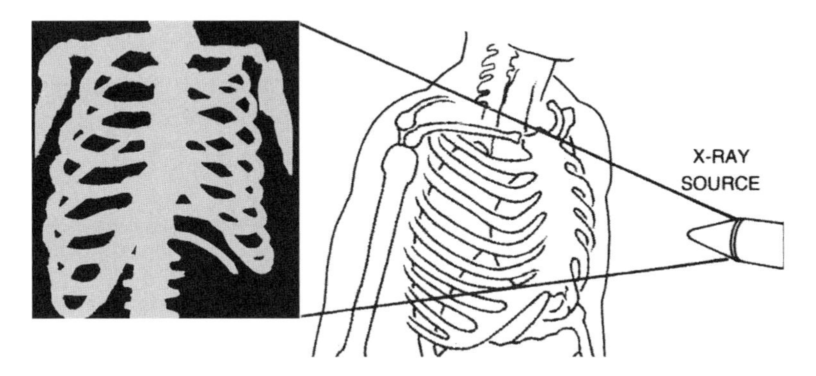

FIGURE 15-7 X-ray projection on the film.

There are three tissues that appear in a chest X-ray: bones, lungs, and soft tissues, such as heart and blood vessels. Bones appear white (high absorption of X-rays in bones), and lungs appear black (lungs will have the least absorption of X-rays due to air in the lungs). The soft tissues appear as shades of gray as X-rays are moderately absorbed by soft tissues.

15.7 VERTICAL BUCKY STAND

A Bucky grid is used in radiography to prevent the scattered rays from reaching the film or the screen. This is an assembly of lead strips or slots that is placed between the patient being X-rayed and the film. X-rays traveling in straight lines from the X-ray tube through the patient will strike the film, but the scattered rays are absorbed by the lead strips. The Bucky grid is part of the vertical Bucky stand. **Figure 15-8a** shows a Bucky stand, and **Figure 15-8b** shows the x-ray projection on the chest. The height correlation scale is attached to the Bucky stand so it corresponds with the height scale on the x-ray tube hanger or stand. The x-ray tube supports and table are installed prior to the installation of the stand. The x-ray tube unit is rotated so that the x-ray beam is horizontal and directed toward the vertical Bucky stand. It is important to verify the vertical and horizontal centering of the x-ray beam on the film at both the minimum and maximum SID points. The tray assembly can be loaded from either the left or right side. Usually the Bucky stand is equipped with a cassette-size sensing tray.

This type of stand requires high-quality electrical and mechanical safety features. Experienced technicians should work on the assembly of this device and follow the Recommendations of the International Commission on Radiological Protection. Excessive exposure to x-ray radiation can cause damage to human tissue.

15.8 COMPUTER TOMOGRAPHY: PRINCIPLES AND SCANS

Computer tomography (CT) scans are basically many x-ray images that are collected and processed by a computer to render a three-dimensional image of an organ or blood vessels or other areas of the body. These scans provide cross-sectional views of body organs and

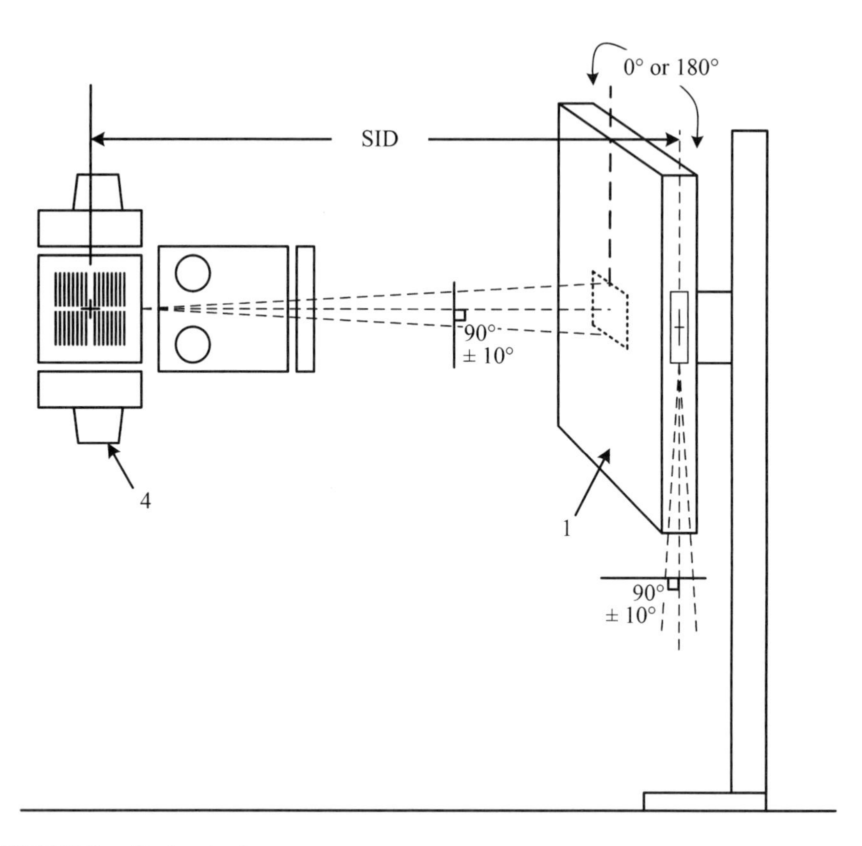

FIGURE 15-8a Bucky stand.

FIGURE 15-8b X-ray field on the chest.

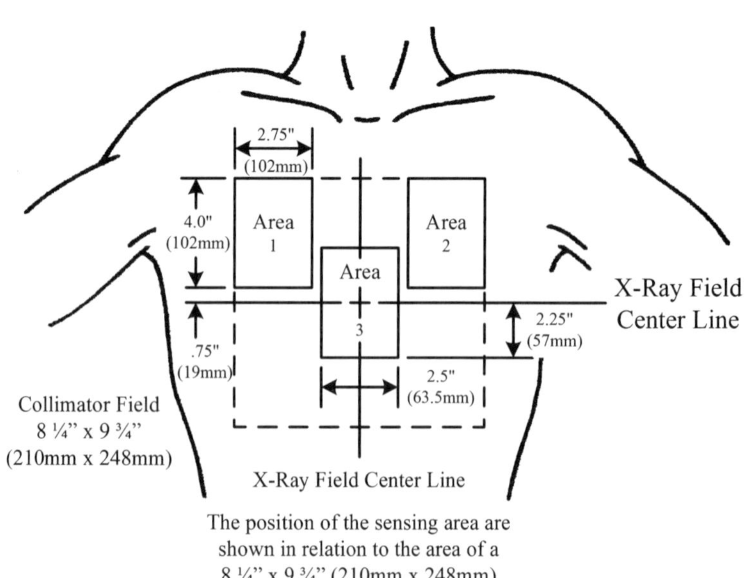

tissues. For example, the depth of tumors can be measured and seen in three-dimensional views using a CT scanner. The three-dimensional image is constructed from a series of two-dimensional X-ray images taken around a single axis of rotation.

The CT system was invented in 1972 by EMI Central Research Laboratories. The first scanner took several hours to collect the two-dimensional raw data and several days to generate the final image.

The three-dimensional images are sharp, detailed, and focused and tissues can be differentiated with more clarity than the standard x-ray images of the same tissues. The data collected is immense as it is taken from different angles around the body. This data is then processed by sophisticated computer algorithms. Computer tomography technology is used in several areas of medicine:

- CT brain studies: a CT scan of the brain can detect the presence of tumor, its size, and precise location. It can reduce the need for invasive procedures such as cerebral angiography. CT scans are also used to detect strokes and certain types of hematomas.
- CT abdominal and pelvic scans: CT can clearly show small bones, surrounding tissues, and blood vessels. In cases of trauma, it can identify injuries to the liver, spleen, lymph nodes, kidneys, and other vital organs.
- CT chest scans: In addition to showing many types of cancers in chest scans, CT technology is useful in showing accumulation of fluid in chest infections.
- Cardiac CT: Excellent imaging of the coronary arteries and aorta can be obtained with multi-slice high-speed and high-resolution CT scanners.

CT Image Derivation

The CT image is derived from a series of measurements of the transmission of X-rays through an object. The image is related to the local linear attenuation coefficients of the object, μ, as x-ray beams traverse the object. Computer tomography numbers relate to the attenuation coefficients, the formula is as follows:

$$\text{CT number} = \frac{\mu(\text{material}) - \mu(\text{water})}{\text{k}}$$

where μ(material) and μ(water) are the linear coefficients for the material and water respectively, and k is a scaling factor. Here, k is computed as:

$$\text{k} = \frac{\mu(\text{water})}{1{,}000}$$

The value of μ (water) is about 0.95 for the x-ray beam. The CT numbers range from about –1,000 to +3,000. (–1,000 corresponds to air, –300 to –100 correspond to soft tissues; water is 0, and dense bones range up to +3,000). These numbers are important in discriminating tissues such as lung tissue and bone tissue, because linear attenuation coefficients estimate the density of the tissues.

Principles of CT Scans

The CT scanner looks like a large doughnut and a gantry or narrow table slides into the center (the ring of the scanner). The basic system configuration of an x-ray CT is shown in **Figure 15-9a.** The scanner ring consists of one x-ray tube at the inside rim of the hole and several (hundreds of thousands!) x-ray detectors are then mounted directly opposite the x-ray tube. **Figure 15-9b** shows third- and fourth-generation detector placements around the x-ray tube. The third generation was called a fan-beam detector system as the tube moves in one direction, the detectors are just opposite to it and also moving in the same direction. However, in the fourth generation of CT scanners, the detectors are around the X-ray tube and are also not moving. The patient lies on the gantry, and the x-ray slice data is generated as the x-ray tube rotates around the patient.

A fifth generation CT scanner is shown in **Figure 15-10.** The patient lies down on the couch and several x-ray beams pass through the body. The focused beam is then collected by the more than one detector. The placements of vacuum pumps, focus and deflection coils, and the target rings are also shown.

CT arrays are shown in **Figure 15-11a** and **Figure 15-11b.** There are 16 detector channels and each channel has 16 diodes. These diodes are spread in the "A" and "B" sides of the patient table. A thermistor is shown as a heat detector.

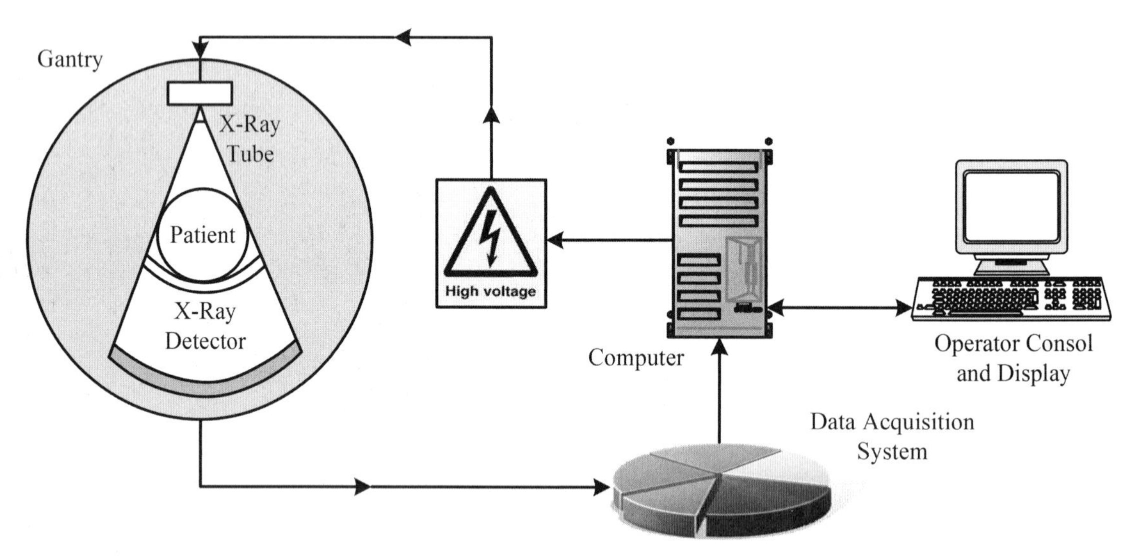

FIGURE 15-9a Basic system configuration of an x-ray CT.

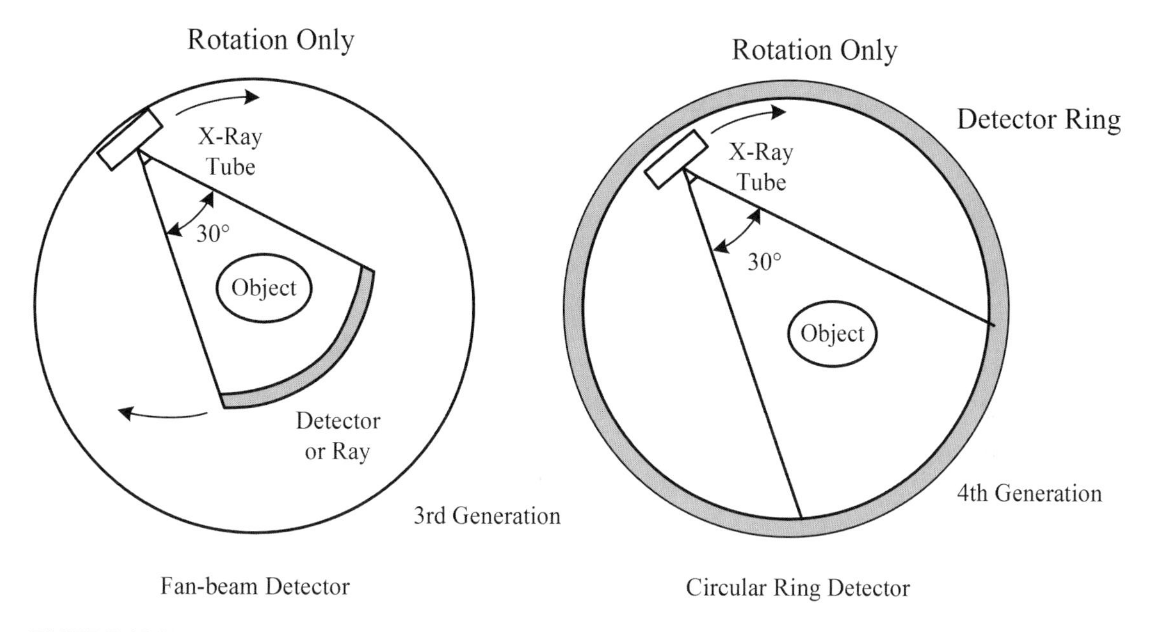

FIGURE 15-9b Third- and fourth-generation beam projection for an x-ray CT.

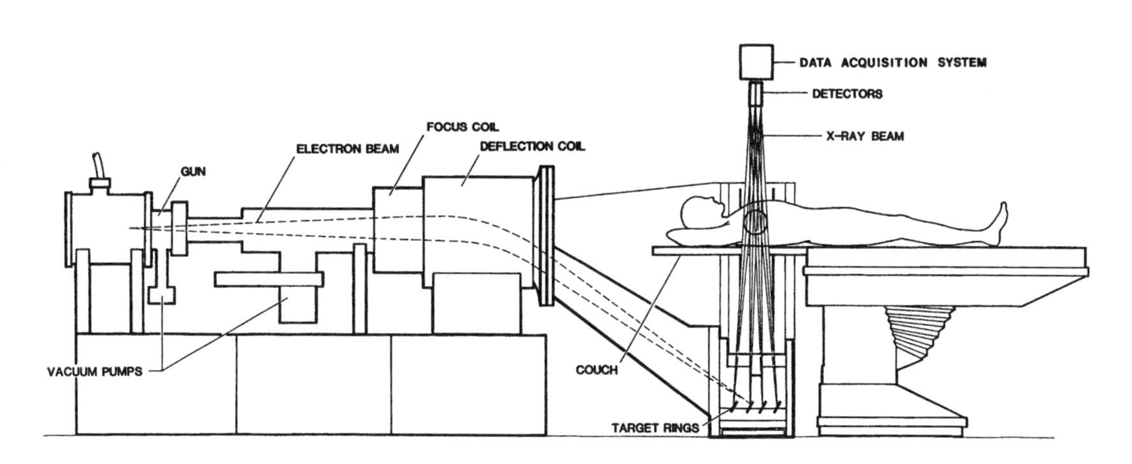

FIGURE 15-10 A detailed view of a CT scanner.

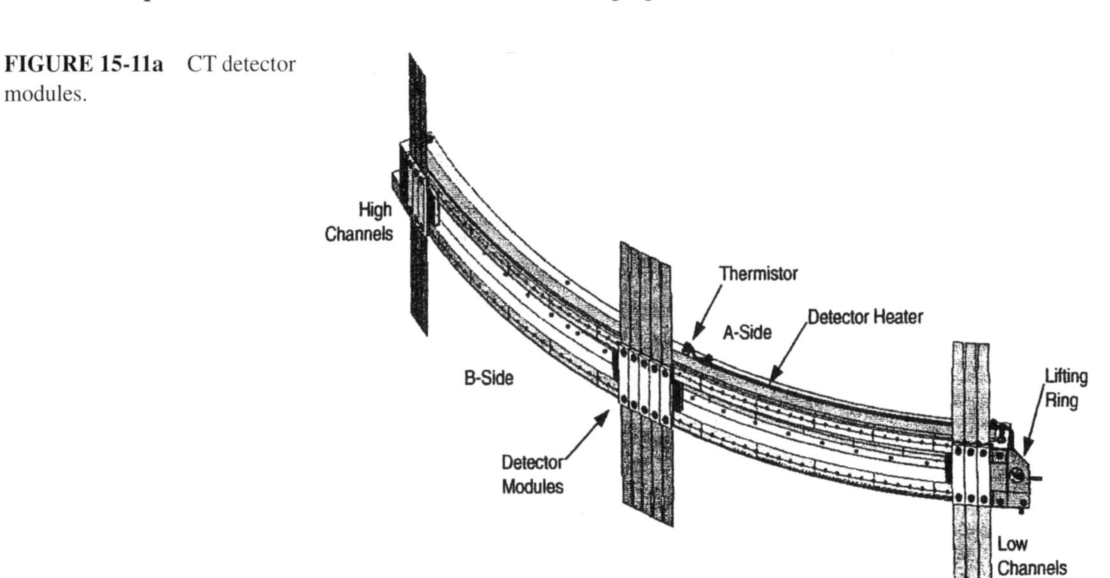

FIGURE 15-11a CT detector modules.

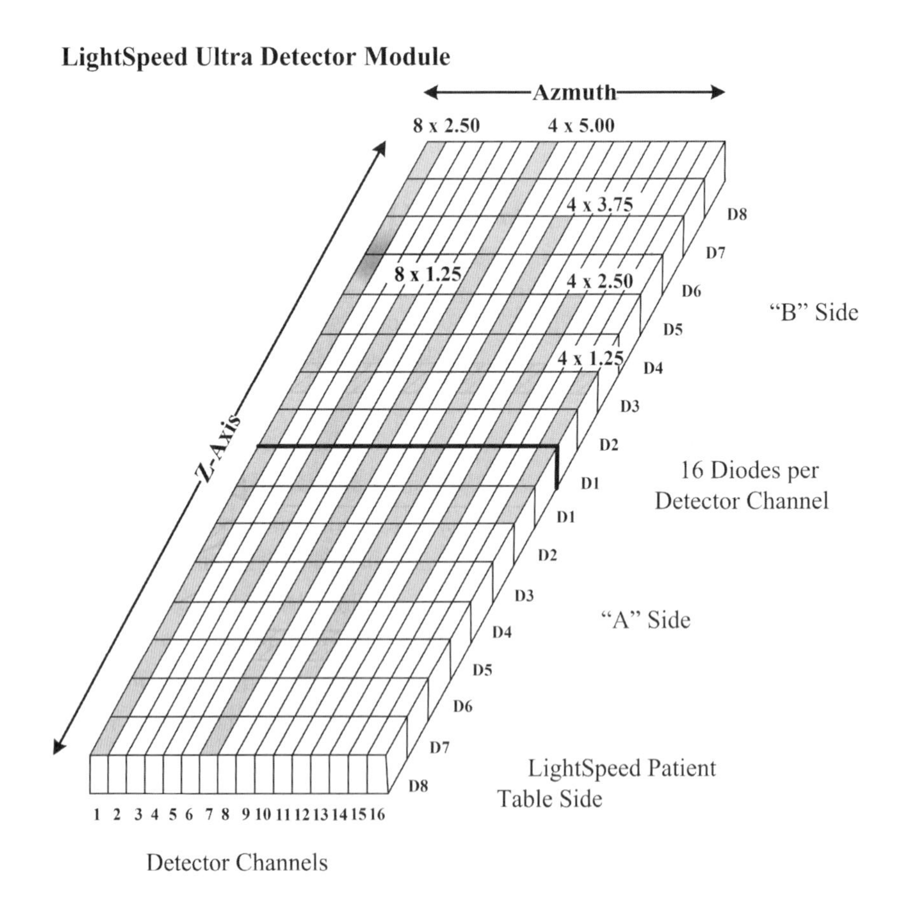

FIGURE 15-11b CT detector channels.

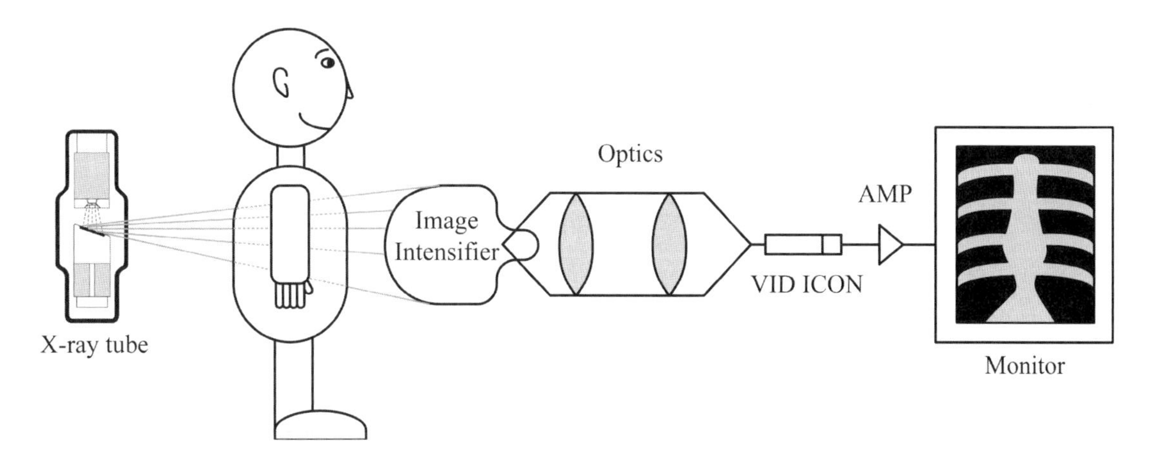

FIGURE 15-12a A fluoroscopy system.

15.9 FLUOROSCOPY

Fluoroscopy involves a dynamic x-ray imaging of physiological functions such as the flow of barium through the intestine or the process of injecting a contrast medium into the heart. The fluoroscopic x-ray tube is different than the regular diagnostic tube in the sense that it operates at lower mAs for longer periods of time. The tube and the image receptor are always aligned on a C-arm at all times.

The image receptor called the fluoroscopic screen can produce the x-ray image in real time. The radiologist can actively diagnose the patient during an examination and does not have to wait for the production of static x-ray film. The C-arm arrangement (also called the carriage) typically includes an x-ray tube (over the table), image intensification tube (under table), foot switch (to move the x-ray tube), tube shutters, spot imaging, cameras, brightness control, and C-arm drivers.

The image intensification tube consists of the photo cathode, input fluorescent screen, G-node output fluorescent screen, and electrostatic lens, all housed in a glass envelope. The electronics in the intensification tube amplify the x-ray image (reception) by almost 600 to 9,000 times and the quantity of photons and electrons in the image gradually increases at each stage inside the glass tube.

In **Figure 15-12a,** x-ray passes through the human body. Some of the intensity is attenuated, and the remaining intensity is collected at the output and intensified in the lenses before the result is displayed on the monitor. An image intensification tube is shown in **Figure 15-12b.** The quantity of photons and electrons is significantly larger at the output than at the input. A mobile C-arm fluoroscopic unit is shown in **Figure 15-12c.**

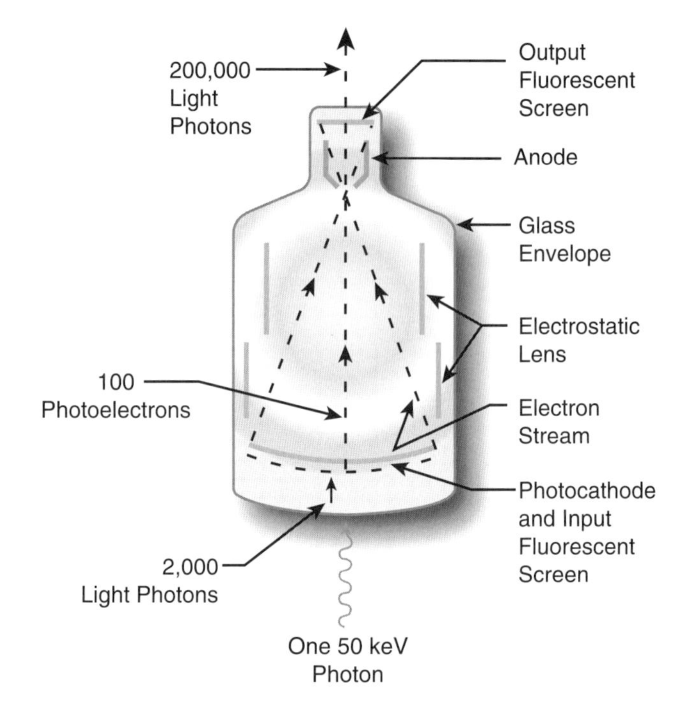

FIGURE 15-12b An image intensifier tube in fluoroscopy.

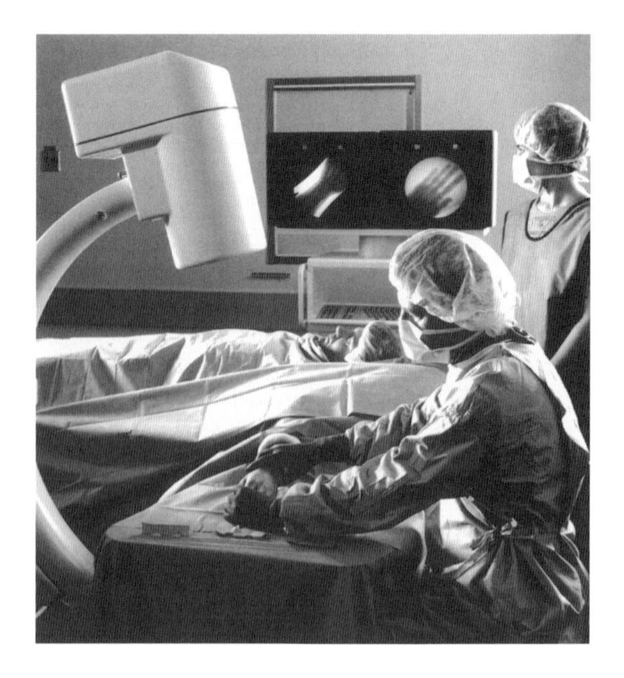

FIGURE 15-12c A mobile C-arm fluoroscopic unit.

15.10 NUCLEAR MEDICINE

In diagnostic procedures other than X-rays, radioactive nuclear medicine, such as a radioisotope, is injected into the human body. The medicine is absorbed by the organs and the surrounding tissues and emits radiation that can be detected and the path and the concentration of the medicine in various parts of the body is traced and determined.

The detection of this radiation produces an image of body organs and their structures.

The radioisotopes most frequently used in patients are Iodine 131, Barium 131, Technetium 99m, and other types; care must be taken to ensure that the radiation dose received by the body falls within safe limits. Interestingly, the radioactivity (the radiation) must be great at the time of measurement, but it should also be reduced as fast as possible when the measurement is completed.

Figure 15-13 shows a block diagram of a radionuclide radiation and reception across an object of interest. The lead collimator collimates (streamlines) the radiation from the

FIGURE 15-13 Block diagram of radionuclide radiation and reception.

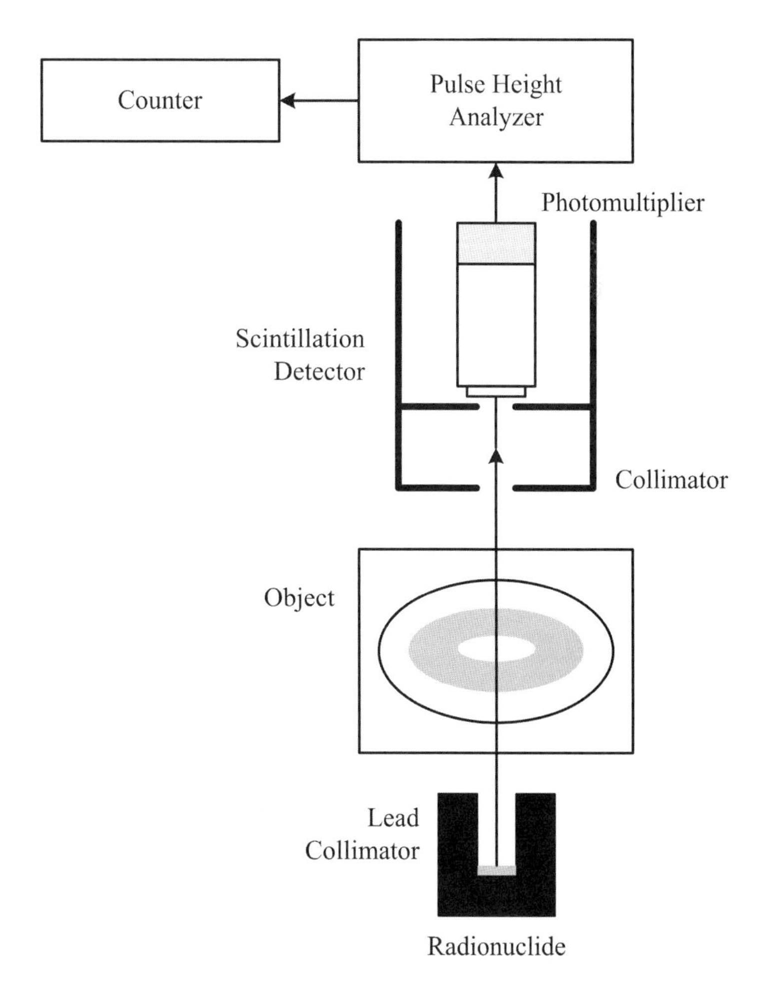

radionuclide crystal and the scintillation detector (such as thallium-activated sodium iodide) collects the remaining radiation intensity after the nuclear disintegrations in the object of interest.

15.11 POSITRON EMISSION TOMOGRAPHY

Positron emission tomography (PET) scanners produce a map of where glucose is consumed in the body. A form of glucose called FDG, which emits positrons, is injected before a PET scan is performed. The scanner then detects where positrons are being emitted from a patient and creates a map. The relationship between the glucose and the positron emission is inseparable and well established and the map, or image, demonstrates the areas of high use of glucose in the body. This high use of glucose helps to determine the presence of cancer. The rationale is that the growing cancer cells consume glucose as a primary source of energy. The faster the cells grow, the more glucose they consume, and the higher their emissions.

The patient receives a small amount of FDG through an IV into the arm. It takes about an hour for the FDG to properly circulate in the body before the PET scan is done. The scan itself takes about one hour to complete. The physician determines the presence of cancer or abnormal biochemistry in the body not solely from the PET scans, but in conjunction with the CT or MRI scans.

15.12 MAGNETIC RESONANCE IMAGING

Magnetic resonance imaging (MRI) is a process that uses a large circular magnet to induce and monitor the resonance of the magnetic moment of nuclei in the presence of static and varying magnetic fields. Hydrogen nuclei are ideally suited for MRI imaging, because they are the most sensitive of the stable nuclei for MRI and also the most abundant nuclei formed in the body.

Step 1 Alignment of Hydrogen Atoms and the Effect of the DC Magnetic Field

When the human body is placed inside the huge circular magnet, the strong magnetic field acts on molecules of the hydrogen atoms in the tissues. These hydrogen atoms align themselves vertically due to the strong magnetic field.

Step 2 Effect of the External RF Signal

Next, the hydrogen atoms are bombarded by external radio waves causing the atoms to change direction.

Step 3 External RF Signal is Turned Off

Finally, the radio waves are turned off, causing the hydrogen atoms to go back to their original direction. In going back to their original direction, they give off energy and radiation, which can be detected.

Step 4 Detection of the RF Signal from the Hydrogen Atoms

The MRI machine measures the time required for the hydrogen atoms to return to their original direction. Hydrogen atoms in the different tissues in the body will take different amounts of time to return back to their original direction; thus an image (based on the differing times) of the body tissues is created by the computer.

Figure 15-14a shows a diagram of an MRI machine. The magnetic field and the generation of the RF pulse are set up by the MRI technician. The MRI machine uses a superconducting magnet and it is well shielded so that the magnetic field does not interfere with other electronic components inside and outside of the machine. It generates a stable and homogeneous magnetic field and any inhomogeneity can be suppressed by the use of electronic shimming coils. The electronic shimming coils are placed outside of the main gradient coils.

Notice in **Figure 15-14a** that the signals to the gradient coils around the magnet and also the RF signal to excite the atoms are all analog signals. The RF signal is modulated by the quadrature phase shift modulation technique. The D/A converters are controlled by the PSG. A photograph of a typical MRI unit is shown in **Figure 15-14b.**

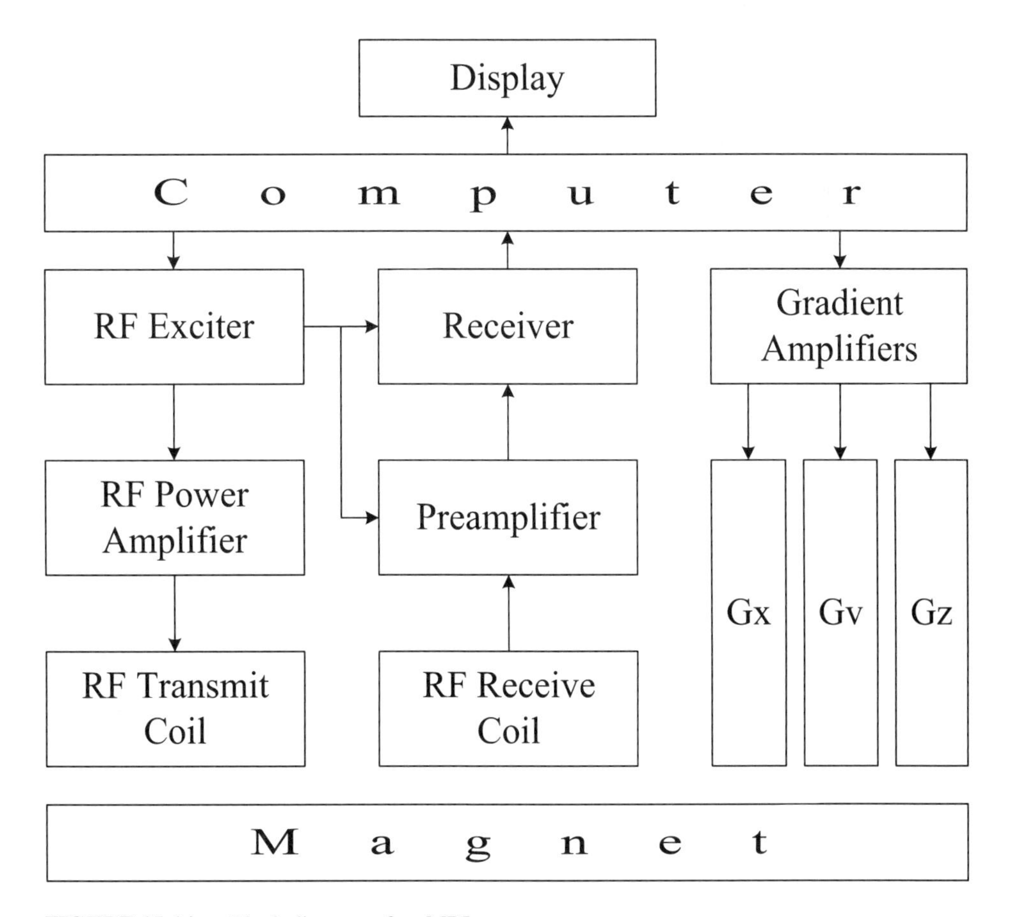

FIGURE 15-14a Block diagram of an MRI system.

FIGURE 15-14b A typical MRI unit.

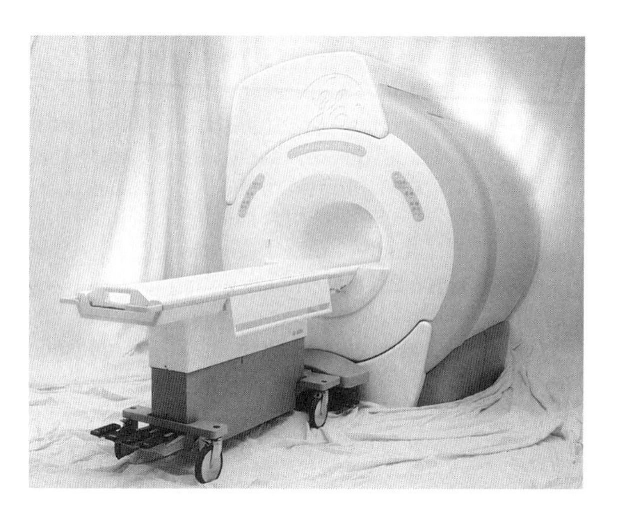

Another cross-section of the MRI coils is shown in **Figure 15-14c.** There is the main coil and the X, Y, and Z coils surround the body tissues for different cross-sectional views. The RF transceiver transmits the RF pulse bombarding on the magnetic vectors of the hydrogen atoms, and receives the RF pulse from the hydrogen atoms.

Next, we explore how steps 1–4 can be explained by MRI math.

MRI Math

The process used by MRI to create images is quite different from the x-ray absorption process. In contrast to the electron density information gained from an x-ray CT, MRI images can extract several different types of information. In an MRI, not only is telemetry from proton density gathered, but also information from T1 and T2 relaxation times, blood flow, fat content, and water content of the tissues. Primarily, the proton density (i.e., number of hydrogen nuclei) imaging is done in an MRI.

Hydrogen protons possess magnetic moments. These moments tend to align with the direction of the DC magnetic field (when the protons are placed in the magnetic field). This is shown in **Figure 15-15a.**

This alignment is disturbed when an external RF interacts with these magnetic moments. When the RF signal stops interacting, the protons relax and emit minute RF signals of their own. These minute RF signals in reverse are the characteristics of proton density and its distribution. These minute RF signals are received as a composite signal shown in **Figure 15-15b.**

The frequency components in this composite signal then indicate the spatial distribution of the protons. The dependence of the composite signal (we can call it now an MRI signal) depends on several factors and can be explained by the following equation:

$$I \propto N(H) \times (1 - 2e^{-(TR - TI)/T1} + e^{-TE/T1}) \times e^{-TE/T2}$$

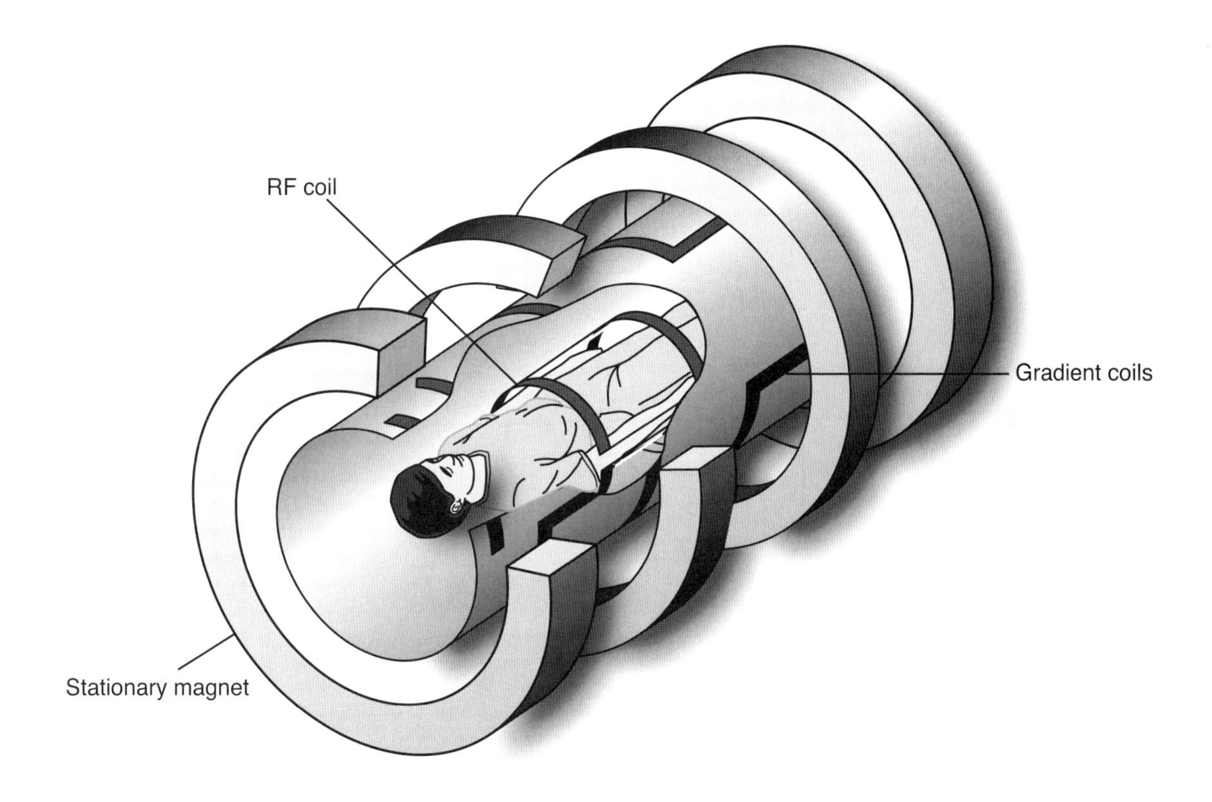

FIGURE 15-14c A stationary magnet, gradient coil, and RF unit in an MRI system.

Where,

I = MRI signal intensity.
N (H) = Proton density.
TR = Time between 180° or 90° pulses.
TI = Time between 180° and 90° pulses.
T1 = Longitudinal magnetic relaxation time.
T2 = Transverse magnetic relaxation time.
TE = Echo delay.

The MRI image contrast is controlled by parameters such as repetition time (TR), echo time (TE), inversion time (TI), longitudinal relaxation time (T1), and transverse relaxation time (T2), in addition to proton spin density. In **Figure 15-15c,** maximum contrast can be obtained when the RF signal strength is at its greatest difference between two tissues and this is shown when the T1 relaxation graphs become farther apart as time increases. Maximum T1 is achieved with a short TR, and a minimum T1 is achieved with a long TR.

Figure 15-15d shows a sagittal MRI image of the head.

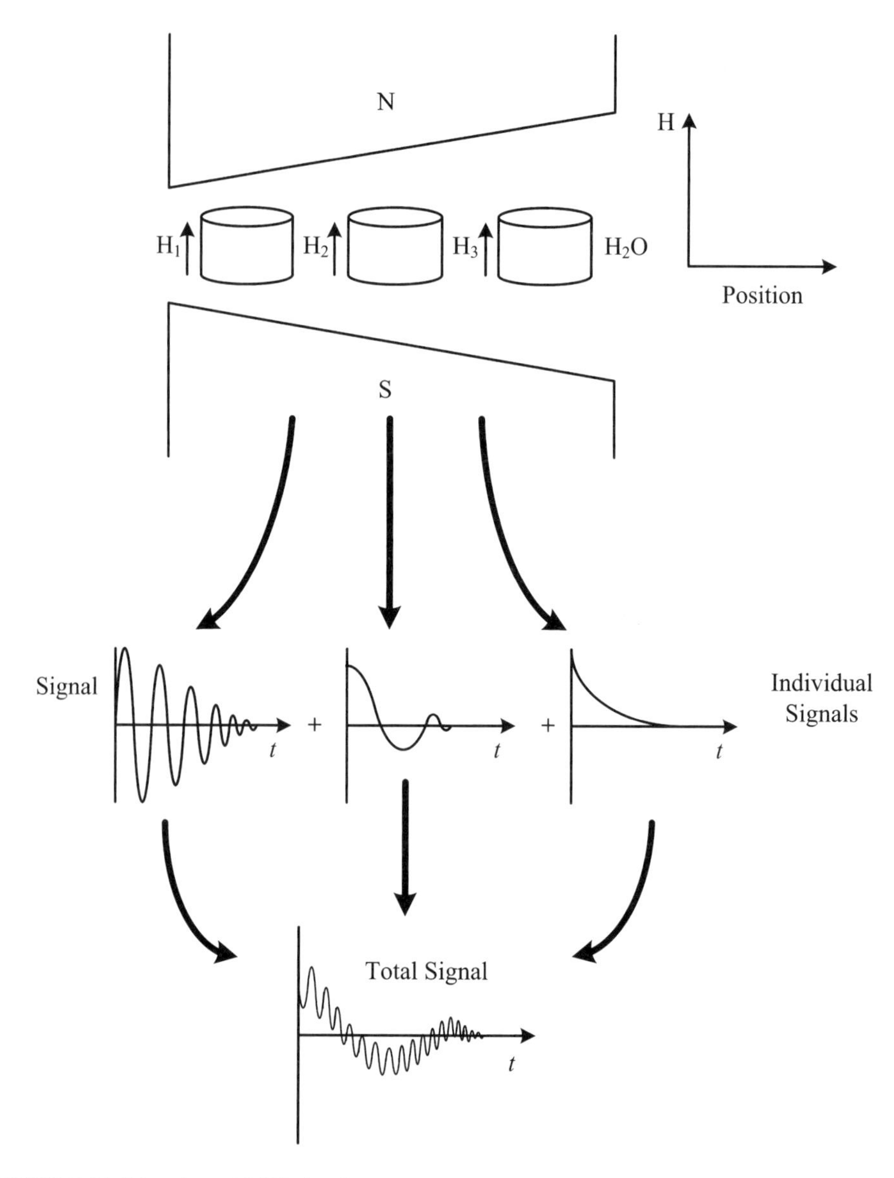

FIGURE 15-15a A total MRI signal.

FIGURE 15-15b Fourier transformation of the MRI signal.

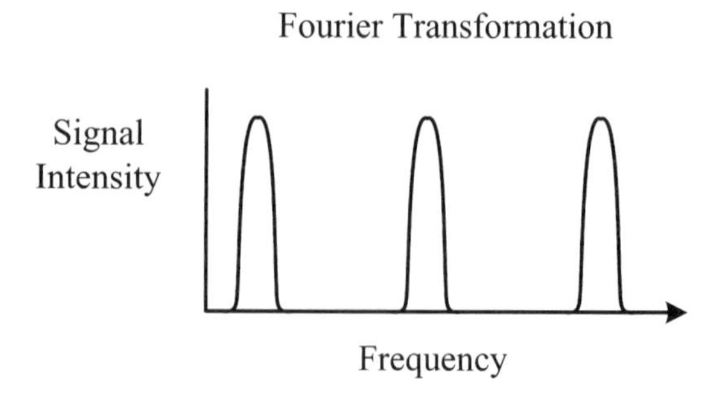

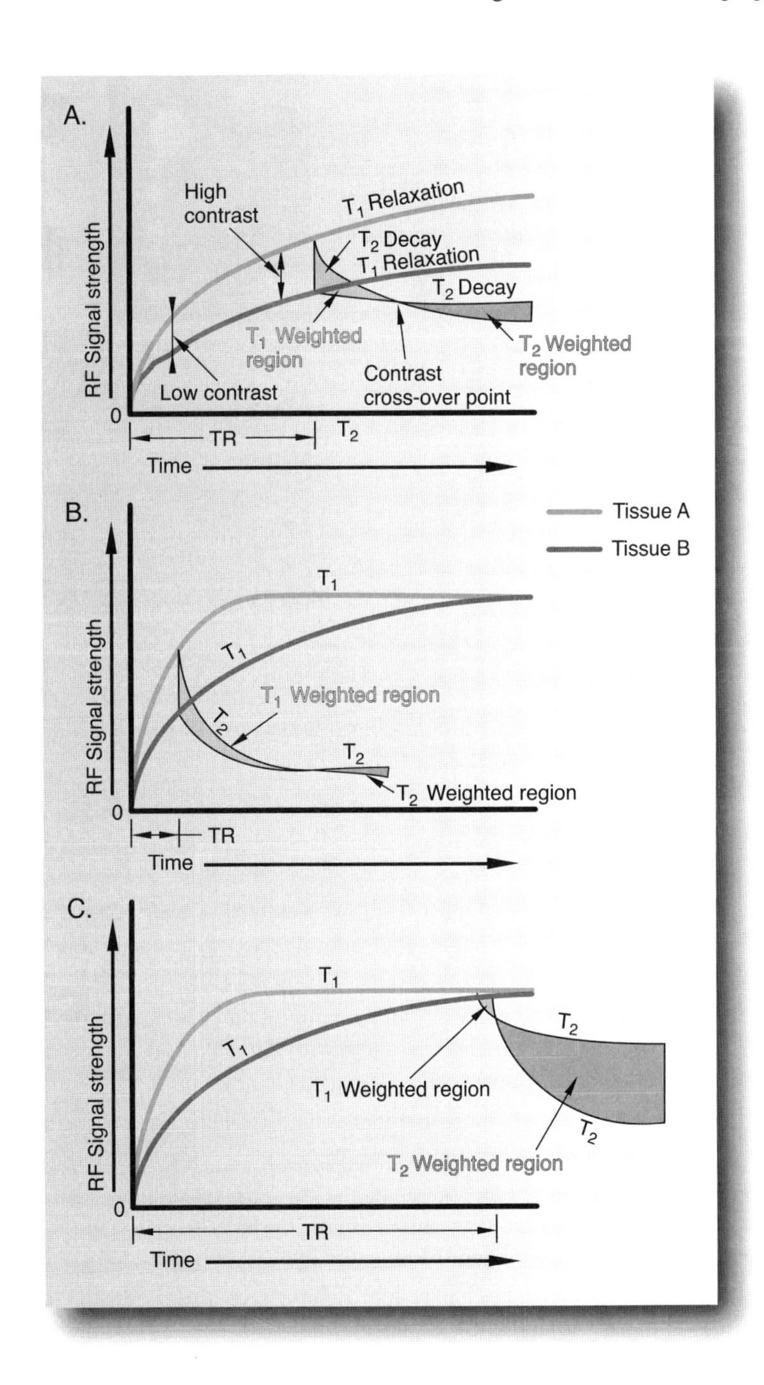

FIGURE 15-15c T_1 and T_2 relaxation times of the MRI signal.

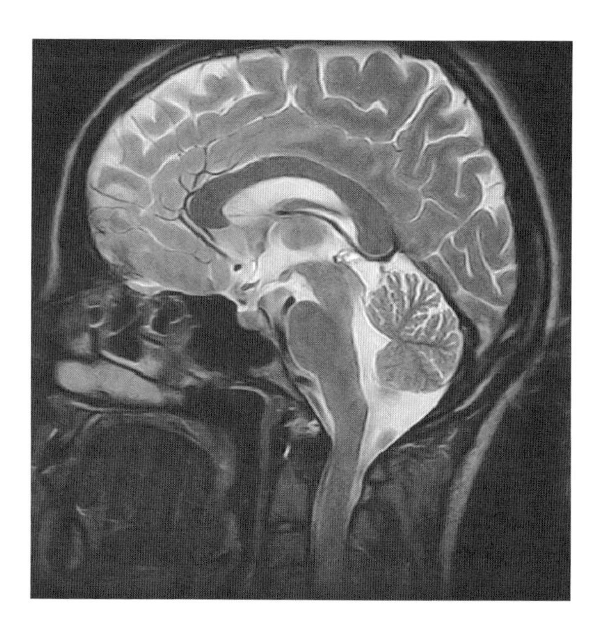

FIGURE 15-15d MRI image of the head.

SUMMARY

Radiology is not only about X-rays; it also covers four other diagnostic imaging systems: CT, fluoroscopy, PET, and MRI.

1. A block diagram is provided of an x-ray machine explaining its function, followed by the physics of X-rays. An x-ray machine consists of transformers, rectifiers, x-ray tube, filament circuit, and exposure and timer circuits. The necessary attributes for x-ray imaging are the x-ray source, object (patient), and the radiation detector.

   An x-ray image shows the variation in x-ray transmission caused by the structures in the object of varying thicknesses and densities.
2. Computed tomography (CT), with its physics and scans, is presented. CT examines body organs by scanning them with X-rays and using a computer to construct a series of cross-sectional scans along a single axis.
3. The theory of fluoroscopy is explained next. Fluoroscopy obtains real-time moving images of the internal structures of a patient through the use of a fluoroscope.
4. The physics of nuclear medicine and PET are also included for discussion in this chapter. The technique produces images of the distribution of radioactive tracers in the body that is emitting gamma rays; the images are recorded by the scintillation camera.
5. As the end of the chapter approaches, MRI principles, MRI scans, and the MRI machine, along with other MRI concepts, are given. MRI uses strong magnets and pulses of radio waves to manipulate the natural magnetic properties in the body.

MEDICAL TERMINOLOGY

The following is a list of medical terminology mentioned in this chapter.

Collimation: process of limiting the X-ray beam from being dispersed in a multitude of directions as it is focused on a particular body part.

Computer tomography (CT): imaging technique using x-ray beams for viewing multiple cross-sectional images of the body.

Fluoroscopy: radiological technique to examine body parts in motion or functions of organs by projecting x-ray images onto a luminous fluorescent screen.

Gantry: housing component for the imaging source composed of the x-ray tube and detectors into which a patient is placed for CT and MRI.

Magnetic resonance imaging (MRI): imaging technique using a strong magnetic field and radio waves to create images of the human body without the use of radiation.

Positron emission tomography (PET): technique using glucose containing a small amount of a radioactive isotope which is injected into a patient's arm. A camera is then used to detect radioactivity in the body where cancer cells will absorb large amounts of the radioactive sugar.

Radiology: the study of the diagnostic use of X-rays in which a radiant energy and radioactive substances are used for diagnostic and treatment purposes.

Scintillation: the discharge that results from radioactive substances. A swift fluctuating pattern of visual disarray often attributed to migraine headaches.

X-ray: an imaging technique that uses high-frequency electromagnetic waves to produce images of structures inside the body. The electromagnetic waves pass through the body and strike a film, producing a picture of the intended structure.

QUIZ

1. The best shielding material against x-ray radiation is:

a) Iron. b) Lead. c) Aluminum. d) Plastic.

2. Beta particles:

a) Can be stopped by a piece of paper. b) Are high-speed electrons or positrons.

c) Are photons. d) None of the above.

3. The power needed in x-ray tubes typically is:

a) 110 V, 10 mA. b) 1,000 V, 100 mA.

c) 110 kV, 500 mA. d) None of the above.

4. An MRI machine uses magnetic field gradients to:

a) Measure T1 and T2 relaxation times.

b) Establish the coordinates in three-dimension.

c) Measure magnetic field strength.

d) Deionize the hydrogen atoms.

5. True or False: In general, an MRI provides good resolution for brain imaging and an X-ray provides good resolution for chest imaging:

a) True b) False

6. What is the main difference between X-ray and radioisotope technique?

a) Soft tissue is imaged better by the radioisotope technique than by X-rays.

b) Radioisotopes are injected into the body as nuclear medicines.

c) Bone is imaged better by X-rays than by the radioisotope technique.

d) None of the above.

6. The technique in which an image intensifier amplifies the image and converts the X-ray into light is called:

   a) Axial computer tomography. b) MRI.

   c) Fluoroscopic technique. d) Nuclear medicine.

7. Calculate the maximum photon energy of X-rays radiated from an anode when 100 kV is applied to the anode.

   a) (100 kV) $\times$ (6.625 $\times$ 10^{-34} J-sec) joules

   b) 100 joules

   c) (100 kV) $\times$ (1.602 $\times$ 10^{-19}) joules

8. The amount of x-ray absorption in the body depends on:

   a) Only the density of the material absorbing it.

   b) Both the density and the thickness of the material absorbing it.

   c) Only the thickness of the material absorbing it.

   d) None of the above.

9. A geiger counter:

   a) Measures x-ray intensity.

   b) Measures radiation from radioactive nuclear medicine.

   c) Counts RF pulses in the MRI imaging technique.

10. The difference between x-ray imaging and CT imaging is

    ____

PROBLEMS

1. Determine the heat units in a single phase rectifier unit, given:

   Voltage = 100 kV_P.
   Current = 150 mA.
   Time = 0.2 sec.
   Convert and give all results in joules.

2. What is the radiation dose limit for a 20-year-old radiology nurse?
3. Calculate the exposure time when an x-ray control panel is set at 200 mA and 15 mA.
4. For a 50 kV anode voltage, what is the maximum photon energy of the x-ray radiation?
5. When we compare patient radiation dose in X-ray versus CT, which modality has a lower dose and why?
6. Calculate the CT number for a liver, given:

   Attenuation coefficient of the measured pixel = 10.

   Attenuation coefficient of water = 20.

7. Make a rough plot of the x-ray intensity versus distance (in centimeters) through the material. Given: the incident x-ray intensity on the muscle = 12 W/m^2, density of the muscle = 1.05 g/cm^3, and mass attenuation coefficient = 0.44 cm^2/g.

8. Discuss the following statements:

   a) Effect of increasing kV_p on the speed and energy of electrons in the x-ray tube

   b) Relationship between kV_p and the density of radiographic film

   c) Changes made independently in kV_p, mA, time, and distance with respect to the patient dose

   d) Relationship of the x-ray absorption characteristics of air, muscle, bone, and fat, along with the resultant radiographic densities

9. Discuss digital radiography and its digital image processing in terms of receptor and detector system, image quality, and the resolution.

10. Discuss TI, TR, T1, T2, and TE in the MRI imaging technique.

CASE STUDIES

1. A 70-year-old man fell off a ladder when he was cleaning the exterior windows of his house. He fell so badly on his right leg that he could not get up due to severe pain. His son called for an ambulance, which immediately transported him to the hospital. At the hospital X-rays were taken and they showed his right femur had fractured. The X-ray also revealed the loss of bone mass in his right hip and femur. Answer the following questions:

   a) What kind of surgery is needed in this case to ease his pain?

   b) How is bone mass related to aging?

   c) How would physical therapy help after surgery?

   d) What did an x-ray image reveal compared to a normal image?

2. Mary repeats the same things over and over not realizing she is doing it. She is 75 years old and in generally good health. Mary finds that she misplaces household items quite often and has been getting more and more dependent on her husband concerning decision making. Her doctor has suggested PET scans of her brain. He thinks that Mary may be suffering from progressive Alzheimer's disease. In this case we may ask the following questions:

   a) Why did the doctor suggest PET scans of the brain instead of an MRI?

   b) How is the brain affected by the Alzheimer's disease?

   c) What will the PET scan show in Mary's case compared to normal scans?

RESEARCH TOPICS

1. In a vast majority of diagnostic procedures, CT scans are done routinely. Radiation and the risk of receiving that radiation are present. Your research paper should contain a collection of information on the recommended dose and the risk of developing cancer as a result of a body CT scan based on worst-case scenarios.

2. Three-dimensional images in the CT and MRI diagnostic modalities require huge data storage. New technologies apply digital compression and imaging algorithms for properly storing this vast amount of data. This research topic may include Diacom data storage and various other recommendations to solve this problem at the present time.

CHAPTER 16

Fiber Optics and Lasers in Bioinstrumentation

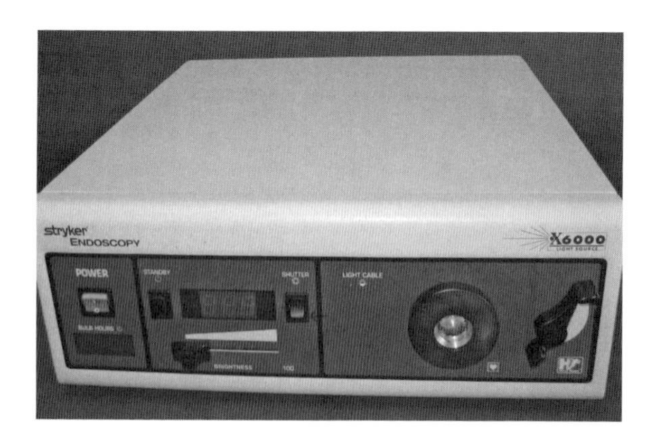

CHAPTER OUTLINE

OBJECTIVES

This objective of this chapter is to explain to the reader the physics of fiber optics and laser technology and their current applications in health care.

Upon completion of this chapter, the reader will be able to:

- Compute the angle of reflection or refraction in a fiber cable for a given light beam.
- Compare the characteristics of different types of fibers.
- Discuss the various applications of fiber optics in the medical field.
- Describe the differences between ordinary light and a laser beam.
- Explain laser therapy and its advantages and disadvantages.
- Describe the safety issues in using laser in a hospital.

■ INTERNET WEB SITES

http://www.laserinstitute.org (Laser Institute of America)
http://www.aslms.org (American Society for Laser Medicine and Surgery)
http://www.panoptic.welchallyn.com (Welch Allyn)
http://www.fda.gov/cdrh/consumer/laserfacts.html (U.S. Food and Drug Administration Center for Devices and Radiological Health)

■ INTRODUCTION

Fiber optics and lasers are technologies used in bar code readers, compact discs, laser printers, and in telecommunications and networking. They also have significant applications in medicine. One such example is in imaging and the illumination components of endoscopes to view internal organs. Flexible or rigid fiber cables with laser emitters and detectors are used to access organs through natural openings or transcutaneously in the body. Surgeons, dentists, gastroenterologists, dermatologists, ophthalmologists, maxillo-facial surgeons, and urologists are some of the specialists who apply these technologies.

■

16.1 PHYSICS OF FIBER OPTICS

Fiber optics rely on thin, transparent fibers of glass or plastic that are enclosed by material of a lower refractive index. These fibers transmit light throughout their length by internal reflections. In the medical field, the technique of fiber optics is commonly used in bioinstrumentation, as for viewing body cavities. The central part of the fibers in this system is referred to as the "core" and the layers surrounding the core are collectively referred to as the "cladding." While each of these components of the fiber-optic system is made of silica material, the core is denser than the cladding. Other components of this optical system are the transmitter, optical repeaters (or regenerators), and the receiver. **Figure 16-1** shows a

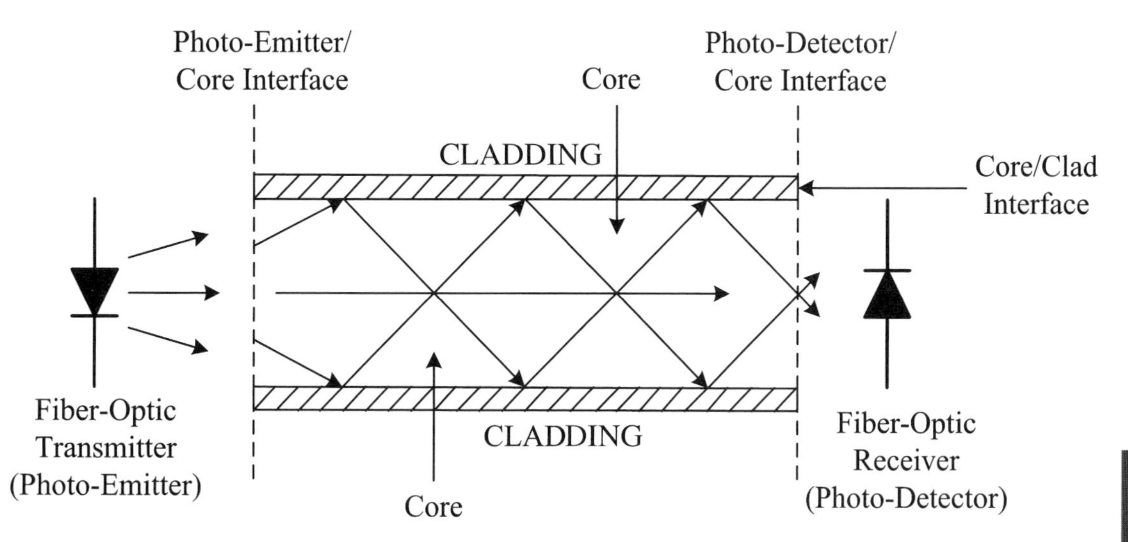

FIGURE 16-1 Fiber link between transmitter and the receiver.

simple diagram of a fiber-optic system. Notice the photo-emitter that transmits the light rays into the core and the photo-detector that receives and detects the light rays from the core at the other end.

Notice that there are mainly three so-called interfaces: photo-emitter and core interface, core and cladding interface, and the core and photo-detector interface. The photo-emitter and the photo-detector are air-coupled media and considered as air interfaces.

The light rays that enter at the photo-emitter and the core interface are guided along the core by internal reflections at the core/cladding interface and finally exit at the other end at the core and the photo-detector interface.

Light Intensity

Figure 16-2 shows the electromagnetic spectrum. The Visible light is a small part of this spectrum and is between the infrared and ultraviolet spectra. The spectrum shows the frequency, wavelength, and photon energy of radio waves, microwaves, visible light, X-rays, and gamma rays. Light is viewed as an electromagnetic wave that travels at approximately 3×10^8 meters per second with a wavelength of approximately 10^{-6} micrometer.

The wavelength and the frequency are inversely related to each other as $\lambda = c/f$, where λ is the wavelength, c is the velocity of light, and f is the frequency.

The light intensity is the photon energy and is measured as electron-volt (eV). This is the energy that an electron gains when it moves through a 1-V electric field.

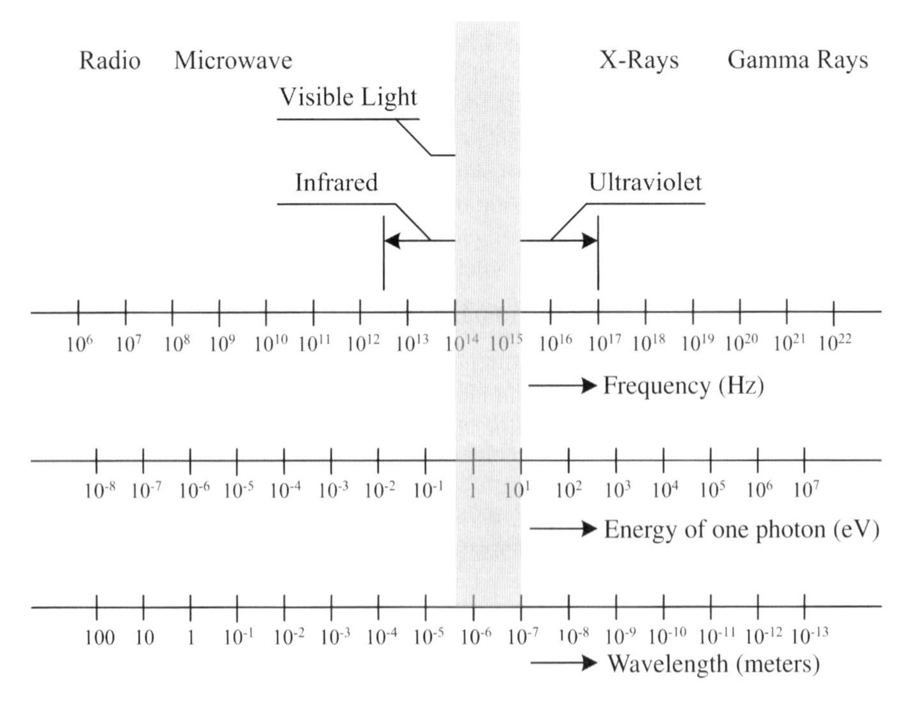

FIGURE 16-2 Electromagnetic spectrum.

Planck's law states the following:

$$E = h \times f$$

where h is the Planck's constant (given as 4.14×10^{-15} eV-seconds), and f is the frequency.

This equation, $E = h \times f$, is the energy of the photon. The magnitude of the momentum then can be derived as:

$$p = E / c = h \times f / c$$

Snell's Law and Refraction

Snell's law is based on refraction, or the bending of light, due to the differences of the refractive indexes of the materials involved. The table in **Figure 16-3** shows the refractive index of various substances. A dense material will have a higher refractive index and the velocity of light will slow down as light passes through it.

In free space, the refractive index is 1 for an air-to-air interface, while in an air-to-glass interface, the refractive index is approximately 1.5.

Figure 16-4a shows the path of a light ray being transmitted to, and received from, a sample medium. The direct path striking the sample returns. Otherwise, it will continue forward reflecting inside the core material, as shown in **Figure 16-4b.** In some cases, the delivering fiber can be different than the receiving fiber, as in the fiber bundle shown in **Figure 16-4c.**

Indices of Refraction for Various Substances

Substance	Index of refraction
Air, dry (STP)	1.00029
Alcohol, ethyl	1.360
Benzene	1.501
Carbon dioxide	1.625
Carbon tetrachloride	1.459
Diamond	2.417
Glass, crown flint	1.575
Lucite	1.50
Quartz, fused	1.45845
Water, distilled	1.333
Water, vapor (STP)	1.00025

FIGURE 16-3 A table for the index of refraction.

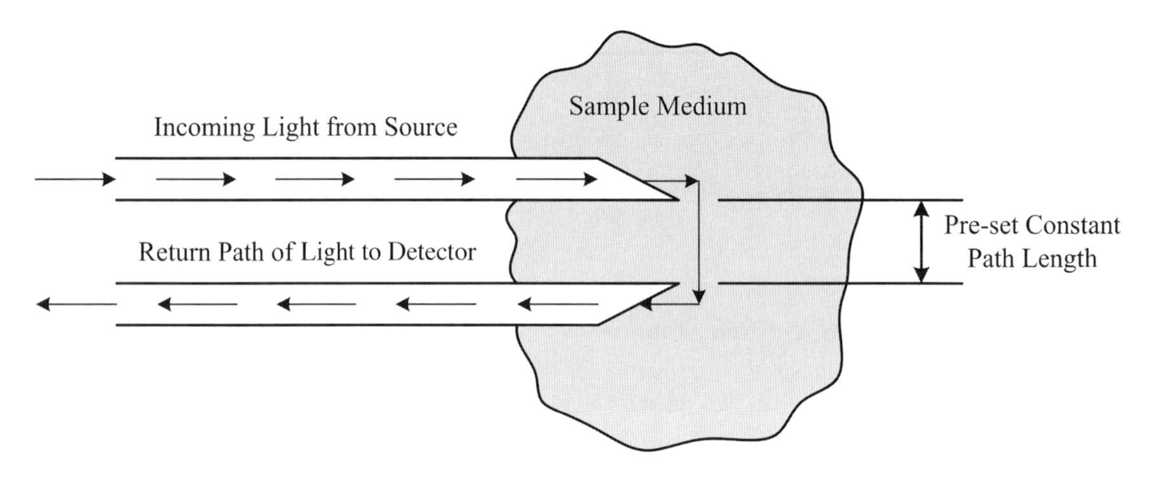

FIGURE 16-4a Light through the fiber material sample.

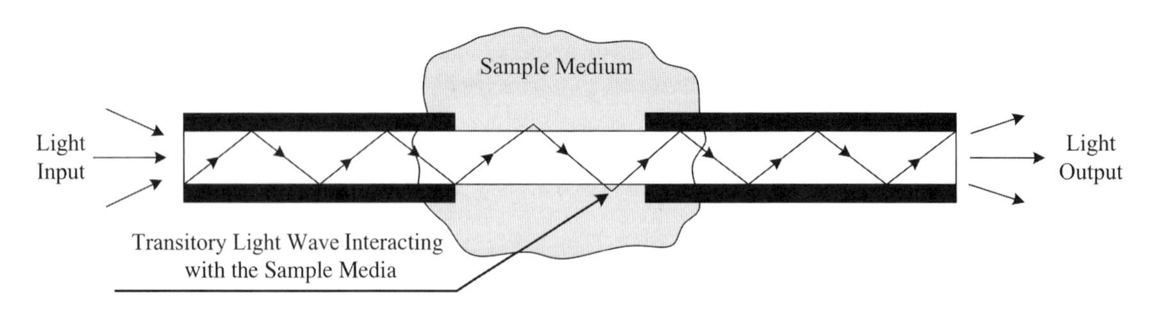

FIGURE 16-4b Light reflection in the fiber core.

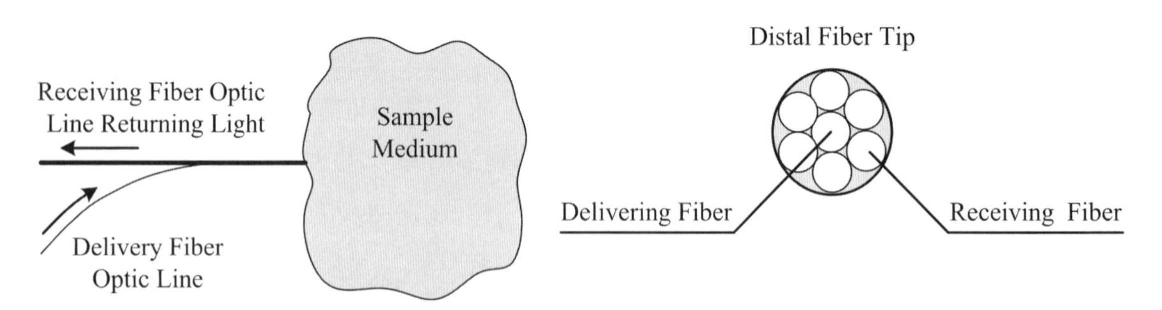

FIGURE 16-4c Light through separate transmitting and receiving fibers.

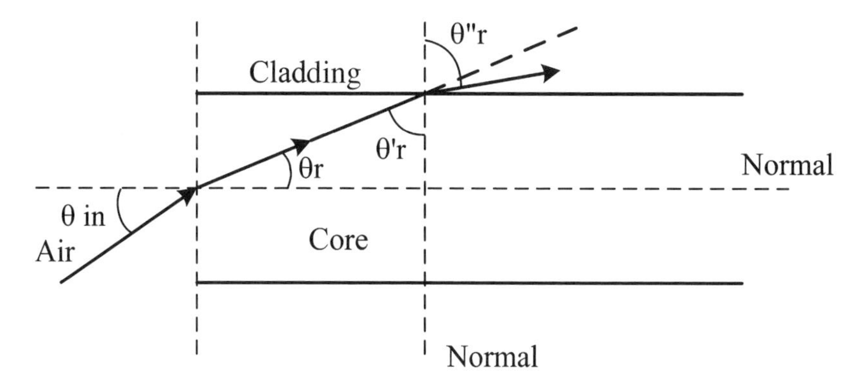

FIGURE 16-5a Air/core interface in the fiber.

For the photo-emitter/core interface, the equation for Snell's law is:

$$\eta_{air} \times \sin\theta_{in} = \eta_{core} \times \sin\theta_r$$

where η_{air} and η_{core} are the refractive indexes of the air and the core material. The angles of θ_{in} and θ_r are the angles at the air/core interface as shown.

In **Figure 16-5a,** the light ray bends toward the normal as the wave travels from the air interface to the dense medium of the core material. However, the ray bends away from the normal at the core/cladding interface shown in **Figure 16-5b.**

For the core/cladding interface, the equation for Snell's law is given as:

$$\eta_{core} \times \sin\theta_r' = \eta_{cladding} \times \sin\theta_r''$$

Where η_{core} and η_{clad} are the refractive indexes of the core and cladding material and the angles θ_r' and θ_r'' are the angles shown at the core/cladding interface.

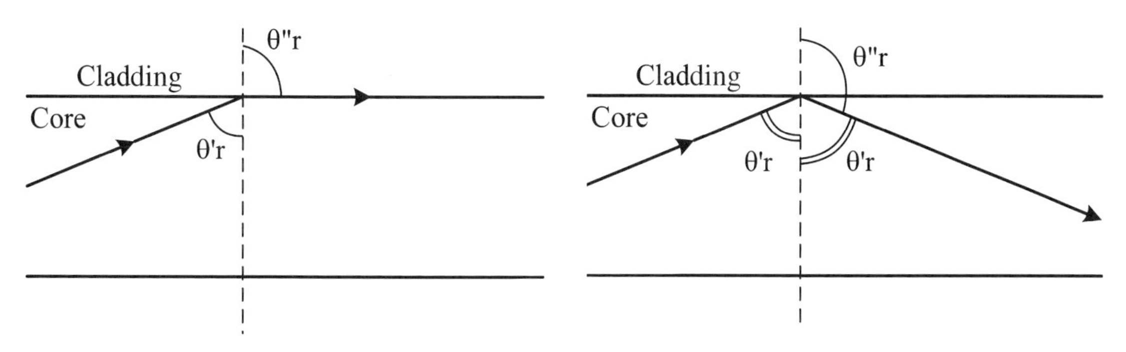

FIGURE 16-5b Core/cladding interface in the fiber.

Example An optical fiber has a core with a refractive index of 1.52 and its cladding has a refractive index of 1.44. What is the critical angle?

The critical angle is computed when the light beam bends 90 degrees at the core/cladding interface.

Using Snell's law:

$$(1.52) \times \sin\theta_r = (1.44) \times \sin(90°) = (1.44)$$
$$\sin\theta_r = (1.44) / (1.52) = 0.947$$
$$\text{Critical angle} = \theta_r = \sin^{-1}(0.947) = 71.26 \text{ degrees}$$

■

Example A light beam is emitted into a single-mode fiber made of quartz. The length of the fiber is 1 meter (m). How long will it take the light to travel through this length? You can assume that the light travels straight along this fiber center.

$$\text{Time} = \text{Distance/velocity}$$

Distance is given as 1 m and the velocity of light in the quartz fiber is 1.94×10^8 meters per second.

$$\text{Time} = \frac{1 \text{ m}}{1.94 \times 10^8 \text{ m/sec}} = 0.005 \ \mu\text{seconds}$$

■

Example A light beam is emitted directly from the air interface into the fiber core with a refractive index of 1.3. The angle of incidence to the air/core interface is 30 degrees. Find the angle of refraction (i.e., at what angle the beam will bend).

Snell's law indicates:

(refractive index of air) × (sin[angle of incidence at the air/core]) = (refractive index of fiber core) × (sin[angle of refraction]) = sin(30°) = 1.3 × sin(angle of refraction)

On solving, angle of refraction = $\sin^{-1}(\sin(30°) / 1.3) = 22.62°$

■

Example For the given **Figure 16-6,** find the incident angle at the air-core interface. ■

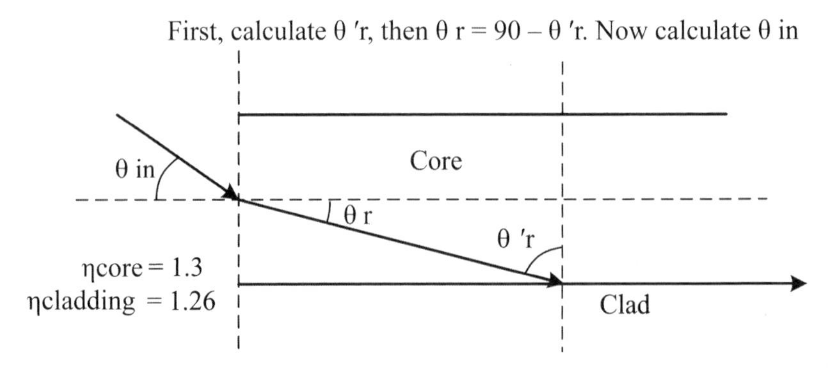

FIGURE 16-6 Critical angle at the core/cladding interface.

Example The index of refraction of water is 1.33. What is the speed of light in the water?

Given: $\eta = 1.33$ and the velocity of light in a vacuum is 3×10^{10} cm/sec.

Therefore, η = (speed of light in a vacuum) / (speed of light in a substance or material)

$$1.33 = (3 \times 10^{10}\ \text{cm/sec}) / (\text{speed of light in water})$$

$$\text{Speed of light in water} = (3 \times 10^{10}\ \text{cm/sec}) / 1.33 = 2.26 \times 10^{10}\ \text{cm/sec}$$

▪

16.2 FIBER MODES, TRANSMISSION, AND DETECTION

The three different fiber modes are single-mode fiber, multimode fiber, and graded multimode fiber. These modes guide the light rays differently. In single-mode fiber, the light travels straight from one end to the other end without any internal reflections. However, in multimode fibers, the wave travel and the useful intensity of the light is due to the internal reflections in the core material.

Photo Emitters and Detectors

There are several parameters in LEDs (light emitting diodes) when used with fiber.

1. **The output power (emitted).** When output power is increased in LEDs, drive requirement is lowered. There is a trade-off; therefore, other losses in the emitting LED are compromised.
2. **Wavelength.** Wavelength emission is based upon the type of optical fiber due to the fact that fibers have attenuation characteristics that vary with the emission wavelength. There are fiber types that can attenuate 10 dB/km (decibels per kilometer) or 800 dB/km. In medical applications, the distance may not be a factor, but how much light is attenuated from one end to the other end is a factor.
3. **Speed in turn-on/turn-off times.** LEDs cannot be turned on and turned off quickly. There is a finite time for LEDs to be switched from on to off. These times vary from 20 nanoseconds (nsec) to 100 nsec.
4. **Emission patterns.** The main goal in the usage of fiber is to couple the fiber to the LED in such a way that almost all the emission (power from the LED) is collimated into the fiber. The LEDs are PN junction diodes constructed of silicon-doped gallium-arsenide or aluminum-gallium-arsenide, where layers of aluminum-gallium-arsenide of p-type semiconductors or n-type semiconductors are grown over the surface of a gallium wafer. The top metal layer has a small opening for light emission. This is shown in **Figure 16-7a.**
5. **Photo detection.** In photo detection, a photon (light) is absorbed by the atom, causing an electron to move from the valence band to the conduction band and become a free electron. These free electrons will become an electrical current when a voltage is applied. This is shown in **Figure 16–7e.**

Figure 16-7b is a graph showing the differences in LED and laser diode emissions. In this output power graph, the laser diode's power increases dramatically after about 200 mA of drive current, while the LED diode's output power is already saturated.

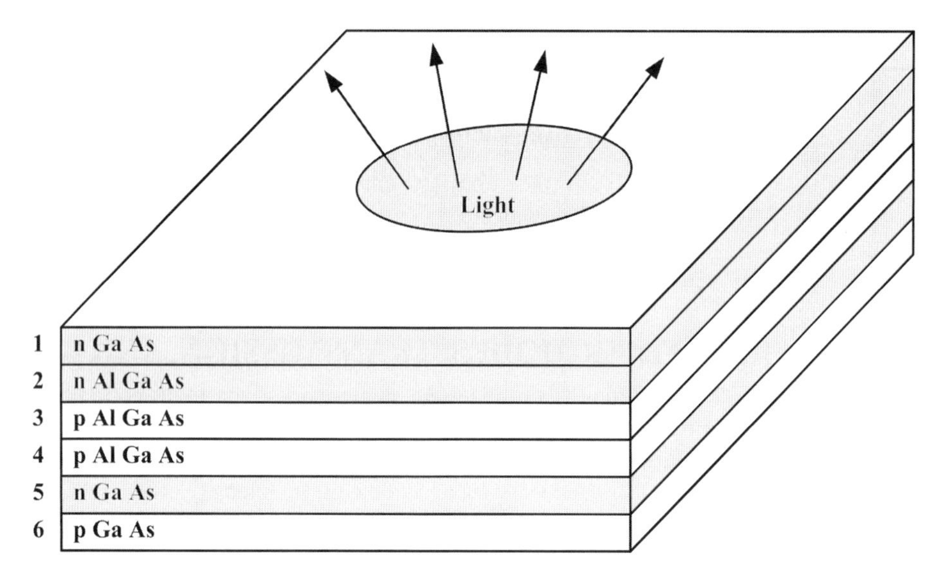

FIGURE 16-7a LED construction.

As illustrated in the graph of the wavelength and output power relationship in **Figure 16-7c,** the spectral width of the laser diode is narrow compared with that of the LED diode. This shows that different wavelengths (known as spectral width) are emitted by the diodes, and the output power is then related to the wavelength.

Because it is important that more light is coupled into the fiber, the emission 3-dB beam width for the laser diode is very small compared with that of the LED diode. The maximum output power in the middle of the emission pattern spreads out and the intensity decreases. The 3-dB beam width is the angle (around the maximum power output) when 0.707 of the maximum power is received or coupled to the fiber. This is shown in **Figure 16-7d.**

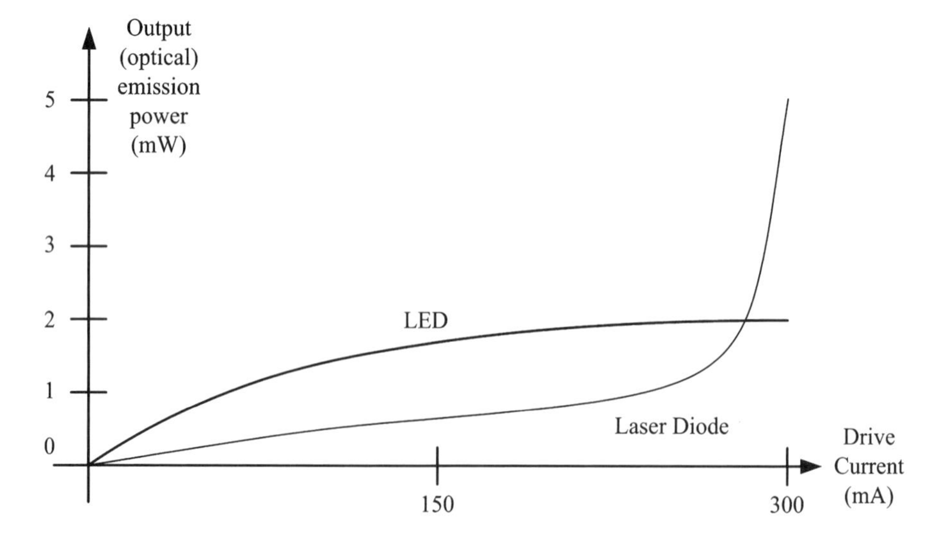

FIGURE 16-7b Output emission power for LED and the laser diode.

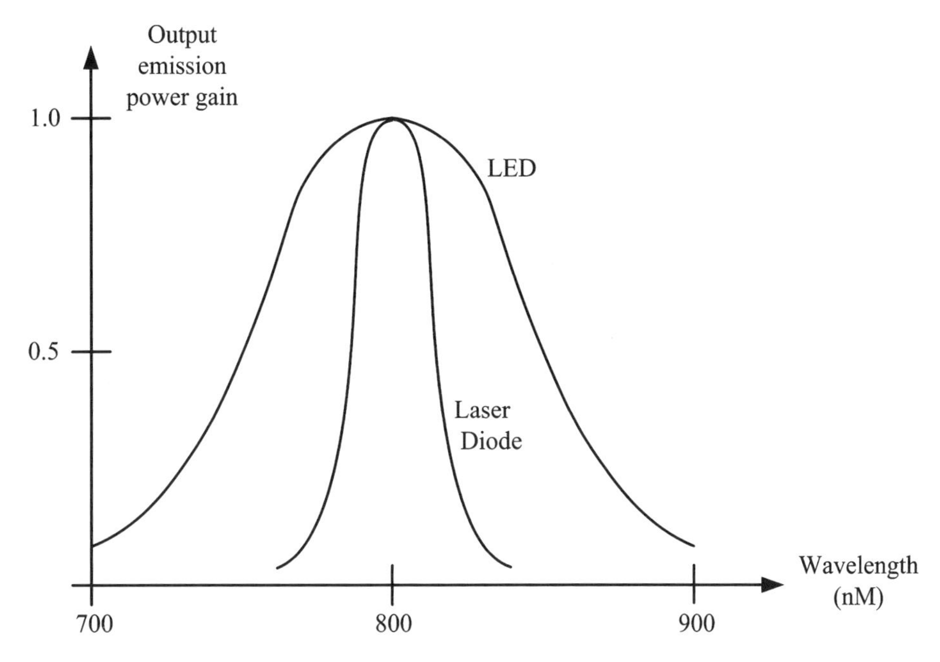

FIGURE 16-7c Output emission power gain for LED and the laser diode with respect to their wavelengths.

Initially, the photo detector diode is reverse-biased and becomes forward-biased due to photon energy absorbed by the atoms of the depletion region. The conventional flow of current is read by the ammeter. Holes move to the negative polarity and electrons to the positive polarity. The depletion width increases as more electrons are depleted due to the photon absorption.

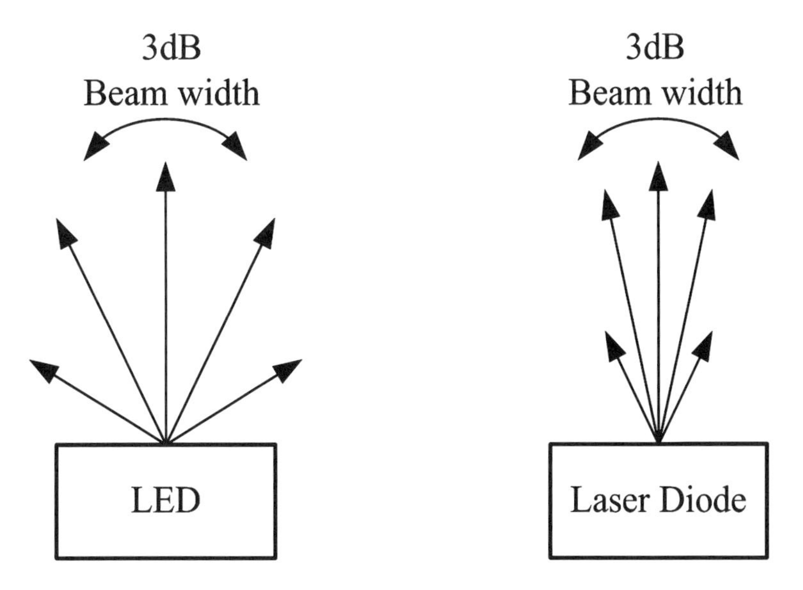

FIGURE 16-7d 3-dB beamwidths of LED and laser diode.

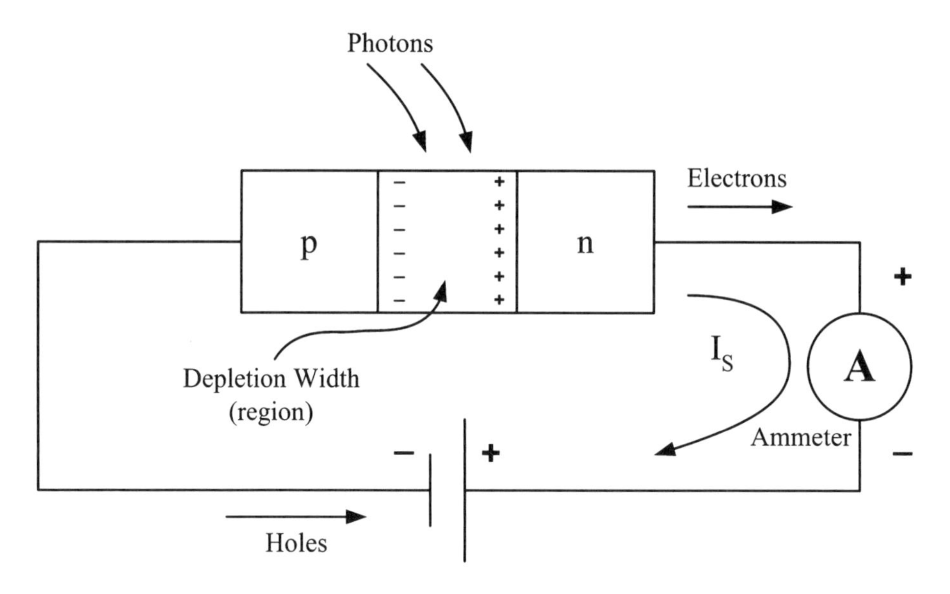

FIGURE 16-7e Photo detection for the reverse-biased diode at the receiver.

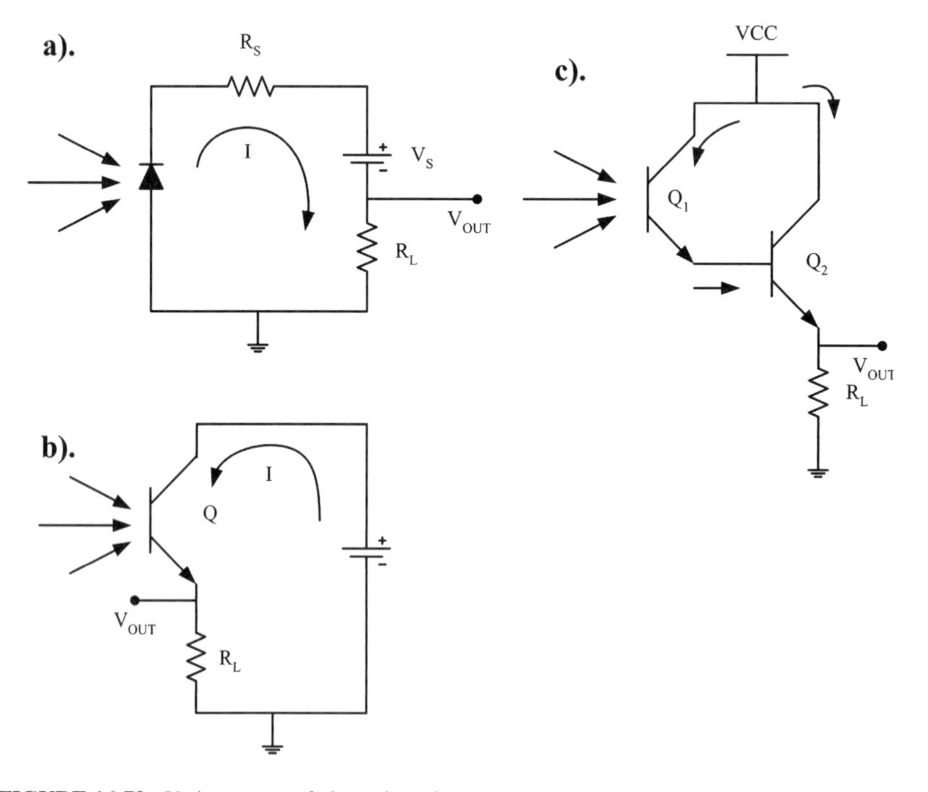

FIGURE 16-7f Various ways of photo detection.

In addition to photodiode detectors, there are phototransistors that can detect the presence of light. A few simple circuits are shown in **Figure 16-7f.** The bipolar transistor and the Darlington pair transistors are only forward-biased. When sufficient light interacts with the base of the transistors, the output is taken at the load R_L.

As previously mentioned in this chapter, the technique of fiber optics is used in several areas of patient care. The following sections discuss how it is applied in the procedure called endoscopy.

16.3 ENDOSCOPY IMAGING

Endoscopy is the examination and inspection of the interior of body organs, joints, or cavities through an endoscope. An endoscope is a device that uses fiber optics and powerful lens systems to provide lighting and visualization of the interior such as organs, joints, or cavities. The portion of the endoscope inserted into the body may be rigid or flexible, depending upon the medical procedure. Fiber-optic endoscopes now enjoy widespread use in medicine and guide a myriad of diagnostic and therapeutic procedures, some of which include:

- Sigmoidoscopy. This is the examination of the rectum and lower portion (sigmoid) of the colon. The most common instruments used in sigmoidoscopy are the flexible sigmoidoscope or the rigid sigmoidoscope.
- Colonoscopy. This is the examination of the inside of the colon and large intestine to detect polyps, tumors, ulceration, inflammation, diverticular colitis, Crohn's disease, and discovery and removal of foreign bodies. The most common endoscope used in this procedure is the colonoscope.
- Bronchoscopy. This is the examination of the trachea and the bronchial trees in the lungs to reveal abscesses, bronchitis, carcinoma, tumors, tuberculosis, alveolitis, infection, and inflammation. Some of the instruments used in bronchoscopy are the bronchoscope and nasopharyngoscope.

Video technology is now widely used in endoscopic instruments. A video chip is positioned at the distal tip of the tube and a video signal is sent to a video processor and to a monitor. The video image may also be transferred from the tip through an array of glass fibers. For example, in a visual examination of the upper intestinal tract, called an esophago-gastro-duodenoscopy (EGD), a lighted flexible fiber-optic cable or video technology-based endoscope is used.

Figure 16-8a and **Figure 16-8b** show a typical endoscope and an endoscope system. Note that one end of the endoscope contains the eyepiece for viewing, whereas the other end is the flexible tip. The control head, tip, and the flexible cable are expensive pieces containing fragile fibers. They should be held firmly and in a vertical position. In addition to transmitting light, the umbilical cord can pass other tubes for delivering air or water and to provide suction. The control head carries the eyepiece and camera for viewing. The image of the body part can be transmitted through fiber cable or a charged–coupled device (CCD) so that the video chip can take the picture.

A mobile cart containing the endoscope connected to the monitor and computer allows the device's operator to move the equipment conveniently throughout the radiology or emergency departments, or wherever necessary.

FIGURE 16-8a A photograph of a flexible endoscope.

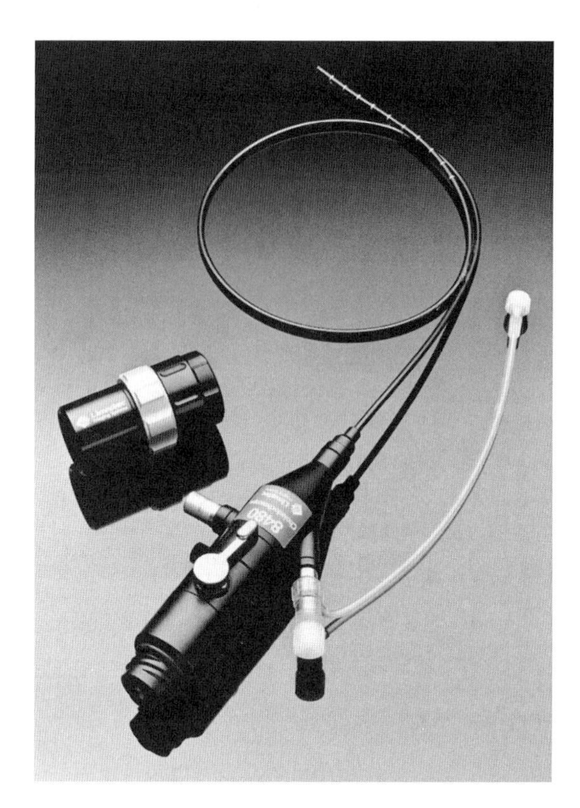

FIGURE 16-8b An endoscope system.

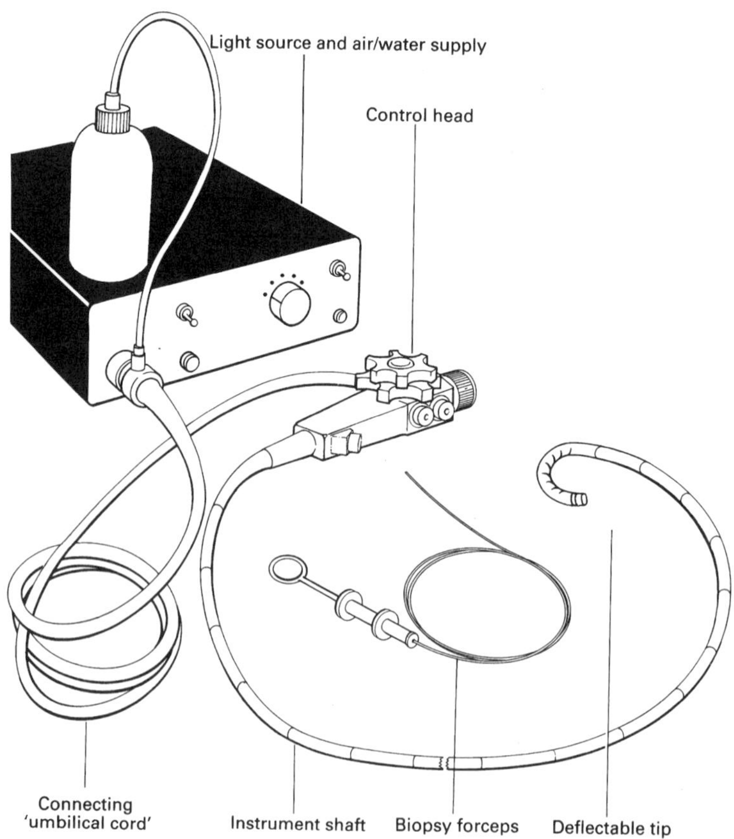

Video Endoscope versus Fiber Endoscope

An image cannot be obtained unless the organ or body cavities are well illuminated by the light transmission from the external source through the fiber cable. Usually, the image is obtained either by the fiber-mode of light reception through the cable or by using a charged-coupled device (CCD). This is a chip mounted onto the tip of the fiber bundle. The electronic wires can then be brought out to the video receiver. In a fiber endoscope, there are different transmitting and receiving fibers side by side in the umbilical fiber cable.

Charged-Coupled Device Chip

A charged-coupled device (CCD) chip has thousands of photocells that receive photons of light reflected from the organs, joints, body cavities, or mucosal surfaces. Charged-coupled device chips can be black and white or various colors, and a high picture resolution can be achieved additionally by the use of filters and optical lens.

In CCD technology, there is an array of light-sensitive capacitors that transform a light pattern (image) into an electric charge pattern (electronic image) by collecting, storing, and transporting electric charges. Each photosensitive capacitor represents a picture element (pixel) and the matrices of these pixels are then connected to the amplifiers. The transfer of the charges from pixel to pixel, line after line in the matrix to the output amplifier then creates a video signal. For example, **Figure 16-9** shows CCD arrays integrating the amount of light after exposure time of one second (table on the left side) and two seconds (table on the right side), respectively. The numbers represent an electric charge proportional to the light intensity at that location.

In medical applications, very high-resolution CCD chips are used and thousands of pixels in micrometers (millionths of a meter) can yield a digital image.

90	82	83	98
80	85	67	65
38	39	42	65
202	300	82	83

182	160	160	197
162	171	140	130
79	82	86	130
400	582	162	165

FIGURE 16-9 A CCD table.

16.4 SIGMOIDOSCOPY

Sigmoidoscopy is the minimally invasive medical examination of the large intestine from the rectum through the last part of the colon (also called the lower gastrointestinal, or GI, tract). There are two types of sigmoidoscopy: flexible sigmoidoscopy, which uses a flexible endoscope (a sigmoidoscope); and rigid sigmoidoscopy, which uses a rigid device. Flexible sigmoidoscopy is generally the preferred procedure. A sigmoidoscopy is similar to, but not the same as, a colonoscopy. (A sigmoidoscopy only examines up to the sigmoid, the most distal part of the colon, while a colonoscopy examines the whole large bowel. We will learn more about colonoscopy in the next section.) The sigmoidoscopy is a very effective screening tool. This procedure is used to screen the body for colon cancer or polyps, tumors, inflammation, hemorrhoids, diverticula (pouches) and the narrowing in the sigmoid colon.

Figure 16-10a shows a photo of a flexible sigmoidoscope, while **Figure 16-10b** shows a diagram of a sigmoidoscope as it is inserted in the intestine. The instrument is about the diameter of your little finger but can extend to 60 cm in length.

There are several symptoms a patient may present that will alert a physician to recommend a sigmoidoscopy:

- History of consistent constipation or diarrhea
- Lower abdominal pain
- Rectal bleeding
- Changes in bowel habits or itching

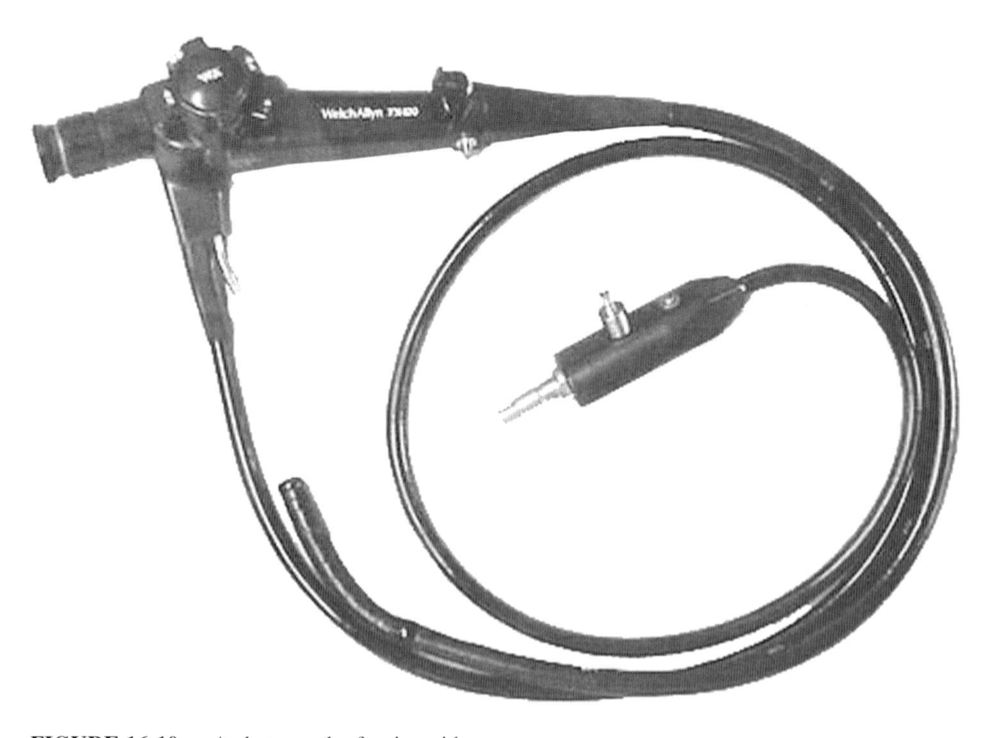

FIGURE 16-10a A photograph of a sigmoidoscope.

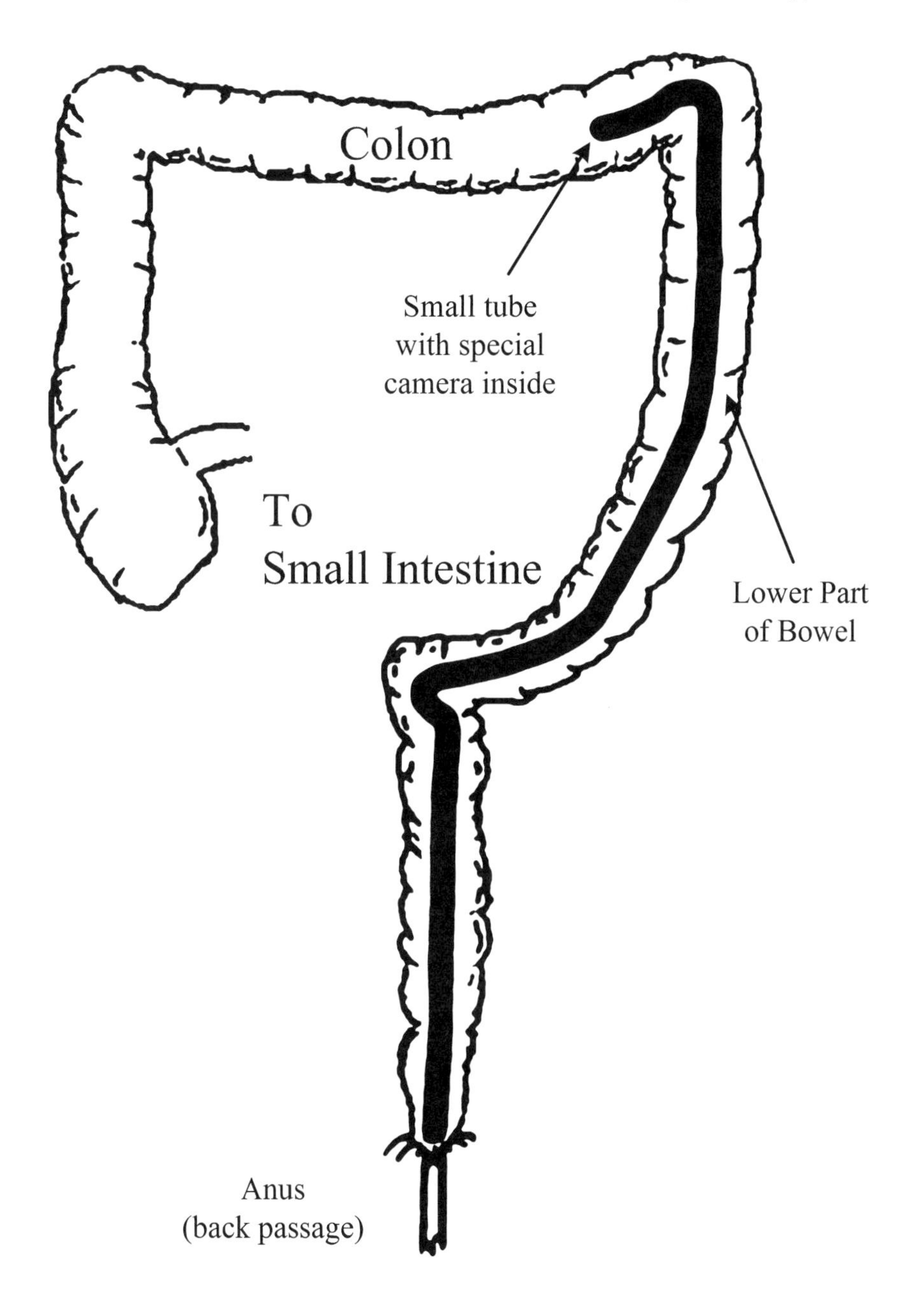

FIGURE 16-10b Sigmoidoscope in the lower part of the bowel.

As the flexible sigmoidoscope follows the natural contours of the intestine, the fiber-optic cable inside the scope transmits light into the colon. The equipment consists of an eyepiece, several buttons for air and water inputs, light source, fiber cable, a suction button, and the biopsy channel. For control, the device is equipped with maneuvering buttons so that the physician can move the scope up and down or left and right for enhanced viewing.

A sigmoidoscopy may be performed on an outpatient basis or as part of your stay in a hospital. Procedures may vary depending on your condition and your physician's practices.

In general, the sigmoidoscopy follows this process:

1. Instructions will be given to you directing you to remove jewelry and other objects that may obstruct the procedure.

2. Instructions will direct you to disrobe as a gown must be worn for this procedure.

3. You will be instructed to lie on your left side on the procedure table with your knees bent towards your chest. Alternatively, you may be positioned in the knee-chest position, on your knees with your head and chest bent down, touching the table.

4. A rectal exam will be executed by the physician to check for the presence of blood, mucus, or fecal matter. This will also help dilate the anus.

5. A lubricated sigmoidoscope will be slowly inserted into the anus and advanced into the rectum and lower part of the colon (distal sigmoid colon). After the sigmoid colon is visualized, the sigmoidoscope will be removed.

6. During the sigmoidoscopy procedure an anoscopy and/or proctoscopy may be performed in combination to avoid multiple procedures. If these procedures are performed, an anoscope and /or a proctoscopy will be inserted to visualize the lower rectum and/or anal canal.

7. Negligible discomfort is associated with the procedure and you may feel a strong urge to have a bowel movement when the sigmoidoscope is inserted. You may experience temporary muscle spasms or lower abdominal pain during the procedure as well. To help alleviate some of the discomfort take deep breaths while the tube is being inserted.

8. Air may be introduced to expand the bowel to aid visualization. During this process, air will escape around the instrument. You should not try to hold in the air. A suction device may be used to remove blood and liquid feces.

9. At some point in the procedure, specimens may be taken from the lining of the large intestine with a special brush or swab.

10. During the procedure, if a polyp is seen, the physician may remove it for biopsy, or leave it for a subsequent operation.

11. After the procedure is completed, the instrument will be removed.

FIGURE 16-11 A typical procedure of sigmoidoscopy.

Figure 16-11 is a list of general procedural guidelines in the use of a flexible sigmoidoscope.

This is an invasive procedure and complications may occur such as persistent bleeding or inflammation of the lining of the abdominal wall. Very rarely, the procedure may perforate the intestinal wall, which can be dangerous and lead to other complications.

16.5 COLONOSCOPY

Colonoscopy is the endoscopic examination of the large colon and the distal part of the small bowel with a CCD camera or a fiber-optic camera on a flexible tube passed through the anus. It may provide a visual diagnosis (e.g., ulceration, polyps) and grants the opportunity for biopsy or removal of suspected lesions. It is the standard diagnostic procedure for most colonic diseases. It demands considerable skill and requires special training and certification exams for the physician who performs this procedure (called gastroenterologists.) Generally, the first line of examination for colon disease is a sigmoidoscopy, which is usually followed by a colonoscopy if further investigation is deemed necessary.

The colonoscope incorporates a CCD chip and an electronics circuit at its tip so that a digital image can be transmitted to a computer and video monitor. The tip of the instrument can be controlled by the control head, which has pull wires, an up-down wheel mechanism, and a right-left wheel mechanism. The head also includes a suction pump, and an air-water jet. The tip has fiber-optic light output, a CCD camera, and the focusing lens. The control head and the tip of the colonoscope is shown in part of **Figure 16-12a.**

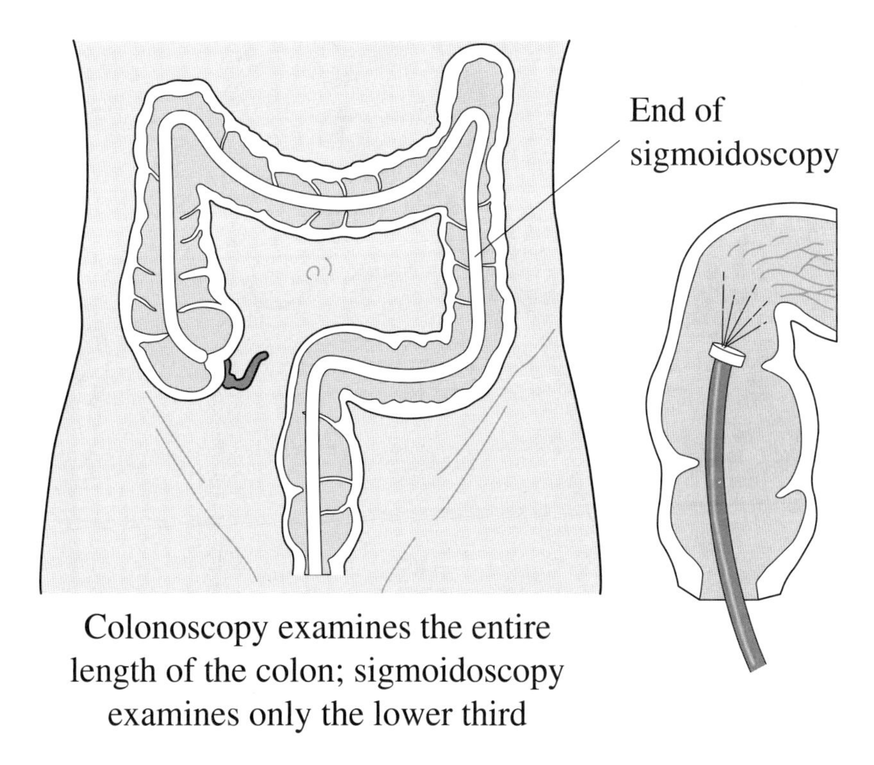

FIGURE 16-12a A colonoscopy loop.

Colonoscopy

General Information

Where It's Done	Who Does It	How Long It Takes	Discomfort/Pain
Hospital or outpatient endoscopy suite.	Doctor (gastroenterologist, some gastrointestinal surgeons) and endoscopy assistants.	20 - 90 minutes, depending on the time needed to reach the colon and whether additional procedures, such as polyp removal, are involved.	Discomfort associated with having the colonoscope inserted into the rectum and colon and having air instilled into the bowel.

Results Ready When	Special Equipment	Risks/Complications	Average Cost
Immediately; 48 - 72 hours for analysis of biopsy samples.	Colonoscope and light source.	Perforation of the colon or rectum in 0.01% to 0.5% of cases, bleeding, infection, dehydration from excessive use of laxatives.	$1300 to $1500

FIGURE 16-12b General information on colonoscopy.

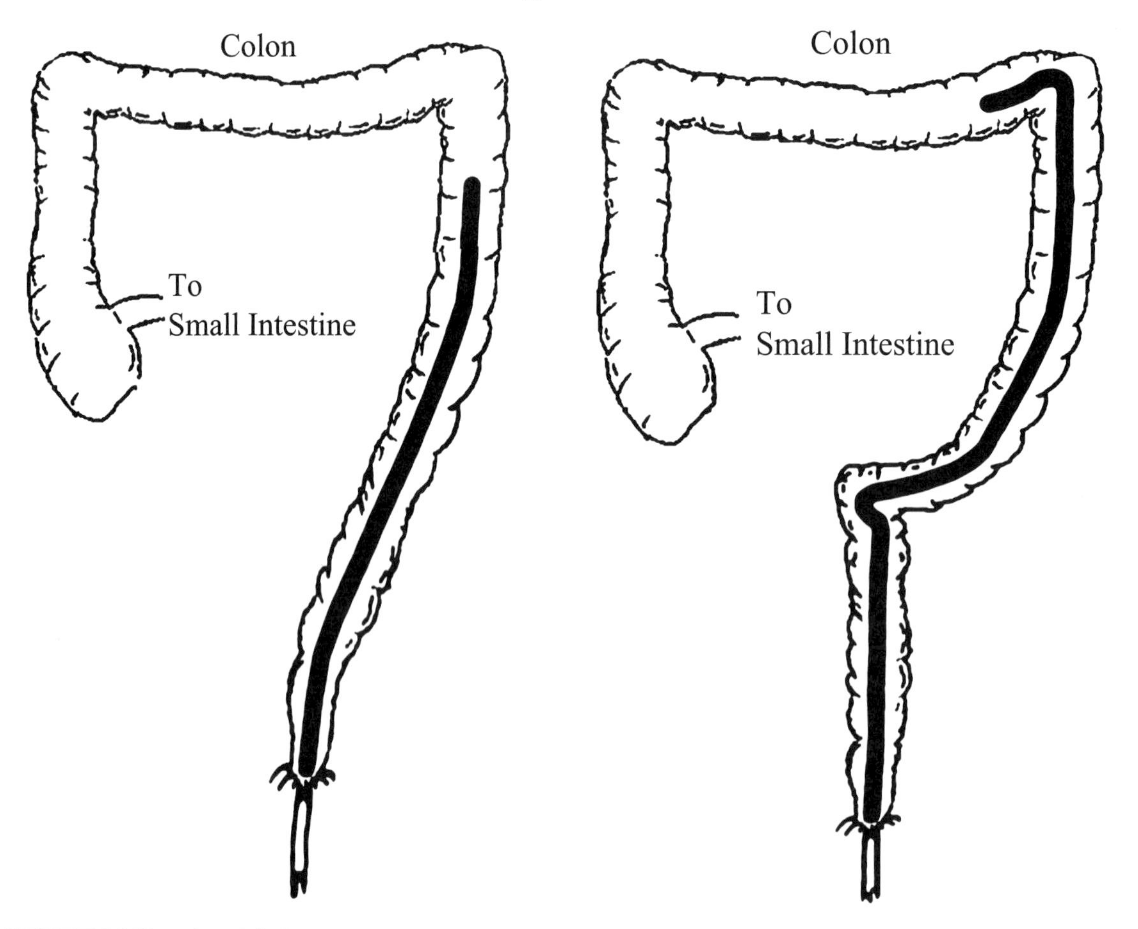

FIGURE 16-13a A straight loop.

FIGURE 16-13b A developing N-loop.

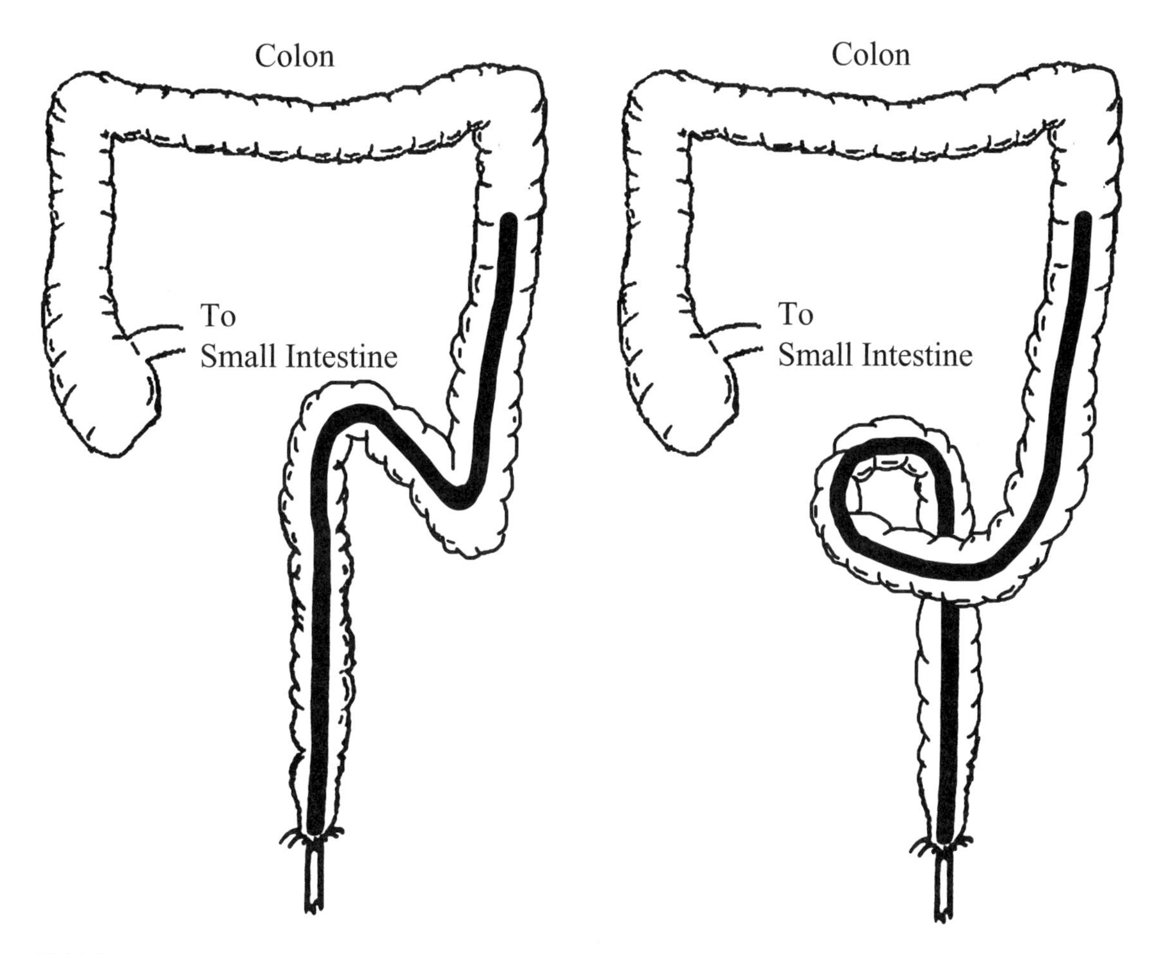

FIGURE 16-13c N-loop.

FIGURE 16-13d Alpha-loop.

The tube of the colonoscope is rotated through the intestine and it can reach the entire length of the colon. **Figure 16-12b** provides additional information about the colonoscopy.

The N-loop or the alpha loop is unavoidable as the colonoscope pushes inward to visualize the inside of the intestine walls as in **Figure 16-13a** through **Figure 16-13d.** The physician has to insert and manipulate the colonoscope tube and typically N-loop is common to develop, however, pushing through any loop is unacceptable if force is required or pain results.

16.6 BRONCHOSCOPY

Bronchoscopy is a procedure during which a pulmonologist or a thoracic surgeon uses a viewing tube, called a bronchoscope, to evaluate the patient's lungs, voice box, vocal cord, trachea, and many branches of bronchi. Bronchoscopy can be used for diagnosis or treatment. The conditions for diagnosis include persistent cough, blood in the sputum (coughed

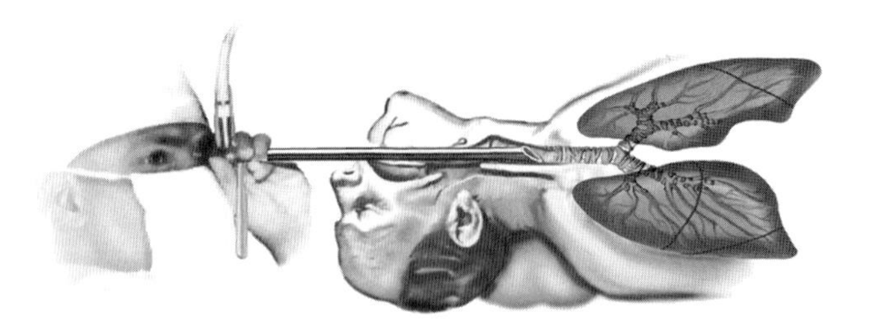

FIGURE 16-14 Bronchoscopy.

up mucus from the lungs) and inflammation in the lung. The treatment includes removing the foreign bodies in the airways, placing a stent (a tiny wire mesh tube) to open a collapsed airway, or removing any growth that is blocking the airway.

In this procedure, the bronchoscope instrument is used for examining, and in some cases taking biopsies from, the interior of the bronchi. **Figure 16-14** shows an image of a bronchoscopy device. A physician examines inside a patient's airway for abnormalities such as inflammation, tumors, bleeding, or even foreign bodies. Both rigid and flexible bronchoscopes are used; however, rigid instruments are less frequently used today.

Xenon Light Source

Figure 16-15 shows a light source designed to illuminate the surgical sites in endoscopic applications. The front panel has a cable port for the light source, which attaches to the fiber cable, and a light intensity meter that indicates the intensity of the light beam from 0% to 100%. The rear panel has video-in and video-out connections. The device is equipped with safety features to prevent the patient from being burned accidentally by an unattended light cable.

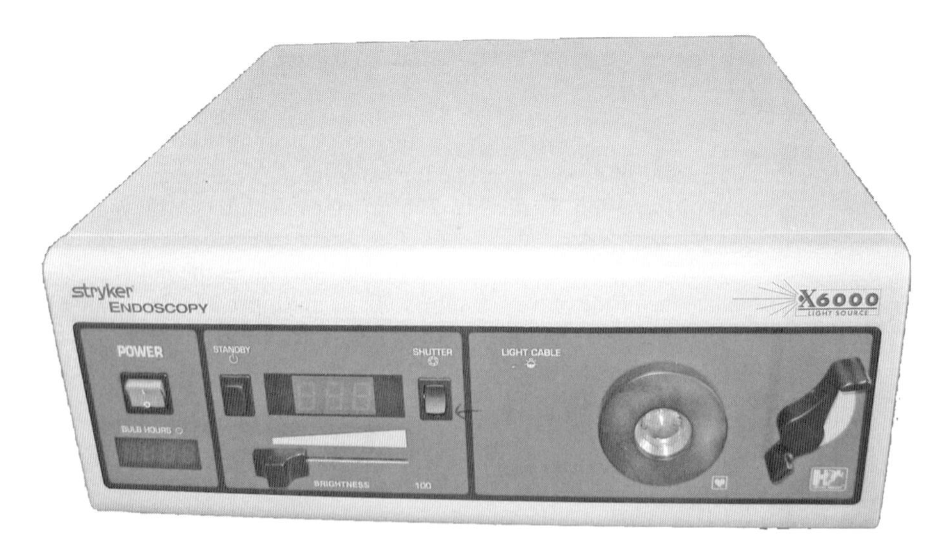

FIGURE 16-15 A light source in bronchoscopy/endoscopy.

16.7 PHYSICS OF LASER

Laser light is coherent and monochromatic. That means that all of its light waves are in phase and of the same frequency. These two properties then make laser light very sharply focused. We know how to burn a piece of paper by focusing sunlight through a magnifying glass; a laser beam is even more focused than that and can be made to focus to the size of a living cell. In eye or brain surgery, a laser beam has a great advantage over other types of surgical electrodes or surgical scalpel because it is sharper, narrower, and more precise in cutting tissue or vaporizing cells. The major disadvantage of laser usage is its cost.

Stimulated Emissions of Radiation

The simple atom consists of a nucleus and one or more electrons that circle in different orbits. Each atom then can be excited by some external medium such as heat, light, or electricity to change its initial energy level to a high energy level. The electrons at lower energy orbits will move to higher energy orbits away from the nucleus. When the same electrons move back to their original energy levels, they release their extra energy as photons (the particles of light).

According to Einstein, when a photon strikes another atom that is already in an excited state, the atom releases a new photon that is identical to the incoming photon. In a way, we have now two photons traveling together in the same direction. We can also think that the incoming light is a wave and when it strikes the excited atom, the atom releases extra energy so the wave becomes a bigger wave. This process is called stimulated emission and is the foundation of how a laser works.

A few examples are given when photons are emitted, or radiated, when electrons of atoms (or molecules) jump from a high energy level to a low energy level. These are the transitions of electrons between various energy levels. In **Figure 16-16a**, an electron drops from a higher energy level to a lower level, and a photon is produced (spontaneous emission); an atomic electron absorbs an incident photon and brings the atom into a higher energy state (absorption), and a photon (on passing through a collection of excited atoms) can stimulate a generation of many more photons creating an avalanche of light (stimulated emission). If the excited atoms are unable to produce photons that match (in wavelength, direction and polarization) the incoming photon, then stimulated emission cannot take place. In **Figure 16-16b,** two photons can be emitted if the electron drops from energy level two to one and follows this with another jump to level zero.

For a laser beam then:

1. Atoms with metastable energy level need to be collected and excited to higher levels.
2. A massive stimulated de-excitation of the excited atoms needs to be held in cavities.
3. Repopulating the excited levels after the photons are contained.
4. Create coherent laser beam of proper use.

Figure 16-17a shows the schematic diagram of a laser beam generator. The most commonly used laser system in the OR is the carbon dioxide laser shown in **Figure 16-17b.**

Example A laser beam emits radiation of wavelength 800 nm and delivers 10 W of power. Calculate the number of photons emitted per second.

▪

FIGURE 16-16a A photon emission.

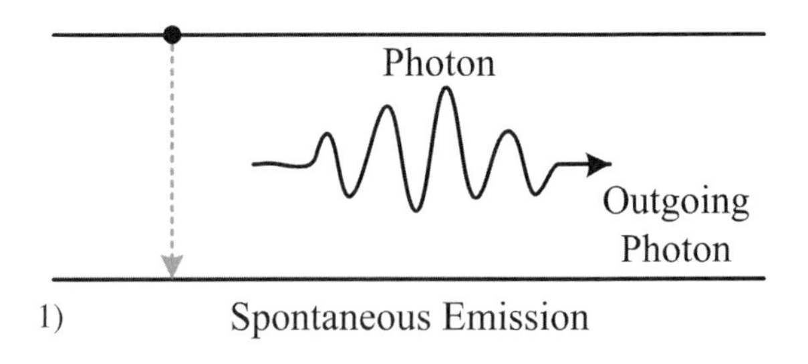

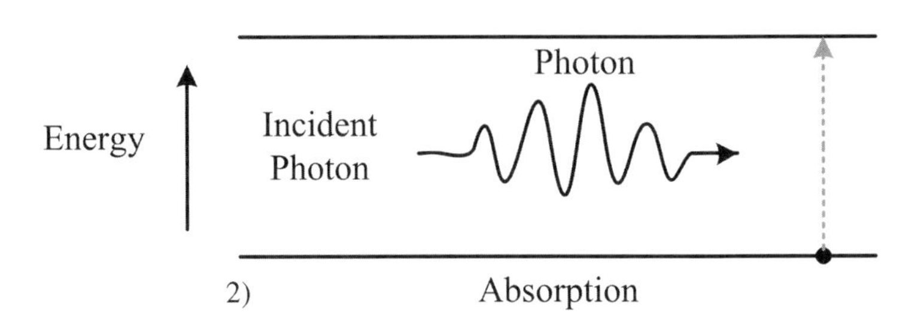

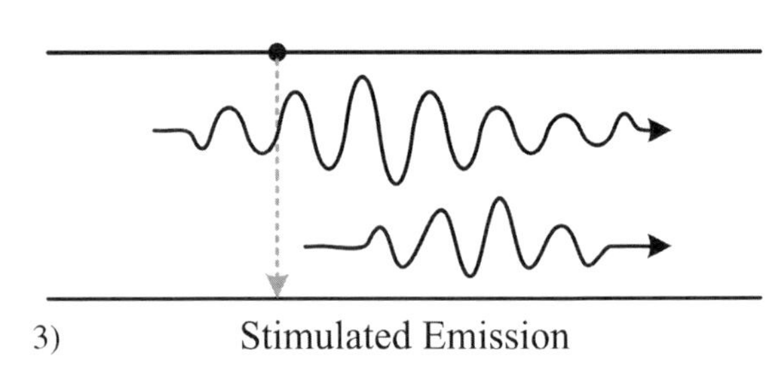

FIGURE 16-16b Emission of two photons.

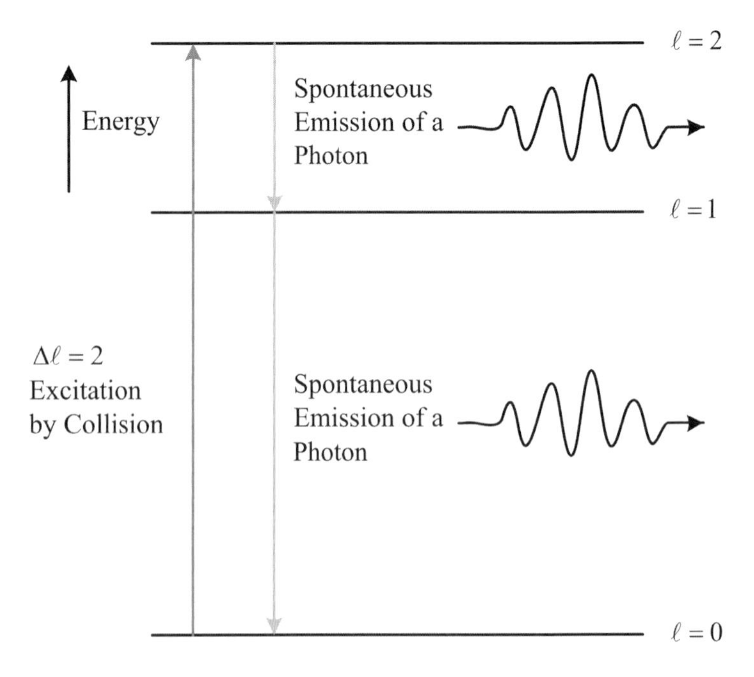

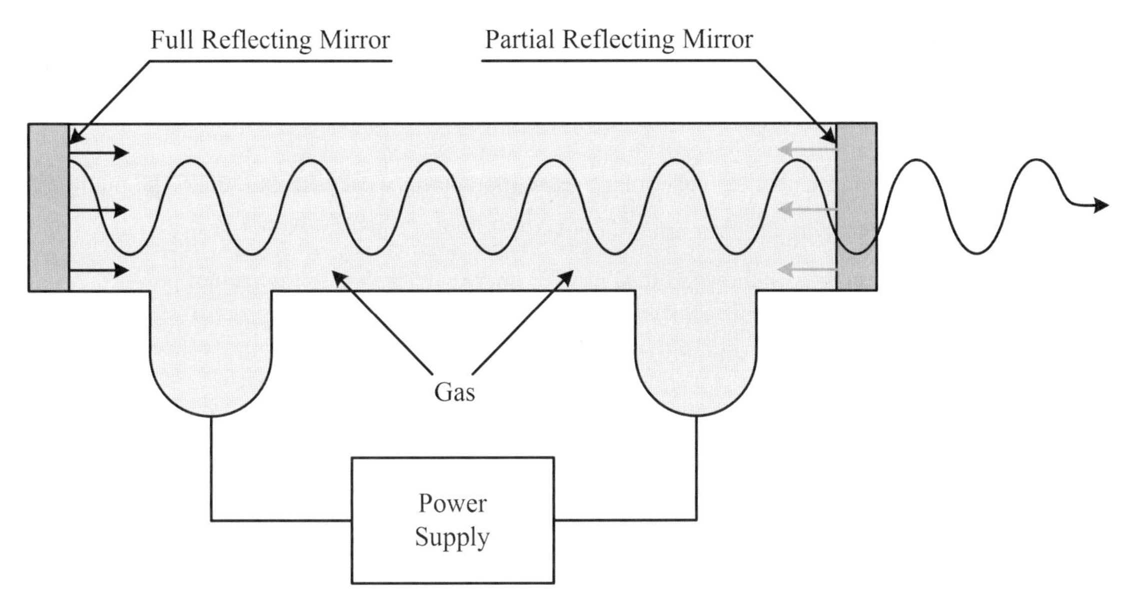

FIGURE 16-17a A laser schematic diagram.

Example In a helium-neon (He-Ne) gas laser, the characteristic red light is emitted due to the stimulated emission occurring between two neon levels at 20.7 eV and 18 eV. Determine the wavelength and frequency of the photon emission.

■

Example Determine the amount of power incident on the laser detector.

Given: the laser wavelength is 632.8 nm; the detector is terminated into 50-ohm load; and the detector produces 22 mV.

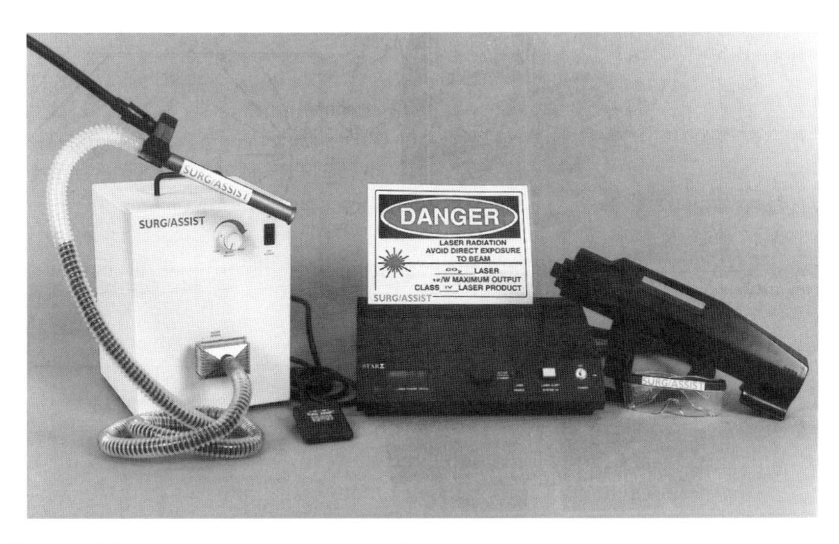

FIGURE 16-17b A photograph of a carbon dioxide laser with plume evacuator.

First, we will calculate the current in the detector circuit when the detector detects the laser beam.

$$I = \text{Voltage across the load / the load impedance} = 22 \text{ mV} / 50\ \Omega = 0.44 \text{ mA}$$

From the responsitivity curve of the laser photodetector data sheet for the 632.8 nm laser:

$$\text{Responsitivity} = \text{Photocurrent in mA / Power of the incident light in watts} = 0.4 \text{ A / W}$$

Therefore: Incident Power = 0.44 mA / 0.4 A/W = 1.1 mW is the amount of power incident on the detector.

■

Example Which laser can be used for the following procedures? Explain.

a) in removing a brain tumor

b) spot welding a detached retina

c) in hair removal

■

The following section discusses types of CO_2 laser; solid-state laser systems, including Nd, and Yag lasers; and laser cooling systems.

16.8 LASER CLASSIFICATIONS

Light transport in tissue, light-tissue interaction, and therapeutic applications must be discussed. A flow chart of the laser and tissue interaction is shown in **Figure 16-18a.** There are two compartments in this interaction: optical and thermo-dynamical.

The laser-tissue interaction consists of a photo-thermal effect, a photo-chemical effect, an electromechanical effect, and a photo-ablative effect. Laser, which is an acronym for Light Amplification and Stimulated Emission of Radiation, concentrates a beam of light to a precise focal point, but the areas adjacent to this focal point are relatively cool by comparison.

In photo-thermal effect, light energy is converted into heat energy. This causes the tissue to heat up and vaporize. The photo-chemical effect causes the target cells to start light-induced chemical reactions. In electromechanical effect, the dielectric breaks down in tissue caused by shock wave plasma expansion resulting in localized mechanical rupture. The photo-ablative effect causes photo-dissociation or breaking of the molecular bonds in tissue.

The energy density, also called fluence, determines the magnitude of the laser interaction. It is calculated as:

$$\text{Energy Density} = \frac{\text{Pulse energy}}{\text{Area of spot size}}$$

As shown in **Figure 16-18b**, the spot size diameter (d) depends on the diameter of the fiber core (d_0) and also the distance between tip of the fiber core and the tissue (h). The smaller is the spot size diameter on the tissue, larger is the magnitude of the energy density for laser interaction.

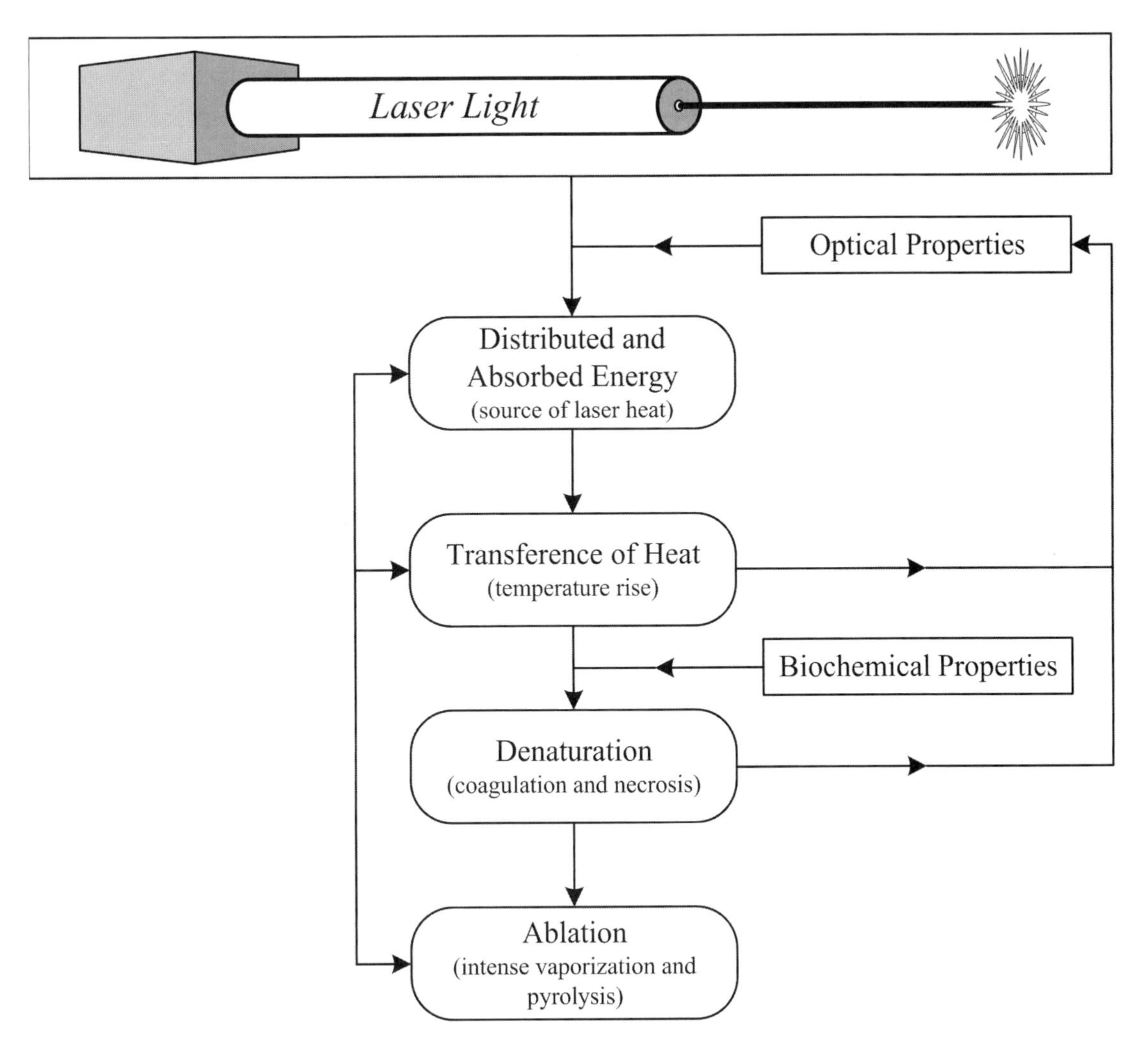

FIGURE 16-18a Process of laser and tissue interaction.

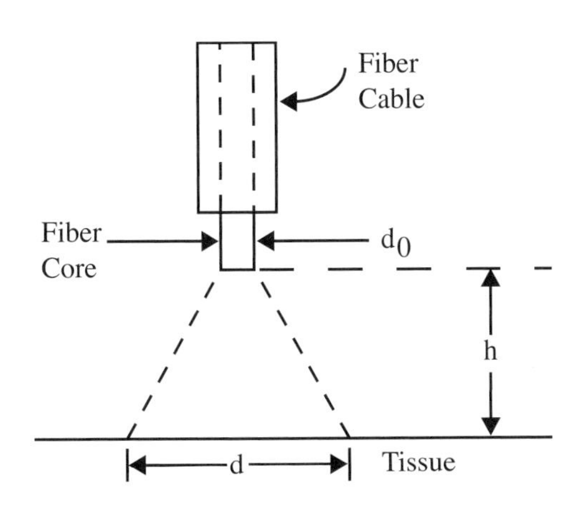

FIGURE 16-18b Laser spot size in laser-tissue interaction.

To generate a laser beam, the machine has at least four major components: an active medium (solid state, liquid, gas); an excitation mechanism (optical, electrical, chemical); a feedback mechanism (resonator mirrors); and an output coupler (partially transmissive mirrors).

16.9 LASER TYPES

Laser beams are strong beams of light produced by electrically stimulating a particular material. A solid, a liquid, or a gas is used. The beam is focused to treat tissues by heating the cells until they burst. There are a number of different types of laser beams; each has a different color and use.

The types of medical lasers in terms of wavelengths (from small to large) can be discussed now. They are as follows:

Argon Laser

The wavelength range of the argon laser is 488 nm to 514 nm. It is a continuous wave gas laser and emits blue-green light and is readily absorbed by hemoglobin and melanin. A fiber-optic cable is used for delivery. Typically argon laser is used for photo-coagulation in ophthalmology.

Ruby Laser

The wavelength is 694 nm and this type of laser emits red light. It is strongly absorbed by blue and black pigments of the skin. It is used for fair skinned patients for hair removal.

Nd:YAG Laser

The wavelength is 1,064 nm or 1,320 nm and emits near-infrared invisible light. It is used for hair removal and is effective on black tattoo ink. These YAG lasers use Yttrium Aluminum Garnet crystal rods doped with the neodymium (Nd) molecules for special types of delivery. This type of laser comes in three types: switched (for tattoo removal), pulsed (for general surgery where tissue coagulation is desired), and continuous wave (for hair removal).

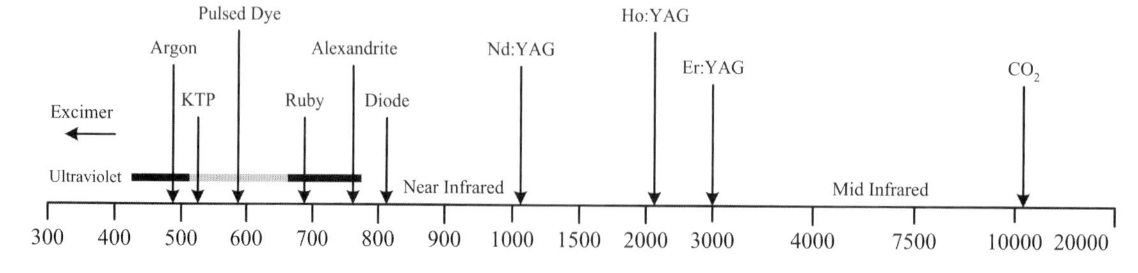

FIGURE 16-19 A wavelength chart (in nanometers) of laser types.

CO_2 Laser

This laser is widely used by surgeons and its interaction with soft tissue is quite visible. Also, as this type of laser beam is absorbed by water, and as soft tissue contains a large amount of water molecules, the interaction between the CO_2 laser and the soft tissue is good for cutting or vaporizing or ablation.

CO_2 lasers can be either continuous wave or pulsed type and can be made to focus into a thin beam. The wavelength of CO_2 laser light is 10,600 nanometers (nm), that is, 10.6 micrometers in the upper infrared range. A wavelength chart is given in **Figure 16-19.**

16.10 LASER MEDICAL APPLICATIONS

A simple list of laser medical applications is given next:

- Cosmetic surgical procedures, including removing wrinkles, eliminating birthmarks or skin discoloration, removing or transplanting hair and skin changes that occur as a result of aging, employing the techniques of photocoagulation and photovaporization
- A tool used in surgical procedures in cardiology, dentistry, dermatology, gastroenterology, neurology, oncology, ophthalmology, orthopedics, otolaryngology, pulmonology, and urology
- Remote spectrophotometry
- Pressure and position sensing
- Scintillation counting
- Intravascular pressure transducers
- In vivo oximeters
- Fiber-optic faceplates, tapers
- Laser imaging (from single molecules to optical tomography)
- Laser-tissue interaction (photochemical, photostimulation, cytotoxicity testing, photothermal, photomechanical, shock and acoustic waves, cavitation, and ablation)
- Laser electrosurgery and oximetry

16.11 LASER RADIATION SAFETY

Laser devices in the United States are subject to Mandatory Performance Standards. They must meet product performance standards and an initial report must be submitted to the Center for Devices and Radiological Health (CDRH) Office of Compliance before these devices can be used in hospitals.

The certification of any laser product means that each device has passed a quality assurance test and the manufacturer assumes the responsibility for the record keeping, notification of defects, and any radiation occurrence on the device.

SUMMARY

This chapter presents basic theory of light and optics in medical devices and then continues with the practical medical applications.

1. We start with the physics of fiber optics discussing light intensity, photon energy, and Snell's law. The interface between core and cladding material is discussed in detail. The optical fiber consists of a core, cladding, and a buffer (a protective outer coating). The cladding guides the light along the core by using the method of total reflection. The cladding has a lower refractive index than the core, but both are made of silica glass or plastic.
2. Various fiber modes, photo-emitters, detectors, and fiber cables are discussed in principle and application.
3. The most significant applications of fiber optics are in the imaging and illumination components of endoscopes. The application of fiber optic imaging in endoscopy procedures such as sigmoidoscopy, colonoscopy, and bronchoscopy is then presented.
4. Next, the physics of a laser is explained, with additional coverage pertaining to the different types of lasers used in medical devices. The types of lasers most often used in medical treatment are the CO_2 laser, the Nd:YAG laser, and the argon laser. The Nd: YAG laser is capable of penetrating more deeply than other lasers.
5. Finally, we finish with a general overview of lasers with particular emphasis on laser radiation safety.

MEDICAL TERMINOLOGY

The following is a list of medical terms mentioned in this chapter.

Dermatologist: physician specializing in diagnosing and treatment of disorders related to the skin.

Endoscope: instrument used for visual examination of body cavities or organs. Used to obtain biopsy samples, control bleeding, and remove foreign objects, as well as for other procedures.

Gastroenterologist: medical doctor specializing in the study of diseases and disorders affecting the gastrointestinal tract including the stomach, intestines, gallbladder, and bile duct.

Ophthalmologist: medical doctor specializing in the treatment of diseases and disorders of the eye.

Urologist: medical doctor specializing in diagnosing and treating diseases and disorders of the female urinary system and the genitourinary system of males (genitourinary refers to both genital and urinary organs).

Maxillo-facial surgeon: surgeon specializing in surgery of the face and jaws to correct deformities, repair injuries, and treat diseases.

Transcutaneously: passing or entering through the skin. For example, transcutaneous electrical nerve supply-pads are placed on either side of the spine and connected to a battery-operated apparatus controlled by the patient for pain relief.

Sigmoidoscope: instrument for visualizing the interior of the rectum, sigmoid colon, and possibly a portion of the descending colon.

Colonoscope: instrument for visual examination of the inner surface of the colon from the rectum to the cecum.

Gastroscope: an endoscope that is used to examine the interior of the stomach.

Bronchoscope: an endoscope that is used for examining and taking biopsies from the interior of the bronchi, as well as for removal of inhaled foreign objects.

Nasopharyngoscope: a device used for viewing nasal passages and pharynx.

Esophago-gastro-duodenoscopy (EGD): the endoscopic examination of the esophagus, stomach, and upper duodenum.

Gastrointestinal (GI): pertaining to the stomach and intestines.

Polyps: mushroom-like growths from the surface of a mucous membrane.

Inflammation: a localized response to an injury or destruction of tissues characterized by heat, redness, swelling, and pain.

Diverticula: pouches or sacs protruding from the wall of a tube or hollow organ.

Hemorrhoid: an inflammation and enlargement of rectal veins; also known as piles.

Photocoagulation: use of a laser to treat macular degeneration by focusing the light source to seal leaking or damaged blood vessels.

Photovaporization: the transformation of a solid or liquid to a state of vapor by light.

Refractive surgery: a surgical procedure designed to eliminate or reduce the dependency on glasses or contacts. The procedure corrects refractive errors by changing the focus of the eye. LASIK and PRK are common procedures.

QUIZ

1. A laser beam can be transmitted via optical fibers in the medical field for what purpose? How is this done?
2. True or False: Light can travel in a curved transparent rod by multiple internal reflections:

   a) True b) False
3. When light travels from one medium to another, does its velocity, wavelength, or frequency change? Explain:
4. Why must aspirin and iron tablets be discontinued one week before a colonoscopy?
5. Endoscopic ultrasonography (EUS) is used as:

   a) An ultrasound attachment to an endoscope to view heart valve motion.

   b) An ultrasound attachment to an endoscope to view the digestive tract.

   c) A straight metal tube with a light beam to view abdominal structures.

   d) None of the above.
6. Wavelength is the distance traveled:

   a) During a half cycle. b) During one second.

   c) During one full cycle. d) During five full cycles.

7. Ultraviolet light has more energy than visible light; X-ray light has ______ than ultraviolet light.

a) Less b) Equal c) More

8. Laser light is monochromatic, that means it is ___________.

a) Of single frequency b) Of single color

c) Both a. and b. d) Either a. or b.

9. Name at least three properties of laser light:

1. ______________________________

2. ______________________________

3. ______________________________

10. A laser beam can be used to _______ bleeding wounds and ulcers.

a) Cut out b) Cauterize

c) Shock d) Weld

RESEARCH TOPICS

1. Medical residents can practice surgical skills on medical simulators before they are allowed to practice on patients. Some hospitals require their residents to master endoscopy procedures on simulators such as the Endoscopy AccuTouch. Write a research paper that emphasizes the importance of medical simulators in general and then compare an array of simulators from a few vendors in terms of their uses and the electronic circuits they contain.
2. Color video images of the GI tract can be transmitted by the wireless endoscopy system. This is done by ingesting a capsule that is propelled through the GI tract and contains a miniaturized transmitter. This new technology is in its trial phase but has immense potential because it does not use invasive endoscopy tubes. Investigate this new technology and write a report on the transmitter and receiver circuits and other components in this wireless endoscopy system.

CASE STUDIES

U.S. Endoscopy is a manufacturer of GI endoscopy accessories. A detailed case study on this new company (started in 1991) is helpful for clinicians, surgeons, and researchers. The home office is located in Mentor, Ohio. The case study should include the various medical-related ventures the company is involved in, and the impact of these ventures on the quality of patient care.

A fragile, small-built woman, age 35, was drinking excessive water in a 24-hour period. She was also vomiting this excessive amount of water. She was not complaining of any abdominal pain, and doctors suspected some kind of foreign object such as a fish bone, as this patient used to have a staple food of rice and fish. X-rays taken several times a day did not reveal any abnormalities, but the ultrasound found the fish bone in the deep stomach. The object was then removed by endoscopy. Several questions can be asked on this case:

- Why was the patient drinking excessive water and then vomiting?
- Why is it that X-rays could not reveal the problem but ultrasound did?
- How do endoscopic scissors cut and remove any foreign objects?

PROBLEMS

1. If the refractive index of water is 1.32, determine the critical angle at the water-air boundary.

2. When a light beam incidentally strikes the surface of water from air, what is the maximum possible value for the angle of refraction?

3. A material with an energy-band gap of 1.25 eV is used in a proton emission; determine the frequency and wavelength of the emitted light.

4. An LED couples-12 dBm of optical power into a fiber bundle. How much is this in milliwatts?

5. Discuss fiber optic tapers in the CCD medical applications in terms of coupling, size, and viewing area.

6. Compute the numerical aperture of the fiber (i.e., the acceptance angle of light entering the fiber from air). Given: core refractive index of 1.35 and cladding index of 1.31. Now, determine the corresponding acceptance angle.

7. Explain the difference between photocoagulating and photovaporizing a tissue using a laser beam and focusing it to achieve high power densities. How does a lens help in focusing?

8. Compare and contrast the three types of laser technology in terms of device, technique, cost, and applications: CO_2 laser, argon laser, and the Nd:YAG laser.

9. Match words in the left column with the description in the right column:

1. Laser output	a) causes cell to vaporize
2. Spot size	b) invisible infrared
3. Safety goggles	c) carries light
4. Precise beam	d) monochromatic
5. CO_2 emits	e) prevent eye damage
6. Argon emits	f) looks inside the body
7. Endoscopy	g) smallest at the focal point
8. Glass or plastic fiber	h) blue light

10. Discuss various applications of laser therapy in terms of the types of laser beam used, the technique, and its cost.

CHAPTER 17

Instrumentation in Intensive Care Units

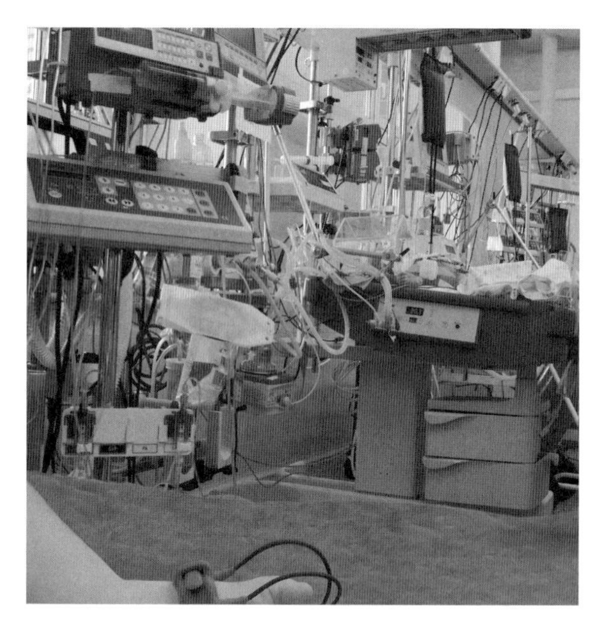

CHAPTER OUTLINE

OBJECTIVES

The objective of this chapter is to introduce the reader to the various bioinstrumentation devices used in hospital intensive care units, such as bedside monitors, patient monitors, telemetry units, and hospital central monitoring systems.

Upon completion of this chapter, the reader will be able to:

- Differentiate various types of intensive care units.
- Discuss the equipment in intensive care units.
- Describe telemetry concepts, such as modulation and carrier.
- Describe bedside monitors and their parameters.
- Describe central monitoring systems used in hospitals.

■ INTERNET WEB SITES

http://www. sccm.org (Society of Critical Care Medicine)
http://www.aacn.org (American Association of Critical Care Nurses)

■ INTRODUCTION

Intensive care medicine, or critical care medicine, is the field of medicine concerned with providing intensive medical care and observation to patients with life-threatening, critical, and/or unstable medical conditions. Most hospitals have departments called intensive care units (ICUs), which are designed especially for the care and treatment of critically ill or injured patients. Patients may come to the ICU for such intensive care because of a malfunctioning organ or organs, for treatment and observation while in trauma or a coma, or for 24-hour post-operative care. ICUs employ specialized and high-tech biomedical monitoring devices, advanced alarms, and highly skilled staff working around the clock to provide comprehensive and continuous patient care. This chapter is a discussion of the various biomedical devices used in ICUs, including bedside monitors, patient monitors, telemetry units, and hospital central monitoring systems.

■

17.1 FACT SHEET FOR INTENSIVE CARE UNIT

Although the purpose of a hospital's ICU is simple, in actual practice an ICU is very complex. Health care professionals who work in the ICU, or rotate through it during their training, provide around-the-clock intensive monitoring and treatment of patients seven days a week. Patients generally are admitted to an ICU if they are likely to benefit from the level of care provided. Intensive care has been shown to benefit patients who are severely ill and medically unstable—that is, they have a potentially life-threatening condition or disorder.

Figure 17-1 shows a possible bed scenario in the ICU of a hospital. A room in the ICU may be small, with only one patient bed, or large, with several beds for different patients.

Here is a typical fact sheet for an ICU:

Capacity:	Approximately 30 beds in 30 rooms
Average daily number of patients:	20
Professional/patient ratio:	1:1 to 1:3 (one staff member for one to three patients)
Patient orientation:	Individualized
Average stay:	4 to 5 days
Team rounds:	Doctors, nurses, dietitians, respiratory therapists, social workers, pharmacists, and case managers may work as a team for the ICU patients.
Commonly used procedures:	Ventilators, Swan-Ganz catheters, central lines, arterial lines, dialysis therapy, continuous renal replacement therapy.
Medical and surgical patients	12–14 beds
RN critical care programs	Adult, neonatal and pediatric acute

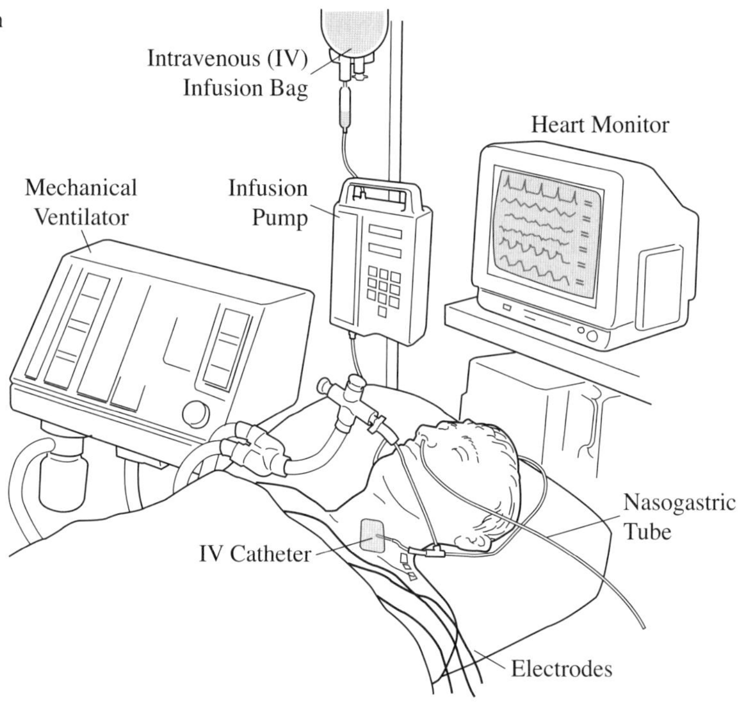

FIGURE 17-1 Intensive care unit in a hospital.

Table 1: How Intensive Care (IC) is Provided	
	Percent (%)
Layout	
Intensive care provided in a separate unit	67% (42)
that has its own nursing station	
Intensive care provided in acute care beds	33% (21)
Mean number of beds (range)	3.5 (1-9)
Equipment Available for IC Patients	
Ventilator	87% (55)
Computerized EKG	92% (58)
Invasive Arterial Monitoring	65% (41)
End of Tidal CO2 Monitor	59% (37)
Transvenous Pacer	40% (25)
Apnea Monitor	33% (21)
Pulmonary Artery Catheter	25% (16)

FIGURE 17-2a A table showing ICU layout and equipment usage.

Table 2: Types of Patients Admitted to Intensive Care Unit or Beds		
Condition	**Percent who would admit patients with the condition to an ICU or IC Bed (N)**	**Percent who report condition as among the most frequent admits (N)**
Chest pain / cardiac event	98% (62)	92% (58)
Diabetic shock / ketoacidosis	97% (61)	41% (26)
Sever COPD / emphysema	95% (60)	78% (49)
GI emergency, e.g., obstruction, GI bleed, appendectomy	92% (58)	49% (31)
Bacteremia / sepsis	89% (56)	30% (19)
Drug / alcohol overdose	89% (56)	54% (34)
Stroke	82% (42)	45% (23)
Asthma (status asthmaticus)	81% (51)	16% (10)
Other respiratory emergency, e.g., pneumothorax,	79% (50)	19% (12)
Foreign body in airway		
Severe allergic reaction / anaphylaxis	76% (48)	0% (0)
Alcoholism with comorbidity	68% (43)	13% (8)
Intractable seizures	37% (23)	3% (2)
Meningitis	32% (20)	0% (0)
Severe fracture	22% (14)	3% (2)
Other severe trauma	22% (14)	2% (1)
Severe mental illness	13% (8)	2% (1)
Severe head injury	8% (5)	0% (0)
Third degree burns	3% (2)	0% (0)

FIGURE 17-2b A table showing the types of patients admitted to an ICU.

Figure 17-2a shows a table of how intensive care may be provided in a hospital and **Figure 17-2b** is a table listing the types of patients who may be admitted to an ICU.

17.2 TYPES OF INTENSIVE CARE

An ICU may be designed and equipped to provide care to patients with a range of conditions, or it may be designed and equipped to provide specialized care to patients with specific conditions. For example, a neuromedical ICU cares for patients with acute conditions involving the nervous system or patients who have just had neurosurgical procedures and require equipment for monitoring and assessing the brain and spinal cord. A neonatal ICU (NICU) is designed and equipped to care for infants who are ill, born prematurely, or have a condition requiring constant monitoring. A trauma/burn ICU provides specialized injury and wound care for patients involved in auto accidents and patients who have gunshot injuries or burns. Following is a more comprehensive list of types of ICUs commonly found in American hospitals:

Intensive care unit (ICU): a specialized section of a hospital containing the equipment, medical and nursing staff, and monitoring devices necessary to provide intensive care.

Cardiothoracic ICU (CTICU): mainly cares for postoperative cardiac and thoracic (heart and lung) surgery patients, providing necessary cardiopulmonary monitoring and assistance.

Surgical ICU (SICU): cares for acutely ill patients in the post-operative phase of major surgery.

Neurosurgical ICU: cares for patients with acute conditions involving the nervous system or patients who have just had neurosurgical procedures and require equipment for monitoring and assessing the brain and spinal cord.

Medical ICU (MICU): cares for critically ill patients with medical conditions related to liver problems, kidney problems, lung problems, blood disorders, and cancers, among other conditions.

Transplant ICU (TICU): cares for transplant patients and donors in various stages of the transplant process, mainly post-operative. It is particularly designed to decrease a patient's susceptibility to infections after surgery.

Cardiac care unit (CCU) or **cardiopulmonary ICU (CICU):** unit that provides specialized care and monitoring for patients with myocardial infarction, severe myocarditis, and other life-threatening heart diseases. Also, pediatric CICU for pediatric patients with congenital heart diseases and other disorders requiring 24-hour observation and care.

Pediatric ICU (PICU): unit specializing in the care of critically ill infants, children, and teenagers.

Neonatal ICU (NICU): unit designed and equipped to care for infants who are ill, born prematurely, or have a condition requiring constant monitoring.

17.3 TYPES OF EQUIPMENT USED IN INTENSIVE CARE UNITS

Biomedical engineering technicians, physicians, and ICU professionals work with many different devices in ICUs. Depending on the type of ICU, these devices can be as common as a catheter (used in many areas of the hospital, not just ICUs) or as complicated as heart-lung machines, respirators, and other life-saving machines. Two of the more commonly used instruments, an intravenous line and nasogastric tubing, are shown in **Figure 17-3a** and **Figure 17-3b,** respectively. **Figure 17-4** shows a more complex mobile bedside monitoring unit with a health care provider at work.

The following list describes some of the more common biomedical instrumentation found in ICUs:

Arterial line: the catheter inserted into the patient's artery, usually in the arm, for continuous direct measurement of blood pressure, oxygen, and CO_2 concentration in the blood, as well as for other physiological parameters. The arterial line is then connected to the bedside monitor.

Bedside monitor: a monitor that is attached to the patient, invasively or noninvasively, by several electrodes and transducers. The most important parameter is the ECG measurement, but blood pressure is also measured indirectly.

Central venous (CVP) line: a thin tube inserted into a vein in the patient's arm or chest in order to measure the venous blood pressure. The other end of the tube is connected to the monitor.

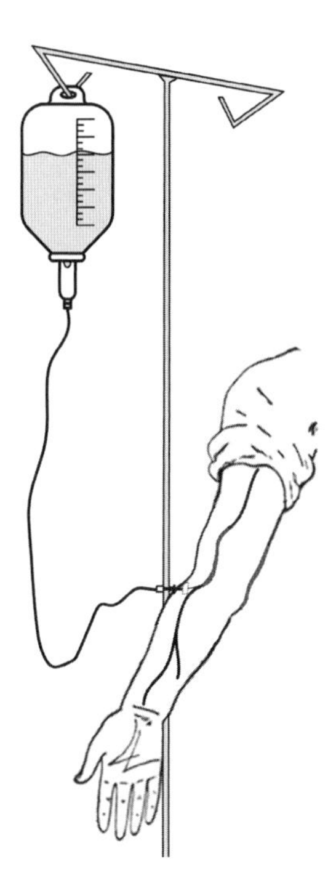

FIGURE 17-3a Intravenous line used in ICUs.

Endo-tracheal tube: the tube connected to a respirator to help the patient in breathing. It is inserted through the nose or mouth and then down the throat and between the vocal chords. The patient cannot speak as long as this tube is connected to the respirator.

IV therapy: the intravenous catheter line inserted into a vein to provide fluids, saline, and medications to the patient.

Nasogastric tubing: a tube is passed through the nose and down through the nasopharynx and esophagus into the stomach. This enables to drain gastric contents, obtain a specimen of the gastric contents or introduce a passage into the GI tract.

Physiological monitor: the comprehensive patient monitoring system that is configured to continuously measure and display ECG, respiration rate, blood pressure, cardiac output, and the amount of oxygen and carbon dioxide in the blood. Each

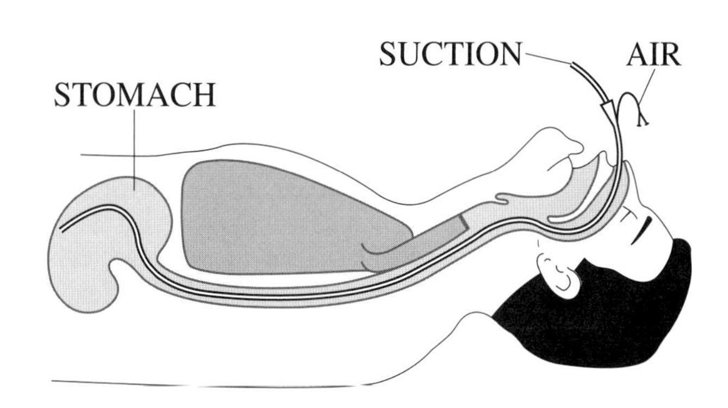

FIGURE 17-3b Nasogastric tubing used in ICUs.

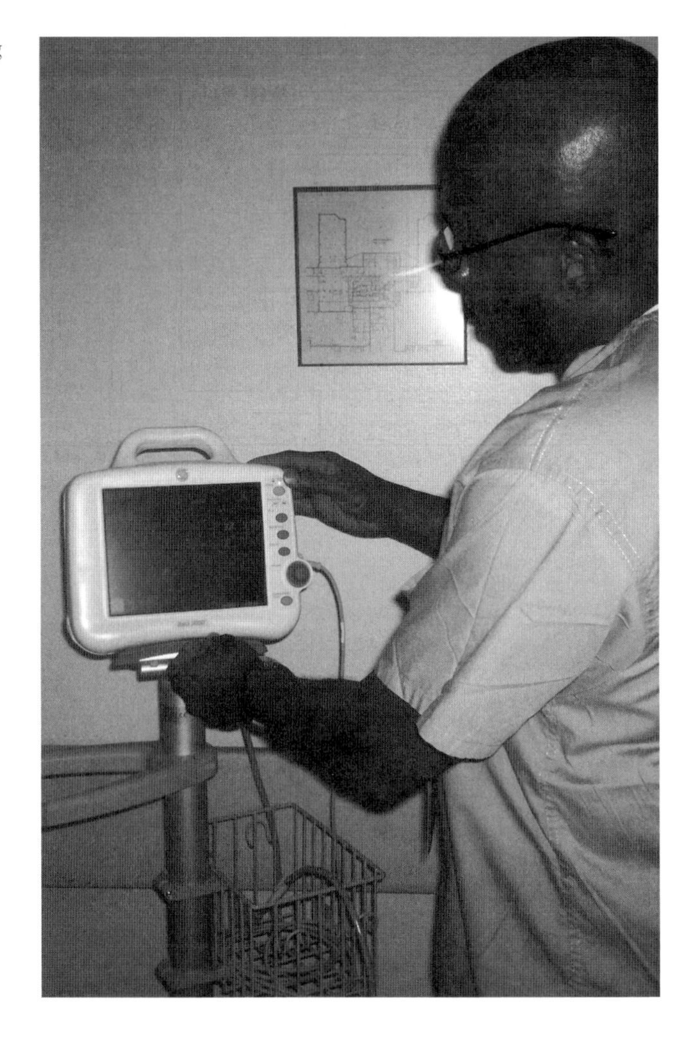

FIGURE 17-4 Health care provider working with mobile ICU monitor.

patient bed in an ICU has a physiological monitor that is connected to the patient via electrodes and sensors, and is also networked to the central nursing station.

Respirator/ventilator: machine that delivers oxygen to the patient's respiratory system in appropriate amount and rate determined by the patient demand.

Swan-Ganz catheter: similar to a CVP line; a catheter that is inserted into the right side of the heart, passes through the lungs and then to the left side of the heart to monitor blood pressure and gas concentrations.

Telemetry unit: connected to the bedside monitor to wirelessly transmit patient information to the central nursing station (CNS). Some telemetry units are independent devices and are directly attached to the patient through electrodes and transducers. The patient data then can be broadcasted to the CNS.

The following sections discuss in more detail several of the instruments that you will find in ICUs.

17.4 BEDSIDE MONITOR

A bedside monitor is a display of the pertinent measurements of the patient's body functions on a TV screen or on a computer monitor. Some of the standard measurements are ECG, respiration, noninvasive blood pressure, pulse oximetry, and arrhythmia analysis. However, some monitors have universal ports for displaying other measurements, such as invasive blood pressure, cardiac output temperature, and $etCO_2$ (end tidal carbon dioxide) in addition to the standard measurements displayed.

The wires or leads of the bedside monitor are connected to sensing devices that are attached to the patient's body. The sensing devices send electronic signals to the monitor for display. **Figure 17-5** shows several modules of a bedside monitor for the display of patient analog data in real time. For the selected module, the input from the patient is amplified, processed, and displayed either as a waveform or in numerical values. SvO_2 and FiO_2 are the abbreviations for saturated venous oxygen and fraction of inspired oxygen (in a gas mixture) respectively. There are alarms on the monitor that will alert the nurse if a particular parameter is beyond the normal readings and the appropriate range. The alarm limits can be adjusted to desired levels to alert nurses or medical staff of a patient's undesirable conditions.

When a patient is admitted to the ICU, a bedside monitor is immediately attached to the patient, with one end of each of the sensing wires connected to the body and the other ends to the monitor. This remains connected for the entire time the patient is in the ICU.

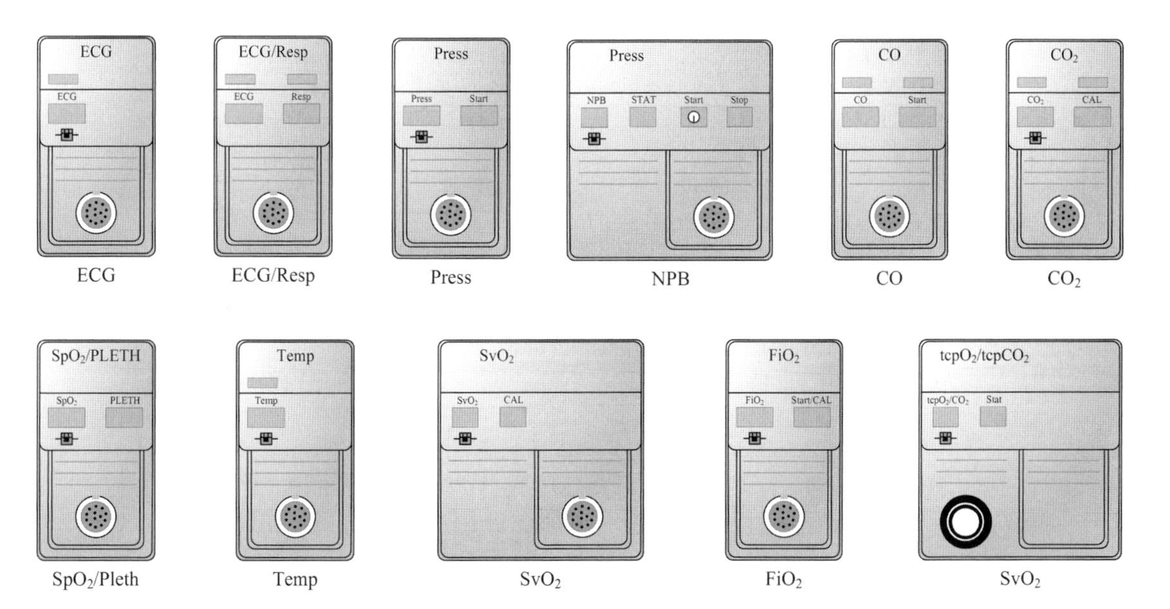

FIGURE 17-5 Various modules of a bedside monitor.

Some of the typical values of bedside monitor measurements are as follows:

	ADULTS:		NEONATES:	
Blood Pressure:	120/80 mmHg		———	
Heart Rate:	50–90 bpm (beats)		120–180 bpm	
Respiratory Rate:	12 bpm (breaths)		40–80 bpm	
Temperature:	37 ° C		37 ° C	
SPO_2:	95–100 %		95–98%	
Cardiac Output:	6 L/min		———	
Expired Gases:	O_2	17%	O_2	17%
	N	79%	N	79%
	CO_2	4%	CO_2	4%

Figure 17-6a shows a bedside monitor and **Figure 17-6b** shows the wireless unit that attaches to the bedside monitor.

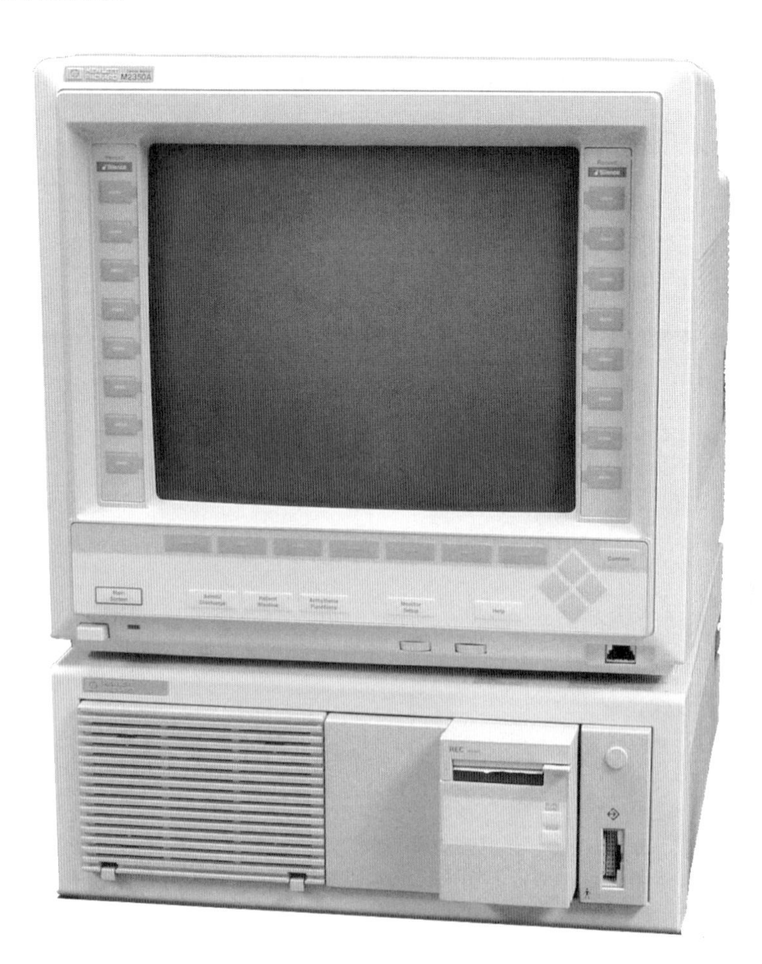

FIGURE 17-6a A bedside monitor.

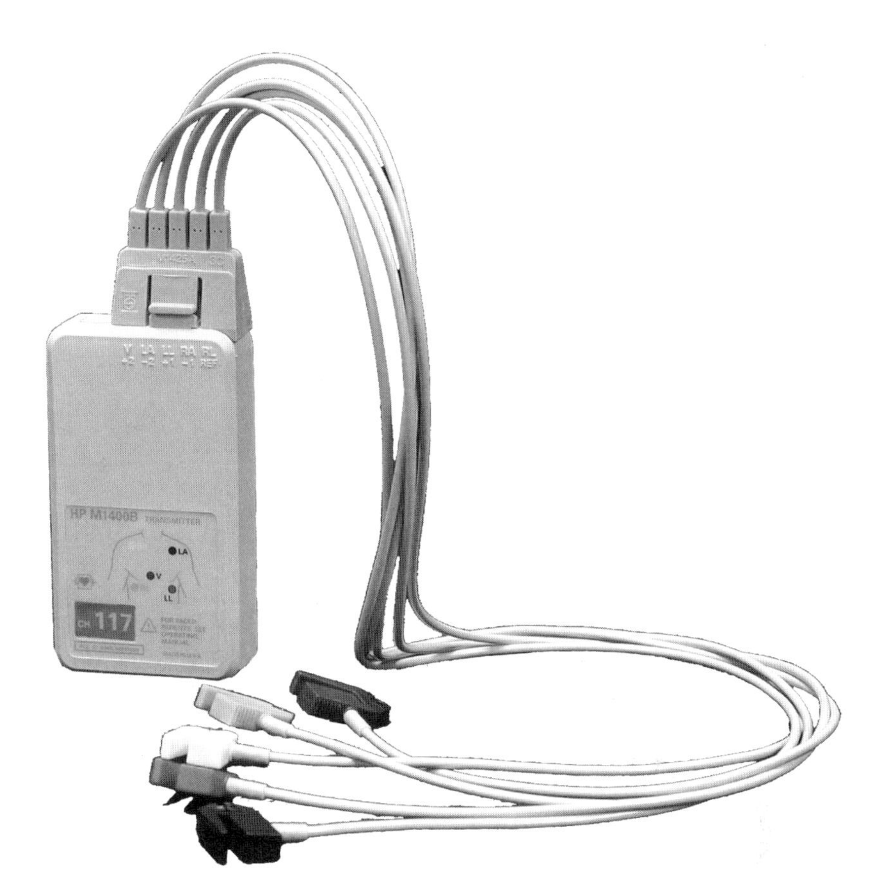

FIGURE 17-6b A wireless unit for a bedside monitor.

17.5 PATIENT MONITOR

The patient monitor used in ICUs displays the fixed set of parameters for the patient's ECG, noninvasive blood pressure, SpO_2, respiration, and temperature. **Figure 17-7a** shows a patient monitor display. Additionally, it can monitor cardiac output, invasive blood pressure, and $etCO_2$, and has features for dose calculations, cardiac calculations, and pulmonary calculations. In a typical monitor display, several parameter waveforms can be selected out of various options.

Figure 17-7b is a block diagram of the components of a patient monitor. Notice the main components are the data acquisition system (DAS) and the processor/power management subassembly. The interface to the patient is through the DAS. The ECG function is a direct connection to the patient and is isolated from the other functions. The monitor has 3-, 5-, and 10-leadwire multilink ECG connectors and can detect heartbeats and arrhythmias.

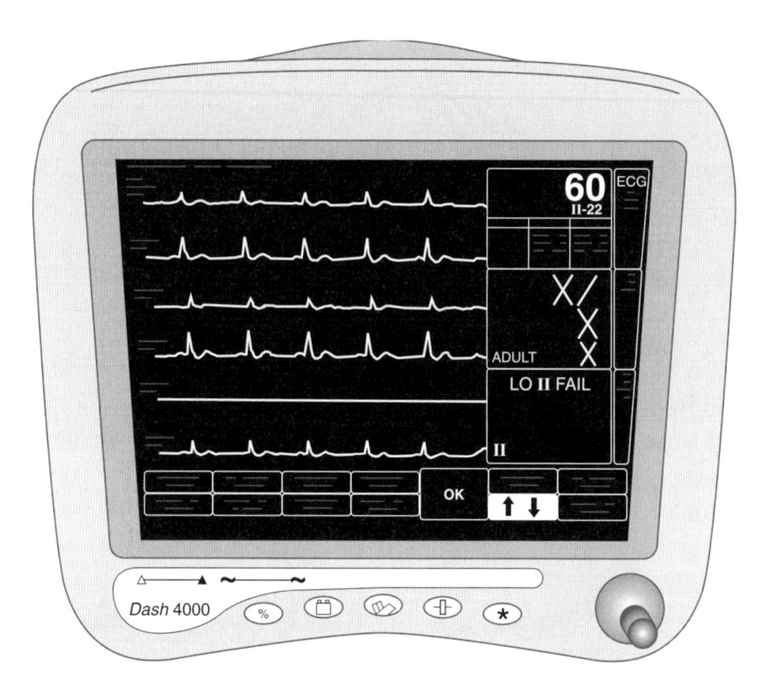

FIGURE 17-7a A patient monitor.

Overall Monitor Block Diagram

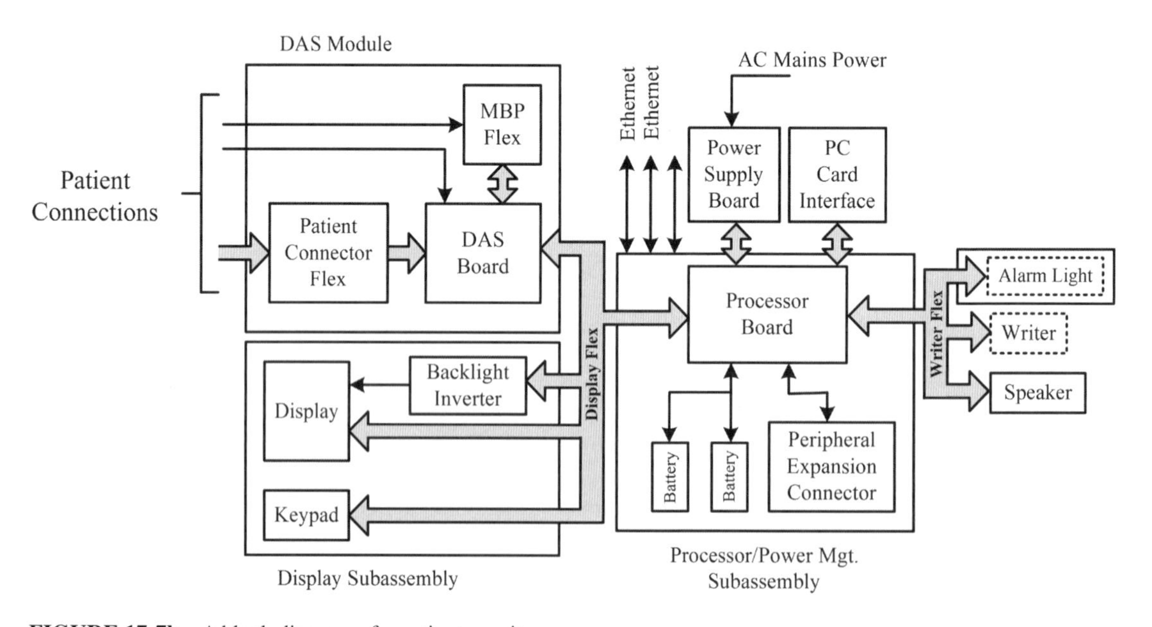

FIGURE 17-7b A block diagram of a patient monitor.

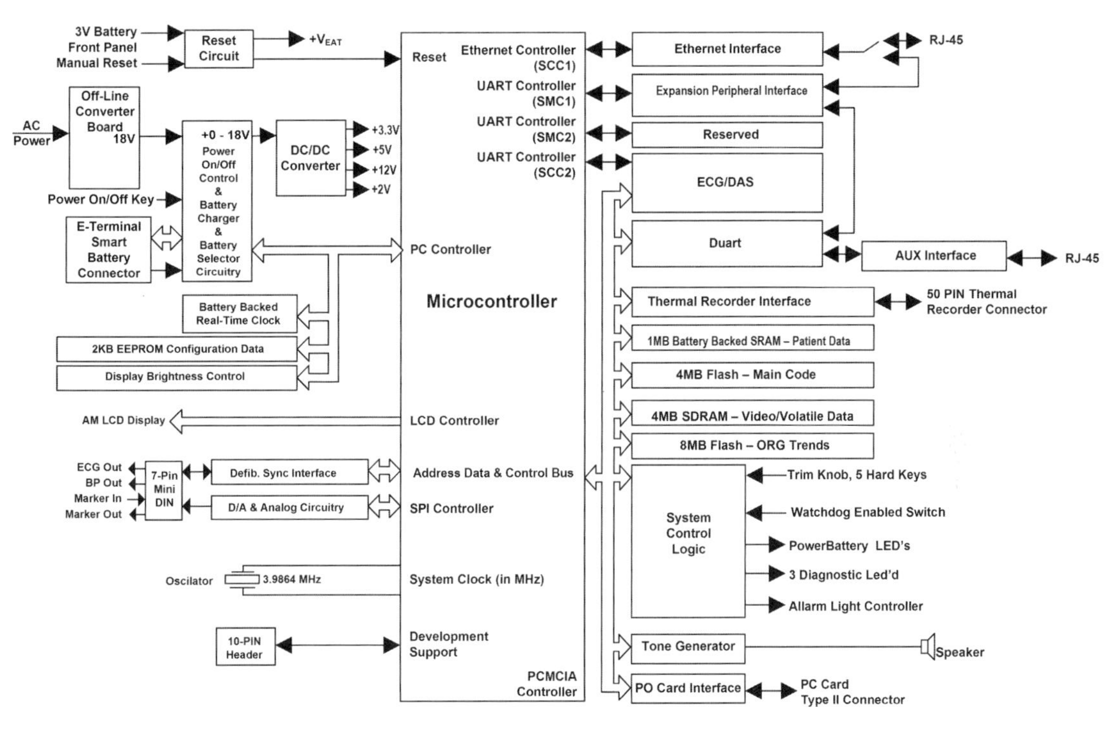

FIGURE 17-8 A block diagram of the main processor in a patient monitor.

The ECG section includes a 7.3728 MHz Motorola MC68HS microcontroller, A/D conversion, and DC-DC isolation converter.

Figure 17-8 shows the block diagram of the processor/power management subassembly. This subassembly provides data processing, communication circuitry, and the display of patient and monitor configuration data, as well as highly integrated electronic devices. The microcontroller has two processors, a 32-bit CPU core, and a communications processor module (CPM). The CPM has an 8 kB dual-port RAM to communicate with the CPU core and, once configured, can also communicate with the external devices.

17.6 MONITORING ALARMS AND ELECTRICAL SYSTEMS IN INTENSIVE CARE UNITS

Critical care often requires that alarm systems be incorporated into ICU devices. These alarms alert the ICU staff of any deviation from the appropriate range of body function parameters designated for each patient. Authorized intensive care health care providers set appropriate alarm limits for the patient's monitoring parameters in ICUs. These limits must be modified as the patient's condition changes. Therefore, daily patient assessments are performed and the alarm limits are set accordingly. It is obviously important to maintain appropriate settings for the patient's welfare; however, it is also important to correctly set the alarms and limits in order to avoid unnecessary nurse calls and interruptions.

The electrical systems in ICUs require stringent guidelines in order to protect patients from electrocution during procedures or treatments and to prevent equipment malfunction. The following list describes a few of these guidelines:

1. All power in ICUs must have backup generator systems to prevent disruption of care in the event of main power failure. There may be a small delay of about 20 seconds before the backup generators are switched on.
2. If a circuit breaker is tripped, the medical equipment is disconnected whenever possible, the circuit breaker is reset, and the equipment is then reconnected. If the circuit breaker trips again, the equipment is replaced and is sent for electrical inspection.
3. No cellular phones are allowed in the ICU. These devices can cause interference with patient monitors and telemetry units.
4. Some power outlets are supported by an uninterruptible power supply (these are usually color coded in green). Devices such as ventilators are connected to these outlets to provide uninterrupted power.
5. The devices used on patients in ICUs have cardiac-protected wiring to avoid any kind of electrical safety hazard. The cardiac-protected wiring is required for medical procedures where an insulated electrical conductor is introduced into direct contact with heart muscle while the conductor is accessible outside the patient's body. Examples of these devices include liquid-filled cardiac catheters, Swan-Ganz probes, and cardiac pacing electrodes.
6. The pulmonary artery catheters, temporary ICD wires, and other types of patient catheters should be connected to proper ground cables.

17.7 TELEMETRY DEVICES AND UNITS

Medical telemetry is the measurement of physiological data over a distance. Transmitting this physiological data from the point of generation to the point of reception can be done in several ways: It can be done via a landline or a wireless medium; it can be sent through the telephone lines to farther distances; or it can be monitored at the CNS close to the patient's room through the wireless link.

The bioelectric potential of ECG, EMG, or EEG and the physiological variables of blood pressure, blood flow, and temperature can be transmitted over a limited range in the hospital. The ICU rooms are equipped with telemetry devices. By attaching a miniature radio transmitter to the patient, the central station can acquire the patient data by the pickup antenna and the receiver circuits. This wireless communication is also called a radio communication or radio frequency (RF) link.

Figure 17-9 shows a block diagram of a typical telemetry transmitter/receiver system. The main component is the modulator, which can be analog or digital. The hospital's use of analog or digital is determined by the needs of the CNS and the requirements of carrier frequency, network interface, power, and wire or wireless media. The central

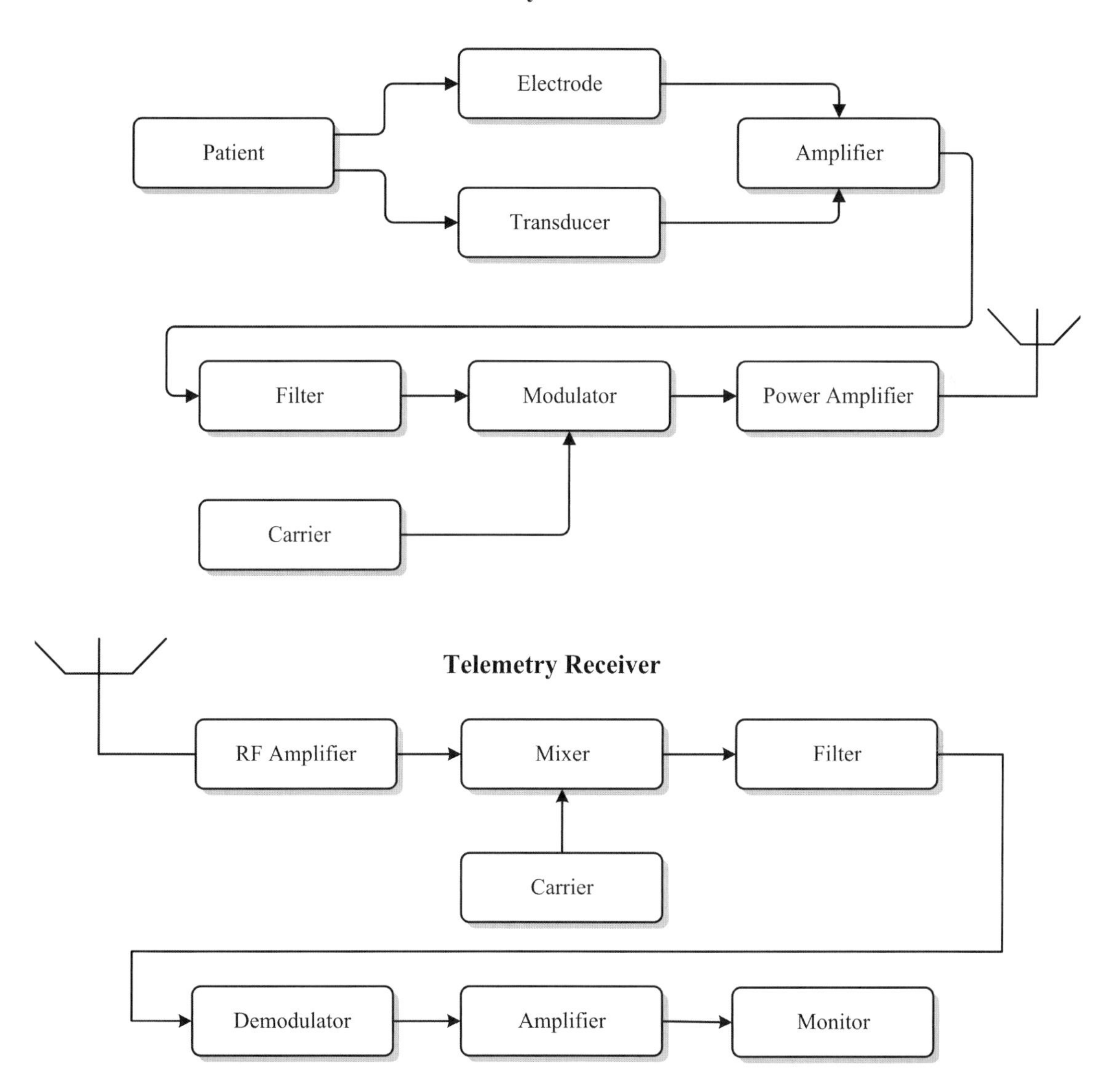

FIGURE 17-9 A block diagram of a telemetry unit.

monitoring of intensive care patients by telemetry significantly reduces the frequency of visits by the nurses to check the various monitors in each room or the condition of the patients.

17.8 TELEMETRY COMMUNICATION CONCEPTS

Telemetry units perform the following steps for RF transmission of patient data (such as ECG signals or blood pressure signals):

Analog Option

1. Determine the frequency and the amplitude of a high-frequency carrier signal.
2. Modulate the carrier by changing the amplitude or frequency of the carrier with respect to the amplitude of the analog physiological patient data. If the amplitude of the carrier changes, then the process is called an amplitude modulation (AM); however, if the frequency of the carrier changes due to the amplitude of the patient signal, it is then called frequency modulation (FM). **Figure 17-10a** shows the AM option and **Figure 17-10b** shows the FM option in a telemetry unit.
3. The modulated carrier then passes through the power amplifier circuits and is radiated in the air through an antenna. The size of a transmitting antenna is typically a half-wavelength $\lambda/2$.

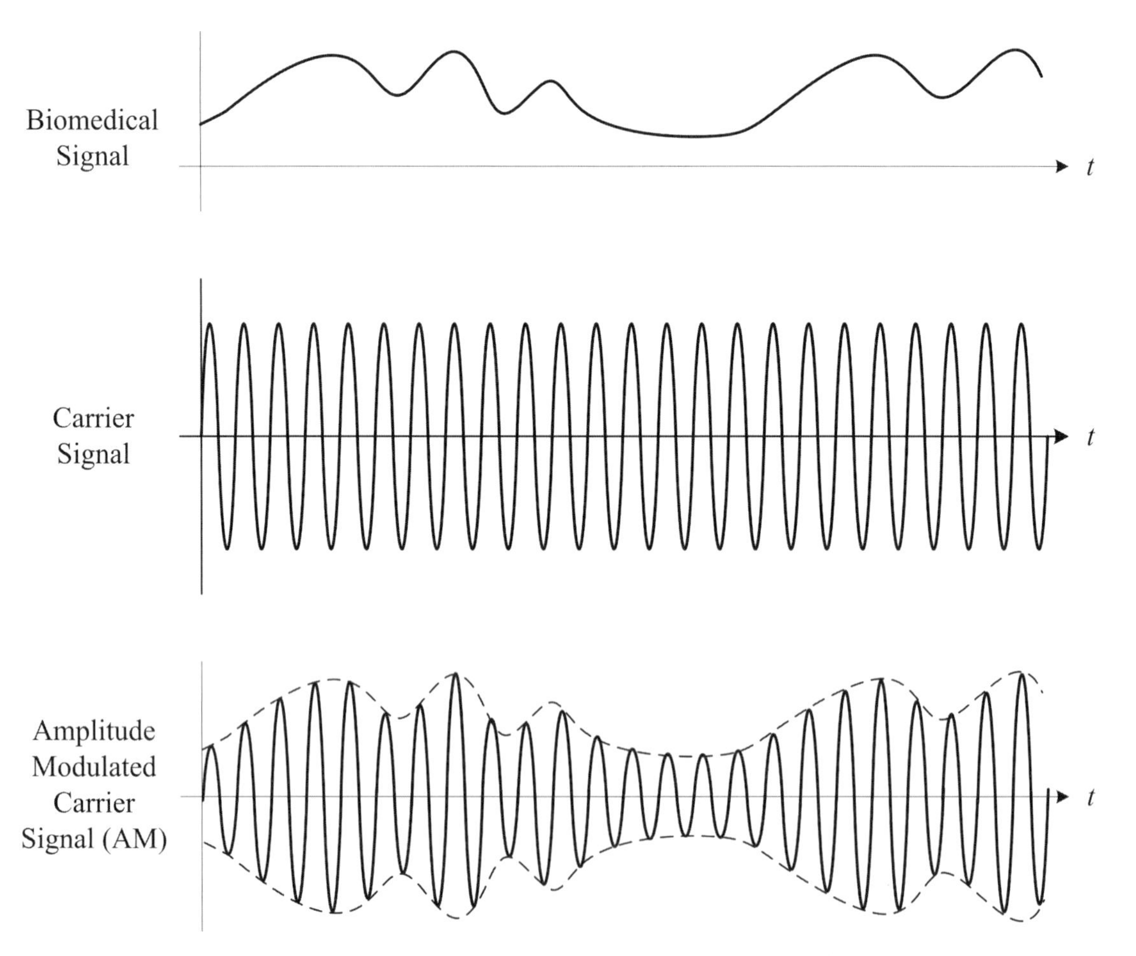

FIGURE 17-10a AM signal in a telemetry unit.

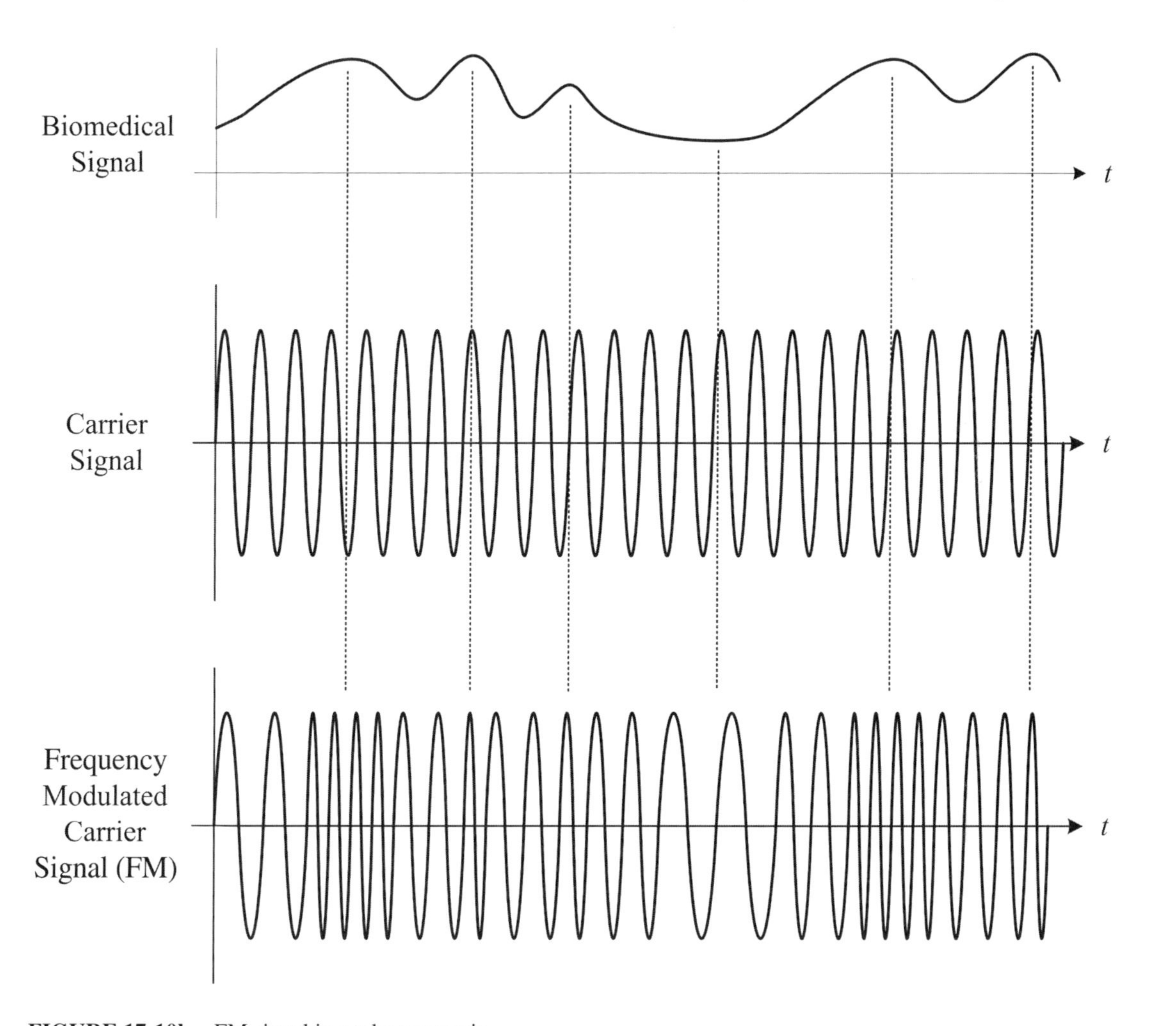

FIGURE 17-10b FM signal in a telemetry unit.

4. The received power, P_R, decreases with the distance, d, between the transmitting and receiving antennas. It is given as:

$$P_R = \frac{P_t}{\pi d^2}$$

where P_t is the transmitted power.

Digital Option

1. The analog patient signal is digitized in an A/D converter based on the number of bits per sample and the sampling frequency.
2. The carrier (frequency and amplitude) is selected.
3. The carrier is modulated with its amplitude changing due to the digitized patient data. This process is called amplitude-shift keying (ASK). If the carrier frequency changes, not the amplitude, the process is then called frequency-shift keying (FSK).

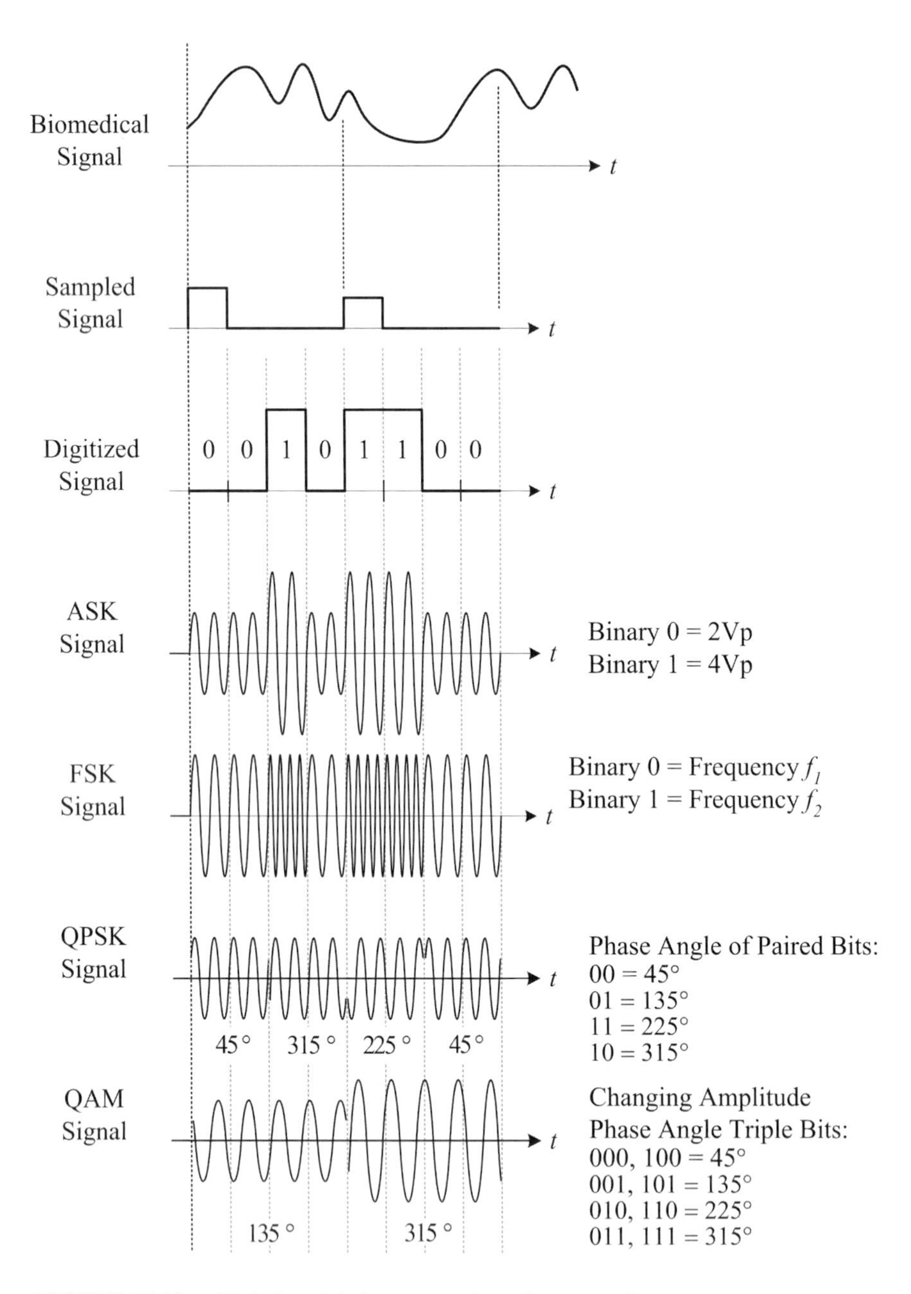

FIGURE 17-10c Digital modulation process in a telemetry unit.

Similarly, if the digitized patient data can change the phase of the carrier, then the modulated carrier is called referred to as a quadrature phase-shift keying (QPSK) process. If both phase and amplitude change in the carrier signal, then this type of modulation is called quadrature amplitude modulation (QAM). This is also shown in **Figure 17-10c.**

4. The power of the modulated carrier is amplified and is fed to an antenna.

Network Option

The wireless medical telemetry service (WMTS) has very specific frequency bands in the upper MHz range. The ranges are 608 MHz–614 MHz, 1395 MHz–1400 MHz, and 1429 MHz–1432 MHz. These bands monitor the ambulatory patients using AM or FM or FSK modulation techniques. The IEEE 802.11b standard is also known as WiFi and is implemented in data transport. It can be interfaced with the hospital computer network.

Bluetooth Technology Option

The newest advance in wireless medical telemetry used in hospitals is Bluetooth technology (standard defined by IEEE 802.15). It uses very little power and its operating radius is

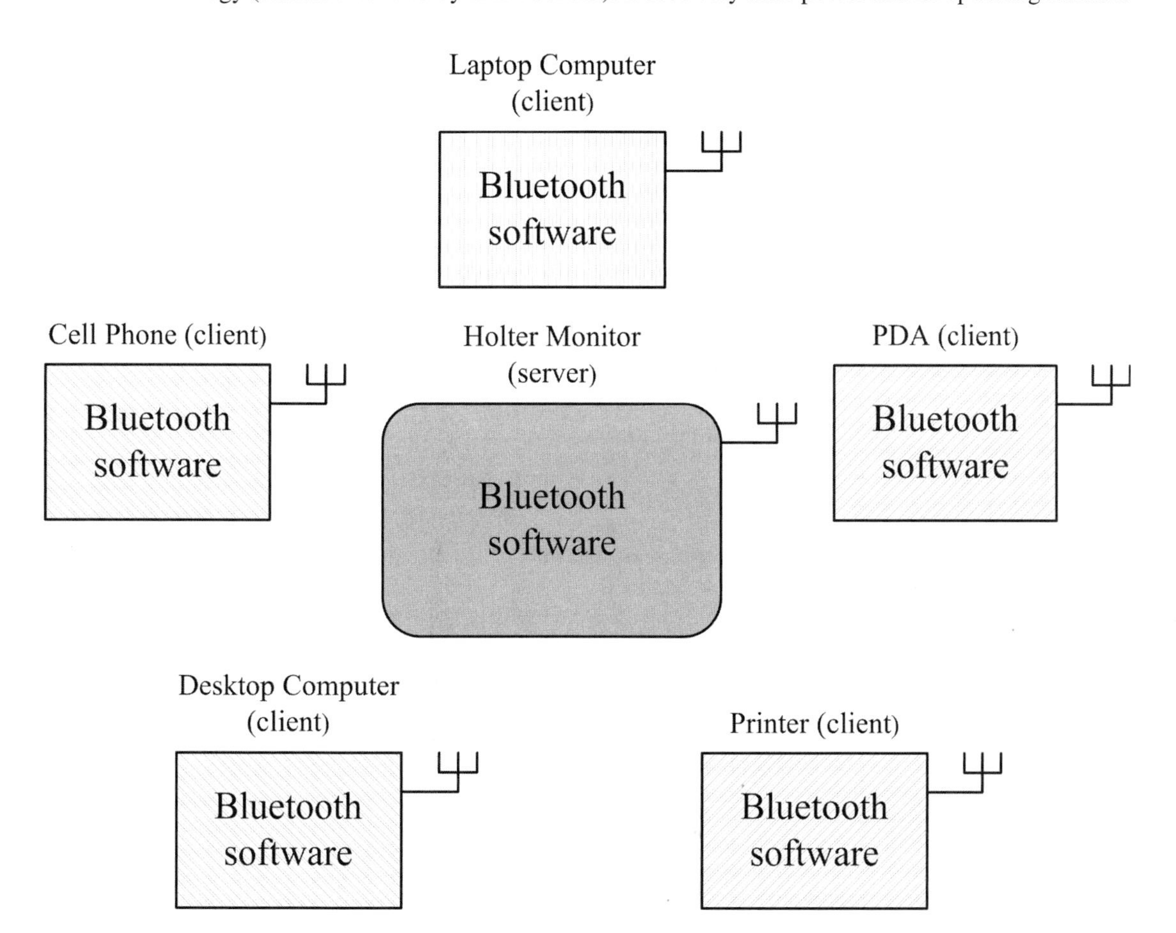

FIGURE 17-11a Bluetooth technology in telemetry.

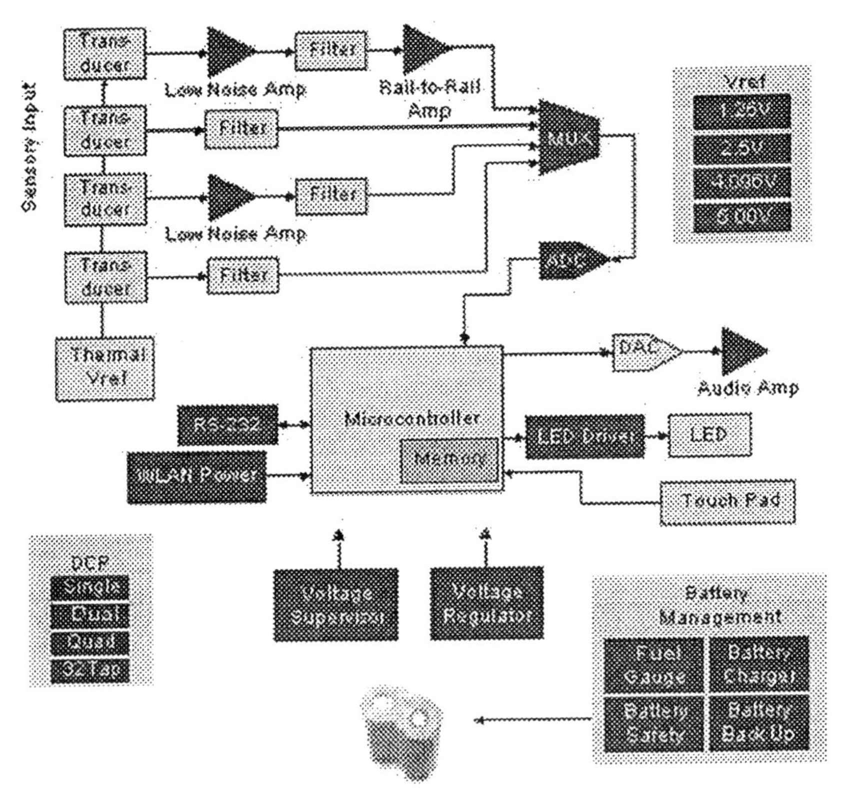

FIGURE 17-11b A commercial medical telemetry unit.

30 feet. This is suited for battery-powered PDAs, medical devices, and short-range communication links. The medical instrument can be considered a "server" and the devices nearby, such as PDAs, laptop computers, and printers are the "clients." Every unit has a transmitting/receiving antenna. This scheme of Bluetooth technology is detailed in **Figure 17-11a.**

A commercial medical telemetry unit by INTERSIL is shown in **Figure 17-11b.** Several transducer outputs are multiplexed and digitized before they are processed and stored in the microcontroller chip.

17.9 CENTRAL MONITORING

Central monitors are remote monitors that display data collected from several patients simultaneously. These monitors are often placed in nursing stations and allow monitoring the status of various parameters from several patients concurrently. The newer technology of central monitoring has evolved into its integration into the hospital information system through telemetry and the computer networks. **Figure 17-12** shows the central monitoring

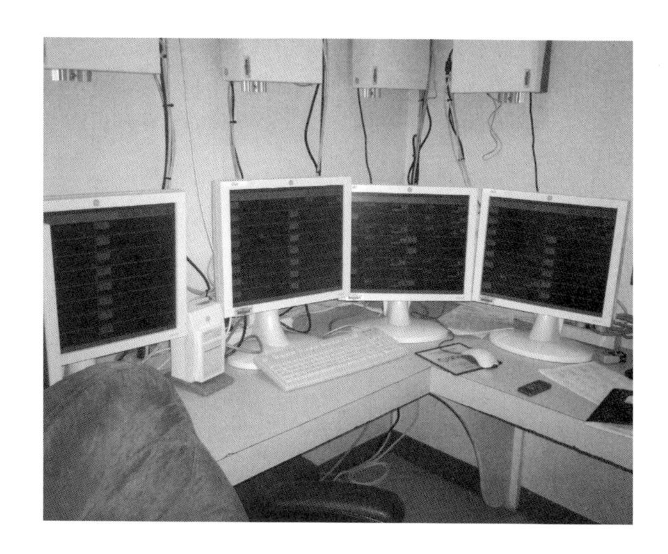

FIGURE 17-12 Central monitoring in an ICU.

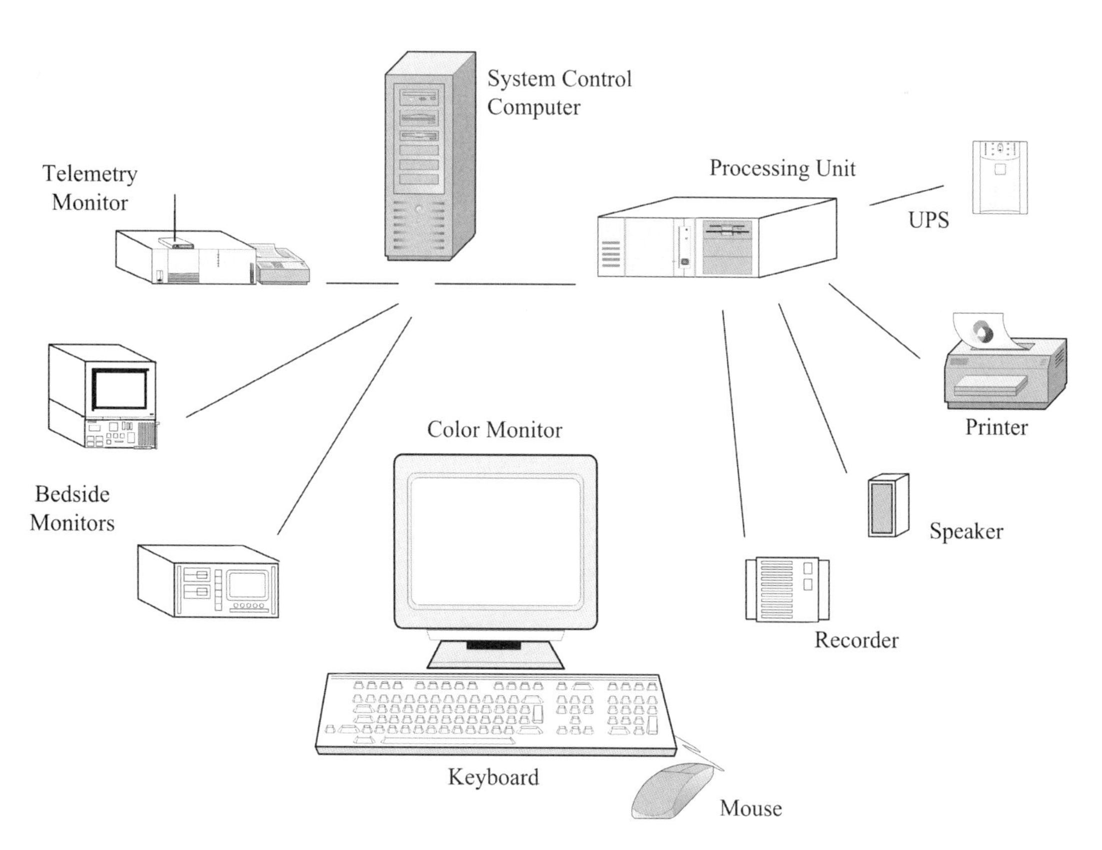

FIGURE 17-13a The information center units.

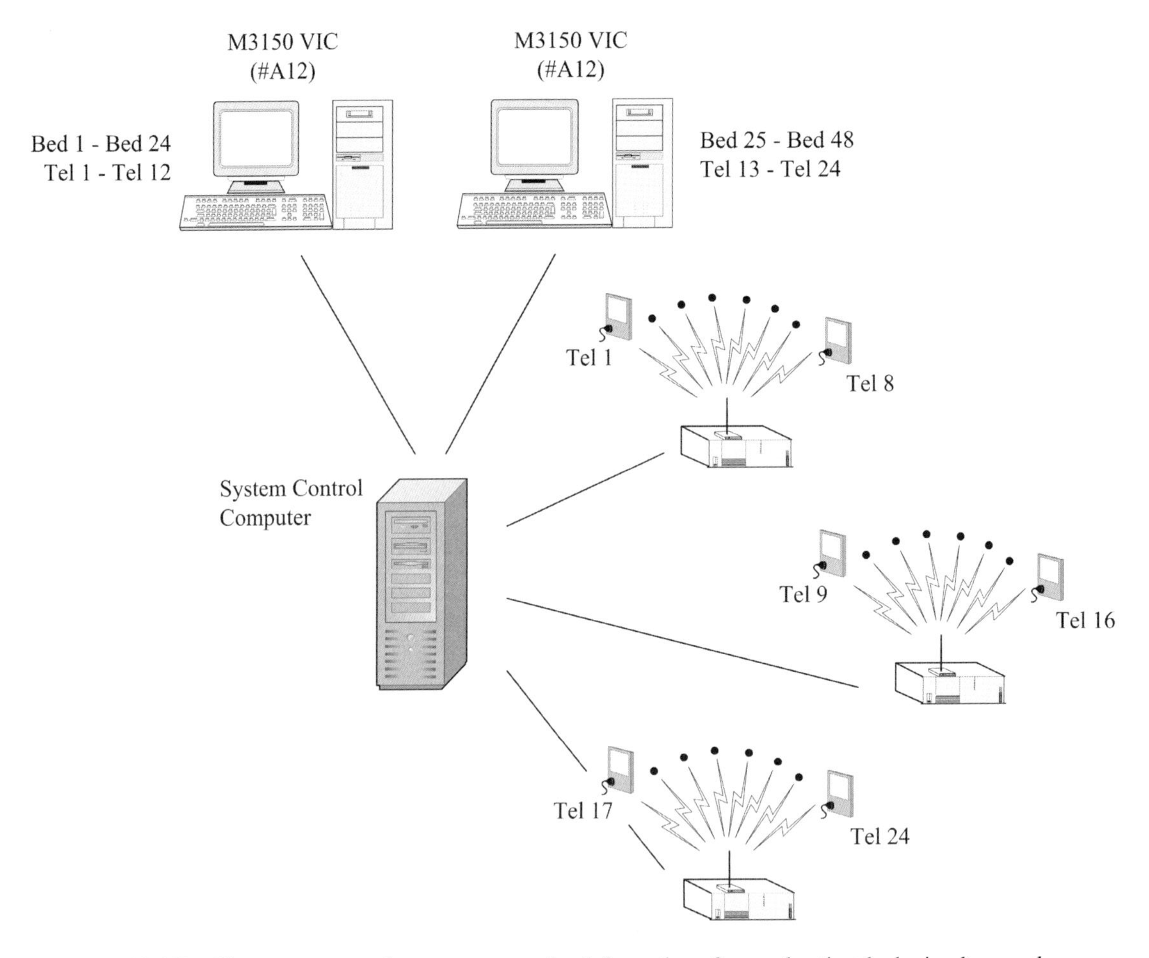

FIGURE 17-13b The system control computer accessing information of several patient beds simultaneously.

location receiving patient information from various patient rooms. In **Figure 17-13a,** an Information Center System receives patient data from a telemetry unit and other bedside monitors. The System Control Computer (SCC) is the main computer that receives telemetry signals and is interfaced to the hospital local area network (LAN). Note in **Figure 17-13b** that the SCC connects to several telemetry units at the same time.

A suggested design of the ICU for the Viridia Information Center connectivity is shown in **Figure 17-14**. Several large hospitals are implementing it.

Another view of the monitor display of data from several patients is shown in **Figure 17-15.**

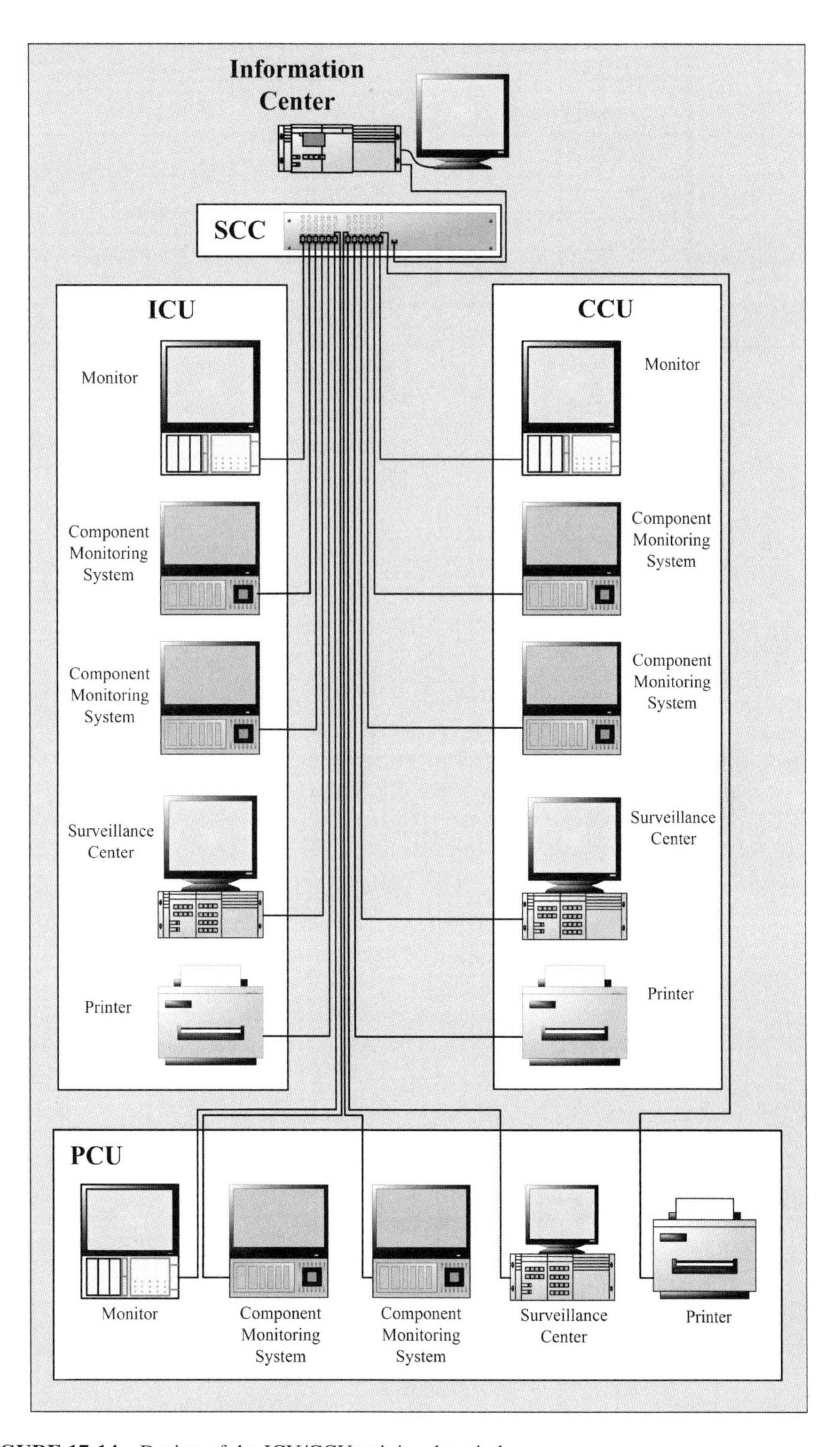

FIGURE 17-14 Design of the ICU/CCU unit in a hospital.

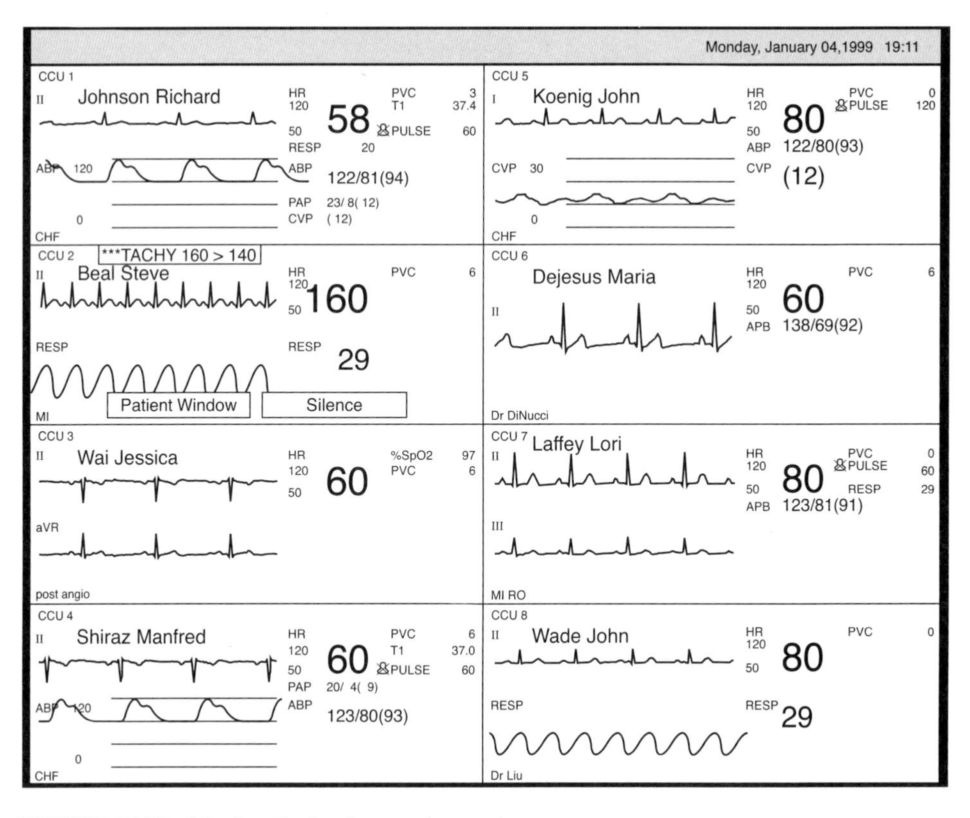

FIGURE 17-15 Monitor display from various patients.

EXAMPLE For the given analog spectrum in **Figure 17-16a,** determine the bandwidth of the amplitude modulated (AM) carrier. The carrier is 425 MHz.

The bandwidth of the modulated carrier includes the upper and lower side bands around the carrier as shown in **Figure 17-16b.** The analog frequencies are added to the carrier frequency in the upper side band and subtracted from the carrier frequency in the lower side band. The total bandwidth of the AM carrier in the example is 200 Hz.

■

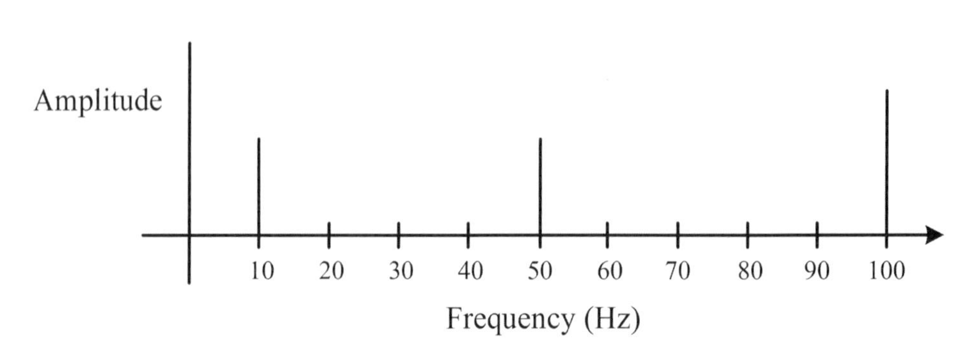

FIGURE 17-16a Spectrum of an analog signal.

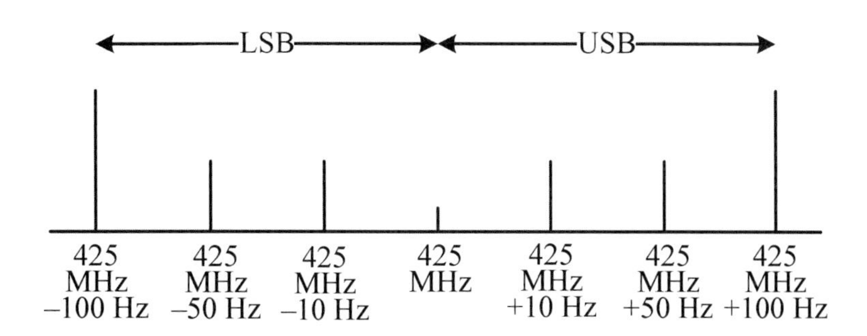

FIGURE 17-16b Spectrum of the AM carrier signal.

EXAMPLE Use the same analog spectrum as in the previous example, but change the modulation of carrier to frequency modulation (FM). Determine the bandwidth of the modulated carrier.

The bandwidth of an FM function carrier is larger than that of an AM carrier. The upper and lower side bands now depend upon the Bessel function frequency changes in the carrier (unmodulated) with respect to the amplitude of the analog signal. Larger is the amplitude of the analog signal, larger is the Bessel function frequency changes given as Bessel order of J_1, J_2, or more. The order can also be fractional. Typically, if the order is two, then the upper side band will consist of (carrier frequency plus times one of all analog frequencies), and (carrier frequency plus times two of all analog frequencies). Lower side band will have the subtracted frequencies.

If the Bessel function frequency changes (i.e., deviation) are of the order of three, then the USB or LSB will continue until three times the maximum frequency of the analog spectrum. This is shown in **Figure 17-16c.** Other analog frequencies are not shown.

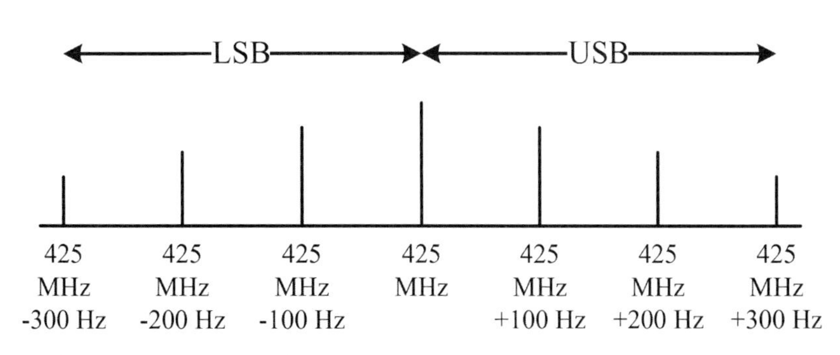

FIGURE 17-16c Spectrum of the FM carrier signal.

EXAMPLE In QPSK modulation, the phase shifts are the following:

00	45°
01	135°
11	225°
10	315°

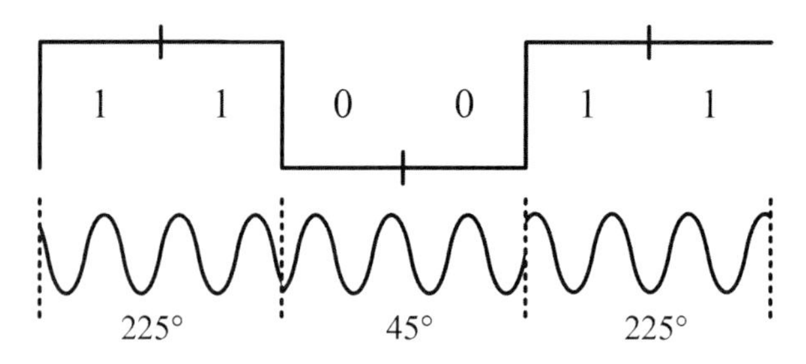

FIGURE 17-16d The QPSK signal in time-domain.

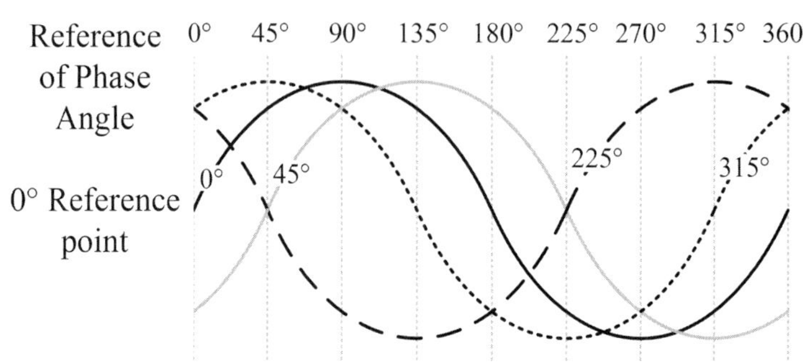

FIGURE 17-16e Phase-shifted sine waves.

Determine the QPSK signal for the input digits of 110011.

The carrier is phase-shifted as in **Figure 17-16d** for the digitized analog signal. The phase-shifted sine waves of 45°, 225°, and 315° (with respect to 0° reference sine wave) are shown in **Figure 17-16e**. In 2-level binary phase shift keying (BPSK), one bit carries two phases (i.e., binary 0 = 0° and binary 1 = 180°), but a 4-level quadrature phase shift keying (QPSK), two bits carry four phases (i.e., 00 = 45°, 01 = 135°, 11 = 225°, 10 = 315°). For more bits, then more phases are being developed. Same scheme can also apply to a 2-level FSK, 4-level FSK, etc. etc. and in doing so, more information can be sent in the same bandwidth.

SUMMARY

An ICU or CCU in any hospital contains rooms and/or beds for patients requiring critical care. Each patient room or bed has several monitors that report patient status (ECG, blood pressure, blood oxygen concentration and respiration) to the unit's Central Nursing Station (CNS). The chapter has covered the following concepts:

1. An ICU fact sheet is included and the chapter discusses the types of equipment used in ICUs. The fact sheet includes the RN-to-patient ratio, average number of patients, number of beds, average length of stay, and medical conditions of the ICU patients. The equipment used in ICUs includes bedside monitors, blood pressure devices, IV pumps, nasogastric tubes, mechanical ventilators, central venous lines, continuous positive air pressure machines (CPAP), and ECG machines.
2. The alarm features and the design criteria of an ICU unit are also discussed.
3. Telemetry devices and the communication carrier concepts are included toward the end of the chapter. The RF carrier is modulated by the patient data in its analog and digital

forms. In AM, the carrier amplitude changes with respect to analog patient data, but in FM the carrier frequency changes.

4. Central monitoring is essential to patient care in an ICU/CCU, and central monitoring is becoming integrated with hospital IT infrastructure, telemetry devices, and clinical information systems.

MEDICAL TERMINOLOGY

The following is a list of medical terms mentioned in this chapter.

Arrhythmia: any deviation from the normal rhythm of the heartbeat.

Dialysis: process of removing waste products from the blood when the kidneys are not functioning properly.

Endo-tracheal: within the trachea.

Intravenous: inside, or into, a vein.

Oximetry: measurement of the blood's oxygen saturation with an oximeter.

Swan-Ganz catheter: flexible catheter containing a balloon near its tip that is used to measure blood pressure in the pulmonary artery.

QUIZ

1. The length of a transmitting antenna in a bedside monitor depends upon the ________.

   a) Transmitted power b) Received power

   c) Transmitting frequency d) None of the above

2. An ICU/CCU is staffed by specially trained nurses who are certified in ________________________________.

3. Name at least three types of patients who are admitted to ICU/CCU units.

   1. ________________
   2. ________________
   3. ________________

4. The frequency of an RF carrier is 500 MHz; its wavelength is:

   a) 3 cm b) 1 cm

   c) 60 cm d) None of the above

5. The main characteristic of an FM modulated carrier is ________________________________.

6. Two bits are needed to generate a QPSK signal, and ____________ bits are needed to generate a 16PSK signal.

7. Name four bio-signals a bedside monitor is used to monitor:

   1. ________________ 2. ________________

   3. ________________ 4. ________________

8. NICU stands for:

   a) Neurological Intensive Care Unit b) Neo-natal Intensive Care Unit

   c) Nephrology Intensive Care Unit

9. Intensive care equipment for life support and emergency resuscitation includes the following: ______

10. The frequency carrier in Bluetooth communication is:

    a) 1.2 GHz b) 2.4 GHz c) 820 MHz d) None of the above

PROBLEMS

1. Compute the distance between the bedside monitor and the central nursing station (CNS), given:

   Transmitter power = 5 mW

   Received power = 10 μV

   Carrier frequency = 470 MHz

2. Sketch the spectral of an FM telemetry unit, given:

   Carrier frequency = 430 MHz

   Bessel order = 4

   Spectrum of the ECG signal is shown in **Figure 17-17.**

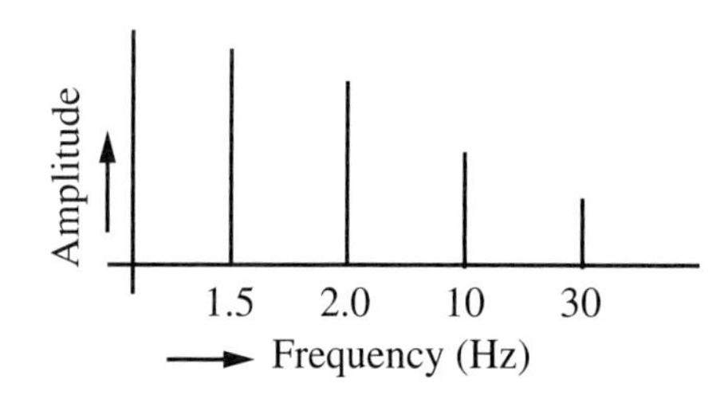

FIGURE 17-17 Spectrum of an ECG signal.

3. Draw a QPSK RF telemetry signal output, given:

   Digitized input signal = 011011

Phase Shift of Carrier	Binary Value
45°	00
135°	01
225°	11
315°	10

4. Draw a simple block diagram of a BPSK modulator using inverter, sine wave oscillator, multipliers or balanced modulators, 180° phase shifter and an analog adder. If data is 1011 at a rate of 1000 bits/second, rough sketch the BPSK signal and also determine its bandwidth.

5. Draw a simple block diagram of 2-level FSK modulator.

6. Draw a simple block diagram of a QPSK modulator.

7. Discuss in detail the operation of the following ICU equipment:
   a) Intracranial pressure monitor
   b) Resuscitation or code cart
   c) Point-of-care analyzers
   d) Chest or thoracostomy tube
8. Discuss warning devices to be used in intensive care units.
9. Design an electronic circuit to indicate when an electrode has become disconnected (due to patient movement) from the patient in an ICU room. The disconnection needs to be transmitted to the central monitoring system.
10. Discuss a mobile X-ray unit required in the ICU for the bedside radiography. Indicate the X-ray power and the needed safety precautions at the bedside.

CASE STUDIES

1. A 62-year-old man with diabetes and complications from respiratory and renal failure was admitted several times to the ICU prior to his ultimate death. Although he had multiple health issues, his religious beliefs allowed him to withdraw from expensive ICU care and he fought with determination until the end of his life. What issues arise with the topics of patient beliefs, prolonged care, distribution of ICU resources, and the cost of intensive care?
2. Some hospitals are employing unlicensed assistive personnel (UAP) or Critical Care Support Technicians in ICUs, NICUs, and other intensive care units. These persons have very limited training and can lack the skills needed in ICUs. Unlicensed personnel are often used, however, because of cost concerns. What issues arise on the subject of unlicensed staff support personnel and what are the opinions of professionals in the field of intensive care medicine?

RESEARCH TOPICS

Infectious diseases in ICUs are a concern to any hospital.

1. The occurrence of catheter-related blood stream infections (CRBSIs) and surgical site infections (SSIs) in ICUs and hospitals is prevalent. As an example, St. John's Hospital and Medical Center in Detroit, Michigan, has collected data on reducing these infections. Write a research paper investigating the causes, the cost in patient care (due to these infections), and the recommendations the Centers for Disease Control (CDC) offers to combat the issue.
2. Telemetry ECG transmitter and receiver modules are attached to the bedside monitors in ICUs. Write a research paper to address the technology used in the transmission and reception of the ECG signals. The research may concentrate on a specific manufacture's unit, and should provide information about transmitted power output, battery type, maximum distance between transmitter and receiver, and the frequency response of the input signal.

CHAPTER 18

Instrumentation in the Operating Room

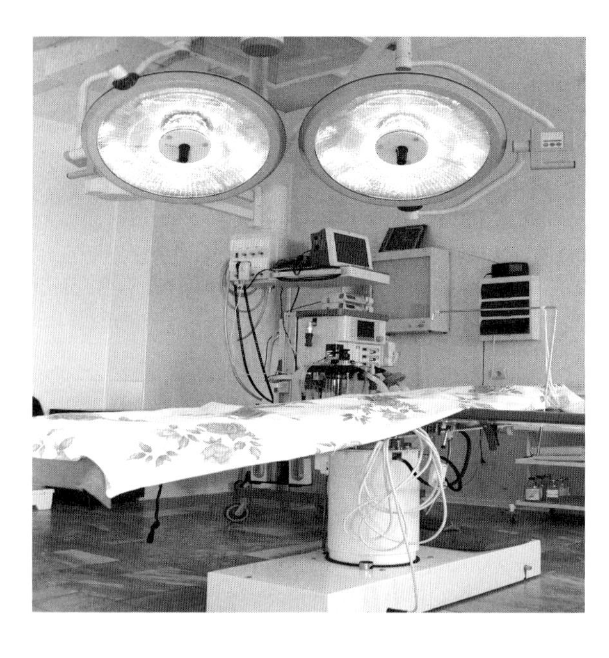

CHAPTER OUTLINE

OBJECTIVES

The objective of this chapter is to familiarize the reader with the environment of the hospital operating room, including the types of patients, the medical staff required in an operating room, and the equipment used, such as surgical and anesthesia machines.

Upon completion of this chapter, the reader will be able to:

- Describe the operating suite environment and the operating room of a hospital.
- Discuss the advantages and disadvantages of the different waveform modes used in surgical machines.
- Describe the various components of an anesthesia machine.
- Describe sterilization processes.

■ INTERNET WEB SITES

http://www.ast.org Association of Surgical Technologies
http://www.mdsr.ecri.org Medical Device Safety Reports
http://www.asahq.org American Society of Anesthesiologists

■ INTRODUCTION

The operating room (OR) is a sophisticated room within a hospital where surgical procedures are conducted. Operating rooms are located within an operating suite in a hospital's surgical department. The design of the OR is specific and must follow strict standards. From anesthesia machines to surgical instruments and from patients to medical staff, the operating room must run smoothly.

18.1 THE OPERATING SUITE ENVIRONMENT

Figure 18-1 shows a standard operating suite plan. In this design, a series of operating rooms (ORs) are located around a clean central area that includes, a supply room, an instrument room, offices with a reception desk, dressing rooms and a post-anesthesia care unit (PACU).

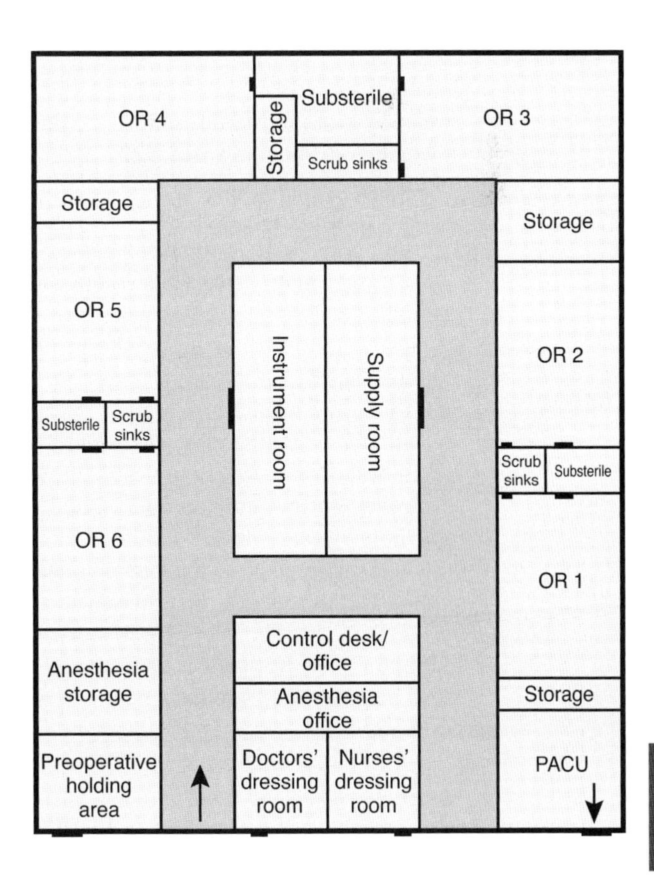

FIGURE 18-1 Design plan of an operating suite within a hospital.

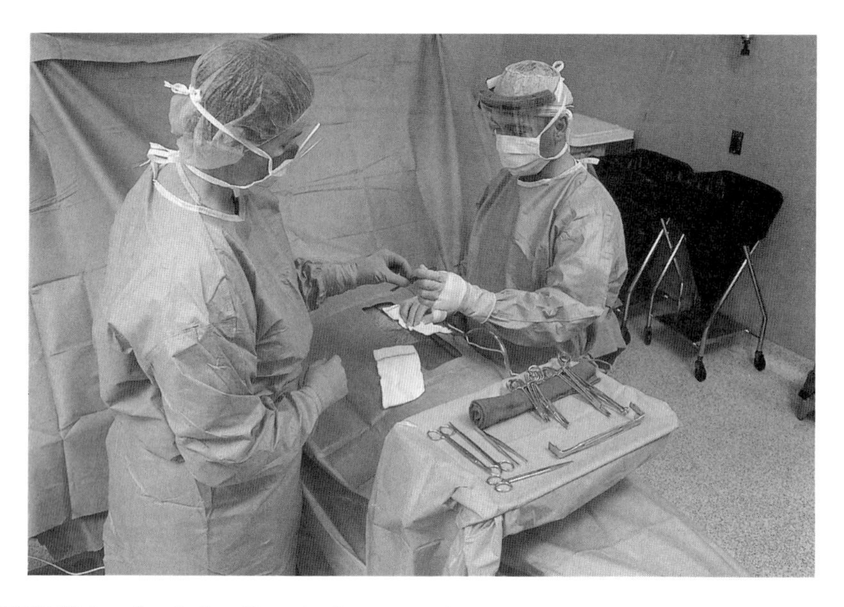

FIGURE 18-2a Surgical staff conducting a procedure in an operating room.

Scrub sinks and substerile sections are situated in the outer corridor. The ORs are the rooms in which surgery takes place. They are restricted and sterilized areas where surgical scrub suits, masks, and hats are required in order to prevent infection and contamination.

Generally, within each OR is the patient operating table, the lighting system, the instruments required for the surgery, an anesthesia machine, and several monitors. The operating table is placed in the center of the room with adjustments to tilt it in any direction. The bright lighting is focused over the table, also with adjustments for proper mobility. The instruments are always sterilized and the anesthesia machine is operated close to the patient. The several monitors display for the surgical team the patient's vital signs such as blood pressure, heart rate, ECG, and respiration. **Figure 18-2a** through **Figure 18-2c** are photos to familiarize you with the operating room environment.

In order for an OR to run efficiently, each room is equipped with electrical outlets, emergency outlets, suction outlets, and gas outlets. The electrical outlets have ground-fault interrupters and are mounted above the floor and on the wall. The emergency outlets are connected to the backup generators in the case of power failure and are usually marked in red. The suction outlets are used for anesthesia and surgery to suction in the sterile field. The suction canisters, as shown in **Figure 18-3,** are connected to the suction outlets. Notice the markings on the sides that enable the staff to estimate fluid use. The gas outlets are designed to bring air, oxygen, and nitrous oxide to the operating room.

Operating rooms also contain instrument stands, such as Mayo stands and double ring stands, as well as kick buckets and several types of back tables. These instruments are shown in **Figure 18-4a** to **Figure 18-4d.**

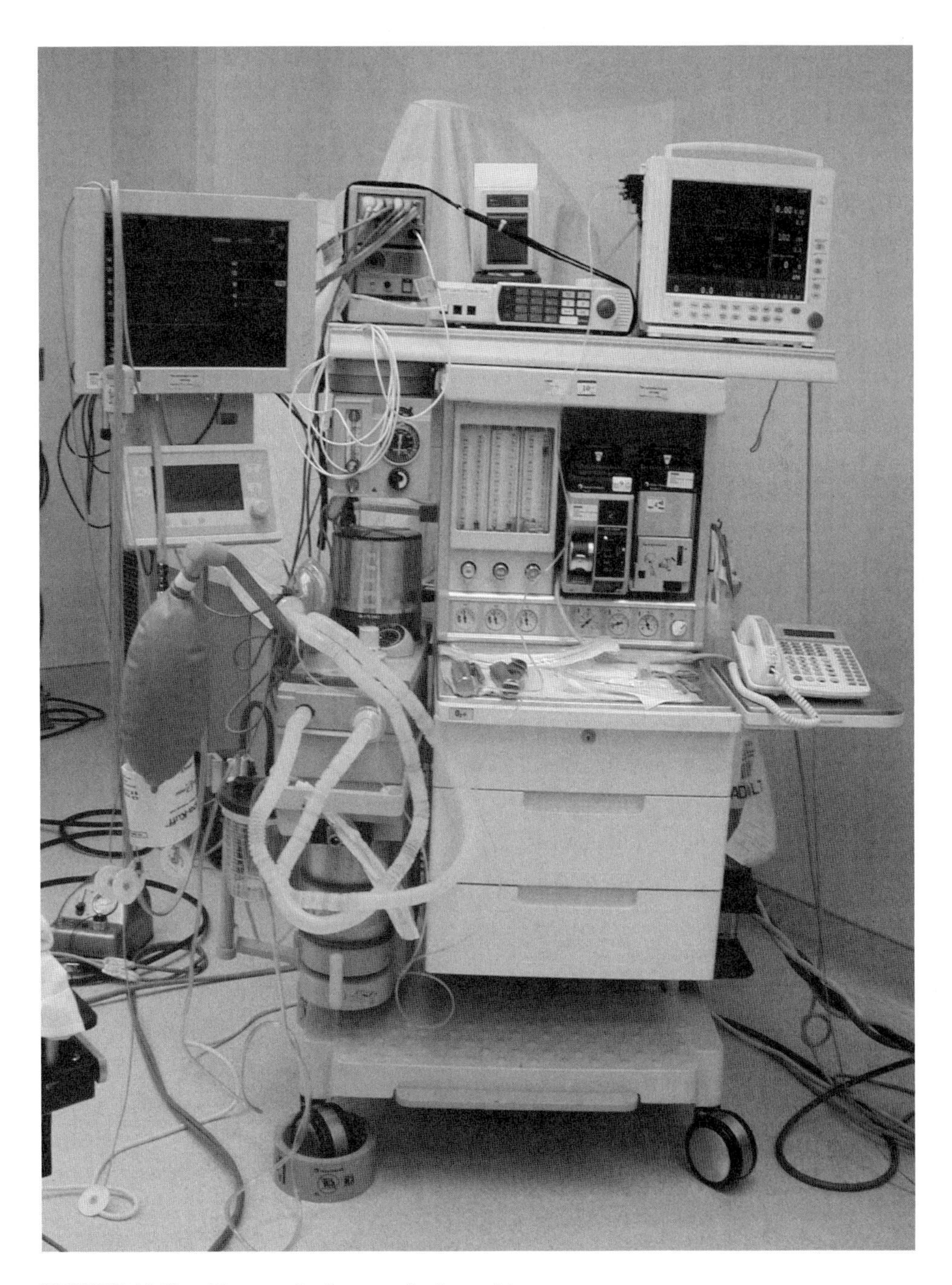

FIGURE 18-2b Photograph of an anesthesia machine.

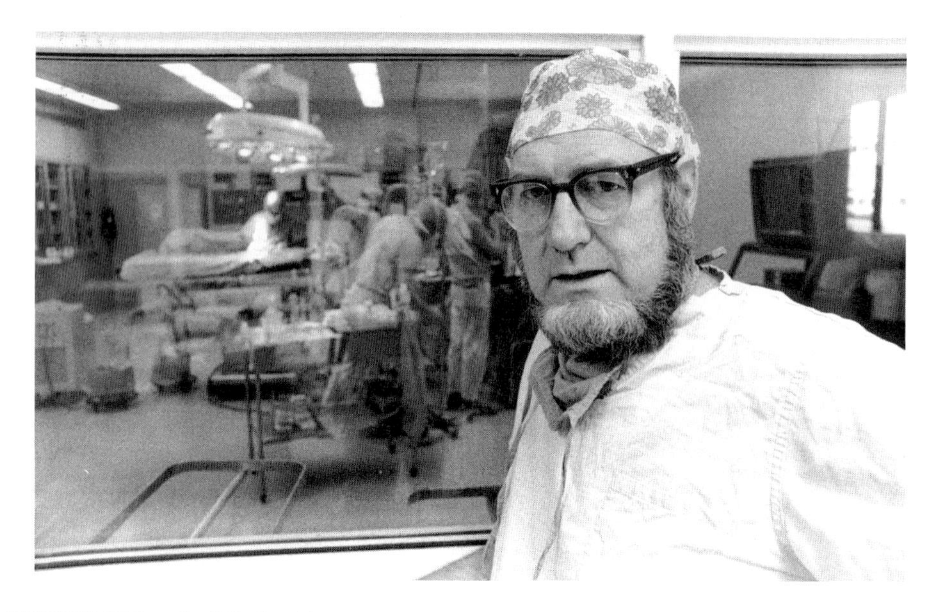

FIGURE 18-2c An OR physician.

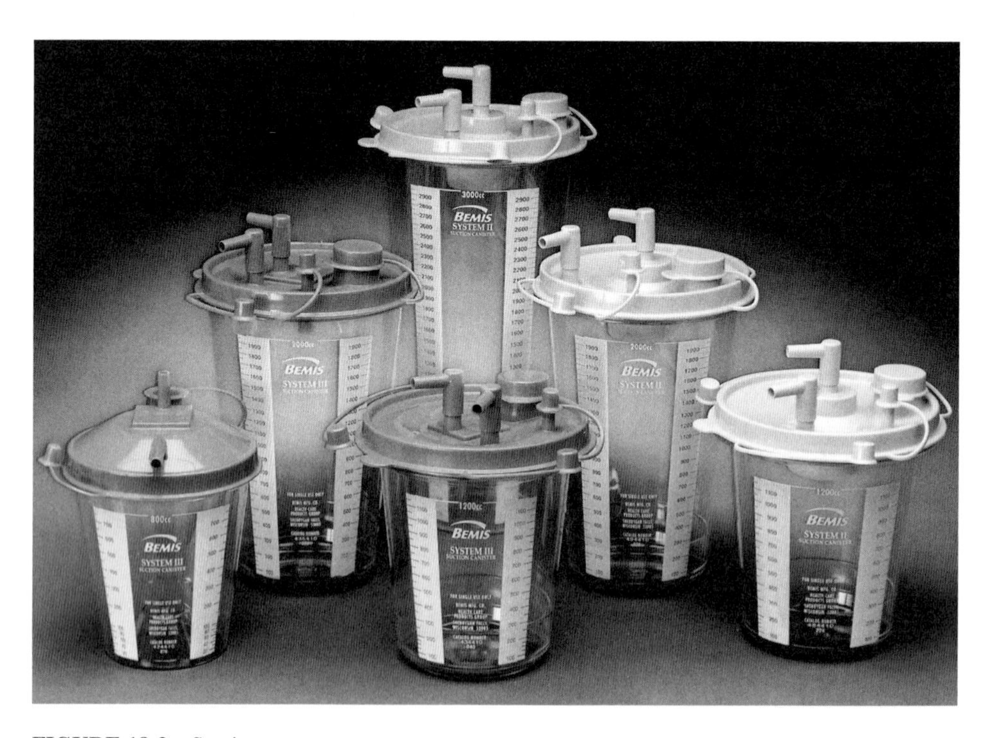

FIGURE 18-3 Suction system.

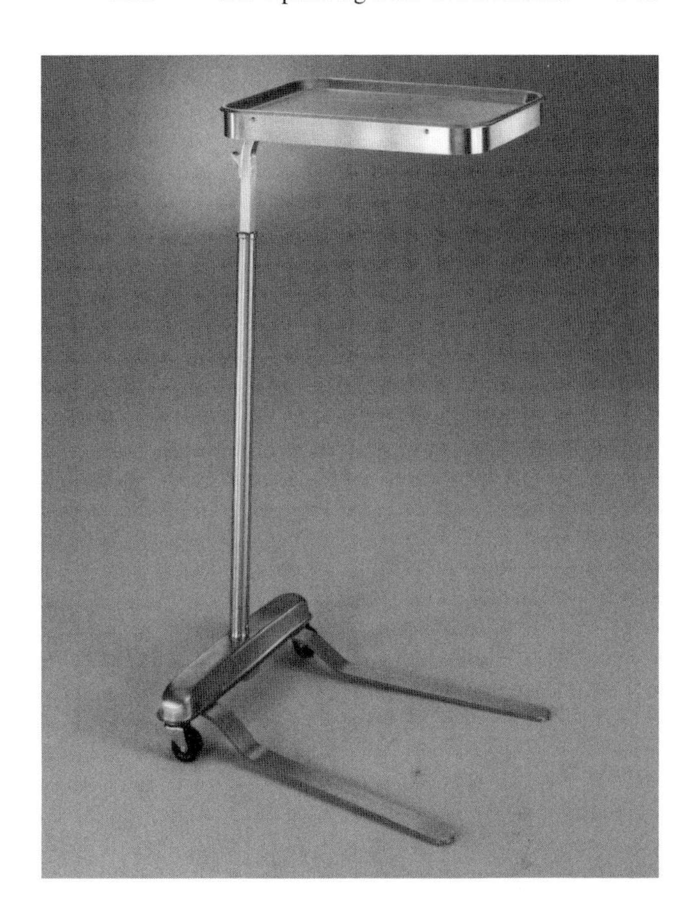

FIGURE 18-4a Mayo instrument stand.

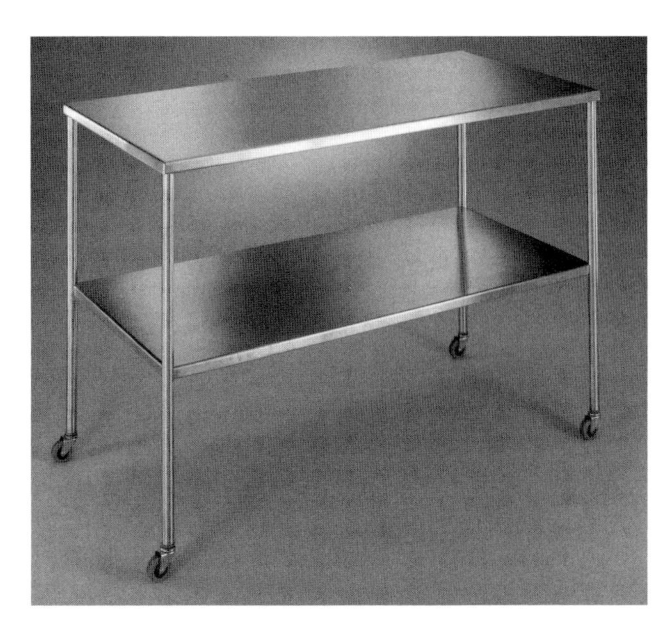

FIGURE 18-4b Double ring instrument stand.

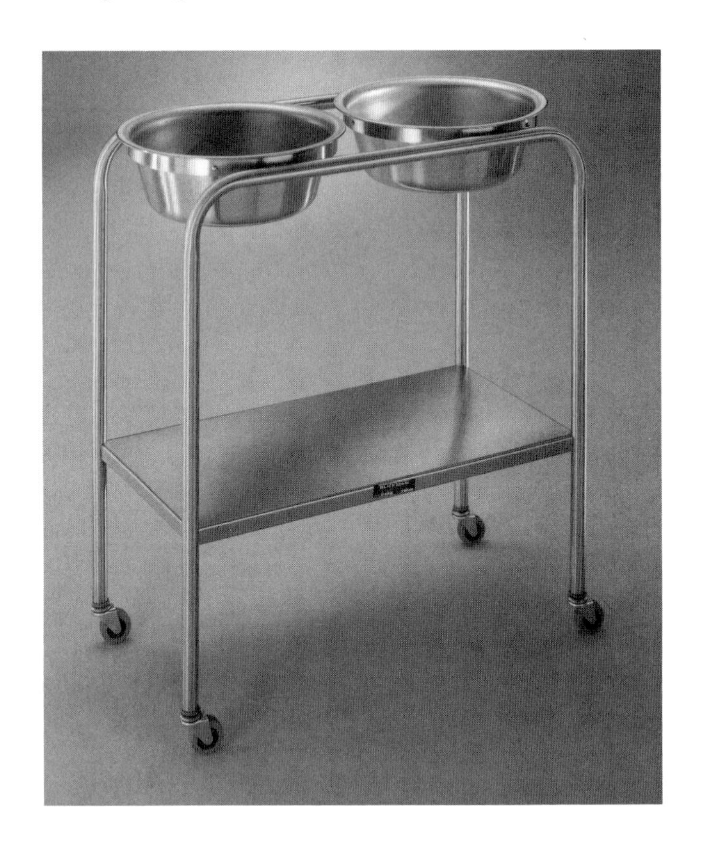

FIGURE 18-4c Back table.

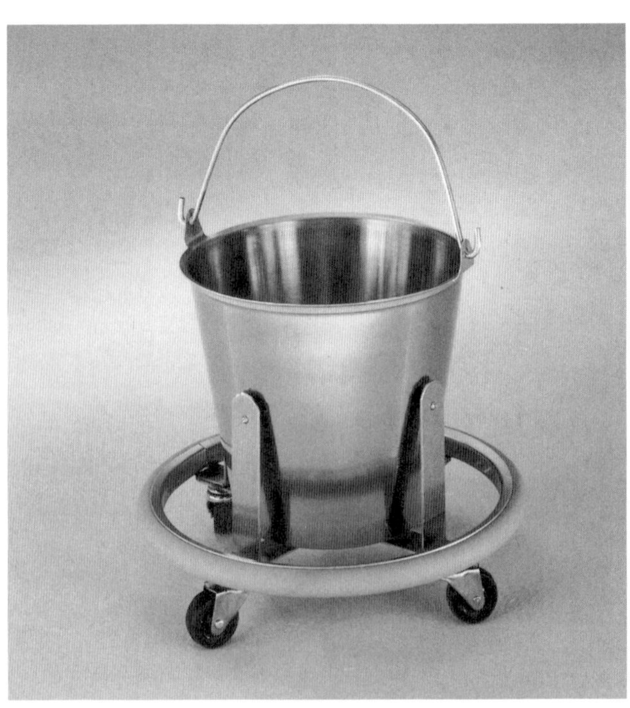

FIGURE 18-4d Kick bucket.

FIGURE 18-5a An operating room.

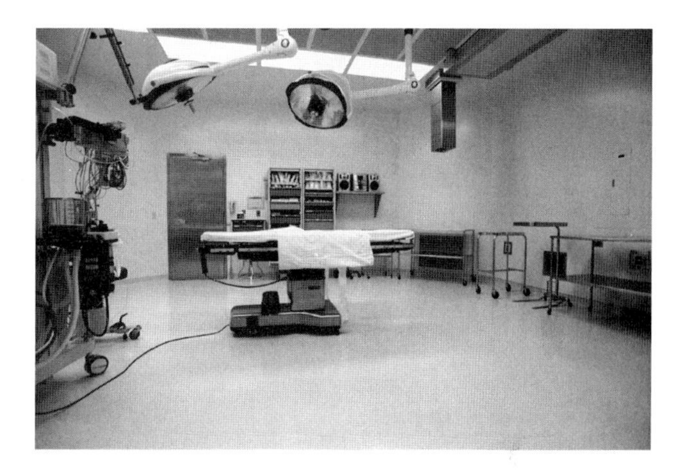

Operating Table

The operating table can be operated manually or electrically, and the patient can lie in supine or prone position. It is a well-padded table with several controls to maneuver and position it as needed for operation, as shown in **Figure 18-5a** and **Figure 18-5b.** Notice the remote control as well. The operating table has break points where the patient's head, waist, or knees can be adjusted or bent for proper positioning prior to surgery.

Surgical Lights

Surgical lights are an important part of the operating environment. They must provide adequate illumination without glare on the patient or any instrument. **Figure 18-6** is a photo of a typical surgical lighting system. The beams from these bright lights emit soothing blue or white radiance and are adjustable so that the surgeon and staff can focus the light exactly where it is needed at all times.

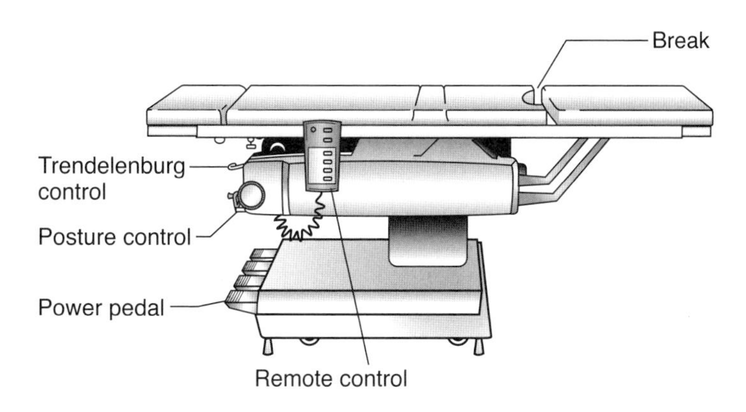

FIGURE 18-5b An operating table.

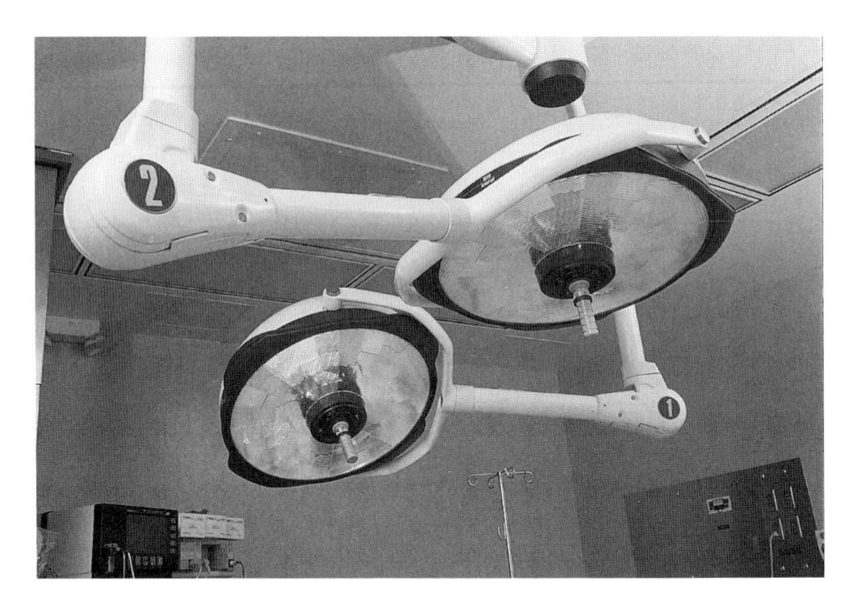

FIGURE 18-6 Surgical lights.

18.2 OPERATING ROOM INSTRUMENTATION

As previously mentioned, the operating room houses a variety of biomedical instruments used to more efficiently perform surgery. There are many types of surgeries and several types of surgical operating rooms (think of cardiac ORs, transplant ORs, obstetric ORs, and so on). Of course, each will be equipped with specific devices and instruments for the required procedure. Generally, you will see the following types of biomedical devices and instruments in a given operating room.

Anesthesia Machine

This machine performs several important tasks and is a vital part of any operating room:

1. Delivers anesthetic gas through a vaporizer
2. Assists breathing during anesthesia through a bag or respirator
3. Monitors vital parameters of the patient such as blood pressure, pulse rate, ECG, oxymetry, and $etCO_2$

Vital Signs Monitors

These are patient monitors and vital information is recorded or displayed from the patient during the entire surgery procedure. They monitor blood pressure, temperature, heart rate, respiration rate, respiratory gases, and many other measurements.

Infusion Pumps

Infusion pumps infuse fluids, medication, or nutrients into a patient's circulatory system during surgical procedures. They are generally used intravenously, although subcutaneous, arterial, and epidural infusions are occasionally used. Infusion pumps can administer fluids in ways that would be impractically expensive or unreliable if performed manually by surgical staff.

Suction Pumps

Suction pumps are pumps used to draw liquid by means of suction produced by a piston drawn through a cylinder. The devices are used to remove air or fluids from the surgical site or from the patient's airway.

Respiratory Ventilators

Respiratory ventilators assist in passing oxygen into the lungs and in extracting carbon dioxide from the lungs. There are various modes of ventilation that control the pressure in the breathing circuit.

Medical Warmers

These are blood or fluid warmers maintained at temperatures between 37° C and 42° C and deliver warm blood or fluid to the patient intravenous line.

Vaporizers

This is usually attached to the anesthesia machine and delivers a given concentration of a volatile anesthetic agent. The concentration depends on the temperature, gas flow, and the agent vapor pressure.

Electrocautery or Electrosurgical Units

These are thermal hemostatic devices used in surgical procedures to coagulate vessels or cut tissues. The unit is connected to special electrodes to generate intense heat.

Defibrillators

Defibrillators deliver a therapeutic dose of electrical energy to the patient's heart and are used to terminate arrhythmia and allow normal sinus rhythm to be reestablished. They are an important component in the OR for emergency shock or for other occasions when the heartbeat needs to be reestablished.

Endoscopes

Endoscopes are either a rigid or flexible tube with fiber optics and a light delivery system used by surgeons and surgical staff to illuminate the internal structures of the body during operations.

Patient Transport

Surgical patients are transported to the OR using a gurney or special bed or by wheelchair. Special care is needed in moving these patients, and all transporting devices must be carefully operated to avoid injuries.

Absorber

An absorber is an instrument that removes carbon dioxide and extra moisture from the mixed gases from within the patient breathing circuit.

18.3 ELECTROSURGICAL MACHINES

An electrosurgical machine (also called an electrosurgical unit, or ESU) produces high radiofrequency (RF) energy sufficient to induce cutting and/or coagulation in body tissues and vessels by an electrode during surgery. It is also used for fulguration and blending of joints and tissues. Its components include a generator and handpiece with electrode blades, sharp electrode needles, an electrode handle, and plates. The device also has several types of alarms for patient and equipment safety and for the proper operation and safety of the OR staff. The instrument is designed to provide the correct electrical waveforms to deliver to the site of surgery in order to coagulate blood vessels and to cut tissues smoothly. Surgeons may use the electrosurgical tool instead of, or in conjunction with, a conventional scalpel. When used properly, the electrosurgical unit damages tissue considerably less than the scalpel, with the added ability to stem bleeding safely. Electrosurgery is commonly used in dermatological, gynecological, cardiac, plastic, ocular, spine, ENT, orthopedic, urological, neuro-, and general surgical procedures. As surgery has become more sophisticated, so too have specialized electrosurgical machines. One recent advancement in this technology requires the surgeon to be trained to perform surgery on the patient while viewing the process on a video screen.

The electrosurgical generator component has different output voltage levels, currents, frequencies, output impedances, and output wattages. The surgeon selects proper specification values of these generators when surgery is either micro or macro electrosurgery. A 25-watt (W) generator may output a large voltage and a small current, or, vice versa. In addition, the RF cable attached to the generator may have significant capacitance depending on the cable length and diameter and may present danger to the patient with the likelihood of capacitive discharge. For example, in laparoscopic surgery, the recommendation is 1,200 V peak-to-peak (p-p) and 100 W maximum for the monopolar generators. Similarly, in endoscopic and ophthalmic surgeries, the recommendation is explained for monopolar and bipolar generators.

There are two modes used in an electrosurgical device: monopolar and bipolar.

Monopolar Mode or Monopolar Electrosurgery

In monopolar electrosurgery, the surgical instrument contains only the active electrode, whereas the return electrode is applied to the patient's body surface as shown in **Figure 18-7a.** The current between the active electrode and the return electrode flows through the patient's body. Used chiefly for coagulation, monopolar electrosurgery may also, however, be used to cut soft tissue, or, in some circumstances, the combination of coagulation and cutting can be achieved in monopolar mode. This procedure will require electrical sparking to the tissue as it cuts or coagulates. Monopolar electrosurgery machines have three main components: the generator, the active electrode, and the return electrode (also called the dispersive electrode). The closed loop of the electric current is from the generator to the active electrode then to the return electrode and back to the generator.

FIGURE 18-7a Monopolar electrosurgery.

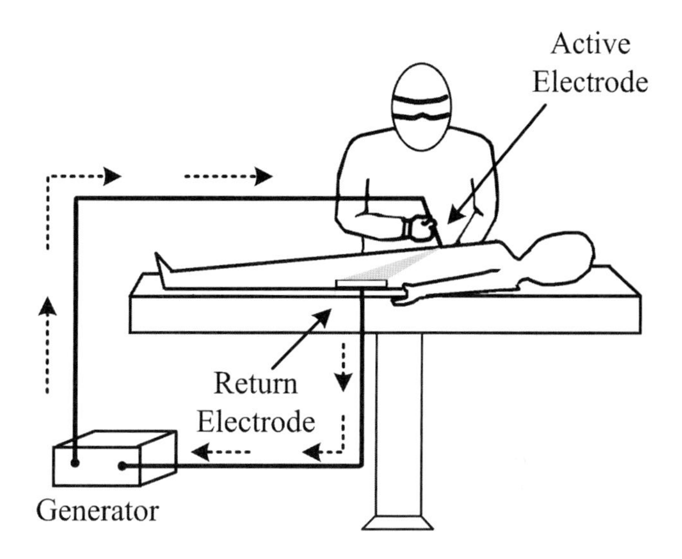

Bipolar Mode or Bipolar Electrosurgery

Bipolar electrosurgery differs from monopolar mode in that the active and the return electrodes are together in a single surgical instrument, as shown in **Figure 18-7b.** The current flows through the active side of the forceps, then through the tissue, and returns through the dispersive side of the forceps to the generator. As the amount of tissue involved in this procedure is limited between the forceps arms, bipolar mode is used only for coagulating tissues.

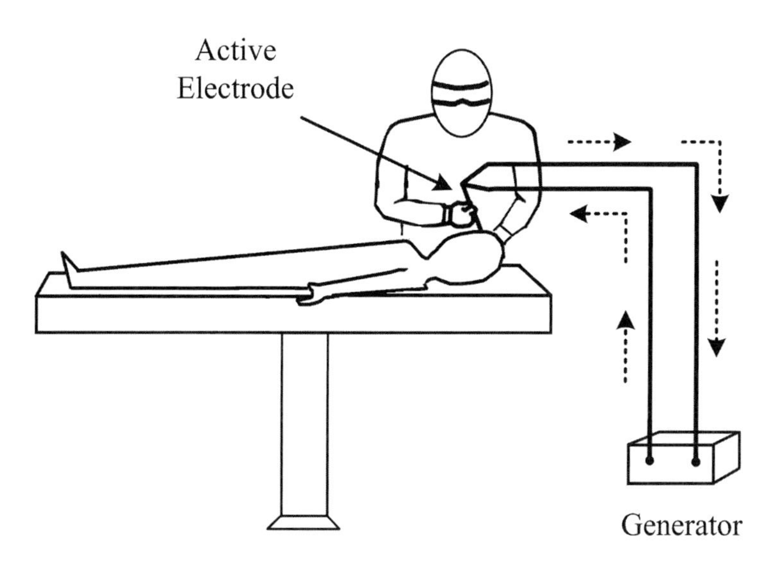

FIGURE 18-7b Bipolar electrosurgery.

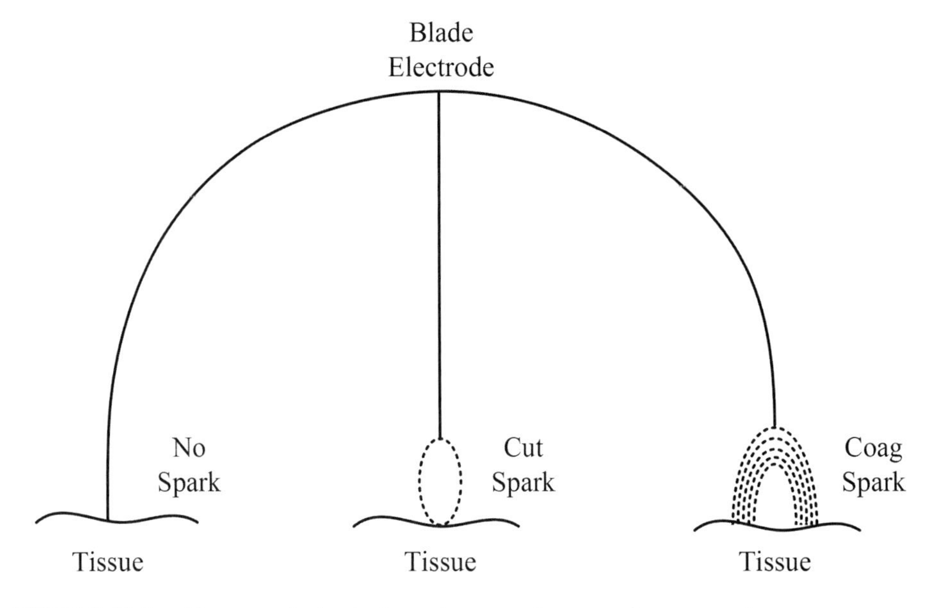

FIGURE 18-8a Electrosurgical unit electrode: no spark, cut spark, coag spark.

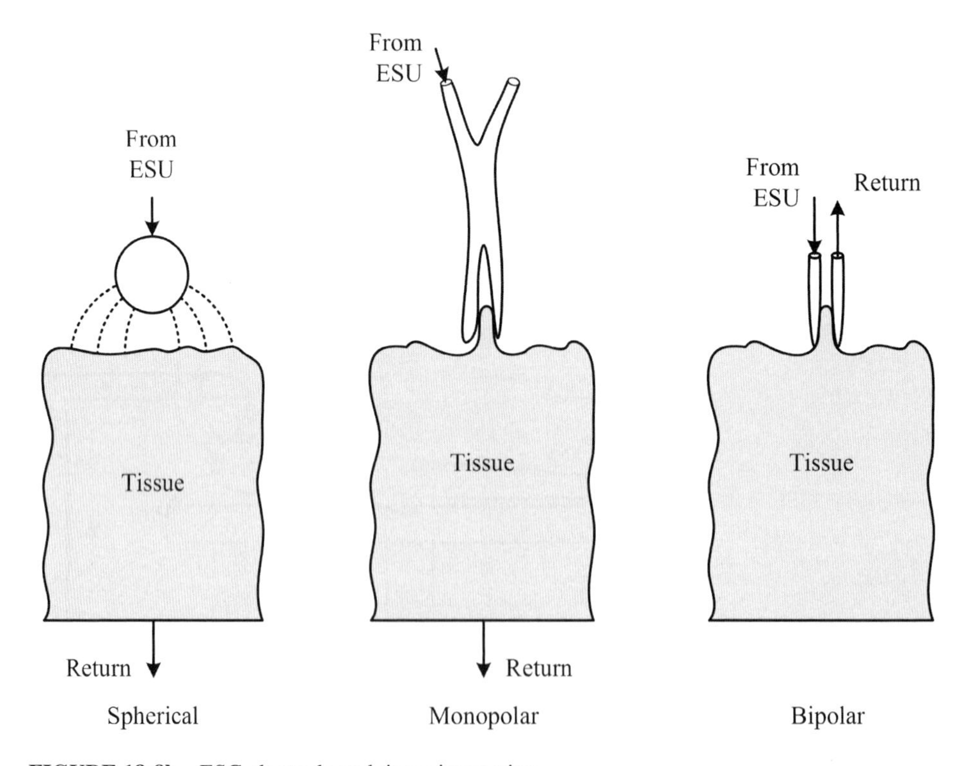

FIGURE 18-8b ESG electrode and tissue interaction.

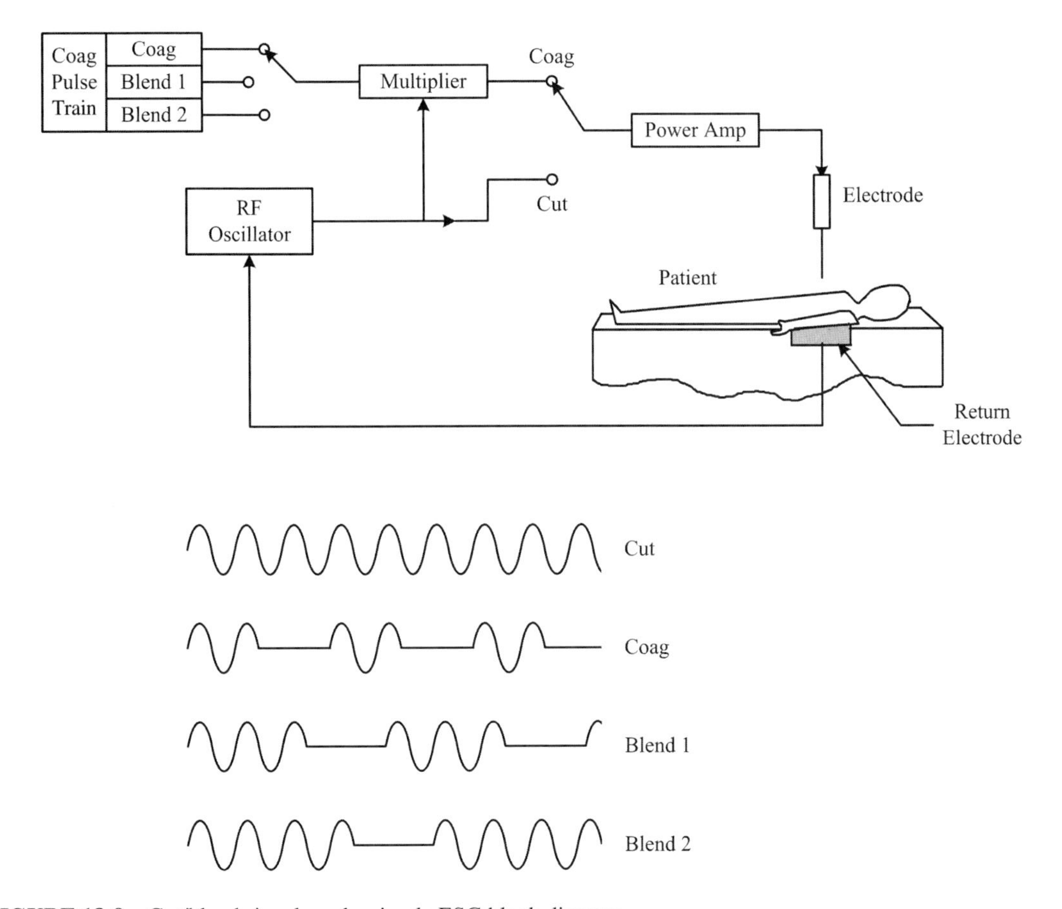

FIGURE 18-9 Cut/blend signals and a simple ESG block diagram.

The delicate procedure of bipolar electrosurgery requires surgical precision. Often, visual magnification of the tissue aids the surgeon to allow minimal damage to the area. This type of surgery is performed on delicate sites such as the spinal cord, the brain, or even the eyes.

Figure 18-8a, Figure 18-8b, and **Figure 18-9** show the configuration of modes, the associated block diagram, and the electronic circuits. **Figure 18-8a** shows electric sparks in cutting or coagulating the tissue compared to no spark on the tissue. In cutting, spark is well-defined and strongest at the tip, but in coagulating, spark is wide over a larger area of the tissue and would cauterize the tissue and coagulate the blood. In the monopolar or bipolar mode compared to the spherical mode shown in **Figure 18-8b**, the electrode grasps and lifts the tissue and various electrical paths are created.

Figure 18-9 shows the various waveforms for cut, coag, and blend modes of ESU operation. The cut mode allows the pure RF sine wave oscillations on the electrodes, whereas the coag mode modulates the RF sine wave oscillations in a multiplier with a pulse train of various duty cycles. Typically, the duty cycles are 30% in coag, 50% in blend 1, and 75% in blend 2.

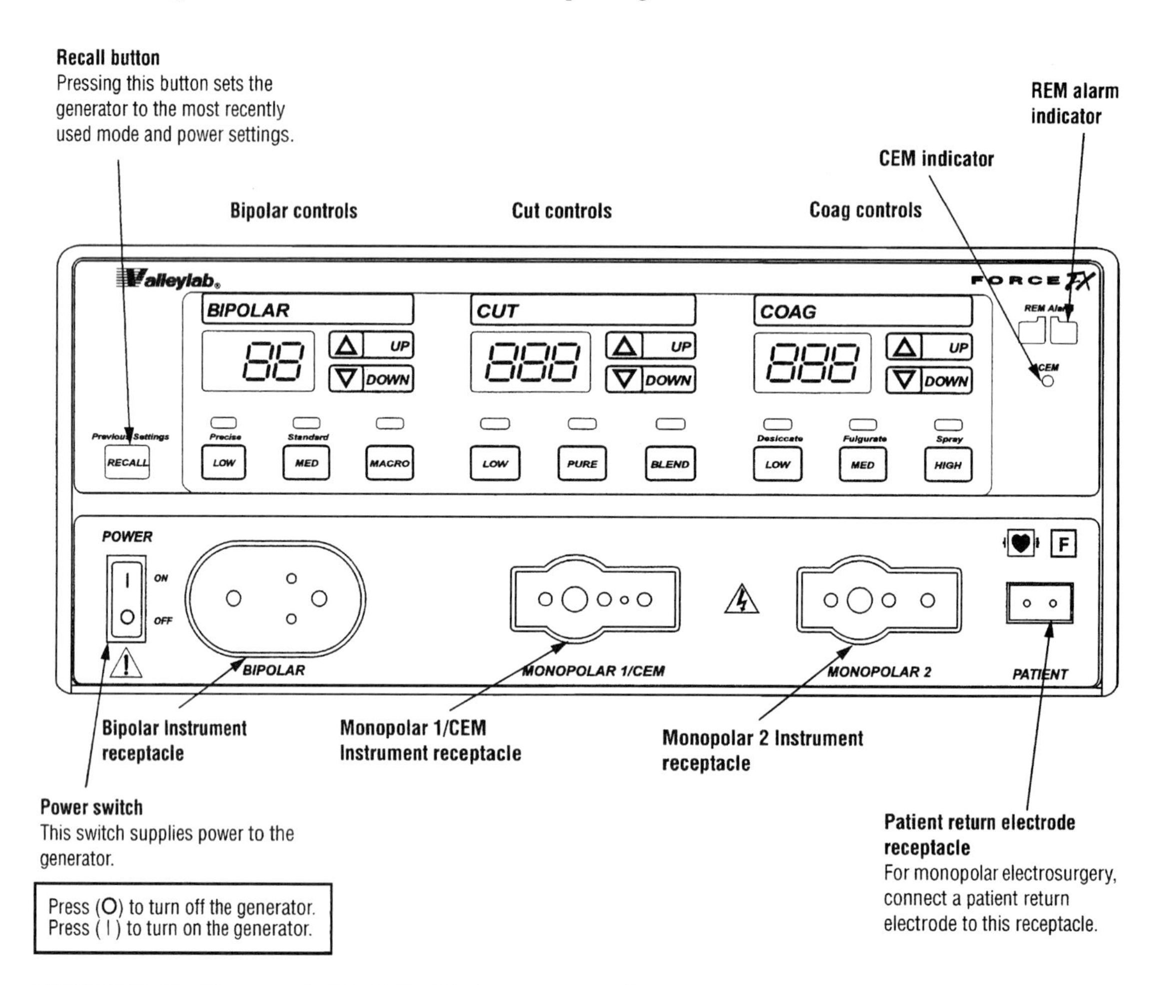

FIGURE 18-10 Front panel of the Valleylab electrosurgery unit.

18.4 VALLEYLAB ELECTROSURGICAL UNIT

Figure 18-10 shows the front control panels of the Valleylab ESU. The front panel has monopolar and bipolar modes. The monopolar mode is divided into the options of cut, coag, and return monitor. The bipolar mode has only a coag option. There are separate switches for hand and foot controls. For the dual pad mode of the return monitor, the resistance indicator displays the patient's resistance. The resistance varies between 10 Ω and 150 Ω.

The return monitor is a safety monitor to guard against patient burns at the dispersive electrode site on the body surface. The microprocessor circuits detect the patient resistance and determine open or short circuit for the return electrode. Once the patient's return electrode site is selected and prepared, the dispersive electrode cable is plugged to the return electrode jack or to an appropriate adapter. For cutting with minimum hemostasis, the pure button in the monopolar cut mode is set, but for cutting with moderate hemostasis, the blend button is pressed. Initially, a low power setting is used for the cut, coag, and bipolar modes, but can be adjusted intraoperatively by the surgeon's requests.

The standard symbols used in electrosurgery are shown in **Figure 18-11.** The pure cut to monopolar and bipolar accessories are also shown in this figure.

Figure 18-12 shows the graphs of the patient resistance and the output power for the various power settings. Each graph can reach a maximum power, such as 300 W or 150 W, and so on. The power levels are adjusted depending on the surgical effects such as electrode size, electrode geometry, waveform, and the surgical technique. In the selection of electrodes, a large electrode without sharp features, such as a ball electrode, will have no tendency to cut, regardless of power level and waveform. But a small and sharp electrode, such as a needle electrode, will cut with minimal mechanical pressure.

The cutting waveforms are continuous (pure) or high-duty cycles with wide pulse widths (blend). However, the monopolar coagulation waveforms are narrow pulse widths with low-duty cycles. It is important to know that when the duty cycle is low, the waveform has less tendency to be able to cut; however, it has a greater tendency to coagulate. The waveform in bipolar coagulation minimizes tissue sticking and popping by limiting the output voltage regardless of any power setting. Compared to monopolar hemostasis, the bipolar hemostasis is more localized, because only the tissue grasped between the forceps tips is affected in the bipolar mode. This localization is desirable in vascular surgeries, plastic surgeries, and neurosurgeries.

Some of the specifications follow:

Fundamental Operating Frequency		Pulse Repetition Frequency	
Pure Cut:	416.7 kHz	Blend:	20 kHz
Blend Cut:	416.7 kHz	Coag:	25 kHz
Coag:	520 kHz	Bipolar	20 kHz
Bipolar Coag:	1.05 MHz		

Max Power		Load Resistance	Max Open Circuit Voltage (p-p)
Mono Pure Cut:	300 W	300 Ω	2,000 V
Mono Blend:	180 W	300 Ω	2,200 V
Mono Coag:	120 W	500 Ω	9,000 V
Bipolar Coag:	50 W	50 Ω	280 V

The output waveform is generated based on the surgeon's input commands. The RF drive passes through the output amplifier, output transformer, and cut/coag buttons. There are several sensors for feedback to the main controller for display and to the serial port. The main micro controller incorporates an eight-input multiplexed eight-bit A/D converter. It is responsible for the overall system control.

The REM system continuously measures resistance at the return electrode site and compares it to a safe resistance (between 5 Ω and 135 Ω). The REM alarm indicator flashes red, a tone sounds, and then the generator stops producing the output power. This is a safety feature.

In cut mode, a sinusoidal oscillating current passes through the tip and shows a spark when the electrode is at a short distance from the skin. However, in coagulation, a wide spark will appear. A larger region of skin will be affected; this is how to cauterize the tissue and coagulate the blood. The electrode is used to lift, clamp, and grasp the tissue. The ESU current can flow broadly through the grasped tissue.

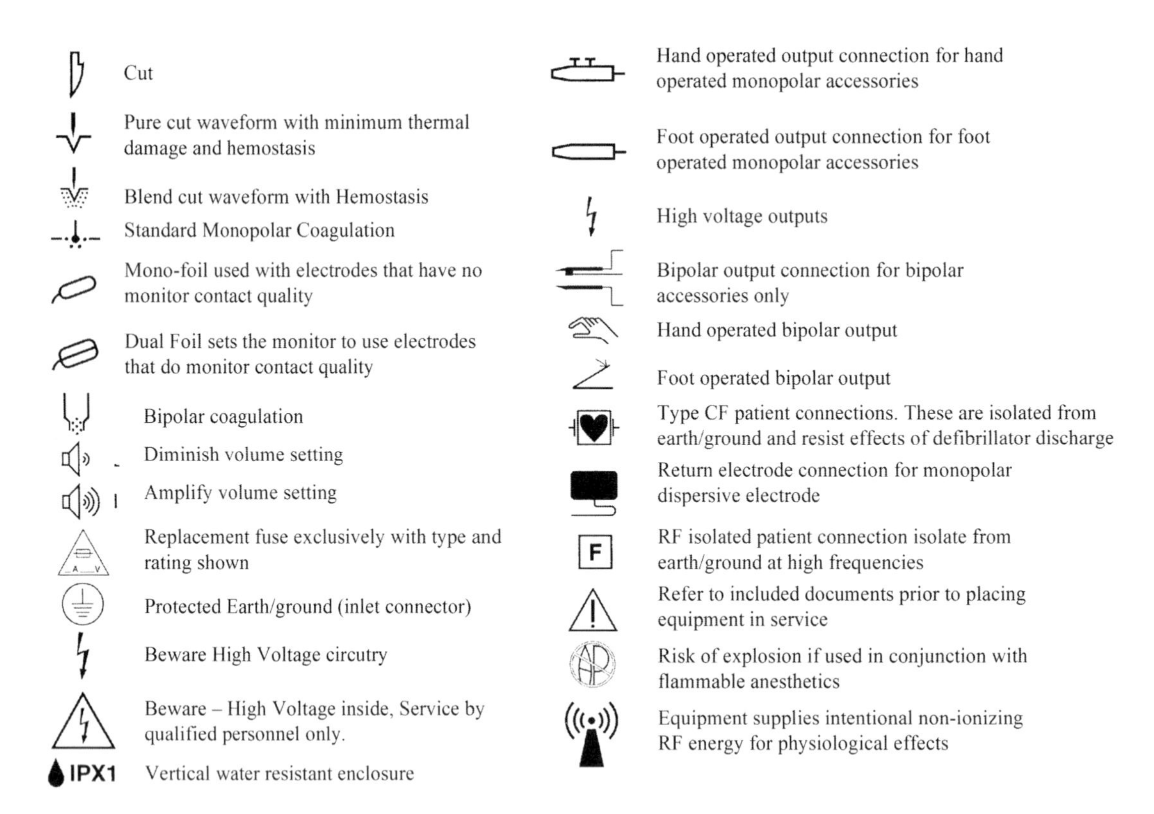

FIGURE 18-11 Standard symbols used in electrosurgery.

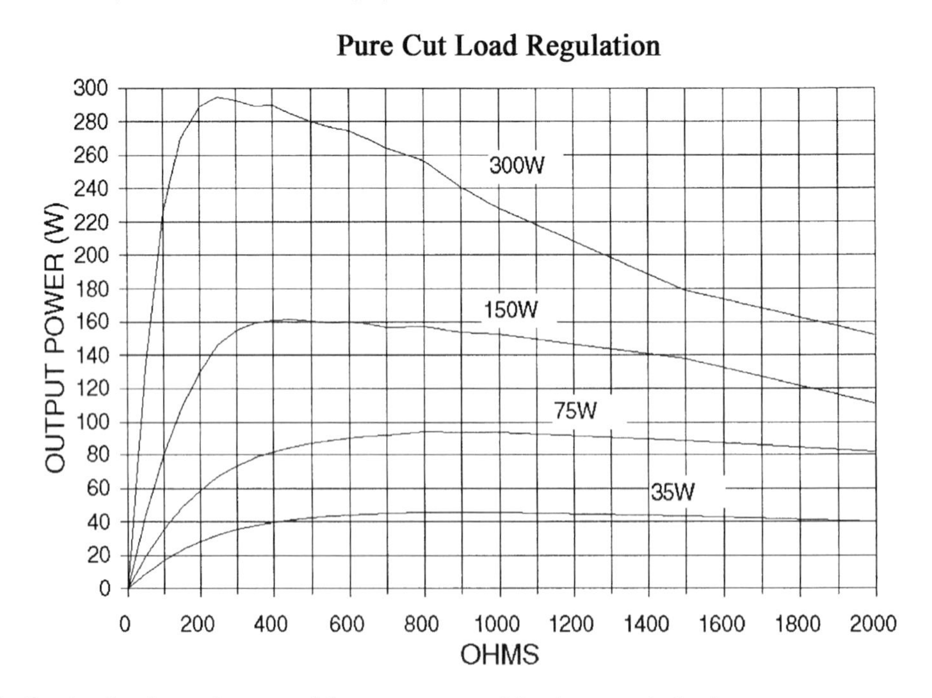

FIGURE 18-12 Graphs of patient resistance and the output power of the electrosurgical unit.

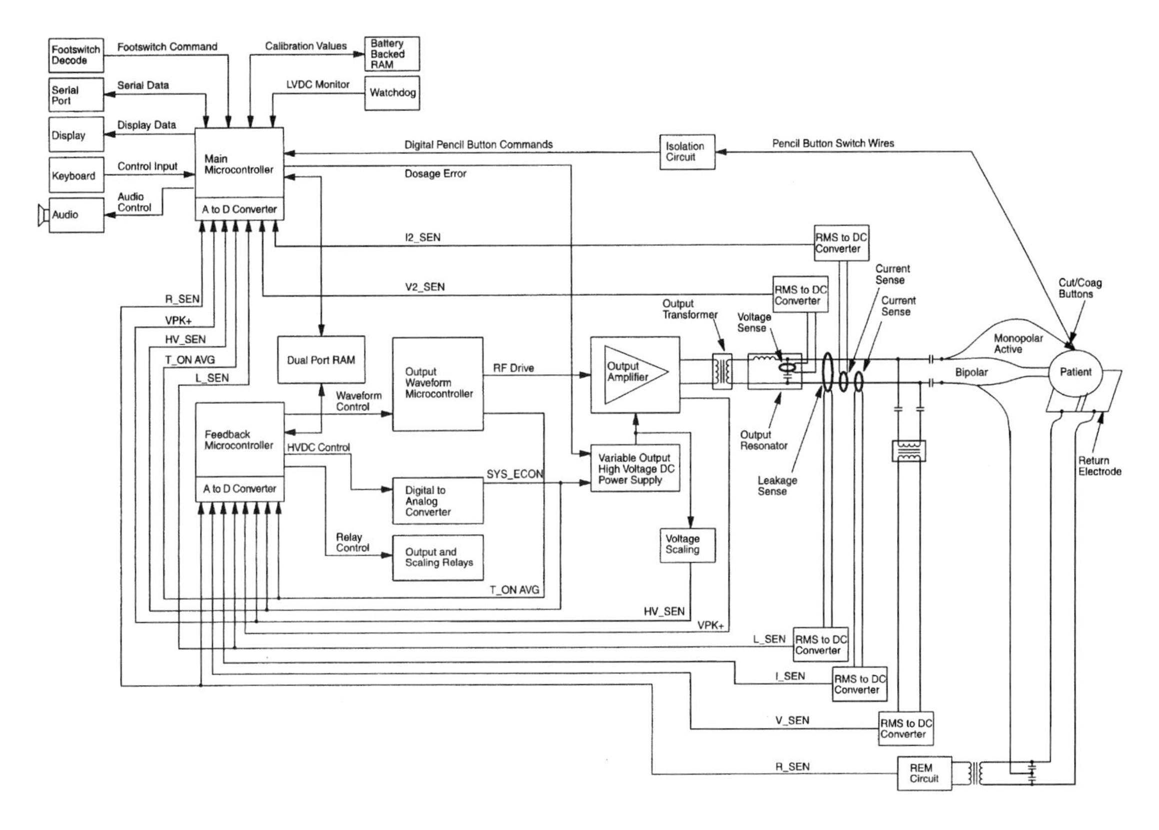

FIGURE 18-13 A detailed block diagram of the Valleylab unit.

Peak-to-peak signals ranging from 1,000 V to 10,000 V can be generated in the open – circuit; however, up to 400 W into a 500-Ω load can be delivered by an ESU unit. A detailed circuit is shown in **Figure 18-13.** It shows the bipolar outputs on the lower right side, and the monopolar outputs in the middle right side with the return path from the patient.

18.5 PRECAUTIONS IN ELECTROSURGERY

Considering the delicate nature of electrosurgery, safe procedure is important. A guideline for ensuring proper safety is presented here.

1. With electrosurgical procedures, the risk of igniting flammable gases and chemicals of any kind is high. Flammable anesthetics and preparation solutions should be stored away from the patient and the site where the electrosurgery is performed.
2. In abdominal surgery, the bowel should be purged and filled with nonflammable gas.
3. The proper placement of the return electrode and its use prevents any burn to the patient. The return electrode must be applied to a clean-shaven surface of the patient and must be dry. Avoid bones and scar tissues. Place the electrode in contact with a conductive surface of the body and close to a good blood supply.

4. The electrosurgical current path should be short and should run longitudinally or diagonally to the body.
5. Needles should not be used for monitoring during electrosurgical procedures.
6. Accessories to electrosurgical procedures should not be connected unless they are needed in the surgery. They should be kept in a nonconductive holster or an insulated location. Examples of the accessories are: forceps, handles, probes, and medical tubing.
7. Precautions should be made when surgery is done on patients with cardiac pacemakers. The pacemaker may be damaged or ventricular fibrillation may occur due to high-frequency electrosurgical output.
8. The electrosurgical leads should not contact the patient or other patient leads.
9. Use only power necessary. The output power should be low and its activation time should be short.

18.6 BASICS OF ANESTHESIA

Anesthesia derives from the Greek *anaisthesis* meaning *without sensation.* The patient is given a measured concentration of gases and drugs through a breathing mask in order to lose consciousness. This is called general anesthesia. The patient will be unconscious for the entire duration of the operation—unaware of his or her surroundings and unable to feel any pain. Once the operation is completed, the anesthesia is withdrawn. The patient will regain consciousness once its effects wear off.

Anesthesia System

The anesthesia system is an anesthesia machine in coordination with gas supplies, ventilators, a carbon dioxide absorber, anesthetic vaporizers, a gas scavenging system, and several types of patient monitors. The anesthesia system performs several functions:

1. It supplies a mixture of gases and anesthetic vapors
2. It monitors gas concentrations from the anesthesia machine.
3. It monitors the patient's vital signs.
4. It controls patient's breath rates, volumes, and pressures in the breathing circuit.
5. It monitors the safety of the patient.

18.7 ANESTHESIA MACHINE

Generally, an anesthesia machine consists of valves and regulators, flowmeters, breathing circuits, vaporizers, and ventilators. **Figure 18-14** shows a block diagram of an anesthesia machine. The anesthesia team is very much familiar with several aspects of an anesthesia system and its delivery mechanism. The patient is given a mixture of gases and anesthetic vapors from the anesthesia machine. The volume of the mixture of the gases, its pressure, and rate are all controlled by the anesthesiologist and the patient is carefully monitored

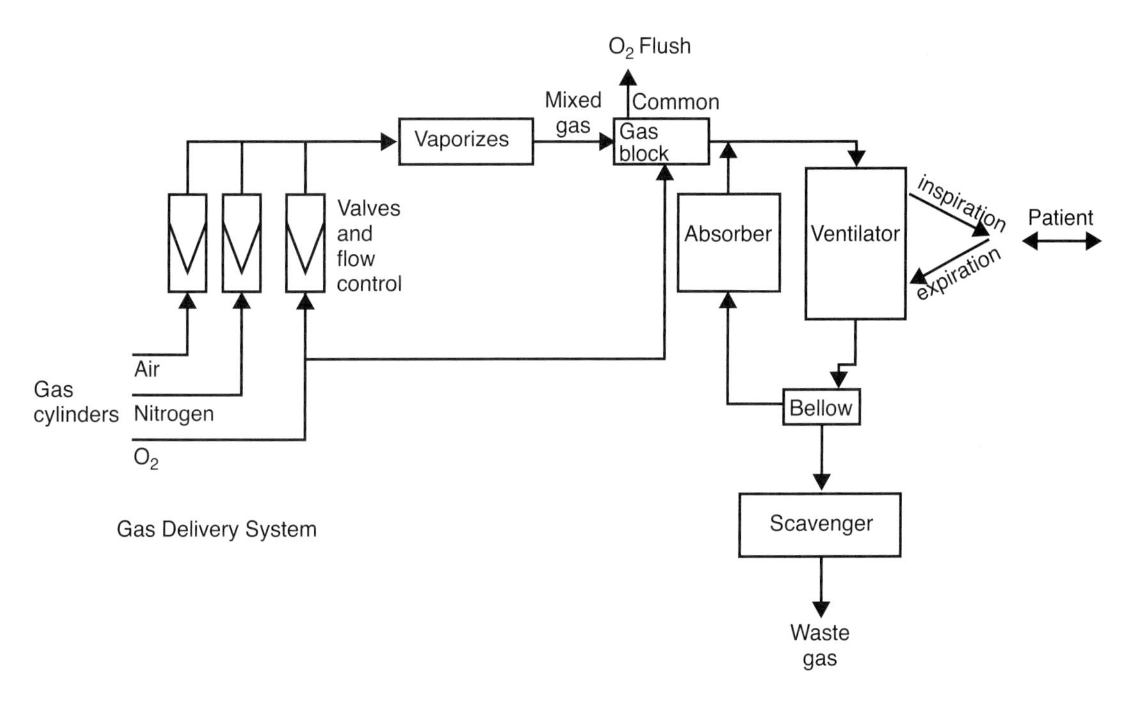

FIGURE 18-14 A simple block diagram of an anesthesia machine.

throughout the operation. There are several safety features to protect the patient and also to remove any excessive gases from the patient's breathing circuit.

There are three gas supply modules: oxygen (O_2), nitrogen (N), and air and each one is connected to a cylinder or a wall outlet. An oxygen flush button and the pneumatic outlets are for the oxygen outlet and a visual oxygen pressure indicator is on the O_2 supply line. There is also an alarm assembly when O_2 is low in the anesthesia machine. The shutoff valves open up when sufficient pressure builds up, and the O_2 and the other gases flow to the vaporizer manifold. The mixed gas passes through the vaporizer and the vapors are now available at the common gas outlet for the patient. The flow control valves control the mixture of the gases and also the exhaust blocks for venting the remaining gases when the system is switched off. **Figure 18-15** shows gas cylinders and **Figure 18-16** shows a functional block diagram of a gas cylinder. The high pressing in the cylinder permit each cylinder to hold a large volume of gas in a compressed state. A gauge connected to the cylinder shows the pressure in pounds per square inch gauge (psig). A regulator connected to the cylinder is used to reduce the pressure of gas as it leaves the cylinder.

The Vaporizer

A vaporizer mixes the vapors of the liquid anesthetic agent with other gases before it sends the mixed gas to the breathing circuit of the patient. The vaporizer keeps the inlet gas in contact with the anesthetic agent until the gas has absorbed all of the agent vapor at the

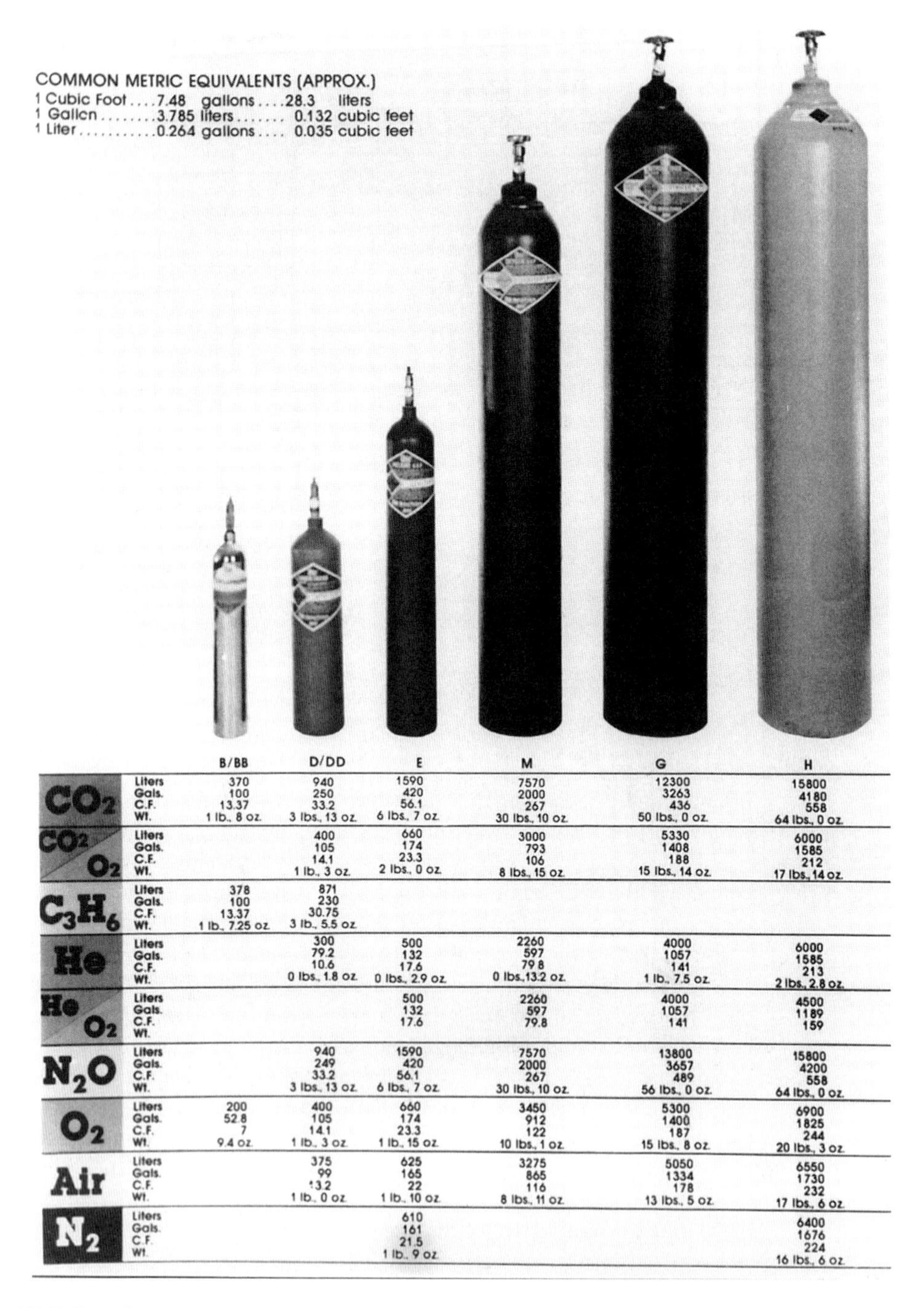

COMMON METRIC EQUIVALENTS (APPROX.)
1 Cubic Foot....7.48 gallons....28.3 liters
1 Gallon........3.785 liters....... 0.132 cubic feet
1 Liter...........0.264 gallons.... 0.035 cubic feet

Gas		B/BB	D/DD	E	M	G	H
CO_2	Liters	370	940	1590	7570	12300	15800
	Gals.	100	250	420	2000	3263	4180
	C.F.	13.37	33.2	56.1	267	436	558
	Wt.	1 lb., 8 oz.	3 lbs., 13 oz.	6 lbs., 7 oz.	30 lbs., 10 oz.	50 lbs., 0 oz.	64 lbs., 0 oz.
CO_2/O_2	Liters		400	660	3000	5330	6000
	Gals.		105	174	793	1408	1585
	C.F.		14.1	23.3	106	188	212
	Wt.		1 lb., 3 oz.	2 lbs., 0 oz.	8 lbs., 15 oz.	15 lbs., 14 oz.	17 lbs., 14 oz.
C_3H_6	Liters	378	871				
	Gals.	100	230				
	C.F.	13.37	30.75				
	Wt.	1 lb., 7.25 oz.	3 lb., 5.5 oz.				
He	Liters		300	500	2260	4000	6000
	Gals.		79.2	132	597	1057	1585
	C.F.		10.6	17.6	79.8	141	213
	Wt.		0 lbs., 1.8 oz.	0 lbs., 2.9 oz.	0 lbs., 13.2 oz.	1 lb., 7.5 oz.	2 lbs., 2.8 oz.
He/O_2	Liters			500	2260	4000	4500
	Gals.			132	597	1057	1189
	C.F.			17.6	79.8	141	159
	Wt.						
N_2O	Liters		940	1590	7570	13800	15800
	Gals.		249	420	2000	3657	4200
	C.F.		33.2	56.1	267	489	558
	Wt.		3 lbs., 13 oz.	6 lbs., 7 oz.	30 lbs., 10 oz.	56 lbs., 0 oz.	64 lbs., 0 oz.
O_2	Liters	200	400	660	3450	5300	6900
	Gals.	52.8	105	174	912	1400	1825
	C.F.	7	14.1	23.3	122	187	244
	Wt.	9.4 oz.	1 lb., 3 oz.	1 lb., 15 oz.	10 lbs., 1 oz.	15 lbs., 8 oz.	20 lbs., 3 oz.
Air	Liters		375	625	3275	5050	6550
	Gals.		99	165	865	1334	1730
	C.F.		13.2	22	116	178	232
	Wt.		1 lb., 0 oz.	1 lb., 10 oz.	8 lbs., 11 oz.	13 lbs., 5 oz.	17 lbs., 6 oz.
N_2	Liters			610			6400
	Gals.			161			1676
	C.F.			21.5			224
	Wt.			1 lb., 9 oz.			16 lbs., 6 oz.

FIGURE 18-15 Gas cylinders.

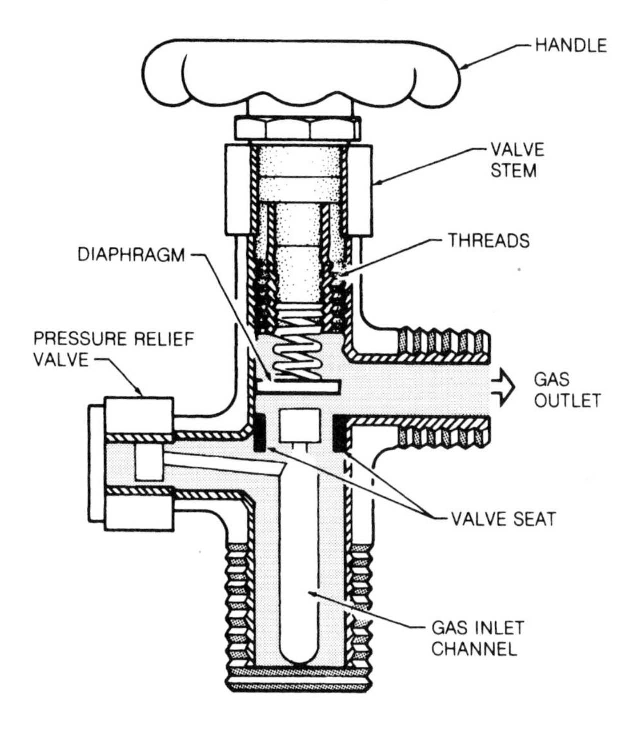

FIGURE 18-16 A functional diagram of a gas cylinder.

proper temperature and pressure. The gas is then considered fully saturated. The output concentration of the mixed gas depends on the flow rate and the amount of the gas flow through the vaporizer chamber of the liquid agent. Temperature changes also affect the output of the vaporizer.

The vaporizer has a liquid level indicator, a control dial and release, and a safety lock lever. The inlet gases of O_2 and nitrogen oxide split into the first and second stream, and only the second stream then passes over the liquid agent and becomes saturated. No agent is added to the first stream and it flows to the outlet of the vaporizer directly. The temperature is kept constant with the use of the thermostat.

Common Gas Block

The common gas block consists of:

- An oxygen flush button to regulate flow of oxygen to the gas mixture.
- A common gas outlet so that gas mixtures can exit from the anesthesia machine.
- A common gas outlet check valve to permit gas mixture to flow in only one direction to the common gas outlet.
- A pressure relief valve to vent gas flow when pressure at the common gas outlet may exceed 5.5 pounds per square inch gauge (psig).

The Ventilator

When the patient is anesthetized during surgery, he or she will require breathing assistance; the ventilator of the anesthesia machine controls the breathing patterns for the patient. This is an electronic ventilator and does not allow any high airway pressure or excess gas in the breathing circuits. It has monitors for pressure, percentage of O_2 in the gas, breath rate, and the tidal volume of the gas.

The Absorber

The absorber is used in any anesthesia system where it removes carbon dioxide and excess moisture. The gas flows are controlled. The absorber includes absorbent granules, gaskets, a locking lever, and canisters. There is a chemical reaction between the absorbent granules and the carbon dioxide (CO_2) from the patient gases and water is produced and moisture is supplied to the patient breathing circuit.

Waste Gas Scavenger

This system removes gas vented from the breathing system and helps minimize venting of waste gas into the OR room. The flow of waste gas from the breathing circuit is directed into the waste gas scavenging manifold. The system connects to the hospital's vacuum system and uses the needle valve to adjust flow through the scavenging manifold. The positive and negative pressure valves behave as relief valves to protect the patient from any pressure fluctuations.

18.8 STERILIZATION

Sterilization in hospitals, particularly ORs, offers protection from contamination and infections. During anesthesia and surgery, the patient can be put in danger of infection if the surgical instruments, electrodes, hands, gloves, and gowns are not completely sterilized. The surgeons scrub their hands and wear sterile clothing. The restricted area in the operating room is a sterile region.

Sterilization destroys all microorganisms including pathogenic and other bacteria by exposure to heat, radiation, chemicals, and gas, or by filtration.

In autoclaving sterilization equipment, a combination of high pressure and steam is applied to decontaminate the instruments and render them sterile. Treatment conditions to achieve sterility varies in relation to the volume of the material treated, moisture content, the level of contamination and volume of the autoclave (i.e., the amount of saturated steam under high pressure).

There are at least four types of sterilization processes used in a hospital OR: wet heat, dry heat, gas, and radiation.

Wet Heat

Wet heat is commonly used and is referred to as steam sterilization. **Figure 18-17** is a photo of a steam sterilizer. The structure of the sterilizer is around the chamber in which an item or a test pack (a medical device or metal surgical instrument) is placed for sterilization. Steam enters the chamber and displaces the air from the pack and allows the steam to

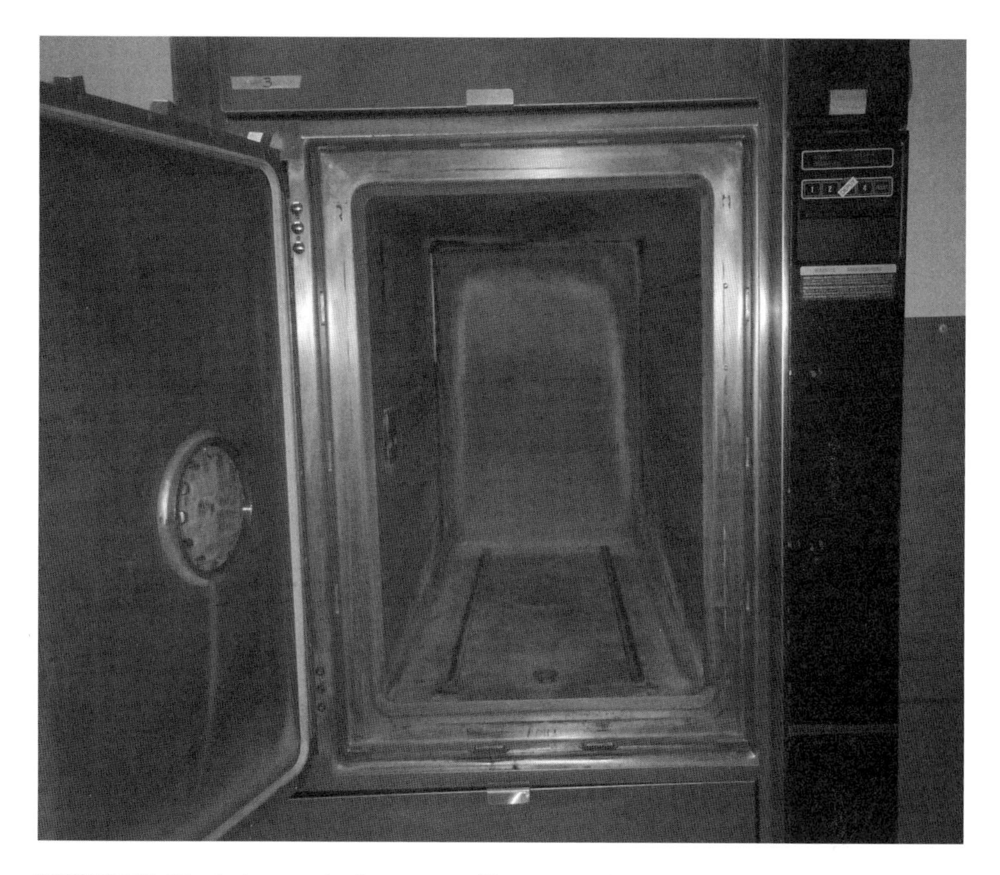

FIGURE 18-17 A photograph of a steam sterilizer.

penetrate the pack. The temperature ranges from 120° C to 135° C, with an exposure time of 10 to 30 minutes. The sterilizer has a vacuum pump, pressure gauge for the pressure setting, and a thermostat for temperature setting. Moist heat in the form of saturated heat under pressure in the enclosed chamber may not sterilize all the devices; however, it is the first step in the sterilization process. The steam can soften the outer layers of microorganisms, allowing the denaturation of proteins inside the microbes, thus destroying and killing the microbes.

Dry Steam

If the water saturation level in the steam entering the autoclave is less than 3 percent, then the steam is called dry steam. The steam becomes superheated and may not sterilize the instruments properly.

Gas Sterilizing

Some instruments are heat-sensitive or moisture-sensitive; therefore, steam or any kind of heat is not a successful method of sterilization. In this case, gas sterilization is the preferred method. The organic and colorless gas ethylene oxide (EtO) is used as a gas sterilizer. It generates a chemical reaction that interferes with the metabolism of bacterial spores and other types of microorganisms. This process of sterilization can take more than 10 hours to complete successfully and can be expensive.

In addition to an expensive and lengthy exposure time, EtO is flammable; therefore, special precautions must be taken to avoid ignition or explosion. It is packaged as 100% EtO in small-chamber cartridges or with the diluted EtO in large cartridges for large-chamber sterilizers. EtO is diluted with chlorofluorocarbon or Freon. Moreover, the EtO-sterilized devices will need proper aeration so that the patient or OR staff is not exposed to toxic levels of EtO.

Similar to steam sterilizers, gas sterilizers depend on several factors, such as:

- Exposure time.
- Temperature.
- Moisture.
- Concentration.

FIGURE 18-18. A table of terminology in the sterilization process.

Terminology of Asepsis and Sterile Technique

Antiseptic: substance commonly used on living tissue to inhibit the growth and reproduction of microbes to prevent infection

Asepsis: absence of microbes, infection

Bacteriocidal: substance that destroys/kills bacteria

Bacteriostatic: substance that restrains the further development or reproduction of bacteria

Bioburden: the number of microbes or amount of organic debris on an object at any given time

Contamination: the presence of pathogenic materials

Cross-contamination: the contamination of a person or object by another

Decontamination: to reduce to an irreducible minimum the presence of pathogenic material

Disinfectant: chemical agent that kills most microbes, but usually not spores; usually used on inanimate objects because compounds are too strong to be used on living tissues

Fomite: an inanimate object on which pathogens may be conveyed

Fungicide: agent that destroys fungus

Infection: the invasion of the human body or tissue by pathogenic microorganisms that reproduce and multiply, causing disease

Nosocomial: an infection acquired within a health care setting

Pathogen: any microbe capable of causing disease

Resident flora: microbes that normally reside below the skin surface or within the body

Sepsis: infection, usually accompanied by fever, that results from the presence of pathogenic microorganisms

Spore: a resistant form of certain types of bacteria, able to survive in adverse conditions

Sporicidal: substance that kills/destroys bacteria in the spore stage

Sterile: item(s) that has/have been rendered free of all living microorganisms, including spores

Sterile field: specified area, usually the area immediately around the patient, that is considered free of microorganisms

Sterile technique: methods used to prevent contamination of the sterile field by microorganisms; protection of the patient against infection-causing microbes preoperatively, intraoperatively, and postoperatively

Sterility, event related: sterility determined by how a package is handled rather than time elapsed; package is considered sterile until opened or integrity of packaging material is damaged

Sterilization: the destruction of all microorganisms, including spores, on inanimate surfaces; the destruction of all microorganisms in or about an object, as by steam (flowing or pressurized), chemical agents (alcohol, phenol, heavy metals, ethylene oxide gas), high-velocity electron bombardment, or ultraviolet light radiation

Strike-through contamination: contamination of a sterile field that occurs through the passage of fluid through or a puncture in a microbial barrier

Surgically clean: items mechanically cleaned and chemically disinfected but not sterile

Terminal disinfection: to render items safe to handle by high-level disinfection

Terminal sterilization: to render items safe to handle by sterilization

Transient flora: microbes that reside on the skin surface and are easily removed

Vector: a living carrier that transmits disease

Virucide: agent that destroys viruses

Ionizing Radiation

Ionizing radiation is a method of sterilization used in hospitals that consists of subatomic particles or electromagnetic waves, such as gamma rays, that are energetic enough to detach electrons from atoms or molecules, ionizing them. It is used to sterilize prepackaged medical devices that enter the OR environment. Gamma rays can generate such thermal and chemical reactions that they can disrupt the DNA of all microbes. Beta rays are also used in radiation sterilization.

A terminology table is provided in **Figure 18-18** for the asepsis (absence of microbes) and the sterile technique. It provides definitions and terms used in the sterilization field. The list provides the types of infections that may occur in the OR room if proper precautions are not taken.

SUMMARY

The OR room is designed with the most sophisticated equipment access in any hospital. The surgeons and even OR nurses are well trained. This chapter provides the following concepts:

1. The beginning of the chapter gives the OR environment and lists various equipment in it.
2. The electrosurgical units are discussed in detail with the types of modes in cutting and coagulating the tissues during surgery.
3. The block diagrams of ESU units are discussed and Valleylab equipment is explained in the next section.
4. The precautions in electrosurgery are also discussed.
5. Anesthesia and sterilization concepts are discussed in detail toward the end of the chapter.

MEDICAL TERMINOLOGY

The following is a list of medical terms mentioned in this chapter.

Electrosurgery: removal or destruction of tissue by using an electric current.

Anesthesia: absence of normal sensation or feeling, especially pain.

Sterilization: procedure that kills or removes microorganisms by utilizing heat, radiation, chemicals, or filtration.

Vaporizer: device used to reduce liquid medication to vapor form; used for inhalation or application to mucous membranes.

Autoclave: device used for high-pressure steam sterilization.

Cautery: application of a hot instrument or caustic substance in order to burn or destroy tissue.

Infusion: therapeutic introduction of fluid flowing by gravity into the body.

Suction: process or act of drawing liquids by means of suction.

Gas scavenger: device for removing gases or other volatile agents, thus reducing personnel to exposure and preventing buildup of potentially explosive combinations in laboratories and hospitals.

QUIZ

1. One of the main duties of the surgical technologist is:

a) To detect odors

b) To sterilize instruments

c) To manipulate surgical instruments

d) To monitor safety in the OR

2. Name at least three ancillary departments in a hospital that directly support the OR and its procedures.

1. ____________________

2. ____________________

3. ____________________

3. Suction outlets in the OR are used mainly to:

a) Decontaminate the room

b) Deliver anesthetic gases

c) Discard OR waste

d) None of the above

4. How can an electrosurgical unit become a fire hazard in the OR? Why?

5. What may happen if high humidity occurs in the OR?

a) Pathogens may grow.

b) An electrical short may occur.

c) Anesthesia may not work.

d) None of the above.

6. What does a pulse oximeter detect?

a) The O_2 saturation level in the blood

b) The hemoglobin saturation level in the blood

c) The CO_2 saturation level in the blood

d) The acidity in the blood

7. Coagulation means:
   a) Cutting the tissue
   b) Burning the tissue
   c) Joining the tissue
   d) None of the above
8. Why are lasers used mainly in electrosurgery?
9. True of False: Monopolar mode electrosurgery is only used in coagulation.
   a) True
   b) False
10. A hazardous vaporized tissue plume (i.e., when a surgical instrument cuts bone, a plume of smoke is produced) in the OR is removed by:
    a) Smoke evacuators
    b) A humidifier
    c) A suction pump
    d) All of the above

PROBLEMS

1. An electrosurgical unit produces an open-circuit voltage of 2,500 V (p-p) across an electrode in the cut mode with a duty cycle of 100%. Compute the power delivered to the load of 250 Ω when the internal resistance of the ESU unit is also 250 Ω.
2. Follow the same instructions as in the previous problem, except the mode is a blend with a duty cycle of 50%. Compute the power delivered to the load.
3. Compute the lateral heat generated in radiosurgery given the following parameters:
   a) Electrode size = 0.1 inch
   b) Electrode contact time with the tissue = 10 sec.
   c) Intensity = 100 W
   d) Waveform = partially rectified
4. Define disinfectant, surfactant, and antiseptic. Compare these agents and provide three products for each.
5. Explain temperature and moisture effects on sterilization. How is autoclave dependent on temperature and moisture controls?
6. How is robotics involved in OR procedures? Name at least three components of robotic technology. Give an example of feedback control in robotics during surgery.

7. Medical gas cylinders store compressed gases such as O_2 and N_2O. Define gas pressures and volumes in these cylinders of various sizes.
8. Identify and describe hazards to the patient in the operating room.
9. Indicate the temperature and humidity range in an OR room. Also, describe the rationale behind it.
10. Identify and discuss basic instruments (type and function) and the special instruments used in the OR room.

CASE STUDIES

1. Minimally invasive surgery has changed the design of operating rooms. Legacy Good Samaritan Hospital in Portland, Oregon, has developed plans for state-of-the-art ORs. These high-tech rooms are digital and "imaging friendly." Conduct a case study of the needs of this hospital's OR by asking and answering the following questions:

   a) What is minimally invasive surgery (MIS)?

   b) How can an OR be made an imaging-friendly room? What does imaging-friendly mean?

   c) What kind of costs and design life span can be expected in the plan?

2. Produce a detailed case study on the preoperative, intraoperative, and postoperative phases of the OR management in hospitals, revealing coordination problems in patient care. The case study may discuss sterile field or safety and equipment issues in the OR. The data can be collected on these three phases of OR management.

3. A 15-year-old boy was brought to the OR for plastic surgery. He had recently been involved in an automobile accident, and his face had suffered severe lacerations. As the surgeon started the surgery, a nurse entered the OR and declared that some of the surgical instruments had not been properly sterilized overnight.

   a) Define "sterile field" and explain why it is important to sterilize everything in the OR.

   b) Who is responsible for sterilizing the instruments overnight?

   c) Indicate the types of instruments the plastic surgeon will require in order to operate on the boy's facial lacerations.

   d) Is the hospital required to report this incident to any regulatory agency? Why or why not?

RESEARCH TOPICS

1. Cardiothoracic surgery is surgery performed on the heart and lungs. There are a number of types of procedures in cardiothoracic surgery.
   a) Make a list of the instruments that may be used in these types of procedures.
   b) Itemize the types of surgical procedures in cardiothoracic surgery.
   c) Discuss the types of surgical instruments needed in various different surgeries, such as general surgery, ophthalmic surgery, reconstructive surgery, and neurosurgery.
2. A research topic may cover the computer networks in operating rooms. Presently, computers are used in all disciplines in hospitals and clinics. Concentrate only on the usage of computers and computer networks when the surgery is in progress. The topic may discuss the use of the Internet during surgical procedures.

CHAPTER 19

Biomedical Laboratory Instrumentation

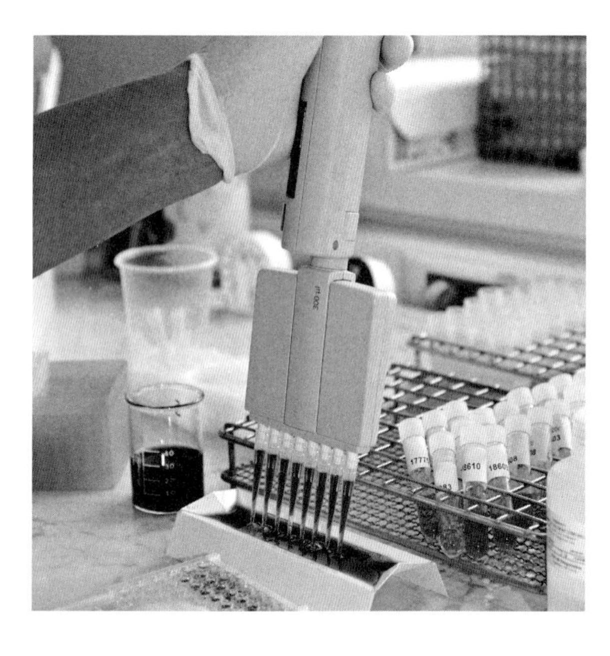

■ CHAPTER OUTLINE

■ OBJECTIVES

The objective of this chapter is to familiarize the reader with the various types of laboratories found in a hospital and the types of biomedical instrumentation a BMET may encounter in the various laboratories.

Upon completion of this chapter, the reader will be able to:

- List the various medical laboratory services in a hospital.
- Identify various equipment in a chemistry lab, hematology lab, microbiology lab, virology lab, and histology lab.
- Discuss sensors for pO_2, pCO_2, and pH in blood gas analyzers.
- Discuss the laboratory personnel in a hospital.

■ INTERNET WEB SITES

http://www.clsi.org (Clinical Laboratory Standards Institute)
http://www.ascp.org (American Society for Clinical Pathology)
http://www.ascls.org (American Society for Clinical Laboratory Science)

■ INTRODUCTION

The department of laboratory medicine of a hospital is a complex and, at times, intimidating department for a biomedical engineer or a BMET technician. Within the department of laboratory medicine, there are many specialized laboratories, each performing specific testing and equipped with specific instrumentation.

This chapter discusses the various services such as chemical and microscopic tests on blood, other body fluids, and tissues done in medical laboratories of a hospital. A medical laboratory may be large, offering sophisticated services and employing many employees, or it may be small with only a few employees.

Figure 19-1 shows the flow chart of the various medical laboratory services in the department of laboratory medicine in the Children's Hospital at Columbus, Ohio. **Figure 19-2** has a list of tests routinely performed at these service laboratories.

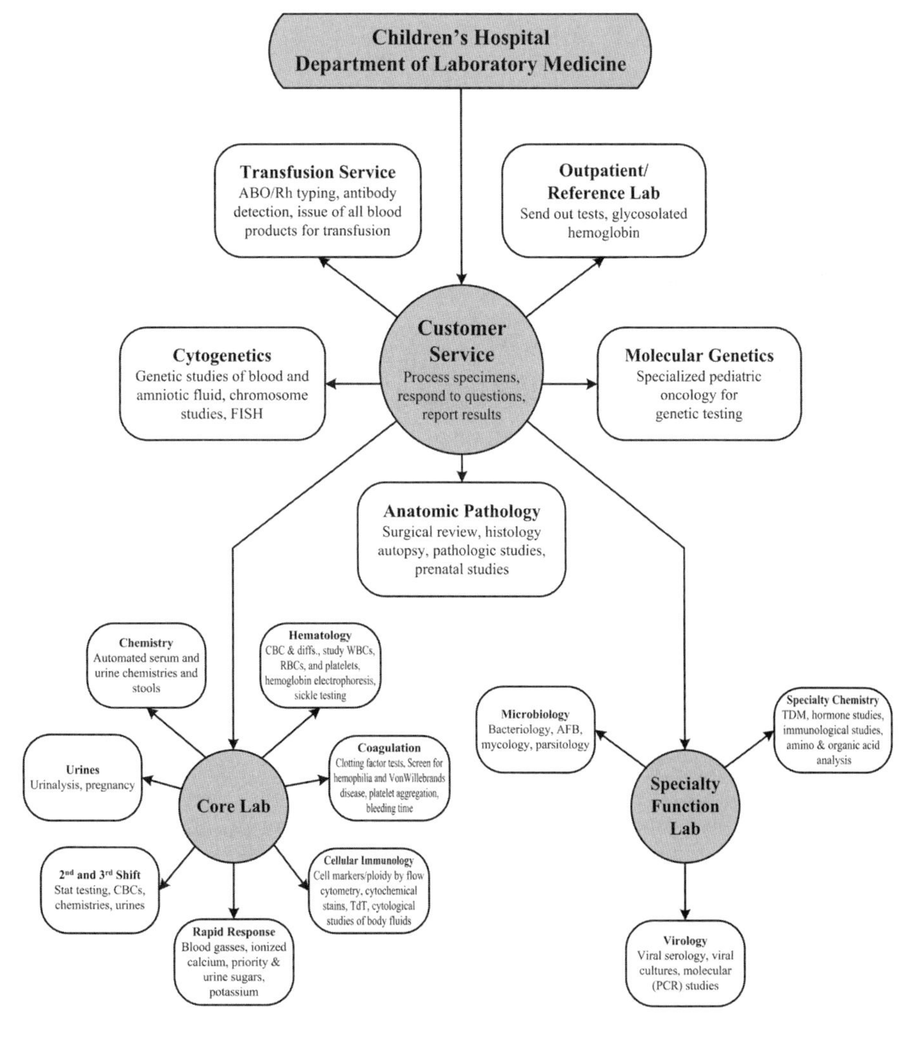

FIGURE 19-1 A flowchart of laboratory services in the Children's Hospital at Columbus, Ohio.

Test / Panels	Tests	Diseases
Microbiology	Cultures on Nutrient Media: · Bacteria · Virus · Fungi · Parasites Microscopic Examination Staining Chemical Reaction Profile Antibiotic Sensitivity	Infections: · Throat · Urinary · Blood · Skin · Intestine · STD
Immunology	Antigen-Antibody Reactions	HIV Hepatitis Chlamydia Gonorrhea
Histology	Study of tissues from surgical procedures and autopsies. · Specimen embedded in paraffin · Sliced on microtome · Fixed to slide · Stained · Sometimes frozen sections for emergencies	Evaluation of any tissue removed in surgery, for example cancer tissue.
Blood Bank	· Type and cross match · Screening for blood born pathogens in blood supply · Preparation of blood components	· Transfusion from blood loss · Blood components for blood disorders

FIGURE 19-2 A list of tests performed in the laboratory. (*continued*)

Test / Panels	Tests	Diseases
Chemistry		
Hepatic	Enzymes: ALT, AST, ALP, GGT, Bilirubin	Hepatitis, liver disease, alcoholism, cirrhosis
Renal (Kidney)	Creatinine, Urea (BUN)	Renal disease
Cardiac	LDH, CK-MB	Heart attack
Electrolytes	Sodium, potassium, chloride, CO_2	Heart attack
Lipids	Cholesterol, triglycerides, HDL, LDL	Arterial disease
Carbohydrate Metabolism	Glucose	Diabetes
Thyroid Panel	T4 (Thyroxin), T-Uptake, Free T4, Free T3, TSH (Thyroid Stimulating Hormone)	Diabetes
Hematology		
CBC (complete blood count)	Red blood cell count White blood cell count Platelet count Red blood cell indices Hemoglobin Hematocrit	Diabetes
Coagulation	Prothrombin Time (PT) Partial Thrombin Time (PTT)	Diseases of the clotting mechanism in the blood such as hemophilia, monitor anti-coagulation therapy such as Coumadin and heparin.

FIGURE 19-2 *(continued)*

19.1 CHEMISTRY LAB

The core laboratory in the Children's Hospital is where technicians perform routine chemistry analysis of fluids such as urine and blood for such elements as sodium, potassium, chloride, calcium, blood gas, and many others. This lab has one of the highest test volumes of any in the department. Every patient admitted to the hospital will have a basic panel of several tests ordered for evaluation of the patient condition. These panels, sometimes called profiles, are performed to determine a general state of the health of the patient. Examples of profiles include renal, hepatic, cardiac, and cardiovascular. Most of these profiles are incorporated into automated or semi-automated analyzers or equipment for the profile analysis. **Figure 19-3a** shows the chemistry

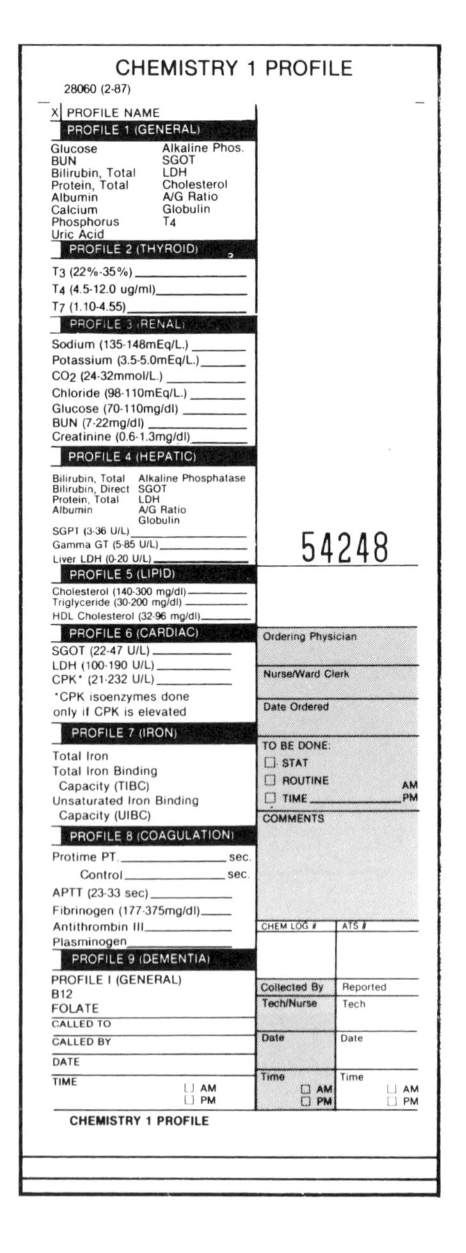

CHEMISTRY 1 PROFILE

28060 (2-87)

X PROFILE NAME

PROFILE 1 (GENERAL)

Glucose
BUN
Bilirubin, Total
Protein, Total
Albumin
Calcium
Phosphorus
Uric Acid
Alkaline Phos.
SGOT
LDH
Cholesterol
A/G Ratio
Globulin
T4

PROFILE 2 (THYROID)

T3 (22%-35%) ________
T4 (4.5-12.0 ug/ml) ________
T7 (1.10-4.55) ________

PROFILE 3 (RENAL)

Sodium (135-148mEq/L.) ________
Potassium (3.5-5.0mEq/L.) ________
CO2 (24-32mmol/L.) ________
Chloride (98-110mEq/L.) ________
Glucose (70-110mg/dl) ________
BUN (7-22mg/dl) ________
Creatinine (0.6-1.3mg/dl) ________

PROFILE 4 (HEPATIC)

Bilirubin, Total
Bilirubin, Direct
Protein, Total
Albumin
Alkaline Phosphatase
SGOT
LDH
A/G Ratio
Globulin
SGPT (3-36 U/L) ________
Gamma GT (5-85 U/L) ________
Liver LDH (0-20 U/L) ________

54248

PROFILE 5 (LIPID)

Cholesterol (140-300 mg/dl) ________
Triglyceride (30-200 mg/dl) ________
HDL Cholesterol (32-96 mg/dl) ________

PROFILE 6 (CARDIAC)

SGOT (22-47 U/L) ________
LDH (100-190 U/L) ________
CPK* (21-232 U/L) ________
*CPK isoenzymes done only if CPK is elevated

Ordering Physician

Nurse/Ward Clerk

Date Ordered

PROFILE 7 (IRON)

Total Iron
Total Iron Binding Capacity (TIBC)
Unsaturated Iron Binding Capacity (UIBC)

TO BE DONE:
☐ STAT
☐ ROUTINE
☐ TIME ________ AM PM

COMMENTS

PROFILE 8 (COAGULATION)

Protime PT ________ sec.
Control ________ sec.
APTT (23-33 sec) ________
Fibrinogen (177-375mg/dl) ________
Antithrombin III ________
Plasminogen ________

CHEM LOG # | ATS #

PROFILE 9 (DEMENTIA)

PROFILE I (GENERAL)
B12
FOLATE

CALLED TO

CALLED BY

DATE

TIME ☐ AM ☐ PM

Collected By Tech/Nurse	Reported Tech
Date	Date
Time ☐ AM ☐ PM	Time ☐ AM ☐ PM

CHEMISTRY 1 PROFILE

FIGURE 19-3a An example of a laboratory requisition form for chemistry profiles.

SUBSTANCE MEASURED	CONVENTIONAL UNITS	SI UNITS
Alanine aminotransferase (ALT)	3–30 U/L	
Albumin	3.8–5.0 g/dL	38–50 g/L
Alkaline phosphatase (AP)	20–130 U/L	
Aspartate aminotransferase (AST)	6–33 U/L	
Bicarbonate (HCO_3^-)	22–28 mEq/L	22–28 mmol/L
Bilirubin (Total)	0.1–1.2 mg/dL	2–21 μmol/L
BUN	8–18 mg/dL	2.9–6.4 mmol/L
Calcium	8.7–10.5 mg/dL	2.18–2.63 mmol/L
Chloride	98–108 mEq/L	98–108 mmol/L
Cholesterol	140–250 mg/dL (desirable level <200 mg/dL)	
Creatine kinase (CK)	30–170 U/L	
Creatinine	0.7–1.4 mg/dL	62–125μmol/L
Gamma glutamyl transferase (GGT)	3–40 U/L	
Glucose	70–110 mg/dL	3.9–6.2 mmol/L
Iron	65–165μg/dL	11.6–29.5μmol/L
Lactate dehydrogenase (LD)	125–290 U/L	
Phosphorus	3.0–4.5 mg/dL	0.96–1.44 mmol/L
Potassium	3.5–5.4 mEq/L	3.5–5.4 mmol/L
Sodium	135–148 mEq/L	135–148 mmol/L
T_3	60–160 ng/dL	0.92–2.46 nmol/L
T_4	5.5–12.5μg/dL	72–163 nmol/L
Total protein	6.0–8.0 g/dL	60–80 g/L
Triglycerides	10–190 mg/dL	0.11–2.15 mmol/L
Uric acid	3.5–7.5 mg/dL	0.21–0.44 mmol/L

FIGURE 19-3b A table of chemistry reference values.

lab requisition form, and the range of tests (reference values) usually performed in the chemistry lab of a hospital is shown in **Figure 19-3b**.

The following are common instruments found in most hospital core chemistry laboratories.

Centrifuges

A centrifuge is a piece of equipment, generally driven by a motor, that puts an object such as fluid in rotation around a fixed axis, applying a force perpendicular to the axis. Centrifuges separate cells and other components in body fluids, such as blood, by placing such force on the fluid. As the speed increases and the radial arm length increases, the centrifugal force increases. **Figure 19-4** shows a photo of a typical centrifuge machine. General purpose centrifuges usually operate at speeds up to 5,000 RPM. There are specialized types of centrifuge devices. Ultracentrifuges operate at much higher speeds and are for specific tests such as to measure molecular weights of solutes or to determine the sizes and shapes of solutes. Refrigerated centrifuges are commonly used to protect samples from the heat generated by the centrifugal force by maintaining approximate temperatures of −15° C to −25° C. A microhematocrit centrifuge is shown in **Figure 19-5.** A microhematocrit centrifuge per-

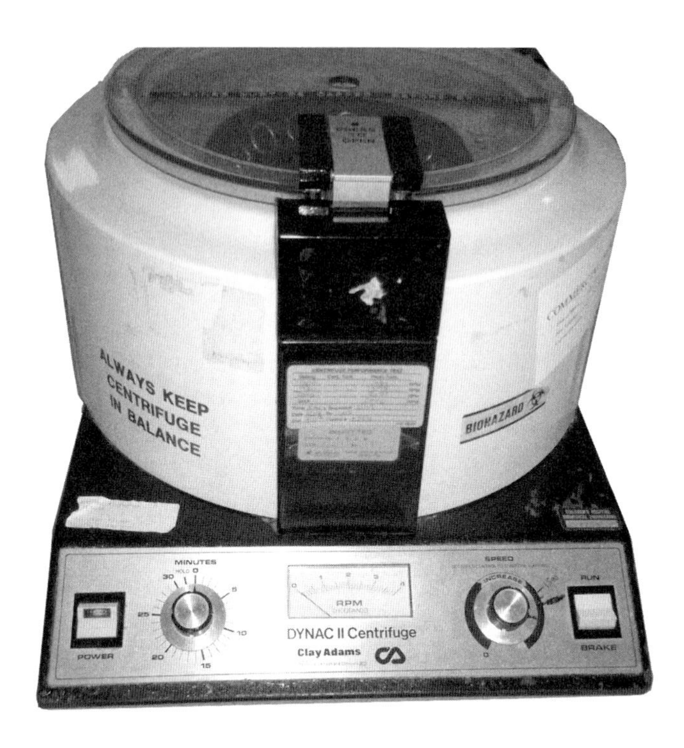

FIGURE 19-4 A photograph of a centrifuge.

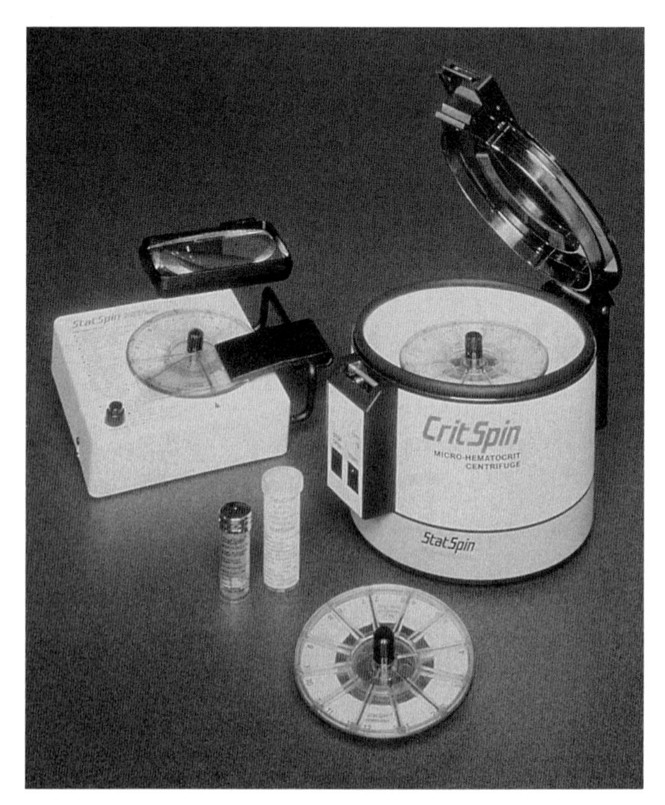

FIGURE 19-5 Microhematocrit centrifuge with built-in reader.

forms separation procedures for blood, fecal, and high-density sedimentation by high-speed centrifugation of blood contained in capillary tubes.

Water Baths

These units are usually filled with deionized water that is maintained at a temperature of 37° C. Most units have the capability of various temperatures and are equipped with an automatic thermostat. These devices are used for carrying out specific seriological or biochemical reactions.

Laboratory Refrigerators and Freezers

Refrigerators in laboratories are used to store reagents used in the analyzers as well as blood, blood products, and other biological samples. Automatic defrosting freezers should not be used if any of the reagents are temperature sensitive. There are some reagents and biological samples that must be kept at a much lower temperature in order to stop cellular growth. These freezers are designed to operate with temperatures ranging from –25° C to –80° C.

Microscopes

There are numerous types of microscopes found in a hospital's chemistry laboratory. They include single-user compound microscopes, 10-user compound microscopes, and fluorescence microscopes. The basic function of any microscope is to magnify an image and project that image for observation. **Figure 19-6** shows a photo of a common microscope and **Figure 19-7** shows details of the components found on most microscopes.

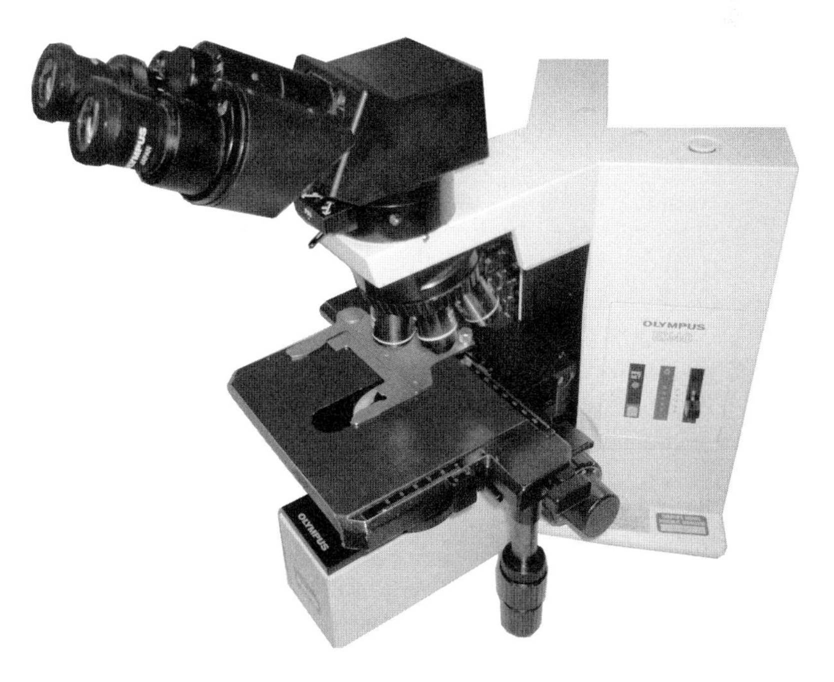

FIGURE 19-6 A photograph of a microscope.

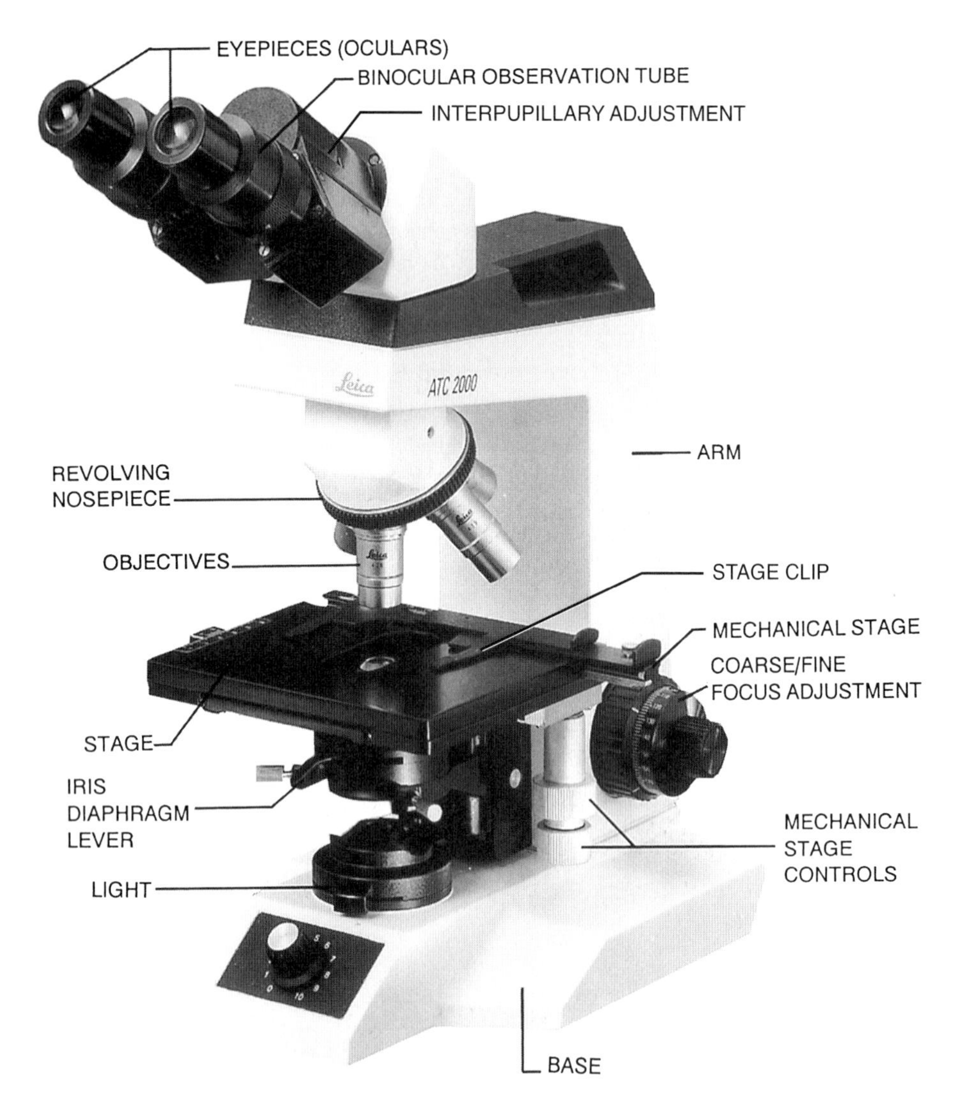

FIGURE 19-7 Components of a microscope.

Incubators

The incubators found in the laboratory are designed to promote the growth of microorganisms. The temperature-controlled incubator is designed to operate at a constant temperature of 37° C. In addition to temperature regulation, some incubators may also have the capability of using carbon dioxide (CO_2) to create a specific atmosphere. **Figure 19-8** shows a photo of an incubator.

Blood Gas Analyzer

A blood gas analyzer is used for the measurement of pH, pO_2, pCO_2, and for calculations of other parameters, such as total carbon dioxide (TCO_2).

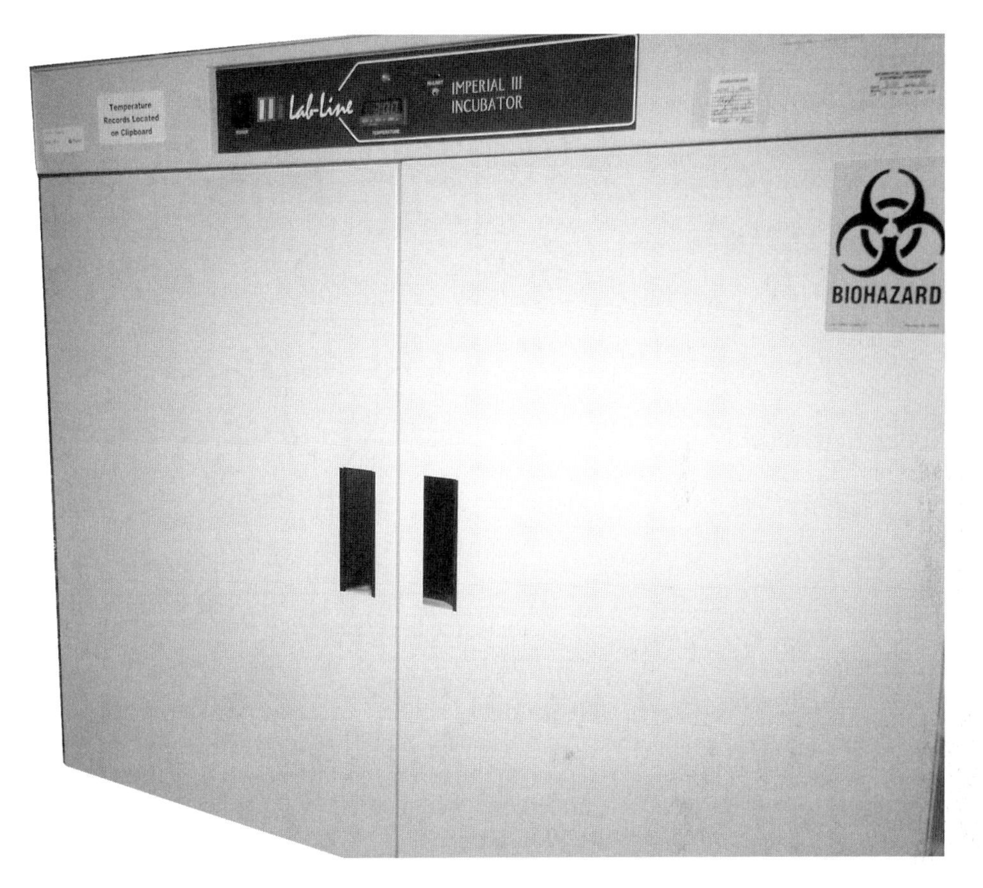

FIGURE 19-8 A photograph of an incubator.

pO_2 Electrode

The pO_2 electrode measurement system is based on the oxygen electrode, which was invented in 1959 by Leland Clark. This electrode measures the current produced by an electrolytic process that takes place because of the oxygen. This pO_2 electrode is made of a platinum cathode, a silver anode, a fill solution, and an oxygen permeable membrane. When the dissolved oxygen from the blood sample diffuses across the membrane into the electrolytic solution, it is reduced at the cathode due to the applied voltage. This circuit is completed at the anode when the silver is oxidized. The resulting current is proportional to the partial pressure of oxygen in the sample. The reactions are as follows:

$$\text{Cathode reaction: } O_2 + 2H_2O + 4e^- = 4(OH)^-$$
$$\text{Anode reaction: } 4Ag^+ + 4Cl^- = 4AgCl$$

The analysis of blood gas values is performed primarily by electrodes. These electrode devices can measure the changes in electrical current or voltage due to electrochemical reactions. **Figure 19-9a** shows the two electrodes in pO_2 measurement. The reference electrode is Ag/AgCl and the electrode is made of platinum (Pt).

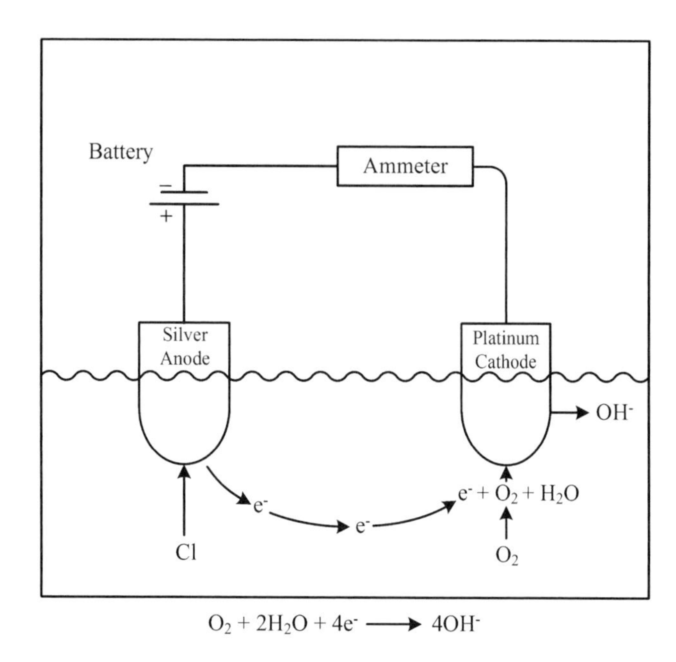

$O_2 + 2H_2O + 4e^- \longrightarrow 4OH^-$

FIGURE 19-9a Electrodes in a blood gas analyzer.

The graph in **Figure 19-9b** shows that the amount of electrical current in the circuit is directly proportional to the amount of dissolved oxygen (that is, the pO_2) at the cathode.

This direct relationship between current and pO_2 is based on how much voltage is applied initially to the cathode. It is important to find a small range of battery voltage when the current and the pO_2 are constant.

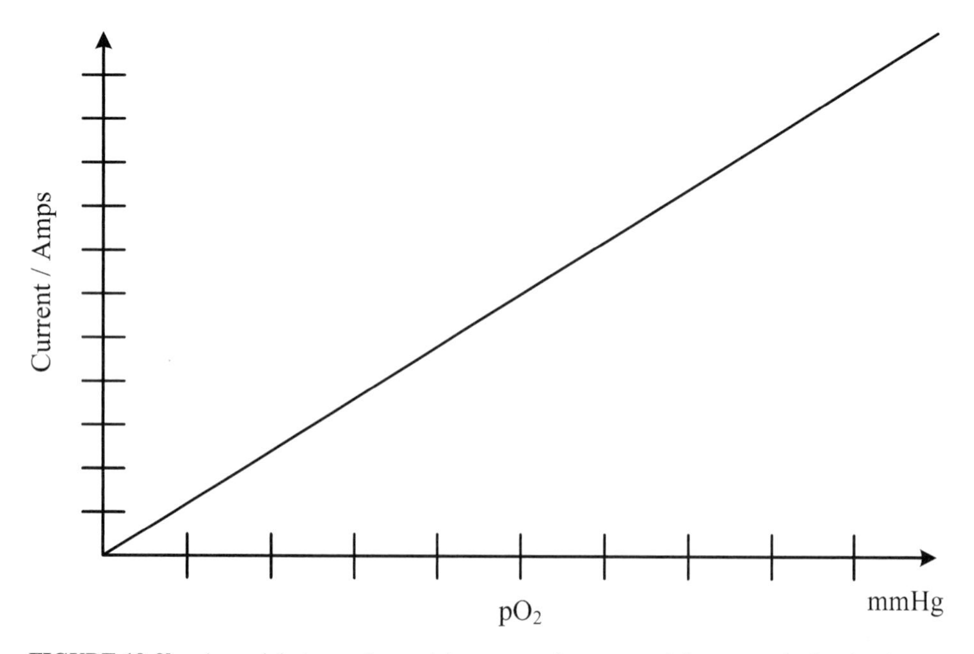

FIGURE 19-9b A graph between the partial pressure of oxygen and the current in the circuit.

A Clark electrode is used to measure blood pO_2 because protein from the blood deposits on the cathode and changes the linear relationship between the current and pO_2. The blood is separated from the electrode terminal by the use of a membrane such as polypropylene, Mylar, or Teflon secured on the electrode by a ring. Oxygen diffuses through the membrane into the electrolyte solution to react with water.

pH Electrode

The acid-base characteristic of blood is described by pH, which is a function of the hydrogen ion activity where:

pH= −log 10 [H+] where [H+] is the molar concentration of hydrogen ions.

In most blood gas analyzers, the pH measurement system consists of a measuring electrode capable of detecting hydrogen ions, and also includes a reference electrode. The pH electrode measures the changes in voltage rather than changes in current, as in the case of the pO_2 electrode. As shown in **Figure 19-9c,** pH electrodes require four electrode terminals. A reference solution of known pH is placed on one side of a glass electrode terminal. Now, the reference voltage is across the Ag/AgC1 and glass electrodes. The other set of electrodes is then between the Hg/HgC1 and glass electrodes. The fluid, in this case the blood, with an unknown pH is around the Hg/HgC1 electrode. The glass electrode allows hydrogen ions to diffuse into it and more hydrogen ions can diffuse from the fluid with high hydrogen ion concentration. The voltages will differ on both sides of the fluids and the pH difference between known and unknown fluids can be determined by the Nernst equation.

The amplifier input resistance is very high and does not allow significant flow of current, but will be able to detect small voltage differences.

The pH electrode itself is a glass electrode that develops a potential difference when the pH of the sample differs from the pH of the electrode fill solution. This potential difference

FIGURE 19-9c pH electrodes.

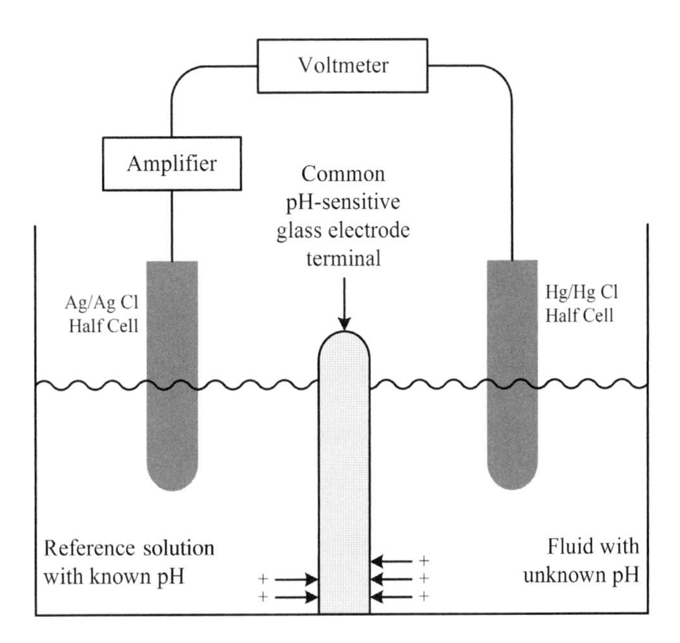

between the two electrodes varies with the hydrogen ion activity in the sample and is measured and converted by the analyzer into pH units.

pCO_2 Electrode

Carbon dioxide is a natural product of the metabolism of cells. Disturbances in the partial pressure of carbon dioxide in the blood normally indicates disorders in the acid/base balance and could indicate difficulties with respiratory exchange of carbon dioxide in the lungs.

In blood gas analyzers the pCO_2 measurement system is based on the electrode described by John W. Severinghaus, the inventor of first blood gas analysis system.

In **Figure 19-9d**, the circuit to measure blood pCO_2 is shown. It is different than the pH electrode in the sense that blood is not allowed to contact the glass electrode, though the blood does contact the CO_2-permeable Teflon membrane. On the other side of the membrane, a bicarbonate solution is placed in direct contact with the glass electrode.

Both electrodes are Ag/AgC1 electrodes; one is immersed into a known pH solution, and the other is immersed into the bicarbonate solution. As blood CO_2 diffuses into the bicarbonate solution, a hydrolysis reaction occurs. As the hydrogen ions diffuse into the glass electrode, the pH of the bicarbonate solution changes. This change is proportional to the pCO_2 and is detected as a voltage. The corresponding pH values of known and unknown fluids develop into voltages, and the voltage difference is amplified and displayed on the voltmeter.

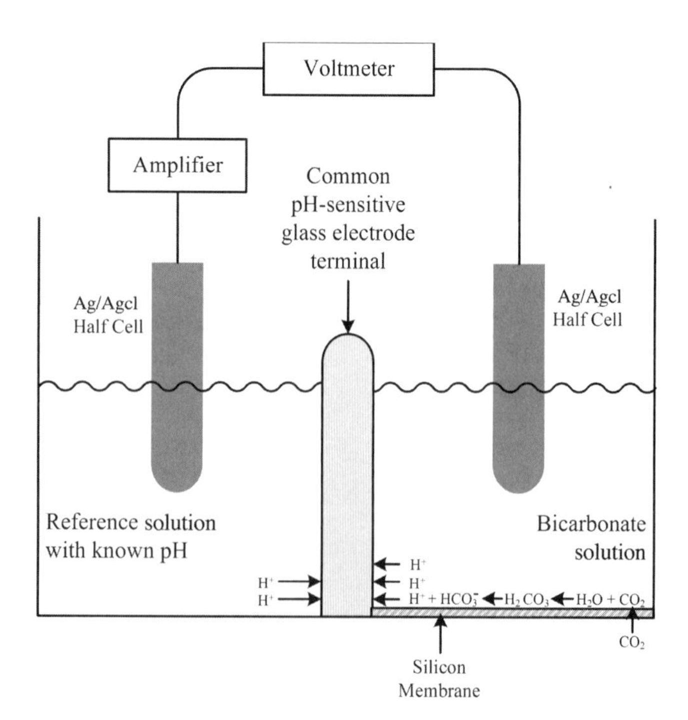

FIGURE 19-9d A circuit to measure pCO_2.

Spectrophotometer

Figure 19-10 shows the diagram of the internal parts of a spectrophotometer. The instrument measures intensities of light in different parts of the light spectrum. A narrow beam of light passes through a colored solution contained in a glass or plastic tube. The tube is called a cuvette. A portion of light is either absorbed by the colored solution or passes through it. The absorbance and transmittance are inversely proportional (that is, the greater the absorbance, the less is transmittance or less the absorbance, more the transmittance).

In **Figure 19-10,** the white light has a wide spectrum (various frequencies, or wavelengths) and the narrow slit isolates one frequency at a time. The monochromatic (one wavelength) light then passes through the colored solution and is detected at the photodetector generating an electrical signal. The signal is displayed as a unit of absorbance or transmittance.

The spectrophotometer is an important chemistry instrument in a hospital or clinic. The amount of light transmitted or absorbed through a specimen (when illuminated by a controlled light source) indicates the characteristic of the specimen itself. The photometer measures the intensity of radiation as a function of frequency or wavelength of the radiation. Several types of drugs are analyzed in the chemistry lab using spectrophotometry.

Urinanalysis

The Iris workstation performs sediment microscopy, urine chemistry, and specific gravity. It is considered the finest urinalysis system used in hospitals. A block diagram of the system is shown in **Figure 19-11.**

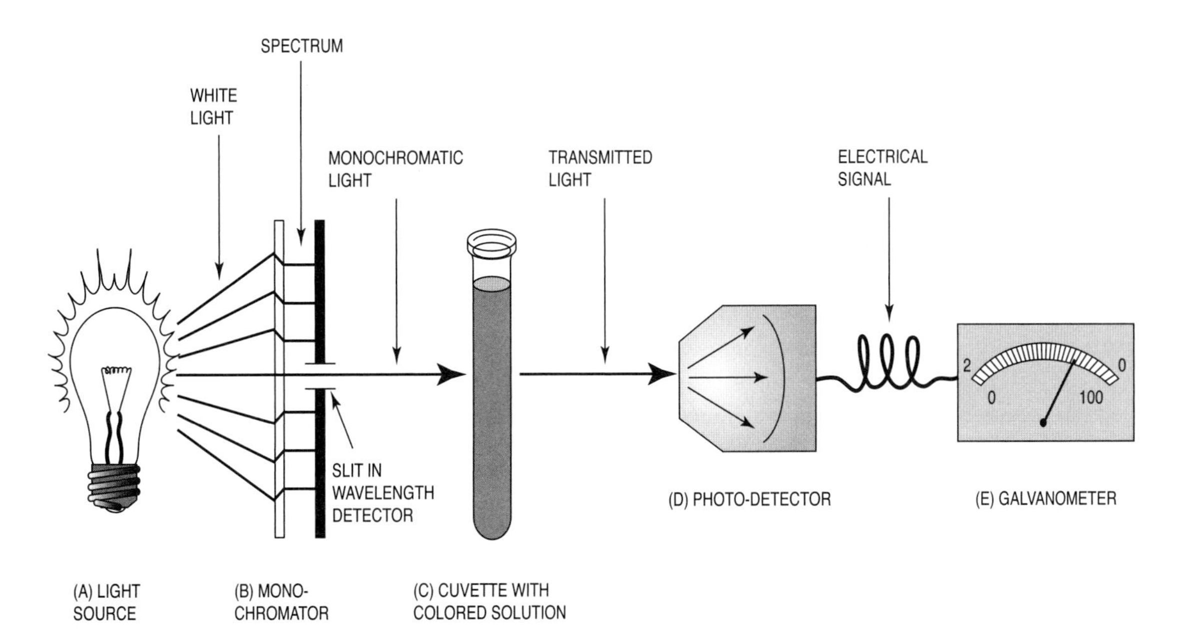

FIGURE 19-10 Internal parts of a spectrophotometer.

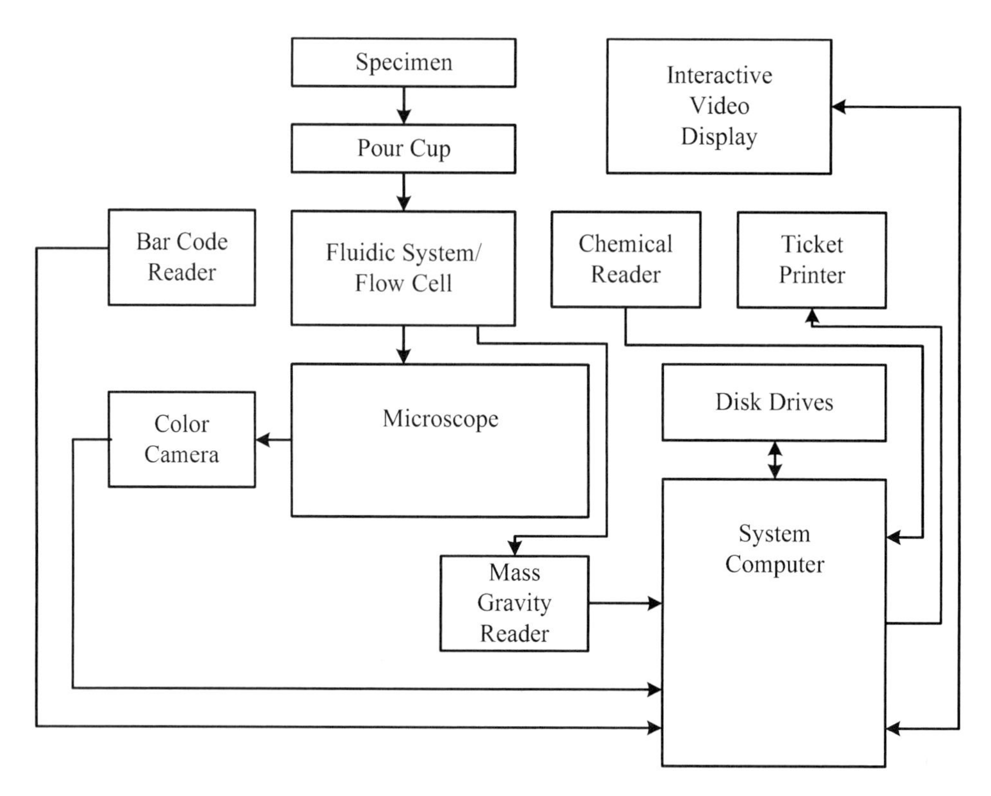

FIGURE 19-11 A block diagram of a urine analysis system.

After pouring the urine sample in the pour cup, the sample is delivered to the fluidics system where it is mixed automatically with stain and then delivered to the slideless microscope. The analytes (chemical constituents) are oriented and imaged by the video color camera. The operator examines the sorted analytes on the interactive video display.

The flow cell is a flow chamber that hydrodynamically focuses particles within the sample for the maximum exposure to the microscope. The stained sample and sheath fluid enter the flow cell simultaneously. The sheath aids in the hydrodynamic focusing of the sample. This sample is illuminated with a strobe lamp and the video camera views it.

Two milliliters of unfiltered specimen is also sent to the mass gravity meter for specific gravity determination. The meter measures the relative density of uncentrifuged urine. When the sample enters a U-shaped borosilicate glass tube wrapped with an electromagnetic coil, the harmonic oscillations (i.e., vibrations) are measured. Any shift in harmonic oscillations is used to calculate the relative density of the solution.

19.2 HEMATOLOGY LAB

The hematology lab in a hospital performs analysis on blood samples including coagulation time and associated deficiencies as well as hemoglobin analysis. A hematology laboratory requisition form for a blood test is shown in **Figure 19-12.** This testing includes the analysis of the concentration, structure, and function of the cells in the blood. This laboratory assists

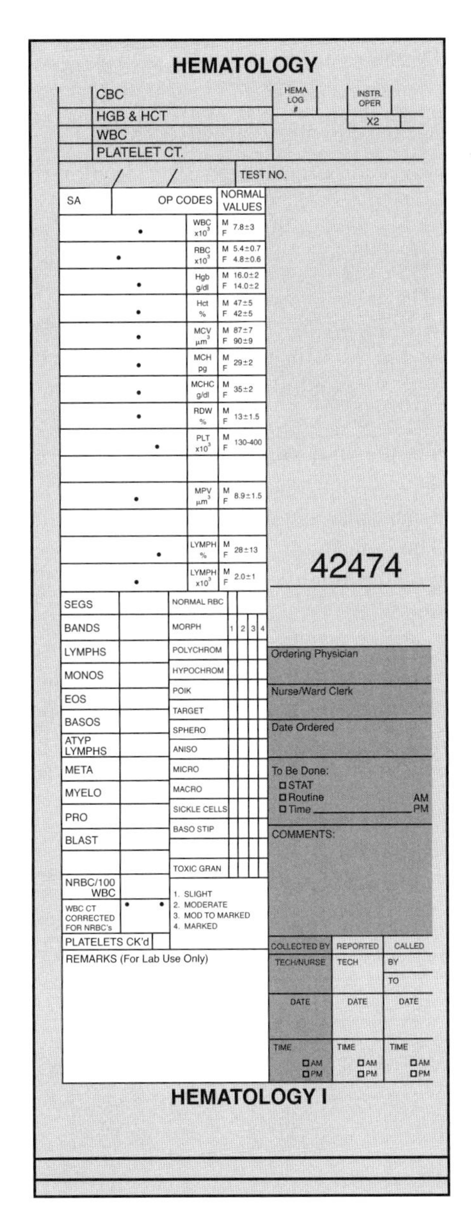

HEMATOLOGY

CBC
HGB & HCT
WBC
PLATELET CT.

HEMA LOG #
INSTR. OPER
X2

/ /
TEST NO.

SA	OP CODES		NORMAL VALUES
	•	WBC x10³	M F 7.8±3
	•	RBC x10³	M 5.4±0.7 F 4.8±0.6
	•	Hgb g/dl	M 16.0±2 F 14.0±2
	•	Hct %	M 47±5 F 42±5
	•	MCV µm³	M 87±7 F 90±9
	•	MCH pg	M F 29±2
	•	MCHC g/dl	M F 35±2
	•	RDW %	M F 13±1.5
	•	PLT x10³	M F 130-400
	•	MPV µm³	M F 8.9±1.5
	•	LYMPH %	M F 28±13
	•	LYMPH x10³	M F 2.0±1

42474

			1	2	3	4
SEGS		NORMAL RBC				
BANDS		MORPH	1	2	3	4
LYMPHS		POLYCHROM				
MONOS		HYPOCHROM				
EOS		POIK				
BASOS		TARGET				
		SPHERO				
ATYP LYMPHS		ANISO				
META		MICRO				
MYELO		MACRO				
PRO		SICKLE CELLS				
BLAST		BASO STIP				
		TOXIC GRAN				
NRBC/100 WBC						
WBC CT CORRECTED FOR NRBC's	• •					
PLATELETS CK'd						

1. SLIGHT
2. MODERATE
3. MOD TO MARKED
4. MARKED

Ordering Physician
Nurse/Ward Clerk
Date Ordered
To Be Done:
□ STAT
□ Routine
□ Time ________ AM PM
COMMENTS:

REMARKS (For Lab Use Only)

COLLECTED BY	REPORTED	CALLED
TECH/NURSE	TECH	BY
		TO
DATE	DATE	DATE
TIME □AM □PM	TIME □AM □PM	TIME □AM □PM

HEMATOLOGY I

FIGURE 19-12 Laboratory requisition form for CBC.

the physician in the diagnosis of diseases of the blood including leukemia, anemia, and many other blood disorders. The most common test performed is a complete blood count (CBC) and is usually performed on an automated system. There are numerous blood parameters of a CBC that are measured by various types of analyzers. They are as follows:

- White blood cell count (WBC)
- Red blood cell count (RBC)
- Hemoglobin concentration (Hgb)

- Hematocrit (Hct)
- Platelet count (PLT)
- Mean cell volume of RBCs (MCV)
- Mean corpuscular Hgb concentration (MCHC)

In the hematology lab, some of the more common cell counters are Bayer Advia, Beckman-Coulter Counters (various models), Abbot Celldyn, SYSMEX, and Beckman counters.

A cell counter is shown in **Figure 19-13.** The automated cell counting instruments are used in the hematology laboratory to count red blood cells, white blood cells, and the platelets. White blood cells (WBC) play an important role in the body's immune response system, whereas red blood cells (RBC), containing hemoglobin, carry oxygen from the lungs to the body cells and tissues. A decrease in hemoglobin will cause anemia, and the patient will show symptoms such as fatigue and shortness of breath. A decrease in platelet count can cause several bleeding disorders.

The hemacytometer, a part of the modern automated cell counter, counts the cells based on the dilution of the blood sample, the depth and area of the counting chamber, and the properties of the diluting fluid. Hematocrit (the packed cell volume), mean corpuscles hemoglobin (MCH), and mean corpuscular hemoglobin concentration (MCHC) are determined from the measured data of cell counts.

An enlarged view of the counting chamber is shown in **Figure 19-14.** "W" denotes the WBC counting area and "R" in the middle denotes the RBC counting area. For counting white blood cells, each corner square is a 1 mm^2 area and there are 16 small squares.

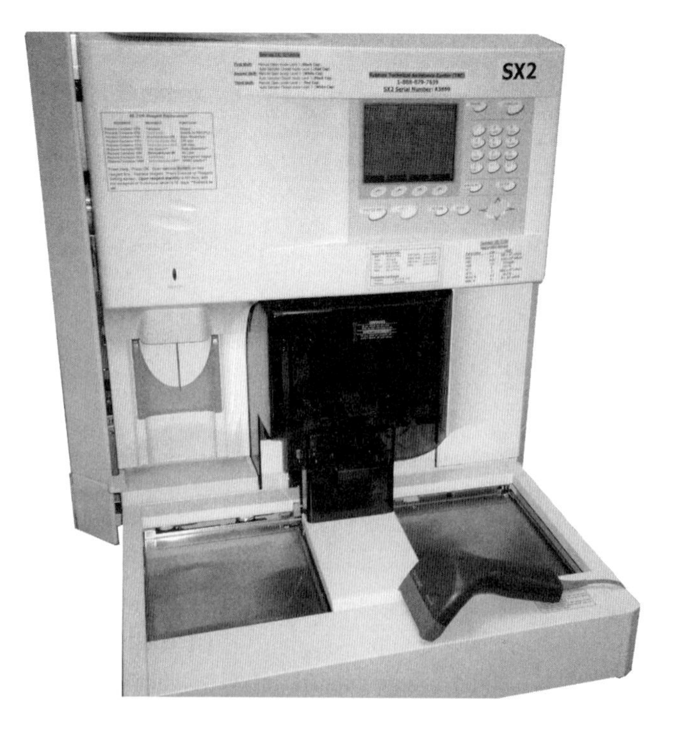

FIGURE 19-13 A photograph of a cell counter.

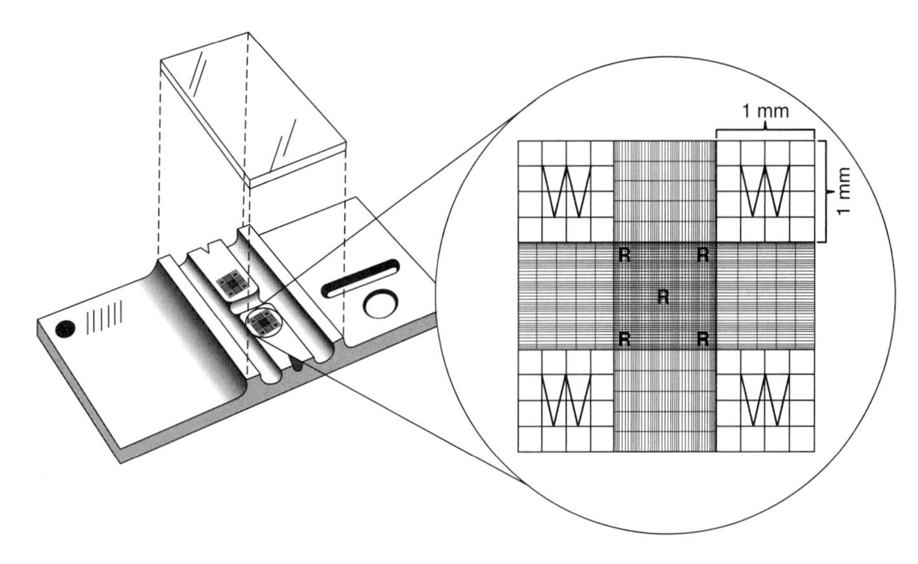

FIGURE 19-14 The hemacytometer.

However, for red blood cell count, the center is divided into 25 smaller squares with an area of 1/25 mm^2. This equals 0.04 mm^2 area.

In general, the total count of either WBC or RBC is given as:

$$\text{Total count (cells/mm}^3) = \frac{(\text{Number of cells counted}) \times (\text{Dilution factor})}{(\text{Area counted mm}^2) \times (\text{Depth 0.1 mm})}$$

The routine ranges of the counts are as follows:

White Blood Cells. . . . . (4 to 11) $\times 10^9$ cells/L

Red Blood Cells . . . . (3.6 to 6) $\times 10^{12}$ cells/L

Platelets. . . . . (50 to 400) $\times 10^9$ cells/L

Hemoglobin . . . . 120 to 180 gm/L

Hematocrit . . . . 0.36 to 0.54 L/L

The three RBC indices are MCH, MCV (mean corpuscular volume), and MCHC. The formulas are as follows:

$$\text{MCH} = \text{Weight of the hemoglobin in the average RBC}$$

$$\text{MCH (picogram, pg)} = \frac{\text{Hemoglobin in g/dL} \times 10}{\text{RBC (cells/L)}}$$

$$\text{MCV} = \text{Average volume of the red blood cell}$$

$$\text{MCV (femtoliter, fL)} = \frac{\text{Hematocrit(L/L)} \times 10^3}{\text{RBC (cells/L)}}$$

$$\text{MCHC} = \text{Average concentration of hemoglobin in a red blood cell.}$$

$$\text{MCHC} = \frac{\text{MCH}}{\text{MCV}} \times 100\%$$

Coagulation Analyzers

When determining coagulation, most automated systems are based on one of three principles: conductivity change as a clot forms, a change in optical density as a clot forms, or a change in viscosity as a clot forms. These tests are commonly known as prothrombin time (PT) and partial thromboplastin time (PTT). These coagulation tests are used to detect blood clotting diseases and also monitor those patients who are on blood thinning medications. Some of the more common coagulation systems are Beckman ACL, Coag-a-Mate, and Diagnostica Stago.

Another example is the Hemochron Whole Blood Coagulation System, which is based on the blood clot detection mechanism. A test tube contains the blood and a precision magnet and is placed into a test well. The magnetic detector is part of the test well. When there is no clot, the detector can detect the magnet, but when a clot begins to form, the magnet is displaced and the detector is no longer able to sense the magnet. The instrument gives a beeping sound and also provides the coagulation time. With this instrument, coagulation testing can be done at bedside; it is also portable. It can provide test results within minutes.

There are special coagulation test tubes and various tests can be performed, such as a whole blood activated clotting time test (ACT), thrombin time test (TT), and heparin response test (HRT).

19.3 BLOOD BANK

The blood bank of a hospital is also referred to as transfusion services. This part of the laboratory medicine department procures, processes, and distributes all blood products that may be given to a patient. Transfusion services is responsible for the type and cross-match of blood to ensure that the donor blood is compatible with the blood of the recipient. They also test for HIV, hematocrit, and several other diseases prior to any transfusion. Some of the more common items of equipment found in this area include centrifuges, cell washers, and blood warmers.

19.4 MICROBIOLOGY LAB

The microbiology lab in a hospital performs numerous tests to diagnose infectious diseases. A small list of microbiology instruments is shown in **Figure 19-15.** All types of bacterial cultures including urine, stool, respiratory, and samples from almost any site in or on the body are performed in the microbiology lab. These samples are then cultured or grown and tested to determine which microbe is causing the infection. These microbes are also tested to determine their sensitivity in order to prescribe the best treatment for the patient. The most common biomedical devices used in this area are incubators, sterilizers, and microscopes. There are also automated systems available for some tests, such as Microscan, Merieux, Vitek, and Phoenix.

The Merieux microbiology instrument is shown in **Figure 19-16.**

Microbiology Instruments

BD Phoenix Automated Microbiology System identifies more than 300 clinically relevant bacteria, assesses the pathogens' resistance and susceptibility to antibiotic treatments.

Veridex CellSearch identifies and counts circulating tumor cells in a blood sample.

Microbeam Walkway of **Dade Behrinh** features automated reagent dispensing, identification of evolving pathogens and windows-based software.

FIGURE 19-15 A list of microbiology instruments.

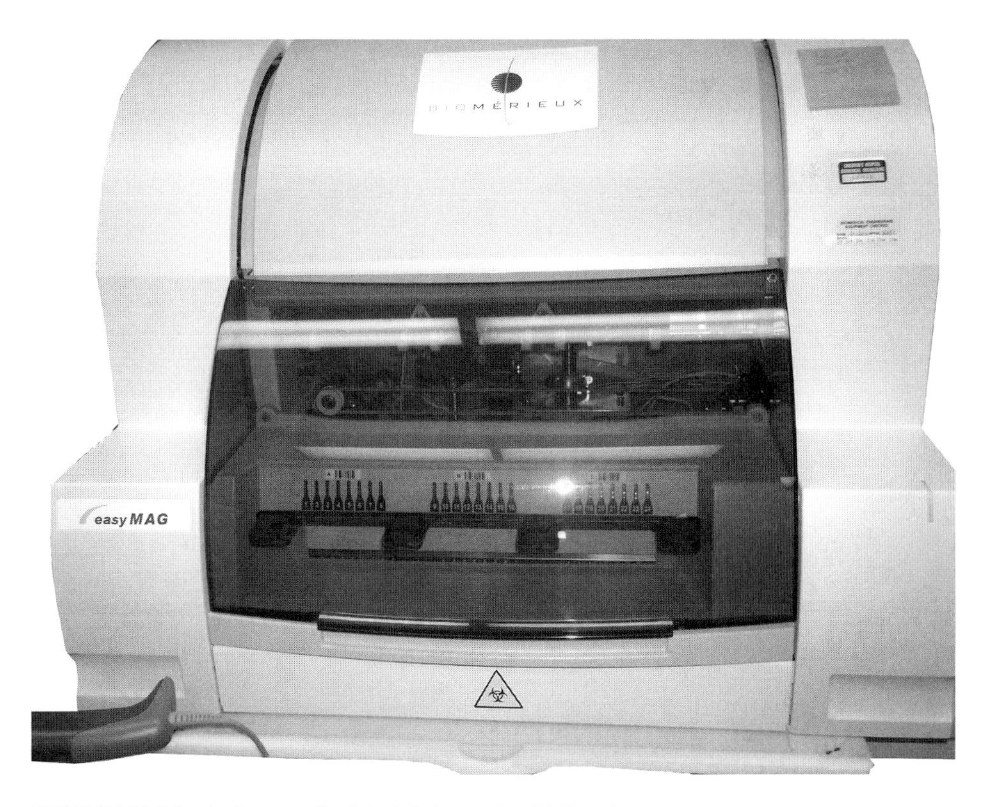

FIGURE 19-16 A photograph of the Merieux microbiology instrument.

19.5 VIROLOGY LAB

The virology diagnostic lab of the department of laboratory medicine in a hospital tests for viral isolation and identification, detection of viral antigens and determination of viral antibody status. Some of the tests performed here include hepatitis, herpes, HIV, Lyme disease, and mumps. The essential equipment in a virology lab are: incubators, electron microscopes, filtration apparatus, centrifuges, water baths, pH meters, autoclaves, and biosafety cabinets.

19.6 SPECIALTY CHEMISTRY LAB

The specialty chemistry laboratory in a hospital often has several distinct testing labs within it. These may include therapeutic drug monitoring (TDM), immunology, and an endocrine area. This laboratory performs testing for quantitative levels of most therapeutic drugs as well as screening for abused drugs. This lab also performs amino acid analysis and provides interpretation of the results for use in the diagnosis and treatment in errors of metabolism and the patient's immune system.

19.7 HISTOLOGY LAB

The histology lab (histology is sometimes referred to as anatomic pathology) prepares tissue and bone samples used for diagnosing many diseases, including cancer. Samples from autopsies are also processed in this laboratory area. The process of preparing the samples requires following several steps. Tissues are first embedded in paraffin, then these paraffin blocks are sliced into very thin slices using a biomedical instrument called a microtome. These slices are then put on a microscope slide and processed through a slide staining system. Once processed, these stained slides are given to a pathologist for examination for any abnormalities.

Microtomes

This is a biomedical machine used for cutting extremely thin slices of tissue or other samples. The most common type is the rotary microtome which is used for cutting paraffin-embedded sections. A cryostat is a specially designed microtome contained in a refrigerated chest and is used to cut frozen sections of samples. After the specimens are obtained they can be processed either by staining or by use of a tissue processor.

Each of these laboratories is dependent on the equipment they use to perform the analysis requested by the physician. Rapid reporting of test results can be instrumental in the treatment of the patient. Should one of the primary instruments fail, many times an older back-up unit must be returned to service. This can be very time consuming and often delays the reporting of test results.

19.8 PERSONNEL

Lab Administrator

The Lab Administrator handles the business portions of the laboratory. Lab administrators are responsible for interfacing with the hospital administration, and, because of their fiscal responsibility, are usually involved in the acquisition process for new laboratory equipment.

Lab Director

The Lab Director is usually an M.D. or Ph.D. and board certified. Many of these directors are specialists in the clinical laboratory including examination of tissues from autopsies or may specialize in the tests performed by the laboratory for the treatment of disease.

Lab Manager

The Lab Manager is responsible for all of the normal operations, including the overall supervision of all operations, and may be involved in personnel performance reviews. Lab managers are responsible for the financial budget in their area of responsibility and are usually involved in the acquisition of new equipment.

Lab Supervisor

The Lab Supervisor is responsible for the daily operation of the lab including scheduling of personnel and will usually perform some routine tests and assist others in the department. The Lab Supervisor is normally the first contact for a manufacturer's sales representatives.

Technologist

The technologists in the laboratory usually have a bachelor's degree or associate degree in medical technology. They are either clinical lab technicians or have the title of Medical Laboratory Technician (MLT). These personnel perform all specialized tests and often assist others in performing routine tests. They may be responsible for training other lab personnel and newly hired personnel. If there is a problem with a piece of equipment or even with a specimen, they may be responsible for troubleshooting and resolving these problems. These technologists are often involved in the equipment evaluation process prior to purchase.

Phlebotomist

A Phlebotomist is a technician who draws the patient's blood and ensures that the samples are submitted to the laboratory for proper testing.

SUMMARY

The clinical laboratory in a hospital has several pieces of specialized equipment and this chapter helps BMETs to gain the perspective and engineering principles of this equipment.

1. The chapter divides the role of a clinical laboratory into several areas such as chemistry lab, hematology, microbiology, virology, and histology. The laboratory personnel examine and analyze body fluids and cells. They look for microorganisms and abnormal cells in blood and body fluids, prepare specimens for examination, count cells, and work with sophisticated equipment.

2. The chapter also includes the blood bank, special chemistry, and the personnel of the clinical laboratory.
3. The main equipment discussed in the chapter are blood cell counter, centrifuge, microscope, coagulation monitor, blood gas analyzer, urine analyzer, and spectrophotometer.

MEDICAL TERMINOLOGY

The following is a list of medical terms mentioned in this chapter.

Blood gas analyzer: device to provide chemical analysis of the blood to measure the concentration of oxygen and carbon dioxide.

Blood gas electrodes: conductor through which a current enters or leaves a medium, as in a gaseous discharge tube.

Cell counter: electronic device used to count cells, especially of blood or other body fluids, in a standard volume.

Coagulation: process of transforming liquid into a solid, especially with blood clotting.

Cytogenetics: study of cells in relation to genetics and the structure of chromosome material.

Hematology: study of blood and blood-forming tissues, including etiology, diagnosis, treatment, prognosis, and prevention of blood diseases.

Histology: study of tissue sectioned microscopically for structural analysis of the tissue.

Immunological studies: study looking at the immune reaction to a particular antigen (protein). A study does not look at the invading organism but the reaction of the immune system to the organism and associated antibodies.

Incubator: enclosed apparatus in which conditions such as temperature, humidity, and protection are provided. Primarily used for premature babies or cultivating bacteria.

Microscope: optical instrument having a magnifying lens or combination of lenses used for viewing objects that are too small to be observed by the naked eye.

Parasites: organisms that grow, feed, and live within, upon, or at the expense of another organism (host) while contributing nothing to the survival of its host.

Serology: study of blood serum to detect evidence of infection or disease by evaluating antigen antibody reactions.

Specimens: representative of a class, genus, or whole, as in a sample such as tissue, blood, or urine used for analysis and diagnosis.

Staining: process of using a dye, reagent, or other substance to produce contrasting color in tissues or microorganisms for examination.

Transfusion: process of transferring blood or blood-based products into the blood stream.

Virology: study of viruses in relation to their structure and classification, ways to infect and exploit cells, reproduction, and techniques to isolate and culture them for research and therapy purposes.

QUIZ

1. Histology is the study of ________________.
   a) Viruses
   b) Parasites
   c) Tissues
   d) None of the above
2. A decrease in hemoglobin count can make a patient ________________.
3. A cell counter:
   a) Separates the cells
   b) Counts the platelets
   c) Counts red blood cells
   d) Transfers the cells
4. Centrifuges are used in hospital labs for:
   a) Separating suspended solids from liquid
   b) Growing microorganisms
   c) Transforming liquid into a solid
   d) None of the above
5. pH is a molar concentration of ________________ atoms.
6. A solution with a pH of 8.5 is ________________.
   a) Acidic
   b) Alkaline
7. Virology is a study of ________________.
   a) Cells
   b) Parasites
   c) Tissues
   d) None of the above
8. The unit of mean cell volume (MCV) is ____________________________.
9. Microtomes are used for:
   a) Counting platelets
   b) Detecting microorganisms
   c) Slicing tissues
   d) None of the above
10. Spectrophotometer is an instrument to study the ________________________.
    a) Frequency of a signal
    b) Intensity of light through a sample
    c) pH of a sample
    d) None of the above

PROBLEMS

1. Calculate RBC indices (that is, MCV, MCH, and MCHC) when given:

   RBC count = 5×10^{12}/L, Hemoglobin = 15 g/dL, and Hematocrit = 40%.

2. WBC count is 3,000 WBC/mm^3. Determine the following: cells/μL, cells/mL, and cells/L.
3. Describe five types of equipment that may be found in a clinical laboratory.
4. Using the Internet for your research, discuss a glucose-monitoring system used in a hospital. Emphasize the sensor and the electronics in the discussion.
5. Describe a colorimetric method of determining chemical concentration.
6. The pH of a solution is 7.3 at 25° C. Calculate pH of the solution at 35° C.
7. A buffer solution has a pH value of 5.1. A pH electrode and a reference electrode are immersed in the buffer solution and the attached voltmeter reads 0.22 V. When the buffer solution is replaced by an unknown solution, the voltmeter now reads 0.41 V. Calculate the pH of the unknown solution.
8. Design an electronic circuit to measure blood cell count. The transducer whose one lead is immersed in the blood sample and the other lead is immersed in the container having a small orifice through which the sample is drawn by a vacuum. The transducer is connected to a Wheatstone bridge, and its resistance changes whenever a white blood cell or a red blood cell or a platelet is drawn into the container through the orifice. You may use a differential amplifier, a timer with start and stop, and a counter to compute the total number of cells.
9. For the scenario of the previous problem, the resistance of the transducer is 0.6 kΩ when there is no blood sample drawn into the container. When a red blood cell is drawn into the container, the transducer resistance changes to 0.8 kΩ. What is the output voltage of the Wheatstone bridge when the D.C. source voltage of the bridge is 10 V.
10. A blood gas analyzer measures the RBC count in the blood sample to be $2 = 10^{10}$ per liter. The mean cell volume is 100 femtoliters. Calculate, in other words, the percentage of the blood volume made up of RBCs.

RESEARCH TOPICS

1. Medical laboratory statistics are not only important for physicians but important for lab technicians as well. Statistics are essential in quality control in lab tests. Your research topic should provide the essential laboratory mathematics (including statistics) needed in data collection and analysis. The research paper should discuss inferential statistics, explaining proper predictions. Important formulas may be included.
2. What are the safety requirements for the laboratory centrifuges? Discuss safety features used in new types of centrifuges and also emphasize the maintenance procedures of these devices.

CASE STUDIES

1. A 60-year-old female was admitted to the emergency room. She was dizzy, complaining of a headache and fatigue. She did not complain of chest discomfort and her blood pressure was slightly elevated. A blood test revealed: Hgb = 6 g/dL, Hct 15%, and sodium = 27. With these values, what could be the diagnosis?

a) Is the patient anemic?

b) What is the normal range of sodium? What does low sodium indicate?

c) What is Hct?

d) What is done to stabilize the patient's condition?

2. An infant needed a solution containing a small amount of potassium chloride. The nurse noticed the dose that was to be administered was four times stronger than necessary and corrected the mistake. This case study requires the individual performing the study to consider the following questions:

a) What would have happened if the overdose of potassium chloride was given to the infant?

b) How did the pharmacist arrive at the point of dispensing this overdose?

c) In similar situations to this error, are there dangerous lab errors where wrong information could be provided about, for example, a patient's blood tests?

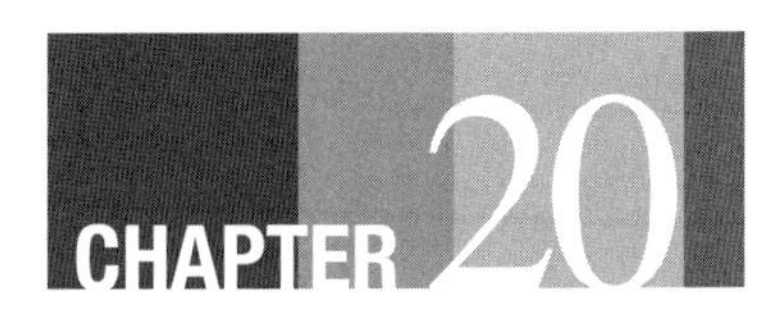

Medical Safety

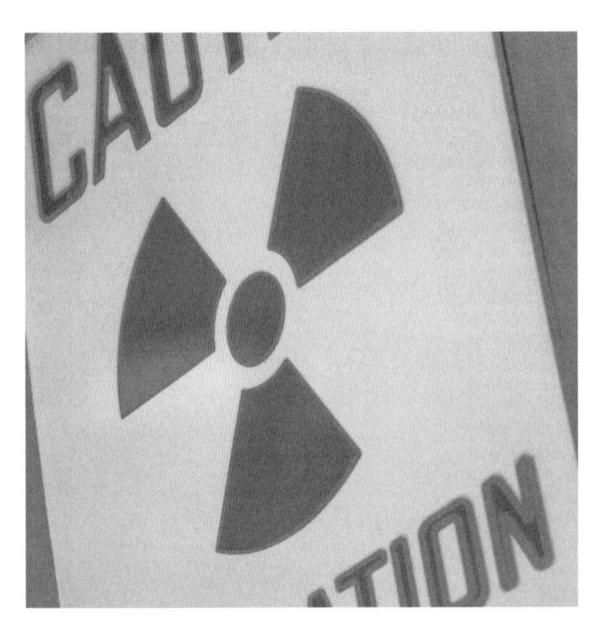

■ CHAPTER OUTLINE

■ OBJECTIVE

The objective of this chapter is to describe to the reader the basics of all types of safety issues in a hospital that every BMET should know and follow.

Upon completion of this chapter, the reader will be able to:

- Identify various types of safety issues.
- Identify the federal and state agencies that regulate the safety and health issues in hospitals.

■ INTERNET WEB SITES

http://www.intertek-etlsemko.com (Intertek)
http://www.safety.duke.edu (Occupational & Environmental Safety Office, Duke University and Duke Medicine)
http://www.hazmat.org (Hazardous Materials Emergency Response Workshop, The Continuing Challenge)
http://www.ecri.org (ECRI Institute)
http://www.nfpa.org (National Fire Protection Association)

■ INTRODUCTION

All biomedical engineering technologists or biomedical equipment technicians (BMET) must be aware of the numerous types of safety hazards that may arise in their daily job functions. Taking the necessary safety precautions must be the highest priority when maintaining and repairing all types of medical equipment. These safety precautions begin with the installation of the equipment and continue through the complete life of the equipment. The most dangerous risk is the failure to recognize and acknowledge these hazards.

The United States of Labor regularly generates a list of potential hazards found in hospitals. It categorizes the hazards as biological, chemical, physical, or environmental, defines them, and provides examples in each category. This chapter discusses the various hazards and safety issues in hospitals.

■

20.1 ELECTRICAL SAFETY

The primary regulatory agencies in electrical safety in hospitals are the National Fire Protection Association (NFPA) and the Joint Commission (JC). The NFPA is an independent nonprofit organization to reduce fire and other hazards in buildings and compiles the National Electrical Code. It was organized to regulate particularly fire safety in health care facilities by advocating codes, standards, training, and education. The JC is also an independent nonprofit organization and certifies health care organizations and programs in the United States for continuously improving the safety and quality of care for patients. In addition, all equipment must meet safety standards as required by the Occupational Safety and Health Administration (OSHA). There are several Nationally Recognized Testing Laboratories (NRTL) that will test the product and verify that it has met the minimum requirements for safety standards. The two most common NRTLs are Underwriters Laboratories (UL) and Intertek's Electrical Testing Laboratories (ETL).

These voluntary standards recommend that every piece of medical equipment that enters a health care facility must be tested for electrical safety. This testing includes proper grounding, checking for leakage currents, and ensuring that all wiring is free of any damage. The electrical plug must also be three prong and of hospital grade. The only exception is equipment that has been designed and manufactured with double insulation.

For equipment that requires an attachment to a patient, such as an ECG monitor, the cables must also be tested and checked for leakage current.

NFPA99 (The NFPA Standard for Health Care Facilities) describes codes concerning the wiring and installation requirements on equipment, the nature of hazards, grounding reliability, receptacles, isolated power systems, and many more types of circuitry. **Figure 20-1** shows NFPA electrical safety guidelines. Some of the codes are discussed below:

1. Double-insulated appliances shall have two conductor cords; however, there are other appliances used in patient care that are provided with a three-wire cord and a three-pin grounding-type plug.
2. The resistance between the appliance chassis and the ground pin of the attachment plug should be less than 0.5 ohms (Ω).
3. The leakage current from frame to ground should not exceed 5 mA in patient care areas for fixed equipment. For portable equipment the tolerance is much lower. The chassis leakage current for portable equipment is not to exceed 300 μA.

4. Beyond 1 kHz, the leakage current limits are multiplied by the frequency (in kHz) up to a maximum of 10 mA.
5. The patient leads connected to the intracardiac catheters or electrodes should be isolated from the appliance's power (120 V) source.
6. The electrical appliances should be tested at least once in 12 months in the general care areas, although the testing of appliances for critical care or wet areas should not exceed 6 months.
7. The primary winding of an isolated transformer is not to exceed 600 V input power and its neutral must be grounded.

FIGURE 20-1 NFPA electrical safety guidelines.

	NFPA-99 1996		AAMI/AAMI ESI-1993	
	Ground Open	Ground Intact	Ground Open	Ground Intact
Chassis source current, cord connected (portable)				
With isolated patient connection	300μa	300μa	300μa	100μa
With nonisolated patient connection	300μa	300μa	300μa	100μa
Likely to contact patient	300μa	300μa	300μa	100μa
No patient contact	300μa	300μa	500μa	100μa
Chassis source current, permanently connected				
With isolated patient connection	5000μa	5000μa	5000μa	100μa
With nonisolated patient connection	5000μa	5000μa	5000μa	100μa
Likely to contact patient	5000μa	5000μa	5000μa	100μa
No patient contact	5000μa	5000μa	5000μa	100μa
Lead to ground current				
With isolated patient connection	50μa	10μa	50μa	10μa
With nonisolated patient connection	100μa	100μa	100μa	50μa
Lead to lead current				
With isolated patient connection	50μa	10μa	-	-
With nonisolated patient connection	50μa	50μa	-	-
Sink current (isolated test)				
With isolated patient connection	n/a	20μa	-	-
With nonisolated patient connection	50μa	50μa	-	-
Ground impedance	0.5 ohms			
Existing system	0.2 ohms			
New construction	0.1 ohms			
Receptacle indicators				
Hospital grade	listed			
Emergency system	red			
Isolated ground	orange			
GFCI trip current	6 mA			

8. Each isolated power system is provided with a continually operating line isolation monitor. The monitor indicates possible leakage current or fault current from an isolated conductor to ground.
9. The voltage and impedance measurements must be done with respect to a reference point. This point is either a grounding point or a grounding contact of a receptacle that is powered from a different circuit.
10. The voltage and impedance measurements should be made with an accuracy of ± 20 percent.

Figure 20-2 shows frequency versus source current limits in electrical safety. Above 1 kHz, the limit is increased proportionally to a maximum value 100 times the limit at 1 kHz.

Every facility has numerous types of equipment that, when maintenance or adjustments are required, could be hazardous to an employee. To comply with the OSHA's Control of Hazardous Energy Source Standard, each facility should have an Energy Control Program. Effective October 31, 1989, OSHA regulations require that any equipment that has undergone major repairs, renovations, or modifications, or any newly installed equipment, must accept some type of lockout device.

This program should:

- Identify all powered equipment and machinery in the facility.
- Identify the sources of energy and associated energy isolation devices.
- Provide procedures for turning off, locking and tagging out, and restarting.
- Contain records of all training completed.

The grounding issue in electrical safety is now settled as every hospital equipment is properly insulated, shielded, and grounded. Due to these efforts, accidental electrocutions in

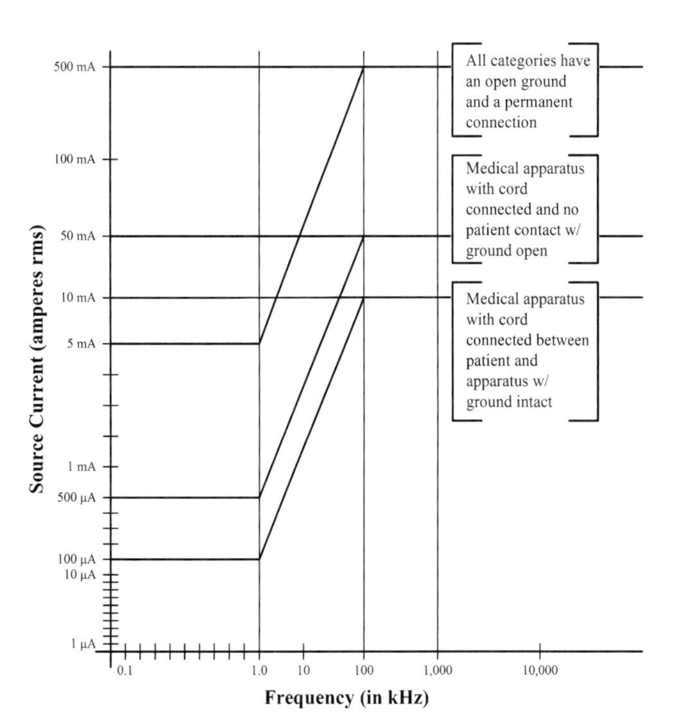

FIGURE 20-2 Frequency versus source current in electrical safety.

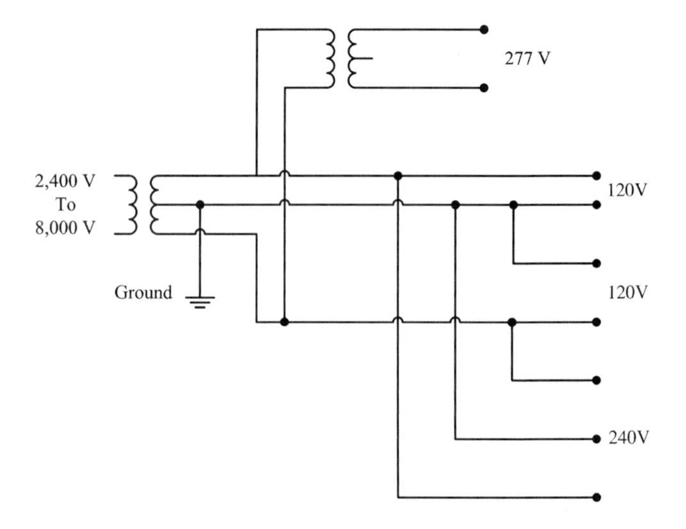

FIGURE 20-3 High-voltage circuit in a hospital.

hospitals are now rare. Electrocution was possible due to contact with the live conductor or the ground conductor. **Figure 20-3** shows the power system in a hospital. The large power from the electrical power station is brought down by step-down transformers to 277 V, 240 V, and 120 V. The electrical system has several fuses and main switches, and almost all hospital diagnostic equipment runs on DC voltages. The 120 V AC is regulated to 3 V, 6 V, 9 V, 12 V, and so on.

Reasons for Grounding

A power cable has three wires: the hot wire (H), which is the black wire at 120 V; the neutral wire (N), which is the white wire and is connected into ground through a pipe as long as 20 feet; and the ground wire (G), which is the green wire. The neutral wire usually carries the return current of the hot wire through the loads, while the ground wire connected to the external parts of equipment carries the leakage current (if any) to the ground.

In case of a short or a fault in the circuit, a high voltage develops into a very large leakage current that must go directly to ground. If not properly grounded, the large current may create undesirable situations with regard to a patient such as heart fibrillation, tissue injury, organ failure, or even death.

Most medical devices have an isolated power supply and a grounding system. Moreover, none of the electrodes are grounded directly. The fuses are also placed in the "live" (ungrounded) side of each circuit.

Types of Shock Hazards (Micro and Macro)

There are two different types of shock hazards:

1. **Macroshock:** occurs when current is applied to the surface of the body, producing tissue injury and unnecessary stimulation. It is a few millamperes through the body and may include the heart. A current not exceeding 5 mA is generally not considered harmful, although the sensation can be rather unpleasant and painful. Currents in excess of about 10 mA can tetanize the skeletal muscle and make it impossible to "let go" of

the conductor if grasped by the hand. Ventricular fibrillation can occur by macroshock at currents above about 100 mA.

2. **Microshock:** occurs when the current is applied to the surface of the heart, also producing tissue injury. The current required for microshock is in the microampere range, which is one-thousandth of the current required for macroshock. Ventricular fibrillation can occur around 100 μA of microshock current in most patients.

Circuits for Protection from Electrical Hazards

There are two types of circuits used to protect against electrical hazards: the ground fault circuit interrupter (GFCI) and the isolation transformer.

Ground Fault Circuit Interrupter The GFCI is a circuit breaker in the sense that the hot wire and the neutral wire do not have equal currents. The circuit will break, that is, the hot wire opens up when an inequality of currents is detected between the hot and neutral wires. **Figure 20-4** shows where the hot wire and the neutral wire pass through the transformer coils on the same transformer core in a GFCI. When currents are equal in these wires, the net flux equals zero. However, when the current is unbalanced (not equal), a net flux is induced across the third relay coil of the transformer. The relay then opens up the normally closed switch to an open position in the hot wire.

Isolation Transformer This circuit offers electrical safety when grounded power is changed into the ungrounded 120-V power. **Figure 20-5** shows that the primary coil of the transformer is grounded, but the secondary coil is not. In a way, this transformer isolates the Line-2 wire from the ground wire. A line isolation monitor (LIM) across the secondary coil monitors this isolation from the ground. Any time there is a short and the ground-seeking current exceeds the safe current, the LIM will provide an alarm signal.

Safety can be improved with only a few modifications in the isolation transformer circuits. **Figure 20-6a** has a static LIM with a balanced fault condition. In a static LIM, the detector can detect faults that occur from either power line. However, the potential of having identical impedances (i.e. Z) to the ground from each power line (that is, a balanced fault) goes undetected. The solution, shown in **Figure 20-6b**, is called the dynamic

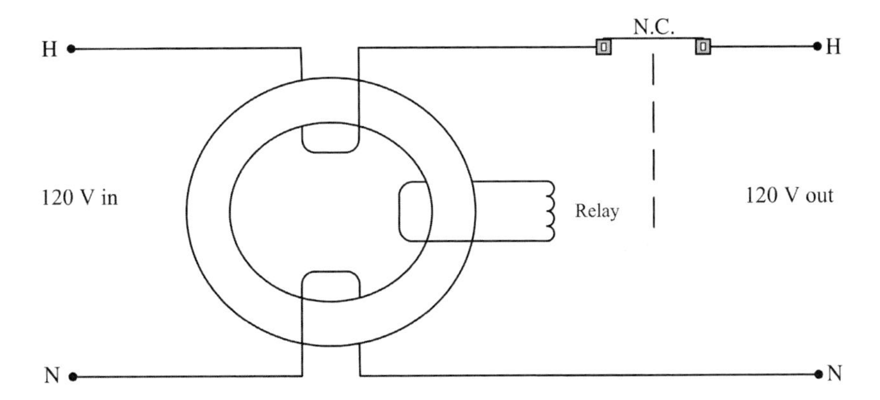

FIGURE 20-4 GFCI circuit breaker.

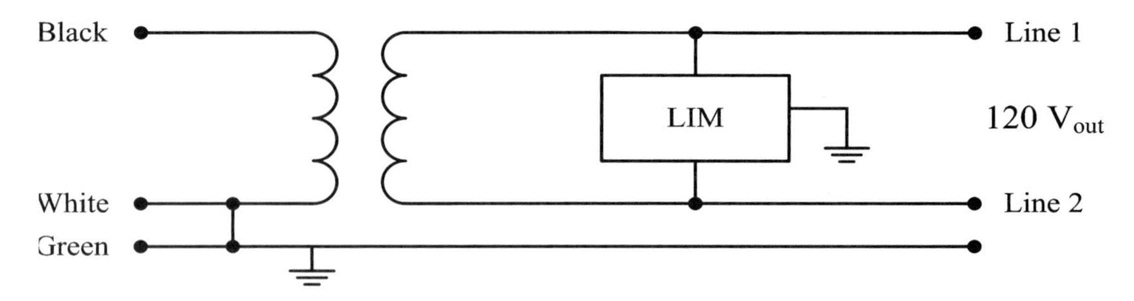

FIGURE 20-5 LIM monitor.

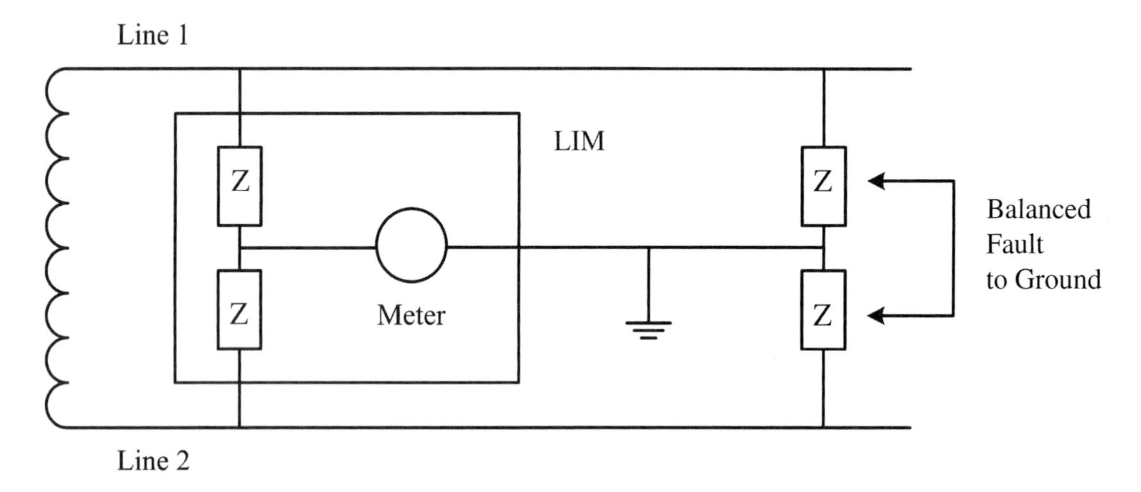

FIGURE 20-6a Balanced fault condition.

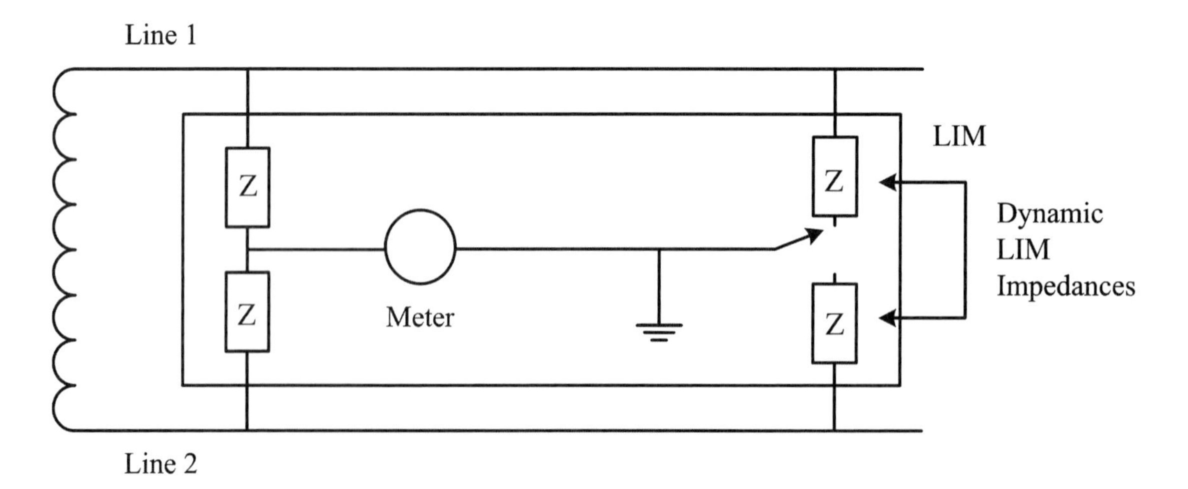

FIGURE 20-6b Dynamic LIM impedance.

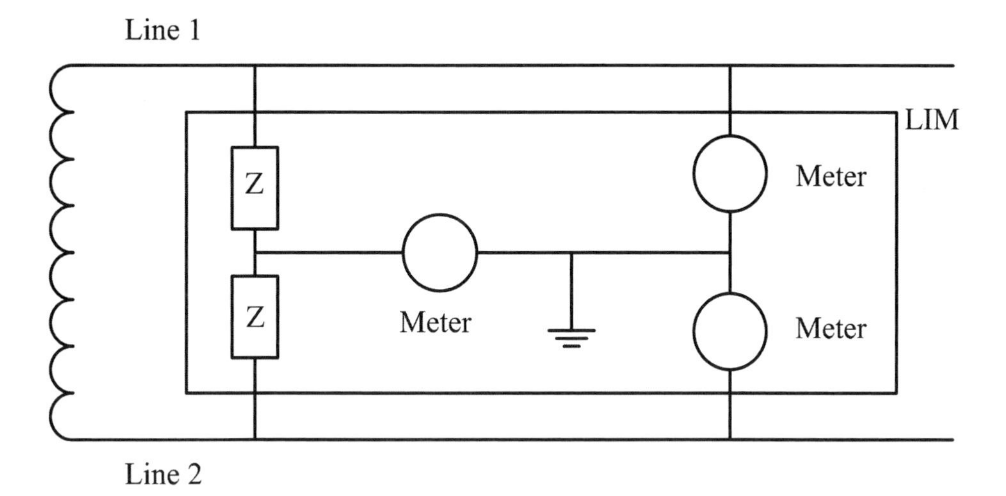

FIGURE 20-6c Several LIM monitors.

LIM. This dynamic LIM can mechanically switch from one power line to another at high speed to check for a balanced condition. One of the best solutions is shown in **Figure 20-6c** where the LIM constantly measures the potential hazard currents between each power line and the ground. Most LIMs will sound an alarm if current detected is in the range of 2 mA to 5 mA. The new types of LIMs are microprocessor-controlled to provide quick and accurate notification of hazardous current situations.

A schematic of a safety tester is given in **Figure 20-7**. The circuit is created by AAMI and NFPA as a standard test load to measure the current that flows between power ground (earth) and any exposed chassis conductive surface or hardware. With the voltmeter connected, the leakage current limit remains constant at 1 mA/mV independent of frequency.

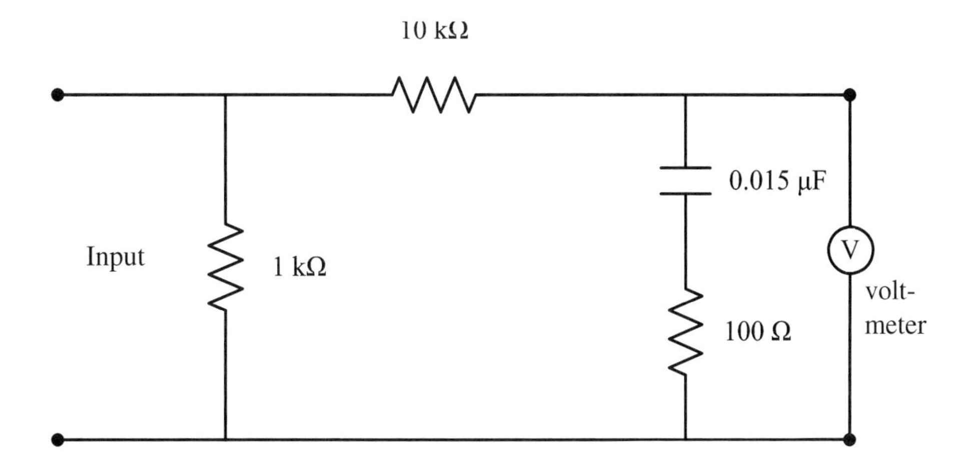

FIGURE 20-7 Schematic of safety tester.

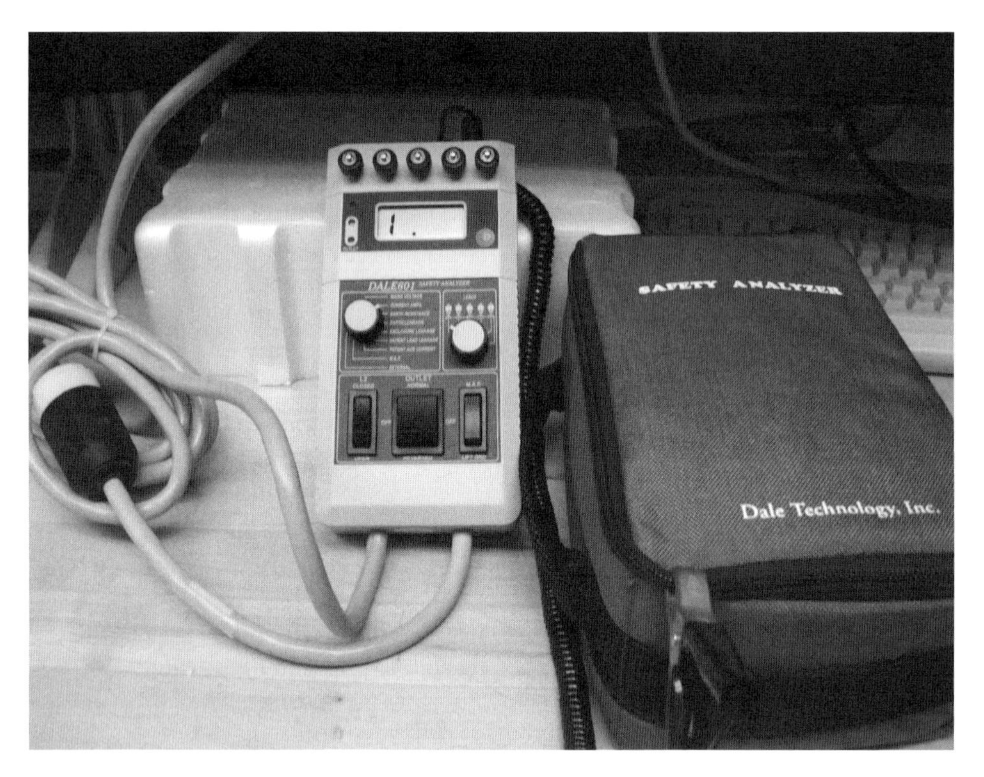

FIGURE 20-8 A safety analyzer.

On a regular basis a biomedical technician measures the power cord resistance and the enclosure leakage current of any equipment using an electrical safety analyzer. The reading of the power cord resistance should not be greater than 0.5 ohm, and the reading of the leakage current should not be greater than 300 μA. **Figure 20-8** shows a photo of a safety analyzer.

20.2 RADIATION SAFETY

Personnel exposure to X-rays over a long period of time can be extremely hazardous. The technician must take appropriate precautions when energizing an X-ray machine, including wearing a lead-lined apron as well as a dosimeter badge. The safety office provides a report to the radiation safety committee regarding each department's compliance with the dosimeter badge guidelines. The dosimeter badge insert is replaced semimonthly and technicians send reports to the facility employers showing the current and total exposure to the X-rays. The technician is provided with an "in-service" if exposure exceeds the maximum safe limit and is queried as to why the X-ray dose was out of the safe range. These types of reports are usually provided to the facility safety committee quarterly.

20.3 CHEMICAL SAFETY

All employees of any company have a right and a need to know the identities and hazards of any chemical that they may be exposed to when working. If protective measures are available, the employees need to know what is available to prevent adverse effects. The Chemical Safety-Hazardous Materials and Communication standard is a requirement under the OSHA standard 29 CFR 1910.1200. In order to be compliant with the standard, every facility must do the following:

- All bottles and containers must be labeled with name and ingredients. Manufacturer's labels must be legible, in English, (or other languages, if appropriate), and conspicuously displayed.
- Every chemical must have a Material Safety Data Sheet (MSDS) on-site or have immediate access to the information (via the Internet) and must be available to all employees. Every MSDS must be in English (or other languages, if appropriate) and must include:
  - The specific chemical identity of the hazardous chemical and the common names:
  - Known health effects and related health information
  - Exposure limits
  - Precautionary measures
    - Emergency and first-aid procedures
    - Identifying who prepared the MSDS
- A written program must be in place with a list of all hazardous chemicals.
- Hazard information must be communicated to employees, including the standard and the requirements of the standard, where hazardous chemicals are present, and where all documentation is kept, including ready access to the MSDS.
- There must be employee training, including how to read and interpret the information on the labels and the MSDS. Training must also include the hazards and measures that employees can take to protect themselves.
- Procedures must be established.

20.4 BIOLOGICAL SAFETY

Infectious diseases are the primary occupational hazard for biomedical technicians. These diseases can be transmitted by direct or indirect contact with an infected individual. Some diseases can also be transmitted through inhaling. All blood and body fluids, secretions, and excretions (except sweat), should be treated as if they are known to be infected with an infectious disease. Every hospital and medical facility has policies and procedures that address infectious materials and additional measures that can be taken to prevent the spread of diseases. A few of the necessary measures to take follow:

- Hand washing is the most effective measure to prevent contamination. Hands should be washed before eating, drinking, or leaving a possibly contaminated area. Additionally, hands should be washed after a restroom break and after working on any type of equipment that has the possibility of being contaminated. Do not rub eyes or any mucous membrane until after hand washing.

- Use of personal protective equipment including gloves, masks, and some type of face shield should the possibility of contact with a bodily fluid exist. Occasionally, a barrier-resistant gown might be appropriate for certain types of equipment repairs.
- Most medical facilities offer a hepatitis B vaccination, which, for biomedical engineers, is highly recommended.
- For those employees who handle infectious waste, annual training is usually a requirement of either the facility or the Department of Health (DOH).

There are numerous medical devices that require added attention prior to any maintenance. These include but are not limited to the following:

- Centrifuges—fragments of glass from broken tubes may be present at the bottom of the bowl area. In addition, it is possible that body fluids may be present.
- Dialysis equipment always presents the possibility of the presence of body fluids.
- Any equipment in the operating room or emergency room that may be kept or used below knee level, such as foot switches, may be contaminated.
- Most clinical laboratory analyzers.

20.5 FIRE AND EXPLOSIVE SAFETY

Fire safety is extremely important regardless of the business or industry. Every employee should know where the closest fire extinguisher is located as well as where the closest pull alarm is located in reference to his or her workplace. Each fire extinguisher should be checked on a monthly basis to make sure that the contents are still contained in the extinguisher. Pull stations, as well as sprinkler systems, should be checked annually.

There are also numerous chemicals used in an institution that could cause an explosion should there be a leak or inadvertent mixing of two or more chemicals. These chemicals should be stored in a separate area from other chemicals or gases.

20.6 ENVIRONMENTAL SAFETY

Many times, the environment in which we work influences what we do and how we do it. Temperature- and humidity-controlled environments are essential for much of the medical equipment used in a health care facility. Many manufacturers specify the high and low limits of acceptability for temperature and humidity, power requirements and space requirements. Many pieces of equipment such as flow hoods also require some type of ventilation and routine cleaning of the filter assemblies.

20.7 MATERIAL SAFETY DATA SHEET

The Material Safety Data Sheet (MSDS) is designed to provide both workers and emergency personnel with the proper procedures for handling or working with a particular substance. OSHA, EPA, and state and local agencies require workers and emergency personnel to keep data sheets. The information in data sheets includes toxicity, storage and disposal procedures, and health effects of exposure to these substances. These data sheets are available in laboratories, universities, businesses, and environmental or occupational health offices.

SUMMARY

- Medical safety procedures and regulations protect not only patients, but people surrounding these patients, including health care professionals such as BMETs.
- Electrical safety concepts are explained in the beginning of the chapter. Some of the NFPA code regulations are also discussed. The equipment is tested for proper ground; the equipment chassis to ground resistance should not be greater than 0.5 Ω. Also, the leakage current should not be greater than 300 μA.
- Safety features in the event of radiation exposure, chemical spill or hazard, and biological and environmental adverse reactions, as well as fire prevention and explosive safety are included in the chapter.
- A paragraph is written on Material Safety Data Sheets (MSDS) as part of safety questionnaires. MSDS are designed to provide hospital workers with the proper procedures for handling hazardous substances.

MEDICAL TERMINOLOGY

The following is a list of medical terms mentioned in this chapter.

Environmental illnesses: term for diseases caused by the human-made environment in which we live. The diseases can have natural or artificial causes.

Ground fault circuit interrupter (GFCI): device used to protect against electric shock should someone come in contact with a live wire and a path to the ground, which would result in a current through the body.

Intravascular catheter infections: significant growth of a microorganism in a quantitative culture of the catheter tip.

Isolated ground: set of interconnected frames that is grounded via only one connection to a ground reference.

Macroshock: passage of current from one part of the body to another. For example, from arm to arm, which results in the current flowing through the heart. A high-voltage, low-current shock is not dangerous.

Microshock: current can flow directly through the electrically sensitive myocardium. Microshock applies to all cases where an electrode or catheter is situated near or in the heart.

Radio Frequency Identification (RFID) tag: A microchip combined with an antenna in a condensed package. The tag's antenna picks up signals from an RFID reader or scanner and then returns the signal.

Underwriters Laboratories Inc. (UL): company that has developed more than 1,000 standards for safety related to the products.

QUIZ

1. The LIM and GFCI are permanently attached to the power lines in order to:
   a) Short the circuit b) Open the circuit c) Both a and b d) None of the above
2. When does GFCI protect a person against a shock?
   ____
3. Microshock occurs when a current applied to the ______________ causes depolarization.
4. An X-ray technician should wear a lead-lined apron and also a ______________.
5. The fire extinguisher in the hospital should be checked ______________.
   a) Annually b) Bimonthly c) Monthly
6. What is the maximum allowable resistance for the ground wire connecting the receptacles to prevent exceeding the safe current limit for microshock in the patient?
   a) 75 Ω b) 300 Ω c) 0.5 Ω d) None of the above
7. In what parts of the hospital are microshock hazards likely to exist?
   a) X-ray area b) Cardiac catheterization lab
   c) OR room d) None of the above
8. Name two different ways in which electricity can harm the body:
   ____
9. Name two types of radiation-induced injury in the hospital:
   ____
10. MSDS stands for:
    a) Microshock distribution system b) Medical supply distribution system
    c) Material safety data sheet d) None of the above

PROBLEMS

1. Compare and contrast the chemical, biological, and environmental safety features in a hospital.
2. Explain at least five NFPA codes or requirements related to the leakage current limits in medical equipment in hospitals. You may access the NFPA Web site for these codes.
3. Draw a ground fault detector circuit and discuss how it works.
4. Discuss the classes of fire extinguishers.
5. Discuss the safety precautions that must be followed when working in a high concentration of oxygen in the hospital.
6. Match the words in the left column with the description on the right column:

1. Leakage current	a. a path for leakage current
2. Grounding conductor in a power cord	b. 5 mA

3. Standard for ground resistance	c. infectious diseases
4. Hazard current LIM must alarm	d. less than 5 mA
5. Current no longer causes sensation	e. damage to eyes
6. Hazard of ultraviolet light	f. stray current to the chassis
7. Color code of the wire in a power cord	g. 0.5 Ω
8. Dosimeter badge	h. contact with the live conductor
9. Occupational hazard	i. white neutral
10. Electrocution	j. radiation safety

7. Discuss the steps in using a safety analyzer to test the safety of medical equipment.

8. Discuss in detail the MSDS procedures for university workers. You may contact your university or find information on the Internet.

9. Make a list of equipment needed for the environmental, biological, and radiation safety in a hospital.

10. Illustrate a microshock and a macroshock situation in a hospital. Sketch (roughly) the electrical circuit for the situation.

RESEARCH TOPICS

1. Sometimes in hospital accidents, patients who are electronically sensitive are at risk for fatal injury. In some hospitals, there are areas designated as "electronically sensitive patient locations," such as ORs or rooms where patients have catheters under the skin. Discuss why some patients are more susceptible to these electronic signals than others. The research paper should include what can be done to avoid fatal injury.

2. The FDA-approved RFID (Radio Frequency Identification) chips that can be implanted on clothes or even under the skin in humans. Some hospitals in Europe have begun implanting patients with RFID tags for patient identification. Accessing medical records and identifying prescription drugs the patient is on becomes faster and more accurate. This is a new technology, so the research paper should include safety issues in patients implanted with the RFID system. The paper should discuss the vulnerability of infectious bacteria to electromagnetic radiation and also privacy issues.

CASE STUDY

Catheter-related bloodstream infections in ICUs are an issue that could be eliminated in hospitals. Cathy, a victim of a catheter-related infection, nearly died because of an infection. In intravascular catheter-related infections, the risk factors include catheter types, location site, and the duration of catheterization. Answer the following questions:

a) What went wrong in this case? Discuss in detail. How could this happen in an ICU?

b) What is the physiology of an infection that can kill someone?

c) How is an infection preventable, particularly in ICUs? What guidelines do ICUs follow?

CHAPTER 21

Regulation and Standards

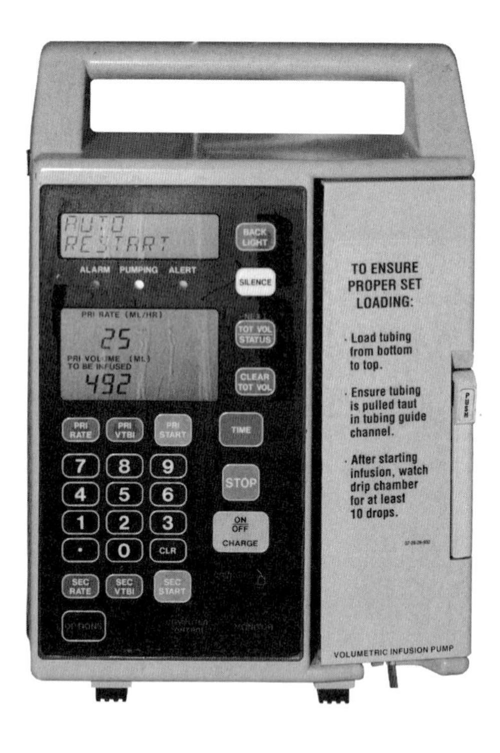

■ CHAPTER OUTLINE

■ OBJECTIVE

The objective of this chapter is to help the reader to identify the various regulatory agencies regarding medical equipment management and to familiarize the reader with standards organizations and their functions and responsibilities.

Upon completion of this chapter the reader will be able to:

- Identify the various regulatory agencies and their functions and responsibilities.

INTERNET WEB SITES

http://www.cms.hhs.gov (Centers for Medicare and Medicaid Services)
http://www.hhs.gov (Department of Health and Human Services)
http://www.ansi.org (American National Standards Institute)
http://www.nfpa.org (National Fire Protection Association)
http://www.cap.org (College of American Pathologists)
http://www.fda.gov (U.S. Food and Drug Administration)
http://www.carf.org (Commission on Accreditation of Rehabilitation Facilities)
http://www.jointcommission.org (The Joint Commission: Helping Health Care Organizations Help Patients)

INTRODUCTION

Medical instrumentation and devices are subject to strict general controls and procedural regulations. The type of device determines the agency or agencies to whose regulation it is subject. Also, standards organizations provide the accepted standards for the function of medical devices. These agencies and standards organizations include, but are not limited to, the U.S. Food and Drug Administration (FDA), Center for Devices and Radiological Health (CDRH), Joint Commission on Accreditation of Health Care Organizations (JC), Clinical Laboratory Improvement Amendments (CLIA), College of American Pathologists (CAP), and Commission on Accreditation of Rehabilitation Facilities (CARF).

In the following sections, each agency or organization is identified in parentheses as being either a regulatory agency or a standards organization.

21.1 FOOD AND DRUG ADMINISTRATION (REGULATORY)

The Food and Drug Administration (FDA) is charged with the oversight and safety of medical devices in the United States and now regulates more than 1,700 types of devices, 500,000 device models, and 23,000 manufacturers. The organizational chart of the Department of Health and Human Services for the FDA structure is shown in **Figure 21-1**.

The classifications of medical devices are defined in section 201(h) of the Food, Drug, and Cosmetic (FD&C) Act as amended in 1976. This section states that a medical device can be "an instrument, apparatus, implement, machine, contrivance, implant, in vitro reagent, or other similar or related article, including any component, part or accessory, which is (1) recognized in the official National Formulary, or the United States Pharmacopoeia, or any supplement to them, (2) intended for use in the diagnosis of disease or other conditions, or in the cure, mitigation, treatment, or prevention of disease, in man or other animals, or (3) intended to affect the structure or any function of the body of man or other animals, and which does not achieve its primary intended purposes through chemical action within or on the body of man or other animals and which is not dependent on being metabolized for the achievement of its primary intended purposes." (See **http://www.emedicinehealth.com** for more information.) These amendments resulted in medical devices being classified in three categories. The device class number is in ascending order of safety risk to the patient in case of device failure.

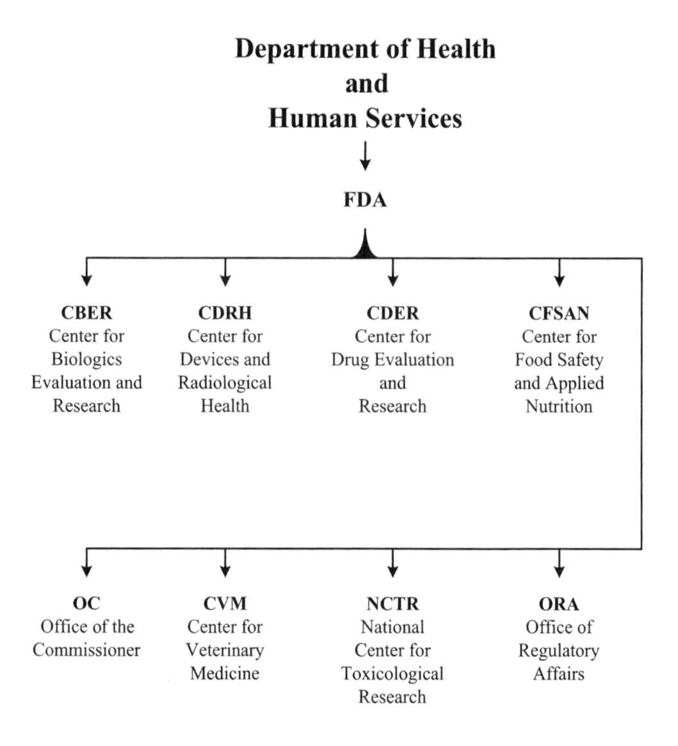

FIGURE 21-1 A list of the FDA departments.

- Class I devices are subject to general controls, which include labeling, registration, reporting and tracking, and adherence to general quality control requirements. Examples of these devices include bandages, medical tape, tongue blades, and gloves.
- Class II devices are subject to special controls, which include clinical trials and performance requirements. A thermometer is an example of a Class II device.
- Class III devices are subject to the aforementioned general and special controls, which require clinical studies and show effectiveness and *safety*. The issue of clinical studies and safety is part of Premarket Approval (PMA) controls. These include implantable devices such as knee replacements and pacemakers.

Each person or company submits a Premarket Notification 510(k) to the FDA for the medical device (in Class I, Class II, and in some cases even Class III), new or modified, before it can be sold. Until FDA approval is given, the person or company cannot market the device. In the case of a Class III device, FDA is strict in requiring the applicant to submit a PMA application in addition to the 510(k) application. The PMA application must contain sufficient scientific data to assure that the medical device is safe. Again, the applicant must receive the approval from the FDA before Class III device can be marketed.

The traditional 510(k) application process has additional approaches for faster approval from FDA. They are the Special 510(k) and Abbreviated 510(k). In the case of the Special 510(k), the medical device has been previously cleared and the modification still follows the fundamental technology. In the Abbreviated 510(k), however, the device follows the guidance and standard document approved by the FDA.

For the Class III PMA application to FDA, the clinical study must include the safety data, adverse reactions and complications, patient complaints, device failures, and many more study the protocols. The applicant must receive an Investigational Device Exemption (IDE) from the FDA during clinical investigations using the device.

As the FDA requires a lot of documentation, the Quality System (QS) includes documentation appropriate to the specific medical device designed or manufactured in accordance to the FDA regulation and standards. There are several elements of QS, but mainly the Document Controls and Design Controls are the written procedures and documented practices required by the FDA.

Document Controls must include medical device specifications, engineering drawings, user's manual, records of any changes, and the signatures of the approving individuals. In the case of Design Controls, the FDA requires the systematic evaluation, revision, and the efficiency of the design for the device during its development with the goal of patient safety.

Center for Devices and Radiological Health (Regulatory)

The tree structure of the Center for Devices and Radiological Health (CDRH) under the FDA is shown in **Figure 21-2**. Under the Office of Compliance, the Division of Enforcement enforces the laws that ensure the safety of medical devices and radiological products. The medical devices are regulated according to the degree of risk they present to the public.

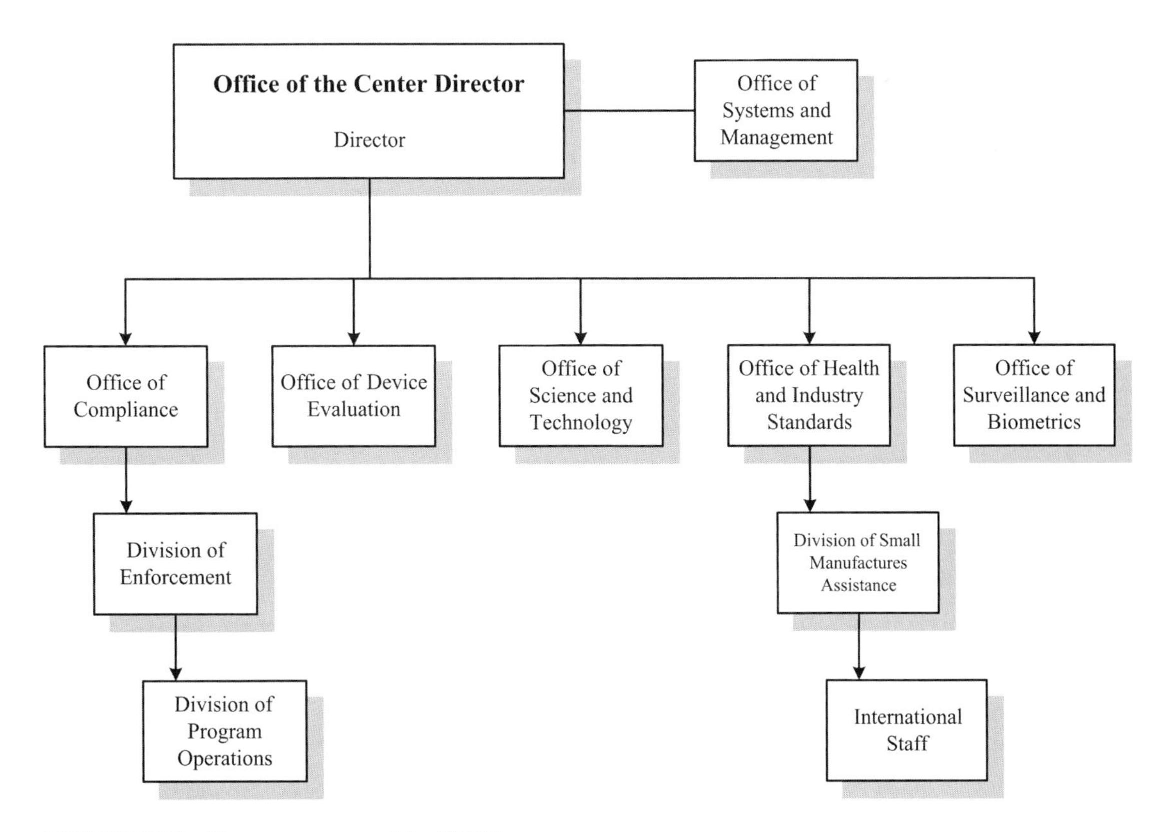

FIGURE 21-2 The tree structure of the CDRH.

The CDRH sets up the "gold standard" for the products being approved and works with the radiological health industry to limit unnecessary radiation emissions.

Office of Regulatory Affairs (Regulatory)

Under the FDA, the Office of Regulatory Affairs coordinates the compliance and fairness aspects of the FDA rules. The structure of this organization is shown in **Figure 21-3**. The ORA is the lead office for all field activities of the FDA and punishes for intentional violations or gross negligence.

Office of Regulatory Affairs (ORA)

FDA is a scientifically based law enforcement agency. Its enforcement activities are coordinated by ORA, whose function is twofold: to safeguard the public health and to ensure honesty and fair dealing between the regulated industry and consumers.

- FDA encourages and expects compliance with the laws and regulations it enforces. To this end, the agency participates in cooperative and educational efforts designed to inform industry, health professionals, and the public of those legal requirements.
- FDA surveys and inspects regulated industry to assess compliance and discover noncompliance. Depending upon the nature of non-compliance, FDA may afford an opportunity for correction by industry. If adequate correction does not occur within a reasonable period, FDA is committed to swiftly initiating action to obtain compliance. Legal remedies include injunction, seizure, and prosecution.
- FDA does not tolerate fraud, intentional violations, or gross negligence, and promptly seeks prosecution to punish and deter whenever appropriate.

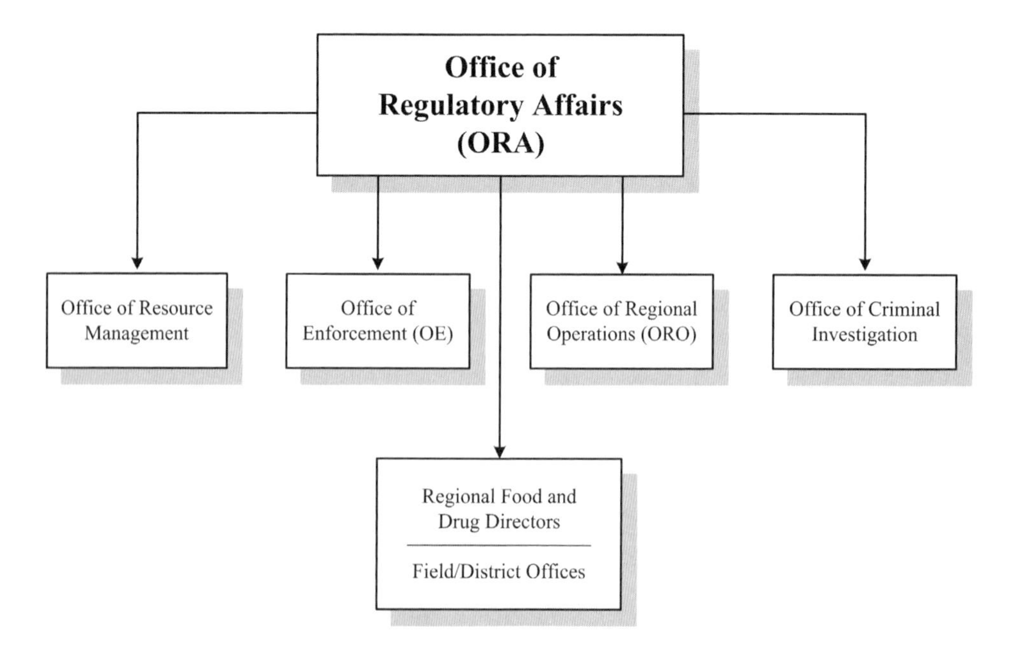

FIGURE 21-3 The tree structure of ORA.

21.2 SAFE MEDICAL DEVICE ACT (REGULATORY)

In 1990, the Safe Medical Device Act (SMDA) amendment was enacted; this legislation requires medical device manufacturers to report adverse events relating to medical equipment and tracking. This was amended further in 1992 to require additional detail regarding these events. These adverse events, known as Medical Device Reports (MDRs) must be reported to the FDA. If the equipment was believed to be related to a death or serious injury, manufacturers and users are required to report that event to the FDA as a MDR. Examples of "Medical Devices" include bandages, sutures, catheters, wheelchairs, ventilators, and patient monitoring equipment. Annually, the FDA receives 80,000 to 120,000 event reports, mostly from manufacturers. Only about 5,000 are reported to be from medical institutions.

21.3 NATIONAL FIRE PROTECTION ASSOCIATION (STANDARDS)

In 1896, the National Fire Protection Association (NFPA) was founded as an international nonprofit standards organization. Today, it is the foremost advocate for public safety and fire protection. Examples of NFPA standards used in medical facilities include:

- NFPA 70 (the National Electric Code—used for all electrical installations)
- NFPA 99 (the Standard for Health Care Facilities—for hospitals, nursing homes, and freestanding facilities such as birthing centers)
- NFPA 101 (the Life Safety Code—used to protect buildings from fires, smoke, and fumes)

The NFPA also sponsors such public programs as Fire Protection Week and Sparky the Fire Dog, among others, to educate the public about fire prevention and safety.

21.4 CLINICAL LABORATORY IMPROVEMENT AMENDMENTS (STANDARDS)

The Centers for Medicare and Medicaid Services (CMS) oversees all aspects of the Clinical Laboratory Improvement Amendments (CLIA) legislation except for research laboratories. Congress passed the CLIA legislation in 1988. This legislation established minimum standards for laboratory testing of samples. Any laboratory that performs testing on human specimens for the purpose of diagnosing, preventing, or treating disease, and for the assessment of general health of a patient, is subject to these regulations. All laboratories must maintain procedure manuals documenting all activities, including QA procedures, equipment preventive maintenance, all repair histories, and record keeping. These manuals must undergo a mandatory annual review by the laboratory administration. The purpose of these amendments was to ensure the reliability, accuracy, and timely reporting of patient results regardless of where these tests were performed. The final regulations were published in 1992. All clinical laboratories must be CLIA-certified in order to receive payments from Medicare or Medicaid.

There are three categories of tests established by these regulations. They are waived complexity, moderate complexity, and high complexity. Waived-complexity laboratories must be part of CLIA and must also follow manufacturers' instructions. For those laboratories performing moderate- or high-complexity tests, CLIA has specific standards for testing, quality control, and personnel qualification. As technology improves and new tests are developed, the CDC and CMS are currently working to develop final CLIA rules and regulations.

21.5 COLLEGE OF AMERICAN PATHOLOGISTS (STANDARDS)

The College of American Pathologists (CAP) is a private, nonprofit accrediting organization that routinely inspects all aspects of a laboratory. This accreditation process is voluntary for every laboratory of which over 6,000 have met these high standards. This organization has been approved by the Centers for Medicare and Medicaid Services (CMS).

CAP is the primary accrediting agency for hospital laboratories and is sponsored by the American Society of Clinical Pathologists (ASCP). Formal routine inspections are conducted every two years, but unannounced random inspections can be conducted at any time. These inspections often include:

- Tours of all areas of the laboratory
- Interviews with the laboratory staff
- Review of quality control procedures and results
- Review of procedures for collecting and handling specimens
- Reviews of any records, including preventive maintenance and repair records

21.6 JOINT COMMISSION ON ACCREDITATION OF HEALTH CARE ORGANIZATIONS (STANDARDS)

The Joint Commission on accreditation of health care organizations (JC) was founded in 1951 as a nonprofit organization. They provide accreditation services for numerous organizations, including hospitals, nursing homes, rehabilitation centers, and some home care service companies. The survey process looks at all aspects of a medical organization from patient rights and treatment, infection control, and leadership, to personnel, life safety, and medical equipment. In the Environment of Care Standards (EC.6) there are numerous Elements of Performance that must be met for medical equipment. Several examples are:

- The organization establishes and uses risk criteria for identifying, evaluating, and creating an inventory of equipment to be included in the medical equipment management plan before the equipment is used. These criteria address the following:
  - Equipment function (diagnosis, care, treatment, and monitoring)
  - Physical risks associated with use
  - Equipment incident history
- The organization identifies appropriate strategies for all equipment in the inventory for achieving effective, safe, and reliable operation of all equipment in the inventory.

The Joint Commission's evaluation and accreditation services are provided for the following types of organizations:

- General, psychiatric, children's, and rehabilitation hospitals
- Critical access hospitals
- Medical equipment services, hospice services and the other home care organizations
- Nursing homes and other long term care facilities
- Behavioral health care organizations, addiction services
- Rehabilitation centers, group practices, office-based surgeries, and other ambulatory care providers
- Independent or freestanding laboratories

FIGURE 21-4 A list of organizations receiving services provided by JC.

Benefits of Joint Commission accreditation:

- Strengthen community confidence in the quality and safety of care, treatment and services.
- Provides a competitive advantage in the marketplace.
- Improves risk management and risk reduction.
- Helps organize and strengthen patient safety efforts.
- Provides education on good practices to improve business operations.
- Provides professional advice and counsel thereby enhancing staff education.
- Enhances recruitment and enhances development.
- Provides deeming authority for Medicare certification.
- Recognized by insurers and other third parties.
- May reduce liability insurance costs.

FIGURE 21-5 Benefits provided by the JC.

- The organization documents maintenance of non life-support equipment on the inventory that is consistent with maintenance strategies to minimize clinical and physical risks identified in the equipment management plan.

The Joint Commission's evaluation and accreditation services are provided to the following types of organizations shown in **Figure 21-4**. Also, the benefits of the JC accreditation are given in **Figure 21-5**.

It is important to note that the JC Elements of Performance can be (and many times are) revised on an annual basis. The Joint Commission also posts on their Web site a complete list of all organizations that have recently completed the accreditation process, which is available to the general public.

21.7 COMMISSION ON ACCREDITATION OF REHABILITATION FACILITIES (STANDARDS)

Another private nonprofit agency is the Commission on Accreditation of Rehabilitation Facilities (CARF). This accreditation process looks at all aspects of a rehabilitation facility, including medical records and physical therapy. The national standards that are used in the accreditation process have been developed with input from many rehab professionals, other organizations and individuals. The agency's goals are to ensure that people with disabilities receive quality care and to find ways to improve patient care. This accreditation process is also voluntary for rehabilitation facilities.

21.8 OCCUPATIONAL SAFETY AND HEALTH ADMINISTRATION (REGULATORY)

Occupational Safety and Health Administration (OSHA) is an agency of the Department of Labor; and its mission is to prevent work-related injuries, illnesses, and deaths by enforcing rules for workplace safety. Every fiscal year OSHA reports on the number of federal inspections conducted, the reasons for these inspections, and the names of the industry sectors. **Figure 21-6** shows a list of inspections by OSHA for the year 2004.

OSHA's authority extends to most nongovernmental workplaces, but it permits states to develop approved plans that cover only public sector workers. A list of occupational hazards in the hospital is shown in **Figure 21-7**. Most areas of a hospital are covered to ensure the safety and health of workers.

21.9 HEALTH INSURANCE PORTABILITY AND ACCOUNTABILITY ACT (REGULATORY)

The Health Insurance Portability and Accountability Act (HIPAA) of 1996 has had a tremendous effect on the medical device service industry. The original goal of this legislation was to make health care information more portable, which means that anyone should

Federal Inspections – Fiscal Year 2004
39,167 inspections

Numbers	Percent	Reason for Inspection
9,176	23.4%	Complaint/accident related
21,576	55.1%	High hazard targeted
8,415	21.5%	Referrals, follow-ups, etc.

Numbers	Percent	Industry Sector
22,360	57.1%	Construction
8,755	22.4%	Manufacturing
378	1%	Maritime
7,674	19.6	Other industries

FIGURE 21-6 A list of inspections done by OSHA in 2004.

Occupational Hazards by Location in the Hospital

Location	Hazard
Central Supply	Ethylene oxide
	Infection
	Broken equipment (cuts)
	Soaps, detergents
	Steam
	Flammable gases
	Lifting
	Noise
	Asbestos insulation
	Mercury
Dialysis Units	Infection
	Formaldehyde
Dental Services	Mercury
	Ethylene oxide
	Anesthetic gases
	Ionizing radiation
	Infection
Food Service	Wet floors
	Sharp equipment
	Noise
	Soaps, detergents
	Disinfectants
	Ammonia
	Chlorine
	Solvents
	Drain cleaners
	Oven cleaners
	Caustic solutions
	Pesticides
	Microwave ovens
	Steam lines
	Ovens
	Heat
	Electrical hazards
	Lifting
Housekeeping	Soaps, detergents
	Cleaners
	Solvents
	Disinfectants
	Glutaraldehyde
	Infection
	Needle punctures
	Wastes (chemical, radioactive, infectious)
	Electrical hazards
	Lifting
	Climbing
	Slips, falls
Laboratory	Infectious diseases
	Toxic chemicals
	Benzene
	Ethylene oxide
	Formaldehyde
	Solvents
	Flammable/explosive agents
	Carcinogens
	Teratogens
	Mutagens
	Cryogenic hazards
	Wastes (chemical, radioactive, infectious)
	Radiation
Laundry	Wet floors
	Lifting
	Noise
	Heat
	Burns
	Infection
	Needle punctures
	Detergents, soaps
	Bleaches
	Solvents
	Waste (Chemical and radioactive)

FIGURE 21-7 A list of occupational hazards in a hospital. (*continued*)

Occupational Hazards by Location in the Hospital (cont.)

Location	Hazard
Maintenance and Engineering	Electrical hazards Tools, machinery Noise Welding fumes Asbestos Flammable liquids Solvents Mercury Pesticides Cleaners Ammonia Carbon monoxide Ethylene oxide Freon exposure Paints, adhesives Water treatment chemicals Sewage Heat stress Cold stress Slips, falls Lifting Climbing Strains and sprains
Nuclear Medicine	Radionuclides Infection X-irradiation
Office Area	Video Display Terminals Air q uality Ergonomic/body mechanics Chemicals Ozone
Operating Rooms	Anesthetics Antiseptics Methyl methacrylate Compressed gases Sterilizing gases Infection Electrical Sharp instruments Lifting
Pathology	Infectious diseases Formaldehyde Glutaraldehyde Flammable substances Freon exposure Solvents Phenols
Patient care	Lifting Pushing, pulling Slips, falls Standing for long periods Infectious diseases Needle punctures Toxic substances Chemotherapeutic agents Radiation Radioactive patients Electrical hazards
Pharmacy	Pharmaceuticals Antineoplastic agents Mercury exposure Slips, falls
Print Shops	Inks Solvents Noise Fire
Radiology	Radiation Infectious diseases Lifting Pushing, pulling

FIGURE 21-7 *(continued)*

be able to go to any health care provider and have his or her medical records instantly available electronically. Under the HIPAA act, the obligation of ensuring patient data security lies with the health care provider. The health care provider is responsible for making sure that anyone working in his or her facility abides by the HIPAA regulations. This pertains not only to employees but also to vendors, manufacturers, subcontractors, and consultants. All health care providers have developed a "business associate agreement" that is a requirement of the HIPAA regulations and must be signed by those vendors.

The deadline for implementing all of the HIPAA regulations was April 21, 2005.

Figure 21-8 shows the HIPAA provisions and **Figure 21-9** provides the detailed documentation for the care of the patient. Figure **21-10** provides the discharge procedure when the patient is discharged from the hospital.

Health Insurance Portability and Accountability Act of 1996 Summary of Administrative Simplification Provisions

Standards for electronic health information transactions. Within 18 months of enactment, the secretary of HHS is required to adopt standards from among those already approved by private standards developing organizations for certain electronic health transactions, including claims, enrollment, eligibility, payment, and coordination of benefits. These standards also must address the security of electronic health information systems.

Mandate on providers and health plans, and timetable. Providers and health plans are required to use the standards for the specified electronic transactions 24 months after they are adopted. Plans and providers may comply directly, or may use compensation, are not covered.

Privacy. The Secretary is required to recommend privacy standards for health information to Congress 12 months after Secretary shall promulgate.

Pre-emption of State Law. The bill supersedes state laws, except where the Secretary determines that the State Law is necessary to prevent fraud and abuse, to ensure appropriate state regulation of insurance or health plans, addresses controlled substances, or for other purposes. If the Secretary promulgates privacy regulations, those regulations do not pre-empt state law that impose more stringent requirements. These provisions do not limit a State's ability to require health plan reporting or adults.

Penalties. The bill imposes civil money penalties and prison for certain violations.

FIGURE 21-8 HIPAA provisions.

Documentation of Patient Care

36	Evaluation of the patient is based on the patient care goals and the patient's plan for care, treatment, and service.	PC.4.10 EP12
37	The goals of care, treatment, and services are revized when necessary.	PC.4.10 EP13
38	Plans for care, treatment, and services are revised, when necessary.	PC.4.10 EP14
39	To the extent possible, as appropriate to the patient's family's needs and the hospitals' services, interventions address patient and family comfort, dignity and psychosocial, emotional, and spiritual needs, as appropriate, about death and grief.	PC.8.70 EP1
40	All quality control test results are documented, including internal, external, liquid and electronic.	PC.16.60 EP1
41	Tests results are documented.	PC.16.60 EP2
42	The hospital's records include documentation in the recipient's clinical record of tissue use, including documentation of the unique identifier of the tissue.	PC.17.20 EP4
43	Monitoring a medication's effect on a patient includes the following: - Gathering the patient's own perceptions about side effects, and when appropriate, perceived efficacy. - Referring to information from the patient's medical record, relevant laboratory results, clinical response, and medical profile.	MM.6.10 EP2
44	Medical record entries are dated, the author identified, and when necessary according to law or regulation and hospital policy, is authenticated wether by written signature, electronic signature, computer key, or rubber stamp.	IM.6.10 EP4
45	The author authenticates either by written signature, electronic signature, computer key, or rubber stamp the following: - The history and physical examination - Operative reports - Consultations - Discharge summary	IM.6.10 EP5
46	Medical records contain, as applicable, the following clinical/case information: - Goals of the treatment and treatment plans - Diagnostic and therapeutic procedures, tests and results - Progress notes made by authorized individuals - Relevant observations - Consultation reports - Medications ordered or prescribed	IM.6.20 EP1
47	Verbal or telephone orders are dated and identify the names of the individuals who gave, received, and implemented the order.	IM.6.50 EP2
48	When required by law or regulation, verbal or telephone orders are authenticated within the specified time frame.	IM.6.50 EP3

FIGURE 21-9 Documentation of patient care.

Discharge Information

55	When indicated and before discharge, the hospital arranges for or helps the family arrange for services needed to meet the patient's needs after discharge.	PC.15.20E P8
56	Written discharge instructions in a form the patient can understand are given to the patient and/or those responsible for providing continuing care.	PC.15.20E P9
57	The hospital communicates appropriate information to any organization or provider to which the patient is transferred or discharged.	PC.15.30 EP1
58	The information shared includes the following, as appropriate to the care, treatment, and services provided: - The reason for transfer or discharge - The patient's physical and psychosocial status - A summary of care, treatment, and services provided and progress toward goals - Community resources or referrals provided to the patient	PC.15.30 EP2
59	A concise discharge summary providing information to other caregivers and facilitating continuity of care includes the following: - The reason for hospitalization - Significant findings - Procedures performed and care, treatment, and services provided - The patients condition at discharge - Information provided to the patient and family, as appropriate	IM.6.10 EP7

FIGURE 21-10 Patient discharge information.

SUMMARY

- In any hospital in United States, the use of any medical equipment has to follow guidelines established by the appropriate regulatory agencies. In addition, there are several standards organizations that periodically upate these guidelines.
- The chapter discusses the role of regulatory agencies such as FDA, CDRH, ORA, and SMDA. The FDA regulates a medical device from the concept to the manufacturing and finally to its use in the hospital. Class I devices are the least complicated and their failure poses little risk. Class II devices are more complicated than class I, but they are non–life-sustaining devices. Class III devices sustain or support life and their failure is life-threatening.
- A 510(k) is a premarketing submission made to the FDA to demonstrate that a device is safe before it is marketed. A PMA is an application submitted to the FDA to request clearance to market class III devices.
- Next, the standards organizations are discussed: NFPA, CLIA, CAP, JC, and CARF. These organizations accredit and certify hospitals that abide by their standards.
- At the end of the chapter, the role of OSHA and HIPAA regulatory agencies in patient care is covered.

MEDICAL TERMINOLOGY

American National Standards Institute (ANSI): coordinates the development and use of voluntary standards in the United States and around the world.

Commission on Accreditation of Rehabilitation Facilities (CARF): an independent, non-profit agency that accredits human service providers in the area of rehabilitation, child and family, community, employment, and aging services.

Center for Disease and Radiological Health (CDRH): Provides independent, professional expertise and technical assistance on the development, safety, and regulation of medical devices and electronic products that produce radiation.

Clinical Laboratory Improvement Amendments (CLIA): In 1988, established quality standards for all laboratory testing to ensure accurate, reliable, and timely patient test results regardless of where the test was performed.

Food and Drug Administration (FDA): Government agency responsible for regulating food, drugs, medical devices, biologics, animal feed and drugs, cosmetics, and radiation-emitting products.

International Organization for Standardization (ISO): is a non-governmental organization that develops and publishes international standards on a variety of subjects including medical equipment.

U.S. Department of Health and Human Services (HHS): United States government's primary agency for protecting the health of all Americans and providing essential human services.

Health Insurance Portability and Accountability Act (HIPAA): 1996 act to improve portability and continuity of health insurance coverage to combat waste, fraud, and abuse in health insurance and health care delivery.

Joint Commission on Accreditation of Health Care Organization (JC): the Joint Commission evaluates and accredits health care organizations and programs in the United States.

Medical Device Regulation: Regulated by the FDA, medical devices must comply with applicable U.S. laws before, during, and after importation.

Occupational Safety and Health Administration (OSHA): Federal agency responsible for ensuring worker safety and health in the United States.

QUIZ

1. The FDA is under the ________________.

a) State Department

b) Center for Devices and Radiological Health (CDRH)

c) Department of Health and Human Services (HHS)

d) IRS (Internal Revenue Service)

2. The organization that is responsible for ensuring the safety and effectiveness of medical devices is ________________.

a) The Office of Health Affairs

b) The Office of Compliance
c) JC (Joint Commission on Accreditation of Health Care Organizations)
d) None of the above

3. HIPAA's privacy rule protects ________________.
a) The privacy of health care provider health information
b) The privacy of patient banking and SSI information
c) The privacy of patient health information
d) None of the above

4. Under HIPAA's Privacy Rule, the patient's health information may be disclosed for:
a) ________________________________
b) ________________________________
c) ________________________________

5. Electronic PHI (Personal Health Information) can be found in:
a) ________________________________
b) ________________________________
c) ________________________________

6. The primary accrediting agency for hospital laboratories is the ________________.
a) FDA
b) CARF
c) CAP
d) CLIA

7. A Premarket Approval Application (PMA) is ________________.
a) A private license granted for marketing a device
b) A process of review of class III medical devices
c) Approved by the Office of Regulatory Affairs (ORA)

8. OSHA is ________________.
a) An agency of the U.S. Department of Health and Human Services
b) Not a regulatory agency but sets up the standards
c) To prevent work-related injuries
d) None of the above

9. NFPA stands for ________________
a) National Fluid Power Association
b) National Federation of Paralegal Association
c) National Fire Protection Association
d) National Foster Parent Association

10. What does the Safe Medical Device Act (SMDA) propose?

____

PROBLEMS

1. What are the required procedures, documents, and records in Medical Device Reporting (MDR) in general, at your local hospital? Provide a discussion with at least one example.
2. Provide an overview of a specific medical device design and its control.
3. Define PMN 510(K), PMA, IDE, GMP, and QS.
4. Through the FDA's Web site, identify the most recent regulatory status of a medical device, and the rationale of the steps taken.
5. Discuss the recommended practices for the safe handling and decontamination of medical devices. Also, identify the appropriate associations and their recommendations in this matter.
6. Provide at least three examples each for Class I, II, and III medical devices.
7. Make a list of information that is required by the HIPAA regulation when a patient is admitted and discharged from a hospital. The reader may use the Internet for collecting information for this problem.
8. Discuss in detail the NFPA hospital safety standards (NFPA 99)and suggest a reference guide for the biomedical engineering staff.
9. Make a list of the OSHA regulations with which hospitals are required to comply. Also, discuss the penalties, if any, of a hospital's failure to comply with OSHA regulations.
10. Make a list of hospital equipment that may emit unacceptable electromagnetic radiation as per CDRH regulations. Also, discuss the penalties, if any, of a hospital's failure to comply with CDRH regulations.

CASE STUDY

A case study is done on the PGP Universal System developed by PGP Corporation in California.

The system implements secure e-mail transmissions for confidential medical data transfers. Even though HIPAA regulations are provided to hospitals, the PGP Universal System claims to have a better encrypting process. The questions to be answered for this case are:

a) What are the HIPAA guidelines in e-mail transfers?

b) What is encryption? Provide examples.

c) How are PGP Universal Systems different from other products?

RESEARCH TOPIC

How are pre- and postmarket medical device clinical studies done? The researcher must collect information from at least two vendors. The research paper should also include a checklist of the guidelines from the FDA on this subject. The collection of clinical data must show the evaluation of safety performance of the device.

CHAPTER 22

Preventive Maintenance

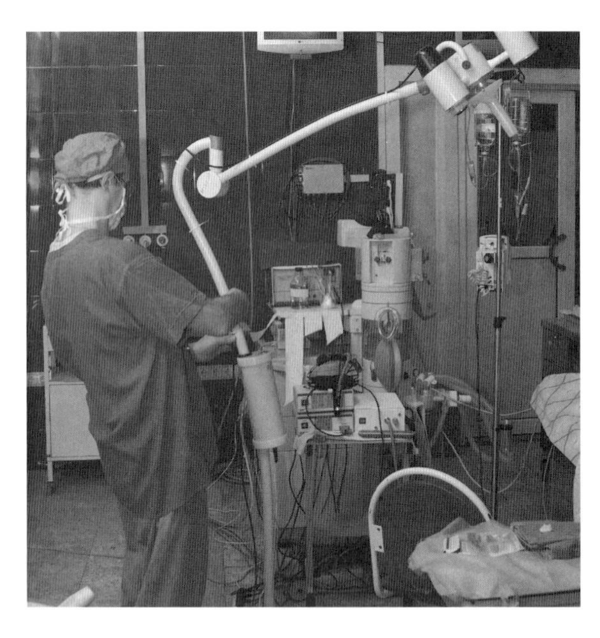

CHAPTER OUTLINE

OBJECTIVE

The objective of this chapter is to familiarize the reader with the scheduled maintenance of medical equipment and to instruct the reader on the basic maintenance of most medical equipment.

INTERNET WEB SITES

http://www.fda.gov (U.S. Food and Drug Administration)
http://www.jointcommission.org (The Joint Commission)
http://www.ecri.org (Emergency Care Research Institute)

INTRODUCTION

All medical equipment in a health care environment should be included in a routine, structured, equipment maintenance plan. The purpose of the scheduled maintenance plan is to perform inspections and calibrations on equipment in order to prevent premature failures. An organizational chart of the biomedical engineering department at the Ohio State University Hospital in Columbus is shown in **Figure 22-1.** The Biomedical Electronics Technician is responsible to managers of both imaging services and biomedical services. In some hospitals, imaging services are done only by outside vendors, such as GE Healthcare or Phillips Medical.

FIGURE 22-1 An organizational chart of the biomedical engineering department at OSU.

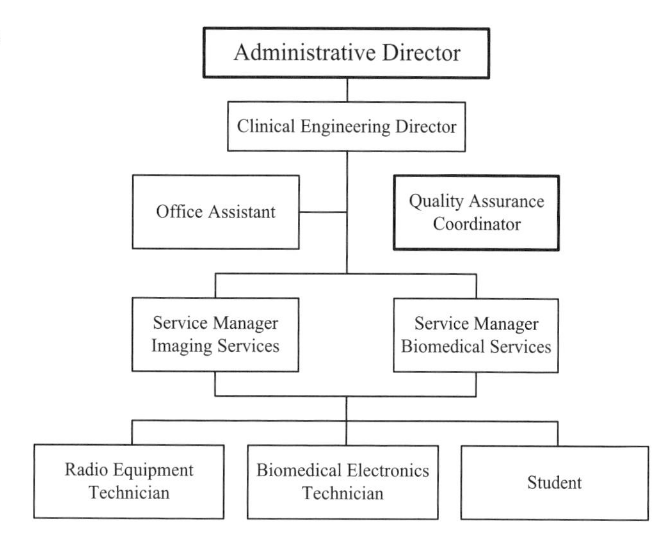

While the FDA classifies medical equipment into Class I, Class II, and Class III in increasing order of risk to the patient should the equipment fail, some local hospitals (including those mentioned previously) classify equipment into three categories called Tier 1, Tier 2, and Tier 3: Tier 1 contains life-support or life-saving equipment, which usually requires frequent maintenance; Tier 2 contains non–life-support equipment that may require only annual maintenance; and Tier 3 contains equipment whose failure can cause no harm to the patient, and whose frequency of maintenance can be reduced to less than once a year if the facility safety committee and the hospital administration both approve.

In addition to the medical equipment maintenance plans in any hospital for BMETs, there is also a hospital maintenance plan for several other essential equipment needs that must be taken care of; the list is given in **Figure 22-2.** The BMET may or may not be responsible for the preventive maintenance (PM) of this equipment.

Hospital Maintenance

- Air Conditioning & Heating
- Appliances
- Autoclaves & Sterilizers
- Carpentry& Cabinetry
- Clocks
- Code 10 System
- Construction Projects
- Electric Service
- Emergency Power
- Equipment Acquisition and Installation
- Exhibits and Special Events
- Fire Protection Systems
- Fume Hoods
- Furniture and Modular Partitions
- Gas Cylinders
- Interior Building Maintenance
- Laboratory and Clinical Equipment
- Light Bulb Replacement
- Masonry
- Nurse Call System
- Painting
- Plumbing
- Pneumatic Tube System
- Preventive Maintenance
- Refrigeration Equipment
- Roofs and Access to Roofs
- Services by Other Departments
- Wall Mounted Items
- Wallpaper and Wall Coverings
- Windows and Window Treatment

FIGURE 22-2 A maintenance plan for equipment in a hospital.

22.1 TIER 1 EQUIPMENT

Tier 1 equipment is life supporting or life saving. Examples of equipment in this tier include defibrillators, ventilators, anesthesia equipment, balloon pumps, and heart-lung machines. The frequency of scheduled maintenance on this equipment is usually dictated by the equipment manufacturer. Often the recommendation is semiannual maintenance; however, this can be more frequent, sometimes monthly or quarterly depending on the equipment and the frequency of nonscheduled maintenance.

22.2 TIER 2 EQUIPMENT

Tier 2 equipment consists of those items that do not fall into the Tier 1 category but still require scheduled maintenance at least once per year based on the manufacturer's recommendation. Examples of equipment in this tier include infusion pumps, syringe pumps, most patient physiological monitors, and infant warmers. The frequency of maintenance for these items can also be adjusted based on the frequency of nonscheduled repairs and with facility safety committee approval.

22.3 TIER 3 EQUIPMENT

If a scheduled maintenance program will have no effect on whether or not a particular piece of equipment fails, the facility may decide to schedule maintenance for this equipment at intervals of several years. This must be done with the approval of both the facility safety committee and the facility administration.

22.4 SCHEDULED MAINTENANCE PLAN

This section uses the Ohio State University Health System's Equipment Management Plan as an example for instruction.

Clinical engineering ensures the accuracy, safety, and proper performance of all electrically powered, as well as nonelectrical, medical equipment. The acquisition, testing, inspection, and repair of existing and incoming patient-care equipment, and the use of borrowed and patient- or staff-owned equipment will be performed in accordance with the established recommendations.

The clinical engineering services department maintains the inventory of medical equipment. The preventive maintenance program for this equipment is risk-based and is approved by the Environment of Care Committee.

- Each device is assigned a unique identification number.
- Each device is assigned a risk level based on recommended list.
- Each device is assigned a degree of injury associated with a malfunction.
- Each device is assigned a stability of design.
- Each device is assigned a performance criteria.

When entered into the database, every device is assigned to a facility, cost center, department, control number, risk level, and preventive maintenance (PM) schedule. PM work orders for the month are generated at the beginning of that month. Work orders are assigned to the technicians responsible for each particular location. On-time completion and problems identified during PM are communicated back to the area manager.

On a monthly basis and upon request, reports are made available to area managers. The report includes:

- An equipment inventory for the area.
- A list of completed PM work orders.
- A list of open PM work orders.
- A list of repair work orders.

The performance standards are routinely monitored and reported to one or more of the following: Clinical Engineering Services Director, Environment of Care Committee, and the affected department director(s)/manager(s).

In **Figure 22-3,** Risk Tier number is between 1 and 7 in the OSU Health System. This is different compared to other hospitals. But, the patient death due to device malfunction is

The Ohio State University Health System

Equipment Inclusion Evaluation Criteria

Equipment Function (FC):		(max score = 5)	Score
Therapeutic:			
	Life Support		5
	Surgical and Intensive Care		4
	Therapy and Treatment		3
Diagnostic:			
	Diagnostic Imaging		4
	Physiological Monitoring		3
Analytic:			
	Clinical Laboratory		4
	Diagnostic Support		3
Miscellaneous Patient Care:			
	Direct Patient Contact		1
	No Patient Contact		0

Physical Risk Associated with Clinical Application (RC):		(max score = 5)	Score
A device malfunction that could result in:			
	Patient Death	Risk Tier #1	5
	Patient or Operator Injury	Risk Tier #2	4
	Inappropriate Therapy or Misdiagnosis	Risk Tier #3-5	2
	No Significant Risks	Risk Tier #6-7	0

Maintenance Requirements (MC):		(max score = 5)	Score
Extensive:			
	Includes equipment that requires routine alignment, calibration or extensive parts replacement		5
Average:			
	Includes equipment that receives preventive maintenance, electrical safety and basic performance testing. Safety training is minimal		3
Operator:			
	Operator function testing		1

Equipment Incident/Failure History (HC)		(max score = 5)	Score
	Objective (on a case by case basis)		

Inclusion Factor = FC + RC + MC + HC. Include equipment in the program if the inclusion factor score is eight (8) or greater. Maintenance requirements of three (3) or greater also require inclusion in the program.

FIGURE 22-3 Equipment evaluation criteria in Ohio State University health system.

Equipment Description	PM Per Year	Risk Level
Alarm Device	0	5
Analyzer, Alcohol, Breath	0	5
Analyzer, Blood Gas, PH	0	3
Analyzer, Clinical Chemistry	0	4
Analyzer, Coagulation	0	4
Analyzer, Electrolyte	0	4
Analyzer, Hematology	0	4
Analyzer, Medical Gas, O_2	0	4
Analyzer, Microbiology	0	4
Analyzer, Platelet Aggregation	0	4
Analyzer, Urine	0	4
Anesthesia Machine	3	1
Anesthesia Ventilator	3	1
Aspirator	0	4
Bath, Dry, Heat	0	4
Battery, Analyzer, Charger	0	4

FIGURE 22-4 A list of risk level for equipment.

always considered Risk Tier 1 in all hospitals. A small list of PM per year and the risk level associated with the equipment is given in **Figure 22-4.**

Several standards are followed on PM completion and safety and a list of such responsibilities is given in **Figure 22-5.** The Clinical Engineering staff receiving less than 12 points requires improvement. This is shown in **Figure 22-6.**

22.5 CALIBRATION

Medical equipment calibration can be done by either the BMETs in the hospital, or by an outside vendor. The calibration must meet the guidelines put forth by the FDA, CLIA, and other organizations. For this reason, outside vendors who offer calibration services will hire some individuals who are certified in this area.

The calibration of electrosurgical units, ECG machines, defibrillators, bedside monitors, ventilators, pulse oximeters, syringe pumps, sphygmomanometers, and others must take place as scheduled. These machines are provided by their manufacturers with product manuals that explain in detail the procedures for proper calibration. For example, the calibration guidelines and procedure for the ESCORT II 3 Trace Patient Monitor manufactured by MDE (Medical Data Electronics) are shown on pages 634–635.

Indicator	Standard	Threshold	Data Source/EC Standard	Report to and Frequency
New Employee Orientation	New Employee will receive orientation in two (2) areas: Hospital and Department	100%	HR Stats (Safety Management)	Director of Clinical Engineering/Annually
Mandatory Training	All Clinical Engineering Service employees will complete annual Safety Education	100%	HR Stats (Safety Management)	Human Resources/Annually
Preventive Maintenance Completion	100% of Life-support equipment scheduled for Preventive Maintence in a given month is completed within 60 days from the end of the scheduled month. Life-support equipment is included in Risk Tier #1	100%	JCAHO, Manufacturer, AHA, AAMI	Environment of Care Committee/ Quarterly
	≥ 95% of Non-life-support equipment scheduled for Preventive Maintenance in a given month is completed within 60 days from the end of the scheduled month.	≥ 95%	JCAHO, Manufacturer, AHA, AAMI	Environment of Care Committee/ Quarterly
Device Alerts	All device alerts will be documented and forwarded to affected users	100%	FDA, Manufacturer, ECRI, (Safety Management)	Environment of Care Committee/ Quarterly

FIGURE 22-5 A list of procedures for clinical engineering staff. (*Continued*)

Occurrence Reports	All Occurrence Reports involving patient care equipment will be reviewed and forwarded to the Risk Manager	100%	FDA (Safety Management)	Environment of Care Committee/ Quarterly
Repetitive Failures	All devices included in the Plan will be monitored for repetitive failures	> 3 failures in 30 days	Clinical Engineering	Environment of Care Committee/ Quarterly
PI Service Documentation Review	Each technician's service documentation will be reviewed annually as noted on the PI Service Documentation Review Form	100%	Clinical Engineering, Patient Care Equipment Management Plan	Director of Clinical Engineering / Annually
Employee Continuing Education / Knowledge	Employee knowledge of clinical and biomedical engineering fundamentals and general safety will be reviewed via observation	100%	Clinical Engineering, ASHE, ICC, (Safety Management Emergency Preparedness)	Director of Clinical Engineering, Envionment of Care Committee / Annually
Customer Satisfaction	Maintain a high level of customer satisfaction as evidenced by the annual customer survey	$\geq$ 85%		Environment of Care Committee/ Annually

FIGURE 22-5 (*Continued*)

Clinical Engineering Service Staff
Performance Improvement Service
Documentation Review

Date: ____________________
Reviewed by: ____________________
Associate name: ____________________

Evaluation Item
Use of appropriate PM procedures
Compliance with program service recommendations
Completion of scheduled service
Completeness of Record

Ratings on a 1-5 scale (lowest to highest). Less than 12 points indicates a need foı improvement and follow-up review.

Comments: ____________________

FIGURE 22-6 Clinical engineering staff performance evaluation at OSU.

- MDE recommends a yearly performance check to verify all functions on the ESCORT II monitor. At the conclusion of the performance check, turn power off and back on again. Ensure that all default settings return.
- The following equipment (or equivalent) is needed to do the performance tests on the ESCORT II monitor. Refer to the manufacturer's operating procedures for detailed information. All test equipment used should be in good working condition and calibrated, if necessary:
  1. MDE Datasim 6000 Patient Simulator
  2. Resistive 3-lead and 5-lead ECG cables and leads
  3. IEC-601.1 Continuity Tester
  4. ECG shorting plug (All leads shorted together)
  5. Ohmic Instruments, Biomedical Electrical Test Set Model BET-300A
  6. Variac/current box
  7. DC power supply with 3.5mm connector
- Begin with a thorough visual inspection of the unit. Inspect the power cord for cracks or exposed conductors. Replace power cord, if defective.
- **Patient Input Leakage**

  Connect the ECG shorting plug to the ESCORT II's ECG input. Set the Biomedical Electrical Test Set to read patient input leakage. Ensure that the leakage current is less than 10 μA. Select CASE to GND and NORM on the Test Set. Ensure that the leakage current is less than 20 μA (the maximum allowable current at the end of the shorting cable).
- **Chassis Ground Resistance Test**

  Connect the AC plug of the IEC-601.1 Continuity Tester to the AC input of the ESCORT II monitor. Using the test probe of the Continuity Tester, make contact to unpainted metal on the monitor. Repeat the chassis ground resistance test to the recorder guide-posts, and other unpainted metal portions on the monitor. The resistance must be no more than 0.5 Ω.
- **ECG Tests**

  Note: When using a patient stimulator, the tolerance factor of the simulator must be considered in determining whether the monitor is within tolerance.
- **ECG Lead Check**

  Connect a 5-lead ECG cable to a calibrated patient simulator. Connect the ECG cable to the ECG connector of the ESCORT II monitor. Press the PAGE HOME function key. Press the softkey adjacent to the ECG label. Set the sweep speed to 25mm/sec. Press the LEAD SEL softkey. Select 5-lead mode. Ensure that an acceptable ECG waveform is displayed.
- **Lead Fail and Baseline Reset Tests**

  Connect a 3-lead ECG cable to the patient simulator. Select 3-lead mode and ensure that Lead II is selected. Remove one lead from the patient simulator. Observe the CHK LEADS message on the screen. Repeat for LL, LA, and RA leads.

- **ECG Calibration**

  Note: Disconnect all parameter cables (except the ECG cable) during the test. Ensure that ECG is set to monitor Lead II.

  Press the PAGE HOME function key. Press the softkey adjacent to the ECG label. Press the NEXT PAGE function key. Press the CAL softkey and verify the calibration pulse on the monitor's screen. Increase the waveform size, using the SIZE softkey, if necessary. Run a recorder strip and verify that the R-wave amplitude is 1 mV peak-to-peak from the isoelectric line to the R-wave peak ± 0.1mV. If the ESCORT II is not equipped with a recorder, press the CAL softkey. Ensure that a calibration pulse is generated on the screen and that the ECG amplitude is within 15 percent of the calibration pulse amplitude.

SUMMARY

The chapter introduces the reader to the schedule of the preventive maintenance of medical equipment and also the responsibilities of the BMETs in a hospital.

1. In the beginning of the chapter, classification of equipment into Tiers 1, 2, and 3 is discussed. Life-saving equipment is Tier 1 equipment, non–life-support equipment is Tier 2, and equipment that, should it fail, will not harm the patient is Tier 3.
2. Next, the maintenance schedules for Tier 1, 2, and 3 types of equipment are explained. Tier 1 equipment requires frequent maintenance, Tier 2 equipment may require annual maintenance, and Tier 3 equipment may require annual or less than yearly maintenance, based upon approval.
3. Finally, the process of calibrating equipment is covered. The simple and pertinent steps of calibration on the ESCORT II Patient Monitor are explained.

MEDICAL TERMINOLOGY

Biomedical services: technical support provided to the health care industry for maintaining and servicing medical equipment.

Biomedical Equipment Technician (BMET): professionals responsible for maintaining a facility's medical and patient care equipment.

Clinical engineer: person that supports and advances patient care by applying engineering and managerial skills to assist the health care industry with developing technology.

Preventive maintenance: a schedule of planned and systematic actions aimed at preventing breakdowns or failures. Designed to preserve and enhance equipment reliability.

QUIZ

1. If the equipment requires frequent maintenance the equipment is ________________.

   a) Tier 1 equipment

   b) Tier 2 equipment

   c) Tier 3 equipment

2. The most important issues of a Medical Equipment Management Plan in a hospital are:

   a) ____________________

   b) ____________________

   c) ____________________

3. In maintaining the inventory of medical equipment, each device is assigned a unique ____________. Also, each device is assigned a ____________.

4. List *at least three* pieces of equipment used in PM procedures:

   a) ____________________

   b) ____________________

   c) ____________________

   d) ____________________

   e) ____________________

5. What are the specific steps recommended in electronic troubleshooting of medical equipment? Explain in detail.

6. When a BMET calibrates medical equipment, what is he or she trying to do?

7. The leakage current must be less than ____________:

   a) 30 μA b) 20 μA c) 10 μA d) None of the above

8. The chassis ground resistance must be less than ____________:

   a) 10 ohms b) 0.5 ohms c) 5 ohms d) None of the above

9. The test equipment needed to measure output in joules:

   a) Oscilloscope b) Defibrillator tester c) DMM

10. The safety analyzer is used for

    ____________________________________.

PROBLEMS

The reader may visit the clinical engineering department of a hospital or use the Internet to answer the following problems.

1. Create a list of the Tier 1 devices used in a hospital. Include the cost of the PM procedure for each piece of equipment in the list.

2. Write the steps in calibrating a(n):

   a) ECG machine b) Pressure monitor

   c) Defibrillator d) Dialysis machine

3. What do BMETs achieve by using a patient simulator? List the advantages and disadvantages of simulation, and also determine simulation objectives in regard to PM procedures.

4. Discuss PM procedures related to clinical laboratory equipment in terms of failures, repairs, and recurring problems. Also, list the routine maintenance steps.

5. Compile a list of questions frequently asked of a hospital's clinical engineering department concerning medical equipment maintenance.
6. Discuss an emergency situation in a hospital in which a piece of medical equipment becomes a possible risk to the safety of either an employee or a patient. Explain what needs to be done in such an emergency.
7. Make a list of test equipment—both specialized and common—that is used to check the correct functioning of medical equipment in a hospital. Describe what each piece of test equipment does.
8. Discuss PM procedures on an anesthesia machine.
9. Write down the calibration steps for an electrosurgical machine and discuss the PM procedures for the machine.
10. Discuss PDAs or any wireless device used by the clinical engineering personnel to repair a piece of medical equipment.

RESEARCH TOPIC

A large hospital may have up to 10,000 pieces of equipment that are used in various departments. Each piece of equipment incurs wear and tear, and certain parts of that equipment will wear more than other parts. Select a group of medical devices and determine the parts that must be repaired or replaced most often. Investigate the reasons for malfunctions and the cost of maintenance. The paper may include guidelines to reduce the malfunctions at the component level.

CASE STUDY

Pervidi and Grand–PM provide hospitals and technicians with computerized maintenance management systems. The combination of PDAs, software, and Web portals is designed to manage maintenance for the biomedical industry. Critical equipment and systems are managed by these software products to provide proper preventive maintenance. The case study should discuss the uniqueness of these products and how they are useful to hospitals.

CHAPTER 23

Computers and Telemedicine

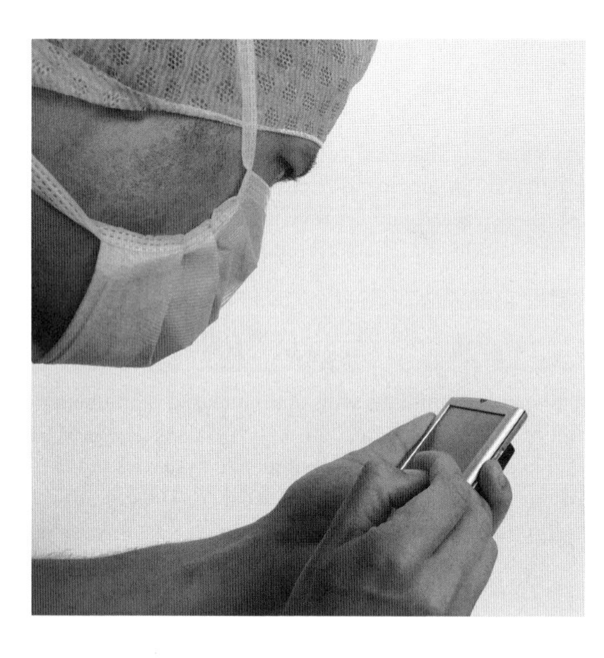

■ CHAPTER OUTLINE

■ OBJECTIVES

The objective of this chapter is to introduce the reader to local- and wide-area computer networks inside and outside of hospitals and the concepts in telemedicine, picture archiving and communication systems, and the Digital Imaging and Communications in Medicine standards.

Upon completion of the chapter, the reader will be able to:

- Describe the computer networks in hospitals.
- Discuss components of local area networks and wide area networks.
- Describe teleradiology.
- Define elements of picture archiving and communication systems.
- Discuss Digital Imaging and Communications in Medicine standards.
- Describe various types of personal digital assistants.

■ INTERNET WEB SITES

http://www.atmeda.org (The American Telemedicine Association)
http://www.hrsa.gov/telehealth (Human Resources and Services Administration/Telehealth)

■ INTRODUCTION

Over the past decade, the implementation of a computer infrastructure that enables hospitals to process and transmit medical data over local area networks (LANs), wide area networks (WANs), and wireless networks has gained tremendous momentum. Networks of Digital Imaging and Communications in Medicine (DICOM), picture archiving and communication systems (PACS), and Health Level Seven (HL7) are used in small clinics and large hospitals worldwide. This chapter explains the concepts of these computer networks, communication systems, as well as the concept of telemedicine, and its standards and protocols in health care delivery.

■

23.1 THE DIGITAL HOSPITAL

'Computer-assisted technology' in medicine covers the computer infrastructure in accessing, visualizing, manipulating, and transferring medical data over both wired and wireless communication networks. Patient care starts with the point of care technology, such as radio frequency identification (RFID) or voice recognition, and progresses to telemedicine as the patient transitions to subacute or to the outpatient status. Often, RFID is superior to bar codes for data capture because it does not require a line of sight; for example, if they are using an RFID reader, nurses do not have to move a patient's arm to match up their wristband as they would if they were using a bar code reader.

The patient is identified with the technology of RFID on the hospital's or clinic's local area network (LAN) called the intranet. The intranet of a hospital works concurrently with the global Internet (the wide area network, or WAN) to allow health care workers and professionals to communicate patient information expeditiously.

In addition to exchanging patient data, the networks allow the exchange of what is called core hospital information services, which include physician documents about the patient, teaching and research information, telemedicine, bioinformatics, and the computer software, among other services. An example of core hospital information services is shown in **Figure 23-1.**

23.2 COMPUTER NETWORKS IN HOSPITALS

The communications network in a hospital can be complex, with larger hospitals utilizing several intranet systems at once. An example of a hospital computer network is shown in **Figure 23-2**. Here you will see that the OR, ICU, and radiology LANs are connected through routers and switches, which allows communication among departments. Notice the WAN connections in the figure showing the data that is to be transferred to the Internet.

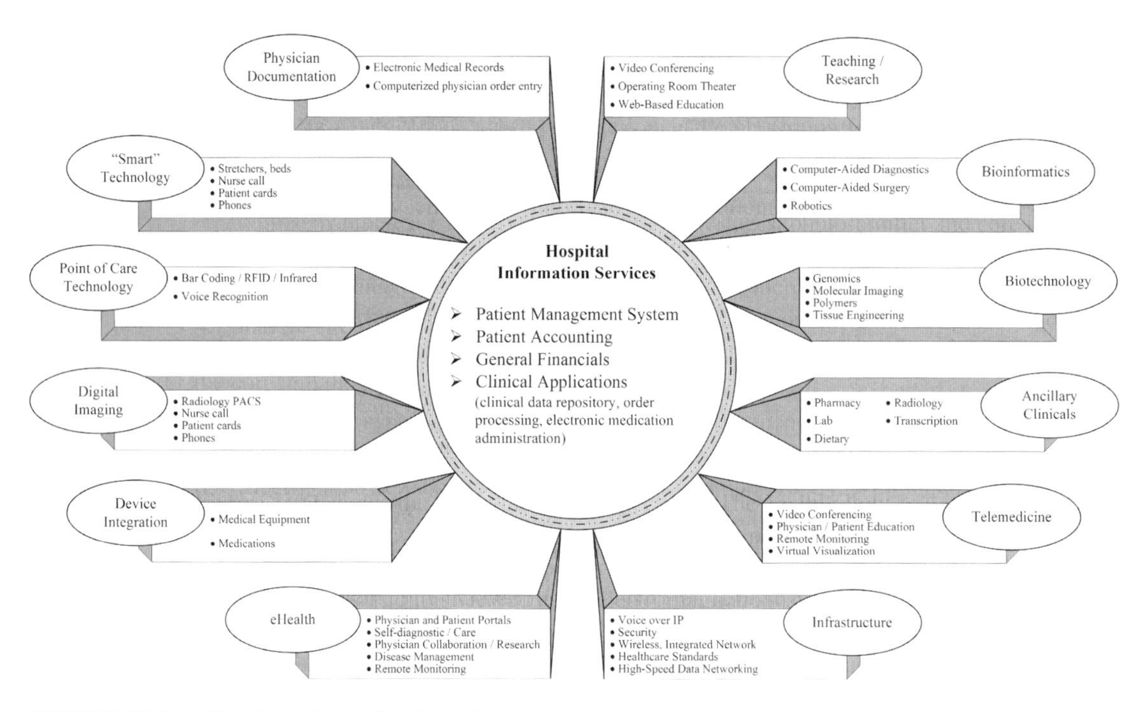

FIGURE 23-1 A list of core hospital information services.

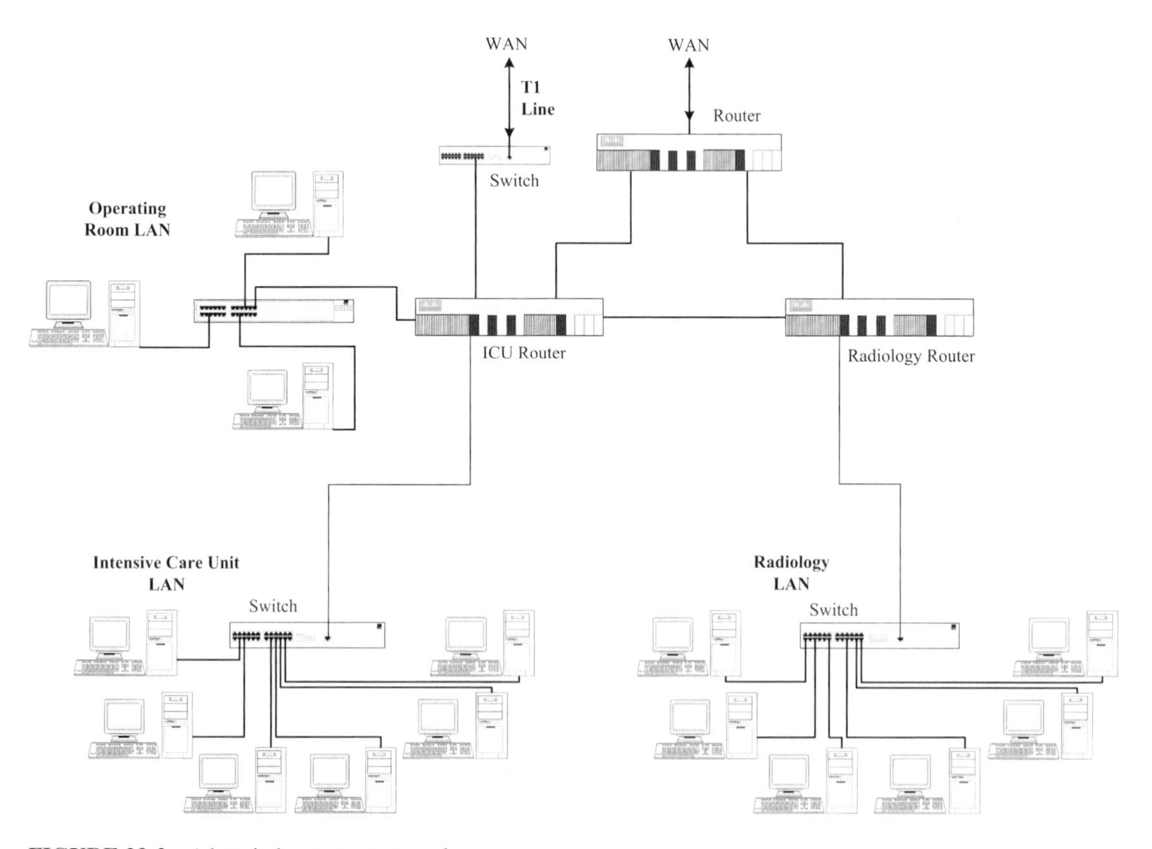

FIGURE 23-2 A hospital computer network.

23.3 COMPUTER SYSTEMS: HARDWARE AND SOFTWARE

The computer hardware used for LAN communication consists of network interface cards (NICs), network cables, hubs, switches, routers, and printers. The main software on any computer is the operating system, such as Windows XP, Vista, Novell Netware, Macintosh, or Linux. The interface to the Internet is then through a private branch exchange (PBX) switch, default gateway (a sophisticated router), modem, and a WAN line such as T1 or Synchronous Optical Network (SONET).

The layout, or topology, of cables in a network is carefully planned and can be categorized as bus-, star-, or ring-types of connections. The cables are expensive; the size of the room and the number of computers it will connect determine which type of topology is suitable.

The most common topology is the star topology, as shown in **Figure 23-3a**. Here, a central node (or hub or switch) is directly connected to the workstations. Because of centralization, troubleshooting the LAN is simple. The copper cable has RJ45 connectors at both ends (i.e., at the computer and also at the hub). The cable is twisted-pair and is graded as 10 Base T, with a speed of 10 megabits per second or 100 Base T with 100 megabits per second speed.

In bus topology, the computers are connected to one common cable (called the bus). Bus topology generally uses more cabling than other topologies because there is no central hub, so each NIC must be connected directly to the bus. Bus topology is uncommon in local area networks; it is used mainly in wide area networks.

Ring topology, as shown in **Figure 23-b,** is based on the process of token passing. It has computers connected in a circle, with each computer having equal access to the network.

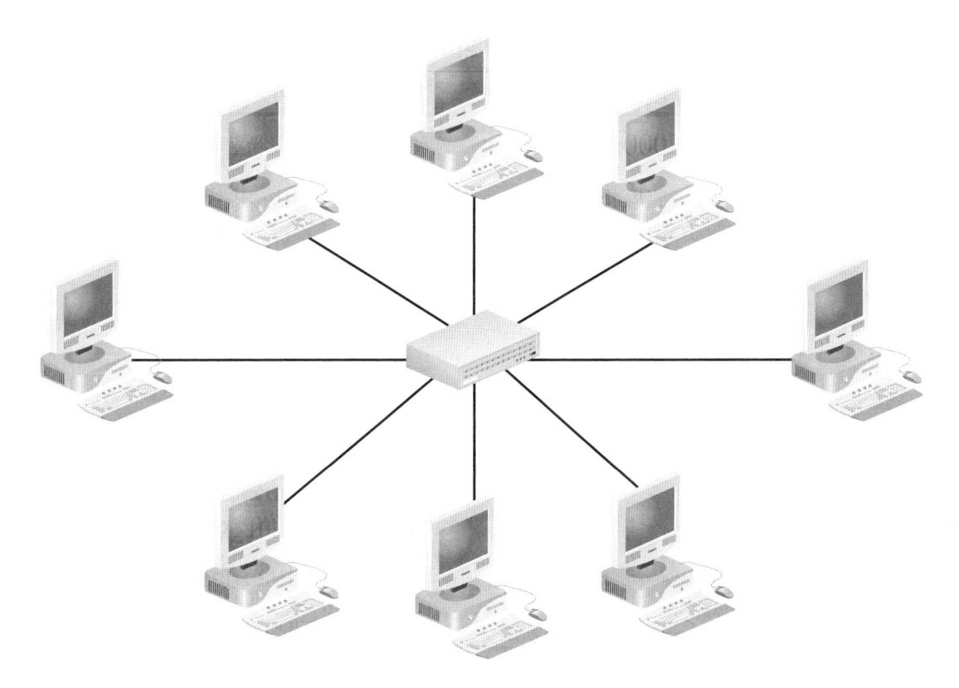

FIGURE 23-3a Star topology.

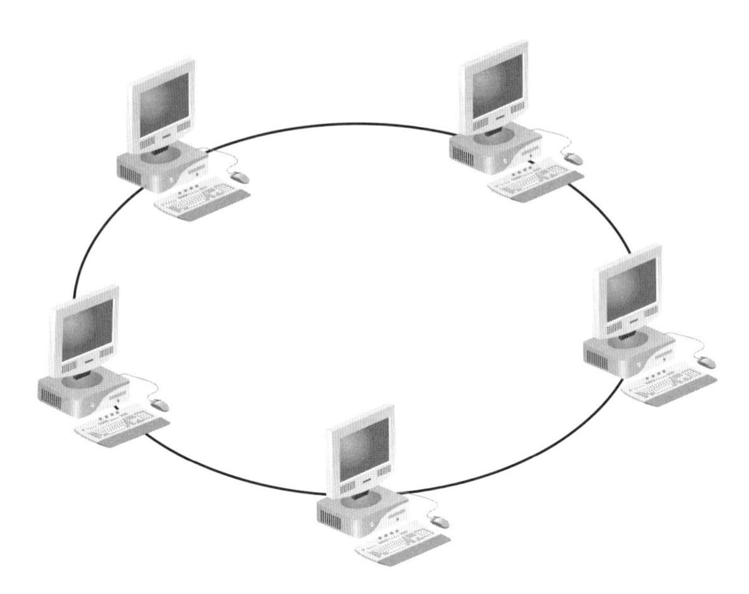

FIGURE 23-3b Ring topology.

A token is a set of a bit pattern that is required when a computer has data that it wants to send to another computer on the network. The token is then passed to the next computer after the data is sent.

The star and bus topologies use carrier sense multiple access collision detect (CSMA/CD). In this process, more than one computer tries to access the network at the same time; the data from one computer collides with the data from another computer, and the NIC cards detect the collision and discontinue sending data for a random time. CSMA/CD compatible networks allow only one computer at a time to access the network.

Transmission Control Protocol/Internet Protocol (TCP/IP) Internet suite consists of four layers: the application layer, transport layer, Internet layer, and Ethernet layer. These layers are part of the operating system and perform specific tasks, such as sending e-mail, transferring files, or accessing Web services on the Internet. One of the important functions of the TCP/IP suite is the addressing scheme for the computers. The scheme includes physical addressing, IP addressing, and port addressing. The physical address belongs to the Ethernet layer, IP belongs to the Internet layer, and the port address belongs to the transport layer. These layers are explained in the following list:

- **Application layer:** This layer supports the applications that the user wants to connect to the network; for example, file transfer services, accessing Web services on the Internet, e-mail services, and remote file access. Some of the protocols of the application layer are file transfer protocol (FTP), hypertext transfer protocol (HTTP) for Web services, and simple mail transfer protocol (SMTP).
- **Transport layer:** This layer divides a transmitting message into smaller data packets and then reassembles it at the receiving end. It initiates "handshaking" between computers and provides port addresses of the transmitting and the receiving computers.

Two of the transport layer protocols are transmission control protocol (TCP) and user-datagram protocol (UDP).

- **Internet layer:** This layer performs routing and deals with the IP addressing of the sending and receiving computers. Some of the Internet protocols are Internet protocol (IP), X.25, and Internet protocol exchange (IPX).

  IP addressing is a four-byte dotted decimal address followed by a four-byte mask. The first byte indicates the class. Class A starts from 0 and ends at 127, class B starts from 128 and ends at 191, and class C starts at 192 and ends at 223. The mask bits start with a sequence of binary 1's (from left to right) representing a network field and then end in binary zeros representing a host field.

  As an example, a class A network is given as 65.0.0.0 and its mask bits are 255.0.0.0. The 65. and 255. are aligned such that the host addresses can be placed in the next three bytes. One of the host addresses in this network can be assigned as 65.10.10.55. The total number of hosts in class network is then $2^{24} - 2$. As all zeros and all 1's are not used, the total number of hosts is reduced by two.

  The address of a small class C network is given as 200.20.20.0 and its associated mask bits are 255.255.255.0. One of the hosts in this network is given as 200.20.20.200. The total number of hosts in this network is then $2^{8} - 2$. Notice the number of hosts in class C is only 254 hosts.

- **Ethernet layer:** This layer is concerned with the MAC (media access control) addressing, issues of voltage levels, bit synchronization, and detecting errors. Some of the Ethernet layer protocols are high-level data link control (HDLC), Ethernet II, and IEEE 802.3. A complete data frame is made with forward and trailing headers at this layer. The forward header consists of synchronization bytes, MAC addresses, IP addresses, port addresses, and the type of data, whereas the trailing header consists of error-detecting code and the ending bytes. An example of an IEEE 802.3 frame follows:

Preamble	SFD	Destination	Source	Length & LLC	Data	FCS

  Number of bytes in each field are: Preamble (7), Start Frame Delimiter (1), Destination (6), Source (6), Length (2) & Logical Link Control (3), Data (43 to 1497), and Frame Check Sequence (4). Length & LLC indicate the length and type of data, whereas FCS indicates the error-detecting code.

A small medical office wireline and wireless networks are shown in **Figure 23-4** and **Figure 23-5**, respectively. In the wireline network, the computers are connected to each other directly through the network cables; however, as you can see, the wireless network connects the computers through the access point, which has transmitting and receiving antennas and the associated electronics circuits.

Even multiple networks can be connected to the Internet, as shown in **Figure 23-6.** A ring topology network is connected to a bus topology network through a router. A gateway is a sophisticated router with a capability of holding a large database of routing addresses.

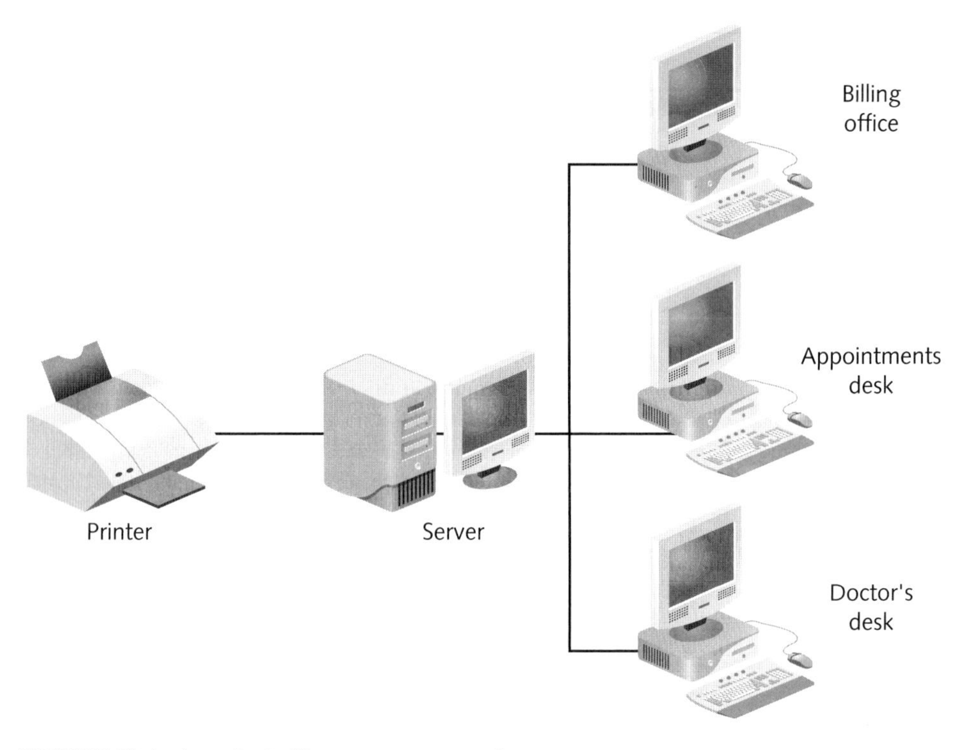

FIGURE 23-4 A medical office computer network.

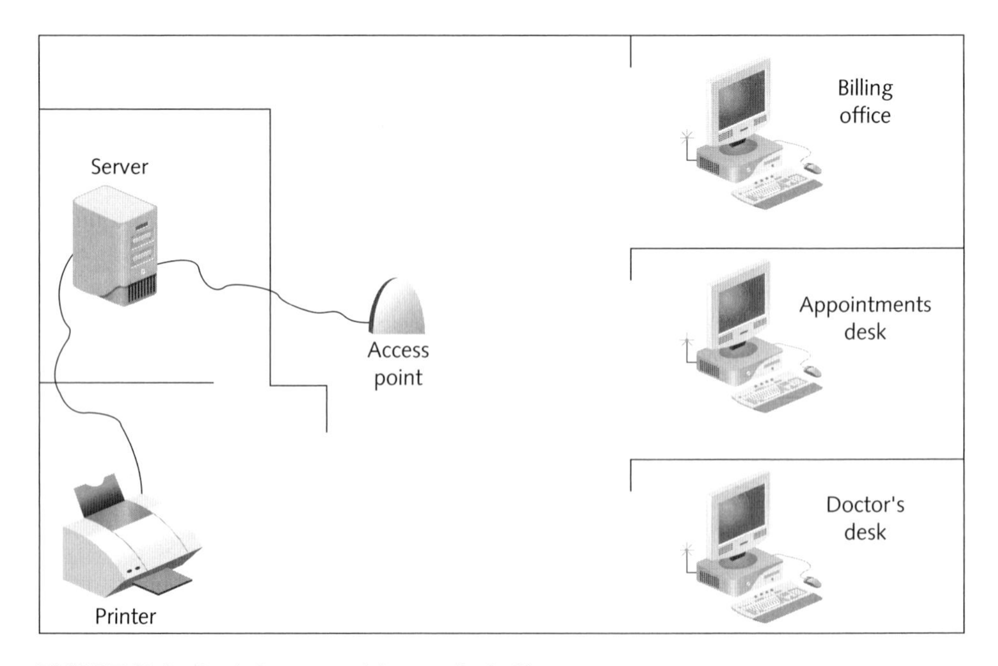

FIGURE 23-5 A wireless network in a medical office.

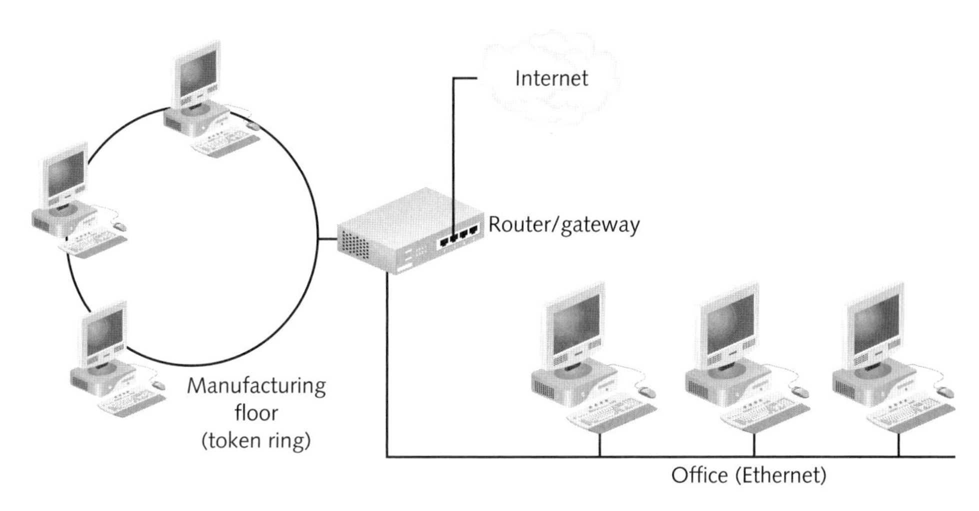

FIGURE 23-6 Medical office connected to the Internet.

EXAMPLE Determine the network address when a host in the network has an IP address of 199.10.20.36 with the subnet mask of 255.255.255.224.

When an IP address with the mask is given, the network address is determined by the ANDING (a digital logic) process.

199.10.20.36

255.255.255.224

ANDING results: 199.10.20.32

■

EXAMPLE For the previous example, determine the first and the last IP addresses of hosts in the network.

The network address is 199.10.20.32 = 199.10.20.00100000.

And the mask bits are 255.255.255.224 = 255.255.255.11100000.

As the mask of binary 1's stops in the fourth byte, there are only five zeros left for the host addressing. The host addresses can start at 00100001, 00100010, 00100011, and so on. Therefore, the first IP = 199.10.20. 00100001 = 199.10.20.33 and the last IP = 199.10.20.00111110 = 199.10.20.62.

■

EXAMPLE A class C network needs to be broken into five smaller networks, or subnets. The address is 199.10.20.0 and the corresponding mask is 255.255.255.0. Determine the total number of hosts in each smaller network.

To provide five subnets, three zeros of the fourth byte are pulled into the network field and correspondingly extend the mask bits by three binary 1's.

The new mask is now 255.255.255.11100000 = 255.255.255.224.

First subnet: 199.10.20.00100000

New mask: 255.255.255.11100000

Similarly, second subnet: 199.10.20.01000000

Third subnet: 199.10.20.01100000

Fourth subnet: 199.10.20.10000000

Fifth subnet: 199.10.20.10100000

Sixth subnet: 199.10.20.11000000

With five zeros of host addressing, the total number of hosts in each network = $(2)^5 - 2 = 30$.

■

Router Configuration

As routers are connected to several small hospital networks, each of them is configured separately for interfaces and routes among themselves. The configuration helps for efficient routing and data flow. Some of these routers can also be firewalled in order to stop or filter data from reaching one LAN from another LAN across routers.

For example, the ICU router, as shown in **Figure 23-2,** can be configured for two interfaces—one to the Intensive Care LAN and the other to the Radiology router. Assume the IP address of the intensive care interface is 200.10.10.1 and that of the radiology interface is 210.10.10.1. Also, the routing Internet protocol (RIP) is used to route packets from the ICU router to the Radiology router.

```
Router ICU > enable
Router ICU > config t
Router ICU (config) > interface ethernet 0
Router ICU (config) > IP address 200.10.10.1 255.255.255.0
Router ICU (config) > no shut
Router ICU (config) > interface ethernet 1
Router ICU (config) > IP address 210.10.10.1 255.255.255.0
Router ICU (config) > no shut
Router ICU (config) > router RIP
Router ICU (config) > network 200.10.10.0
Router ICU (config) > network 210.10.10.0
Router ICU (config) > exit
```

Generally, each router is configured by one of the hosts (called a console computer) on a LAN. As each router connects to the several switches and LANs, several LANs are connected to each other, and a large hospital network is established.

23.4 WIRELESS NETWORKS IN HOSPITALS

Contemporary IT infrastructure in hospitals includes a wireless network to access patient history, diagnostic information, and drug interactions any time the patient receives care. Wireless laptops, PDAs, and tablets are part of this wireless technology. This "point-of-care charting and ordering" enables hospital medical staff to enter and access records of doctor's orders and patient test results almost immediately.

23.5 PERSONAL DIGITAL ASSISTANTS (PDAs) IN HEALTH CARE

Health care providers, such as BMETs and physicians, use medical PDAs for a variety of tasks. Providers can access medicine lists, lab results, and patient records or equipment records, among other data. With access to the Internet or hospital intranet(s), these data can be updated regularly. Physicians can download information from the Internet or look for information on drugs or medical treatments using PDAs. BMETs can access the database for learning the equipment error messages, or even directly access an ECG machine for diagnostic messages! **Figure 23-7** shows a set of devices such as PDAs and text messaging cell phones, while **Figure 23-8** shows a PDA circuit block diagram.

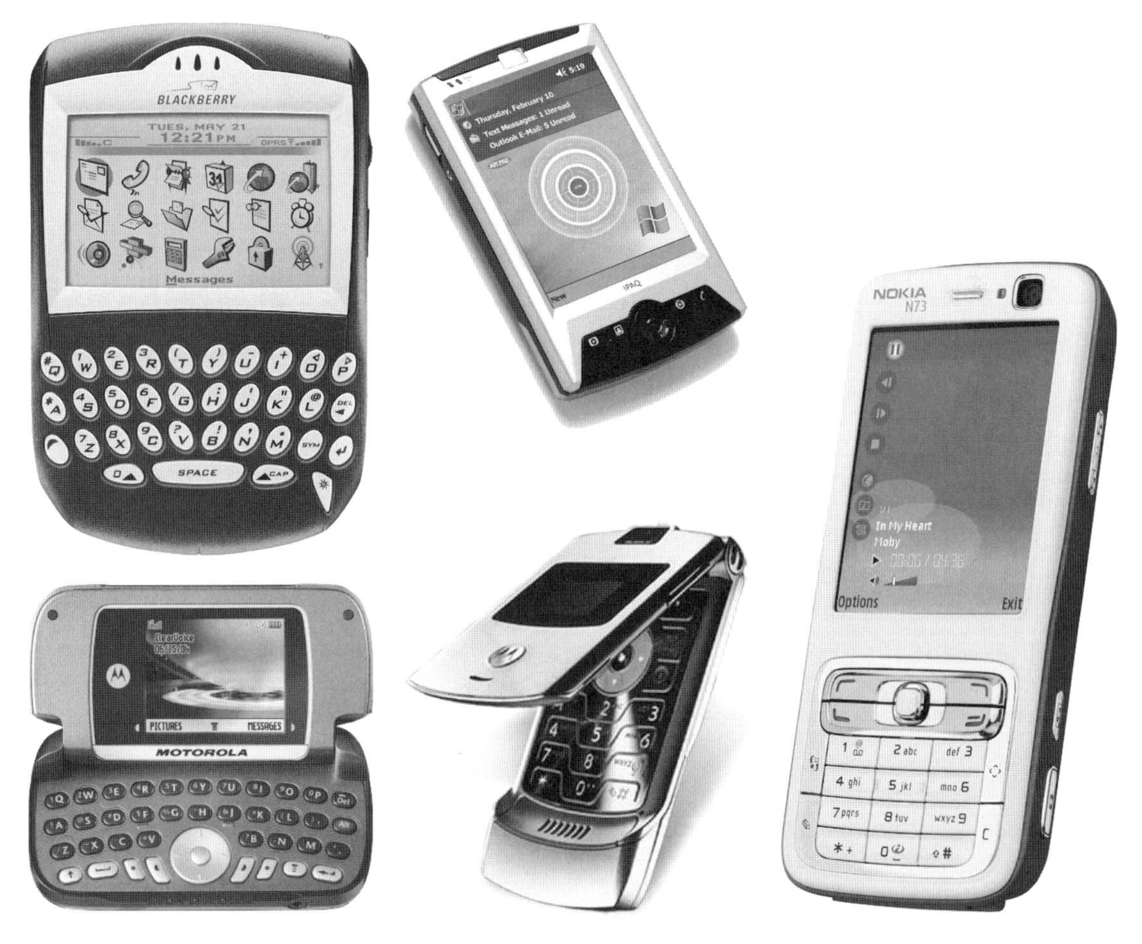

FIGURE 23-7 Medical PDAs.

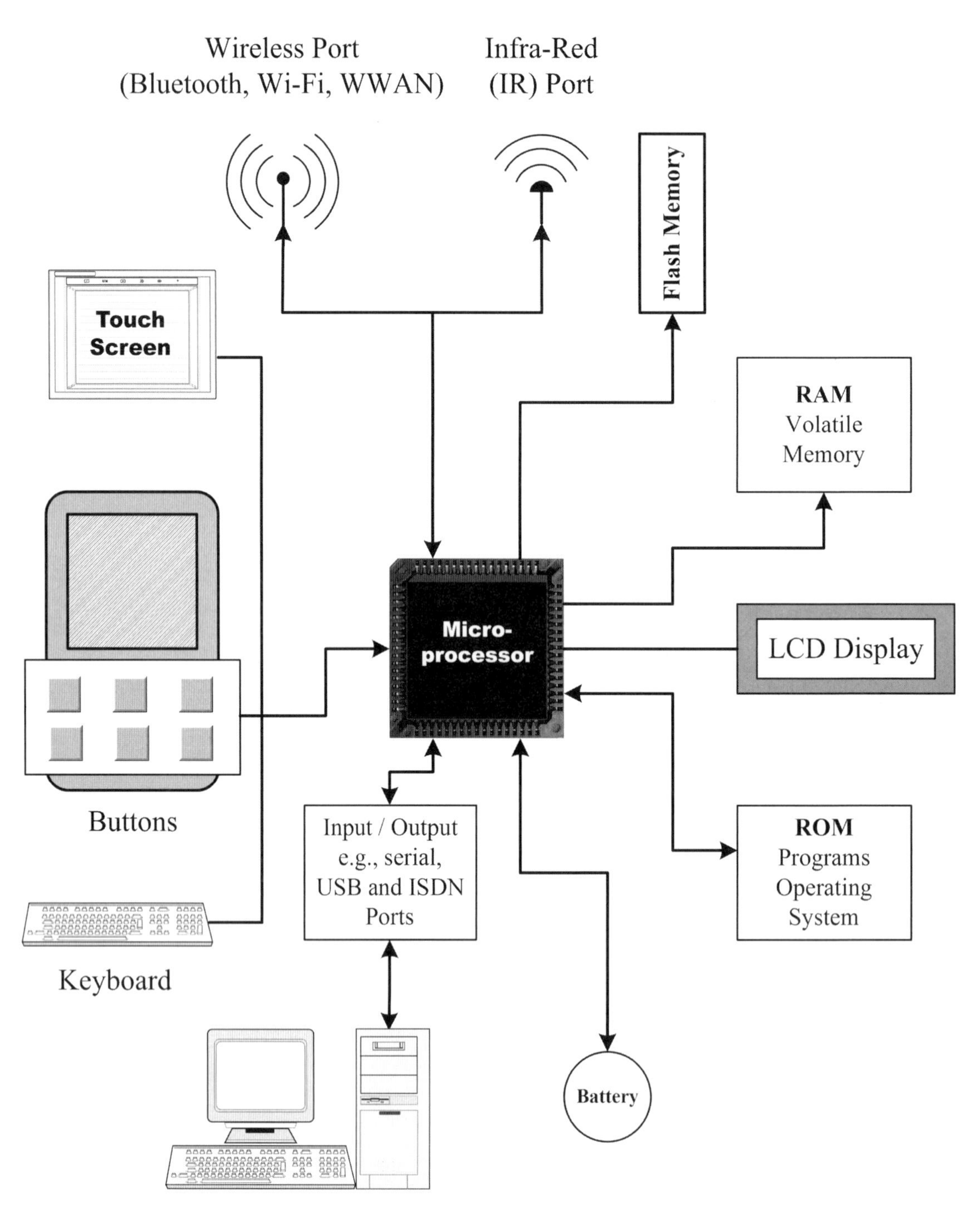

FIGURE 23-8 A block diagram of a PDA device.

23.6 PICTURE ARCHIVING

As soon as an image is scanned, it is immediately available to be reviewed or used electronically by doctors, other health care providers, and outpatient clinics. In some hospitals, large, high-resolution monitors can display these images immediately. This type of digital Web-based imaging is called picture archiving and communication systems (PACS). There are PACS protocols for hardware and software interfacing to the medical imaging equipment and to the computer and telecommunication network.

Figure 23-9 shows the PACS network of the Cayuga Medical Center (CMC). The PACS is available to hospital radiologists and other physicians as a filmless radiology system where the use of X-ray film, chemicals, and the processor equipment is minimized and the computer imaging is enhanced.

The expansion of PACS in partnership with manufacturers has been exponential in recent years. **Figure 23-10** shows various components in PACS network architecture (University of California, San Francisco Medical Center) that includes the PACS internal network, ATM network, and the WAN gateway. Various servers are connected to the PACS central node. The images are stored centrally; however, they are also stored separately at local servers. This is not only to safeguard the database, but also to acquire

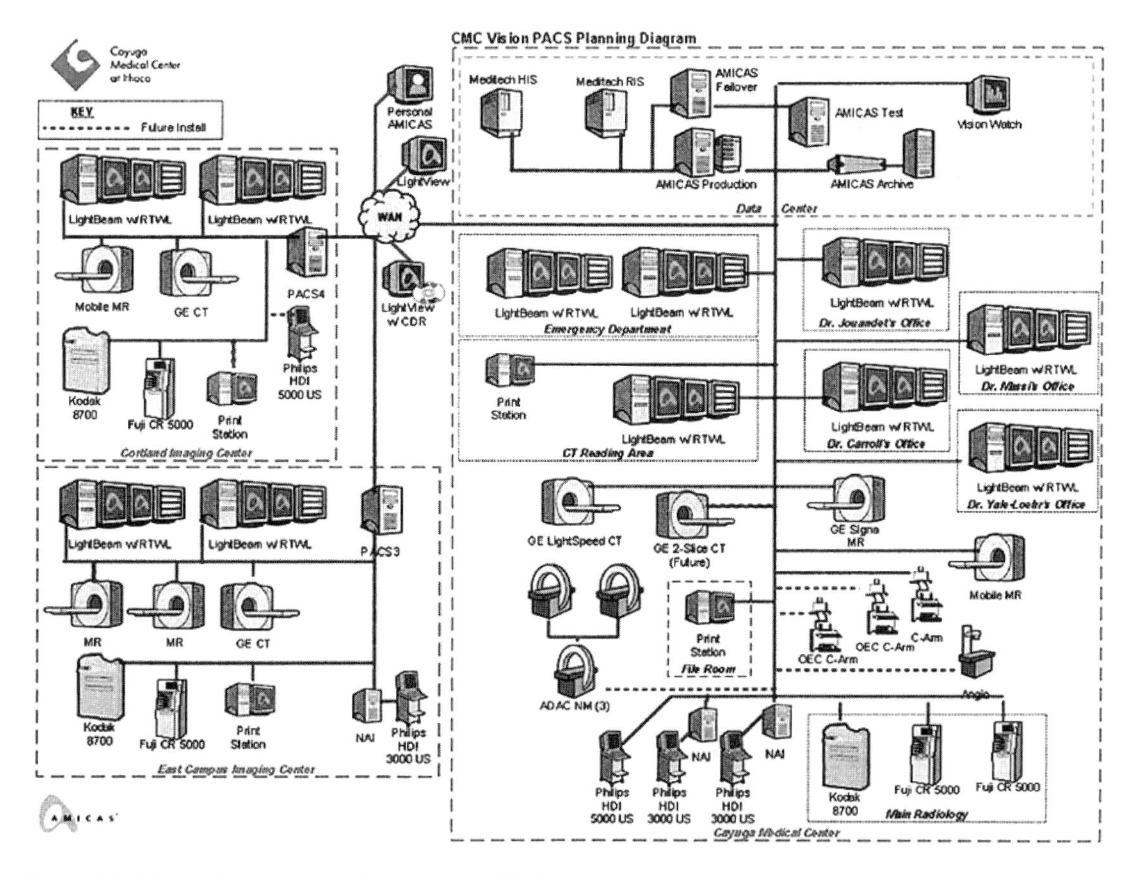

FIGURE 23-9 PACS network of the Cayuga Medical Center.

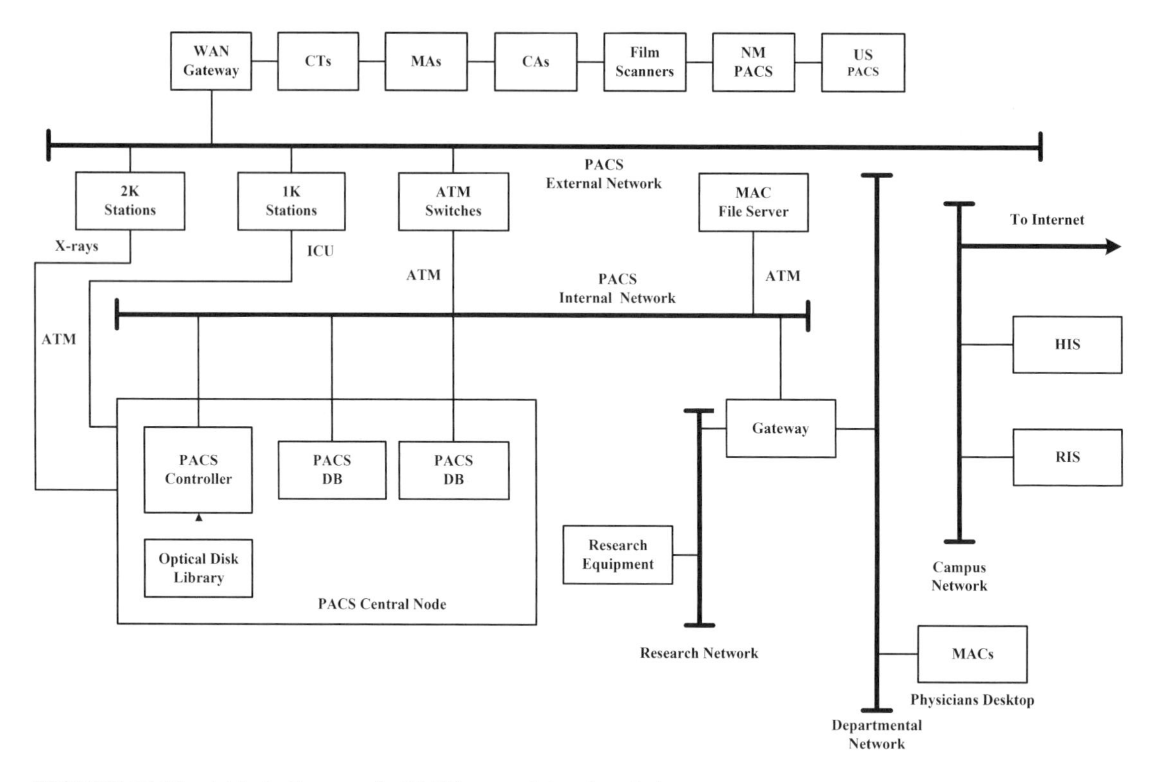

FIGURE 23-10 A block diagram of a PACS network in a hospital.

data when servers are down. The fault tolerant method of redundant array of inexpensive disks (RAID) is implemented widely, particularly at the server site.

The acquisition gateway computer (that acquires the patient images), the hospital information system (HIS), and the radiology information system (RIS) all send their data directly to the PACS controller (that is, the main server in the PACS system). **Figure 23-11** shows a PACS database server. This is a bi-directional communication between a variety of computers and the controller.

The newly generated studies on patient images can be sent to the destination workstations by the PACS controller. **Figure 23-12** shows the DICOM network interfacing with the PACS network.

An intensive care unit PACS module is a good example of a department operating its own module. Important radiological patient information in the ICU can be immediately sent to everyone through the PACS system using a fast-speed ATM switch. High-resolution monitors are placed in the ICU as well as in the radiology department.

A radiologist can read these images and instantly report to the ICU via digital voice dictation. As a three-dimensional rendering of images uses complex computational techniques and mass storage, the hospital-integrated PACS (HI-PACS) integrates the three-dimensional rendering capabilities to the acquired images so that everyone involved can access them. This is shown in **Figure 23-14.** The MAC server and image workstations can visualize and interpret these three-dimensional images.

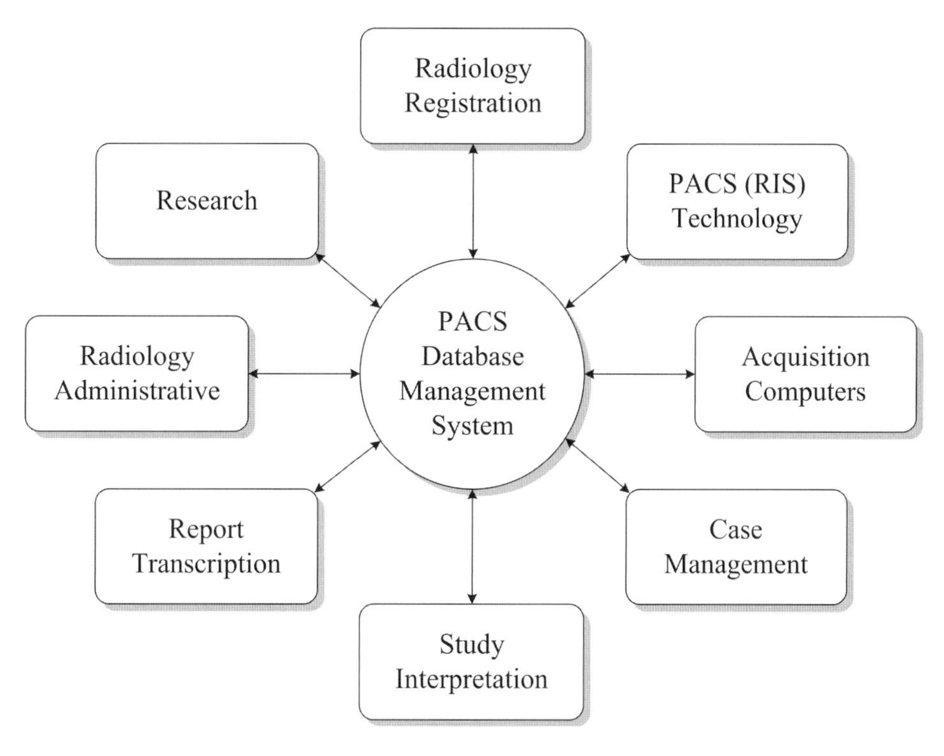

FIGURE 23-11 PACS database management.

One of the applications in the PACS plan is teleconsultation (real-time) service. It can simultaneously manipulate images at local and remote sites. The teleconsultation interfaces to the PACS database and retrieves images through the DICOM network. The set-up is shown in **Figure 23-13.** Also, **Figure 23-14** shows teleconsultation connection to the WAN in more detail.

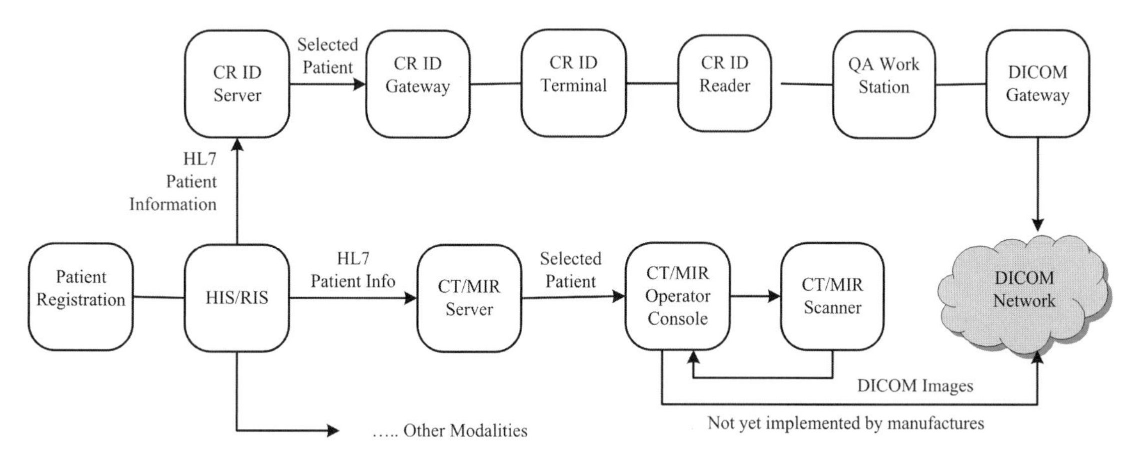

FIGURE 23-12 DICOM network.

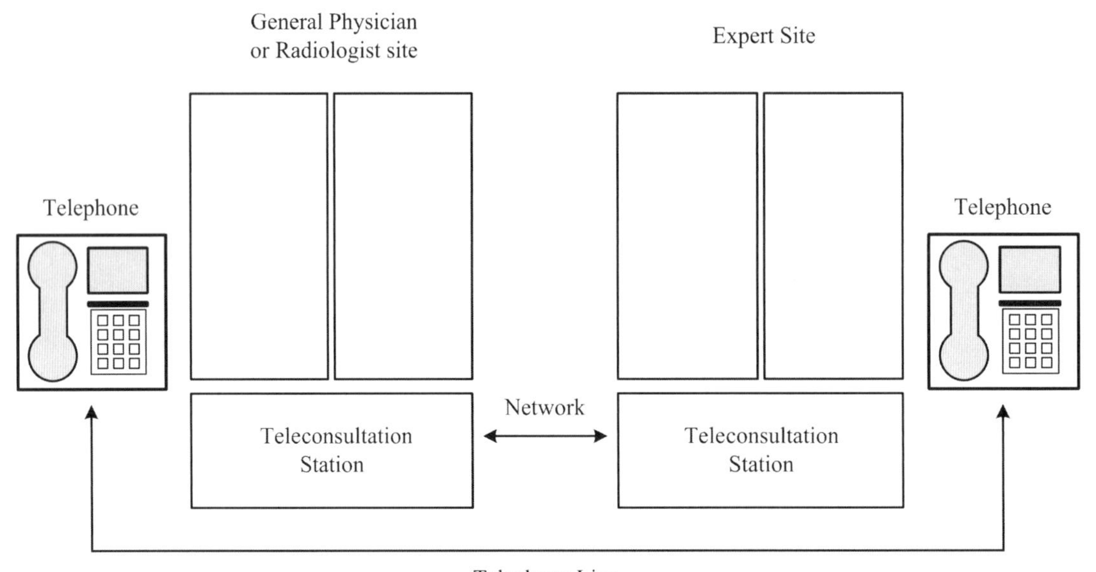

FIGURE 23-13 Teleconsultation in a hospital PACS network.

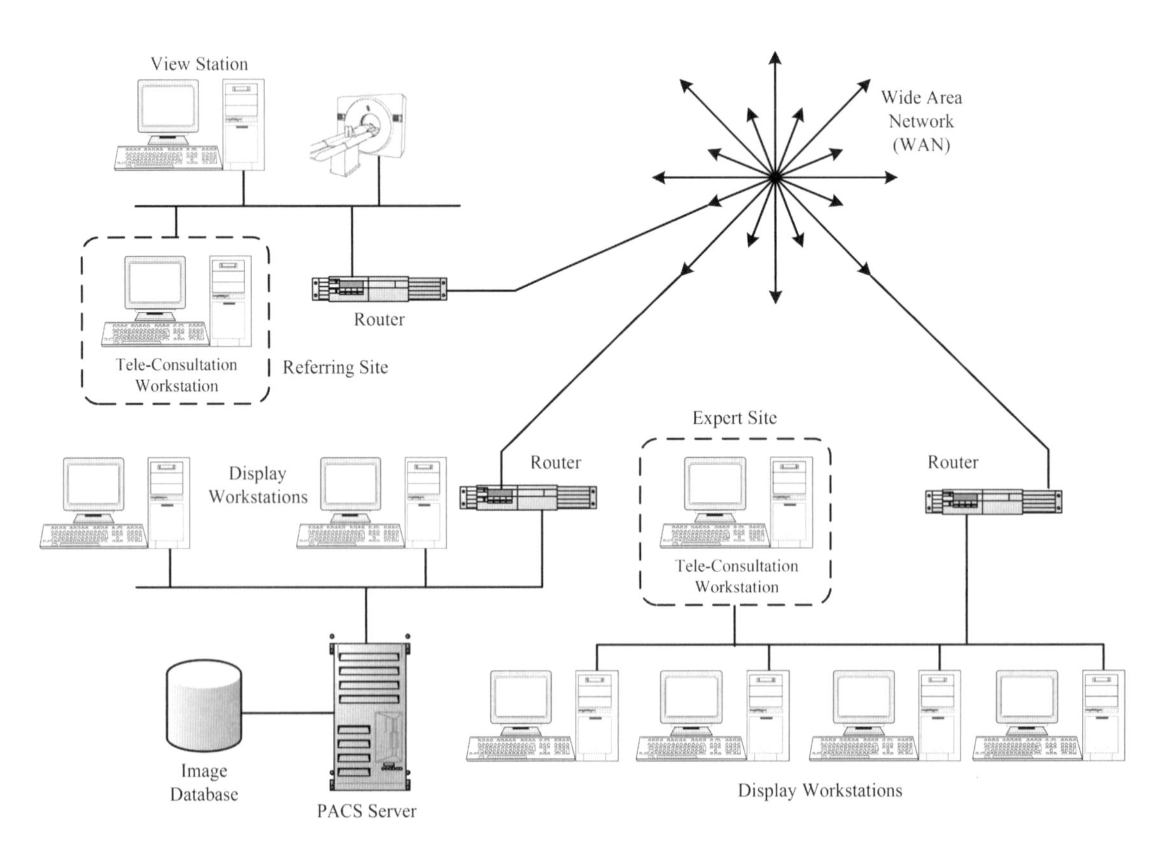

FIGURE 23-14 Teleconsultation outside of the hospital PACS network.

23.7 DIGITAL IMAGING AND COMMUNICATIONS IN MEDICINE (DICOM) STANDARDS

Digital Imaging and Communications in Medicine (DICOM) promotes a single standard communication method (or, protocol) for the wide variety of imaging systems existing in hospital machines (such as MRI, X-rays, CT, and ultrasound) and the transfer of their images through PACS network. The manufacturers can then claim that their machines are DICOM compatible for the DICOM-compliant PACS servers.

DICOM specifies the commands for the devices claiming conformance to the standard. It describes the definition of entities such as graphics, images, reports, texts, and the various studies.

The object class and the service class are the two DICOM classes of information embedded in the standard. An example of object class is the patient (an object). Then attributes of the patient are described, such as name and date of birth. The other objects are study, report, results, digitized film image graphics, MRI image, and so on. The information contained in the object class is precise, well defined, and without any ambiguity.

The service class in DICOM describes services such as how to print the standard image or how to manage network data storage resources. The other service classes are queries about image data, retrieval of images, and storage service.

DICOM uses the TCP/IP standard to transfer images over the network between computers. All the devices from various manufacturers conform to DICOM standards. The query and retrieve service has the priority over send and receive service. For example, the communication is established between a client ultrasound machine and the server PACS controller. **Figure 23-15** shows a DICOM interface.

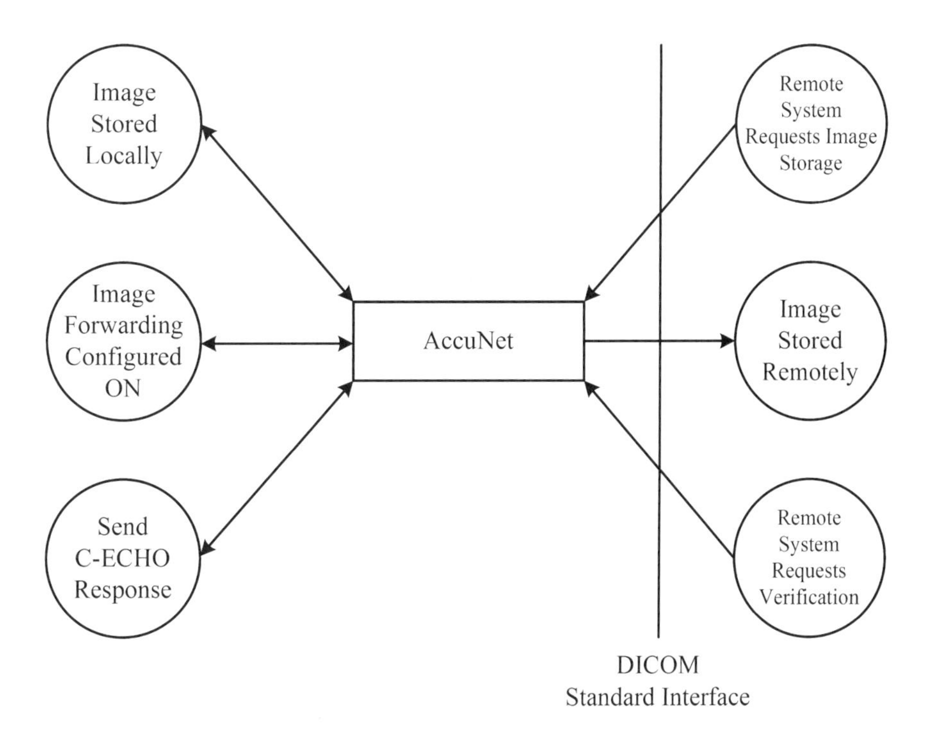

FIGURE 23-15 DICOM interface.

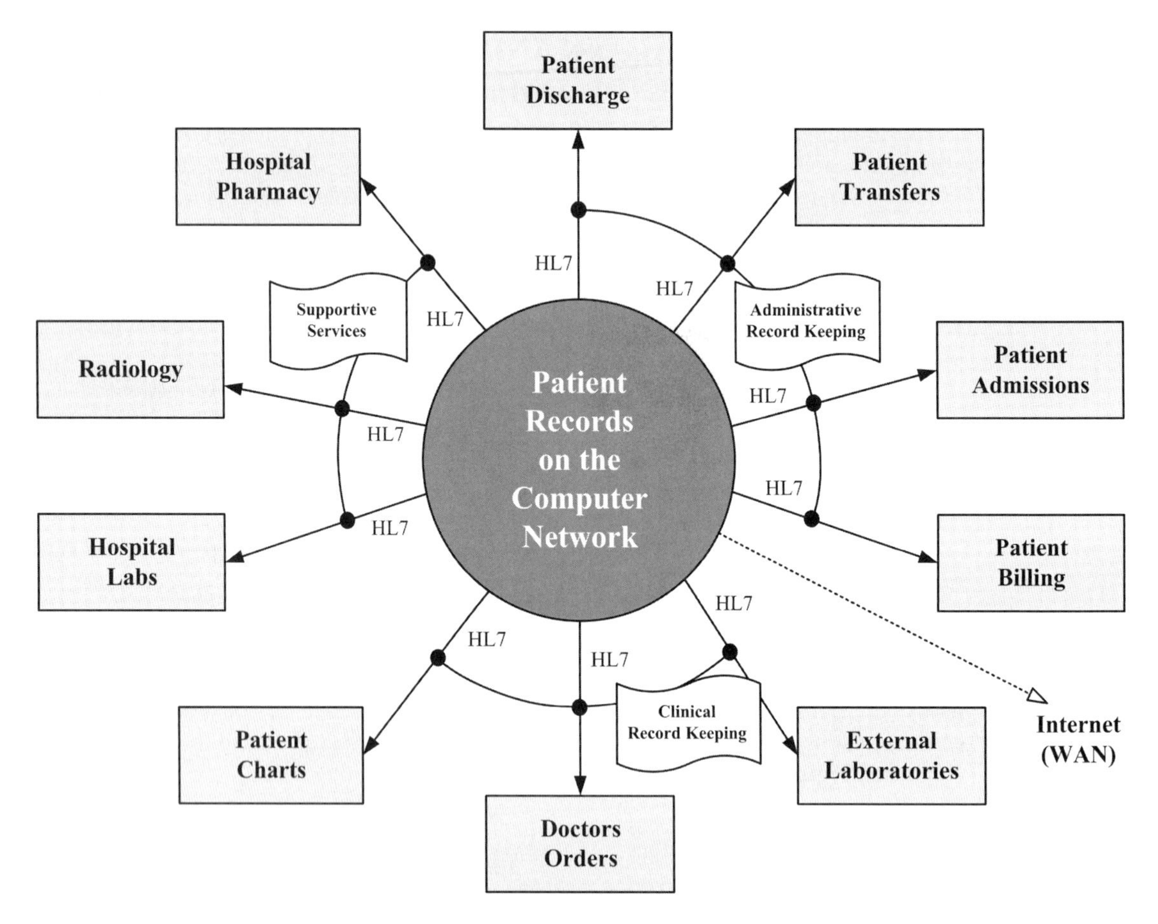

FIGURE 23-16 HL7 interface.

23.8 HEALTH LEVEL SEVEN

Health Level Seven, Inc. (HL7) is an all-volunteer, nonprofit organization involved in the development of international health care standards for sharing clinical data of a patient on the computer network. Health Level Seven is now the standard of the patient's medical insurance coverage information exchanged over intranets and the Internet. It provides inpatient or outpatient information regarding billing, hospital admissions, discharges, laboratory, and radiology tests. Health Level Seven develops software applications designed to support hospital workflow and health care informatics by incorporating different vendor software products into one standard product. Such standards set the language, structure, and data types required for seamless integration from one system to another. **Figure 23-16** shows the HL7 implementation in several areas.

SUMMARY

A digital hospital is an infrastructure of computers, routers, switches, and PDAs to provide a complete, up-to-date, and efficient transfer of patient data electronically.

1. The intranet involves the computer networks of various hospital departments. The computers in these networks are connected to switches and the switches are then connected to the routers.
2. Each computer has an IP address, which is a dotted decimal address of four bytes.
3. A subnet mask of four bytes follows the IP address and consists of 1's representing network field and the remaining zeros representing the host field.
4. Subnets are created by borrowing zeros from the host field and extending 1's in the mask bits.
5. PDAs and wireless laptops are connected to the hospital network though access points.
6. PACS is a communication standard for sending and receiving digital images of X-rays, MRIs, and ultrasound.
7. DICOM is a protocol of formatting digital images of various vendors into a single standard.
8. HL7 is a digital standard of patient and hospital records.

MEDICAL TERMINOLOGIES

Communication carrier: information carried out on specific RF signal similar to AM and FM radio station carriers.

Digital Imaging and Communications in Medicine (DICOM): a set of standards for handling, storing, printing, and transmitting information in medical imaging. Standards include a file format definition and a network communications protocol.

Health Level Seven (HL7): a nonprofit volunteer organization with an interest in the development and advancement of clinical and administrative standards for the exchange, management, and integration of electronic health care information.

Local area network (LAN): a computer network covering a local area linking private telecommunication equipment on a site. LANs normally have much higher data rates, smaller geographic area, and do not require leased telecommunication lines in comparison to WANs.

Picture archiving and communication systems (PACS): computers or networks for the storage, retrieval, distribution, and presentation of images for diagnosis. Examples include MRIs, mammography, and radiography.

Personal Digital Assistant (PDA): a portable, lightweight, handheld electronic device used to store data and perform specific tasks related to software applications and the Internet.

Telemetry: technology enabling remote measurement and reporting of information related to the interest of the system operator. Typically used with wireless communication but can be utilized over telephone, computer network, or optical link.

Teleradiology: electronic transmission of radiological images, such as X-rays, CTs, and MRIs, from one location to another for the purpose of interpretation. Images can be sent to parts of a hospital or locations around the world.

Wide Area Network (WAN): a communication network that uses equipment such as telephone lines, satellite dishes, computers, and so on, over a large geographic area. WANs are used to connect LANs so users can effectively communicate in multiple locations.

Wireless network: a telephone or computer network that communicates (enabling file sharing, printer sharing, Internet connection, etc.) without cabling. Wireless networking hardware uses radio frequencies to transmit information between equipment.

QUIZ

1. A network interface card (NIC) has a media access control (MAC) address of ________________.

   a) 32 bits length b) 48 bits length c) 128 bits length d) None of the above

2. Internet protocol (IP) addressing has a length of ________________.

   a) 48 bits b) 32 bits c) 128 bits d) None of the above

3. An example of wide area network (WAN) is ________________.

   a) CSMA/CD b) Ethernet c) ATM d) ARCNET

4. True or False: PACS is a medical communications standard like DICOM.

   a) True b) False

5. What is the main difference between HL7 and DICOM?

   ____

   ____

6. Routers operate at what layer of OSI?

   a) Data link layer b) Network layer c) Application layer d) Transport layer

7. The data speed on a fiber link is ________________.

   a) 100 Mbits per second b) 10 Mbits per second
   c) 1.5 Mbits per second d) 1 Gbits per second

8. The most common topology in the hospital network is a ________________.

   a) Star b) Ring c) Bus d) Mesh

9. The wireless network in a hospital connects to the ________________.

   a) Hub b) Switch c) Access point d) None of the above

10. HIS and RIS differ in ________________.

PROBLEMS

1. Make a list of protocols in each layer of the TCP/IP suite and discuss their characteristics.
2. Discuss advantages and disadvantages of LAN topologies in terms of cable length, number of hosts, data speed, bandwidth, and its performance.
3. Make a list of LAN equipment needed for a hospital computer network. Indicate the corresponding layer or layers they belong to.
4. Show the Ethernet Frame with a raw data of 11001100.
5. Determine the subnet address when one of the host addresses is given as 210.20.20.38 and its mask is 255.255.255.240. Also, determine the range of host addresses in the subnet.

6. Create five subnets when a large network is given as 200.10.10.0 with a mask of 255.255.255.0. Determine the range of host addresses in the first subnet.
7. Configure a router for a small clinic. The hub/switch is connected to five computers and also to the router. The network is 192.10.10.0.
8. What are the possible ways you can connect a router to the Internet? Discuss in detail.
9. Show the communication steps between HL7 client and the PAC server.
10. Discuss the performance of a protocol analyzer or LAN analyzer and indicate the number of bytes in each header when it captures a data frame. You may use the Internet.

RESEARCH TOPICS

1. In the future, telemedicine will bring health services to individual homes. The concept is to create automatic health stations for the home environment for chronically ill patients. Meeting the high bandwidth requirements, noninvasive sensors are placed in strategic locations throughout the home to monitor glucose, creatinine proteins, and even detect lesions. The research paper should include the most recent efforts in this area and should describe the types of sensors used in patient monitors at home. Then, evaluate the telecommunication network that sends and carries the sensor data collected from the shut-in patient.
2. Malfunctions of image acquisitions when using PACS can result in failure to transfer patient data, and the results could be calamitous. There could be several reasons for this failure, including human error or network design error. The research paper should distinguish between the errors at the device site and the bottleneck on the PACs network. The paper may include the steps taken to correct these problems.

CASE STUDIES

1. An elderly woman does not want to dial a phone to contact her son; instead all she wants to do is push a single button to be connected through a wireless transmitter/receiver. She has medical conditions involving several heart problems; moreover, she has a fear of small things. Although there is a caregiver when her son is not home, her son thinks the electronic communication problem can be cumbersome. The individual or group performing this case study must answer the following questions:
   a) What are the devices that are available at present?
   b) How can the home communication network be separate from the outside telecommunications network?
   c) Why can't the elderly woman be provided with what she wants? Is her request that unreasonable?
2. The U.S. Department of Commerce has done several case studies in recent years on the evaluation of telemedicine systems in hospitals. The researcher can select one of these case studies and determine the various aspects (good and bad) of telemedicine projects. The study should focus on the type of community settings, the question of digital divide, and the application of new technologies in telemedicine.

CHAPTER 24

New Technologies and Advances in Medical Instrumentation

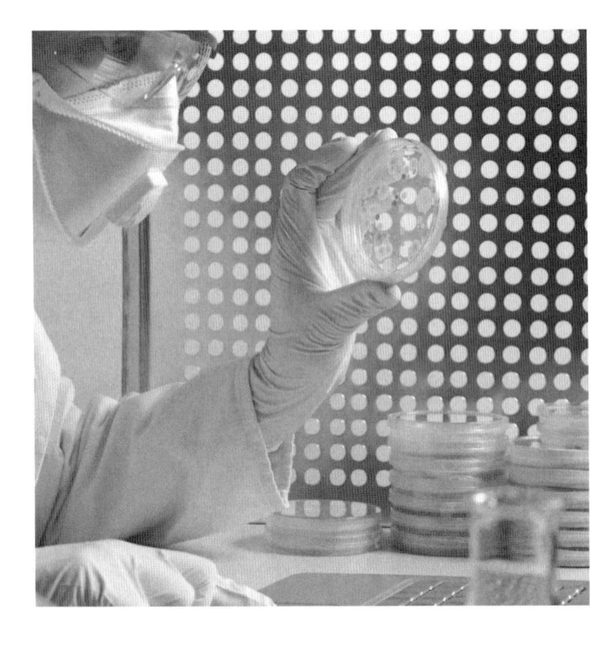

CHAPTER OUTLINE

OBJECTIVE

The objective of this chapter is to introduce the reader to the emerging concepts in biomedical nanotechnology and tissue engineering, including nano materials, tissue regeneration techniques, as well as the companies involved in the fabrication and manufacturing in nanotechnology.

Upon completion of this chapter, the reader will be able to:

- Describe nanoscale.
- Describe elements of a nanotechnology.
- Discuss tissue engineering.
- Identify organizations in nanotechnology or tissue engineering.

INTERNET WEB SITES

http://www.nano.asme.org (Nanotechnology Institute, American Society of Mechanical Engineering)

http://www.tissueengineering.gov (National Science and Technology Council)
http://www.mems.utah.edu (State of Utah Center of Excellence for Biomedical Microfluidics)
http://www.tissue-engineering.net (Tissue Engineering Pages, Biotissue Technologies)
http://www.tissueeng.net (Tissue Engineering Network)
http://www.nano.gov (National Nanotechnology Initiative)

■ INTRODUCTION

Twenty-first century nanotechnology and tissue engineering has provided quantum leaps in molecular- and cellular-level medicine. Nanomedicine is a development of nanotechnology used to repair damaged tissue at the molecular level with molecular size of a thousandth of a thousandth of a millimeter! In the field of tissue engineering, living cells are harvested, grown in a laboratory, and stimulated to form specific tissues or organs. They then can be injected or implanted into a patient's body as needed to create new, healthy tissue or organs. As a comparison, tissue engineering deals with the construction of natural living tissue products, whereas an artificial heart is a bio-engineered, man-made product.

24.1 NANOSCALE AND NANOTECHNOLOGY

A nanometer is one-billionth of a meter. To conceptualize this, consider that the diameter of DNA is approximately 2.5 nanometers (nm), while the thickness of a sheet of paper is about 100,000 nm! Nanotechnology concerns nanometer dimensions of cells and biological molecules. The dimensions are so small that even the conventional lab microscope cannot be used to see them. Presented here is a list of measurements for reference:

One meter is 3.28 feet.

One-thousandth of a meter is a millimeter.

One-thousandth of a millimeter is a micron.

One-thousandth of a micron is a nanometer.

One meter is one billion nanometers.

Figure 24-1 shows how nanosize is compared in nanometers to give some perspective on the size of nanoscale components. The size of a water molecule is about 10^{-1} nanometers whereas bacteria size is about 10^3 nanometers.

Generally nanotechnology, shortened to "nanotech", deals with structures of the size 100 nanometers or smaller, and involves developing materials or devices within that size. At the nanoscale, materials behave quite differently from those at larger scales. The following list describes some of the changes in materials at nanoscale:

- It is possible to vary the fundamental properties of materials such as melting temperature, magnetization or charge capacity without changing the chemical composition of the material.
- It is possible to make materials at nanoscale incredibly harder and less brittle.
- It is possible for materials to start absorbing light and turn that light into heat (optoelectronic applications).

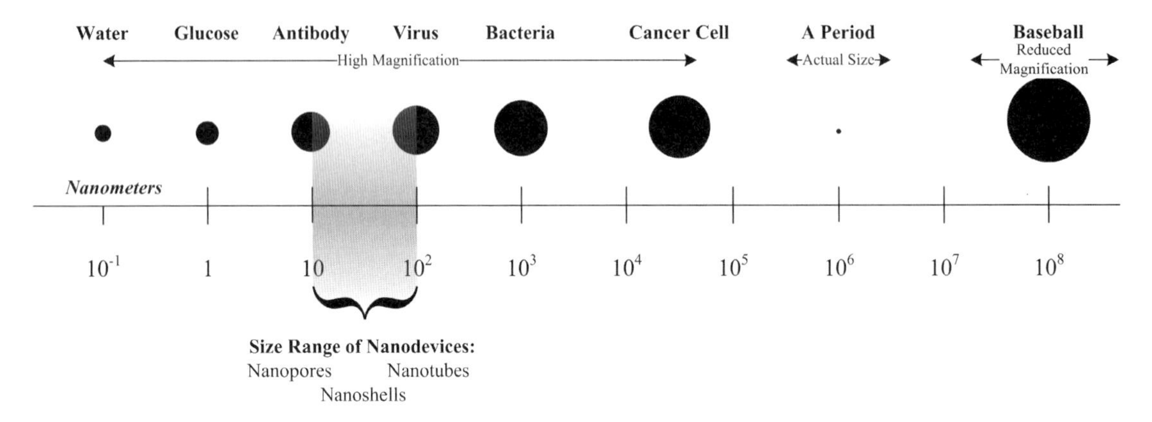

FIGURE 24-1 Nanosize.

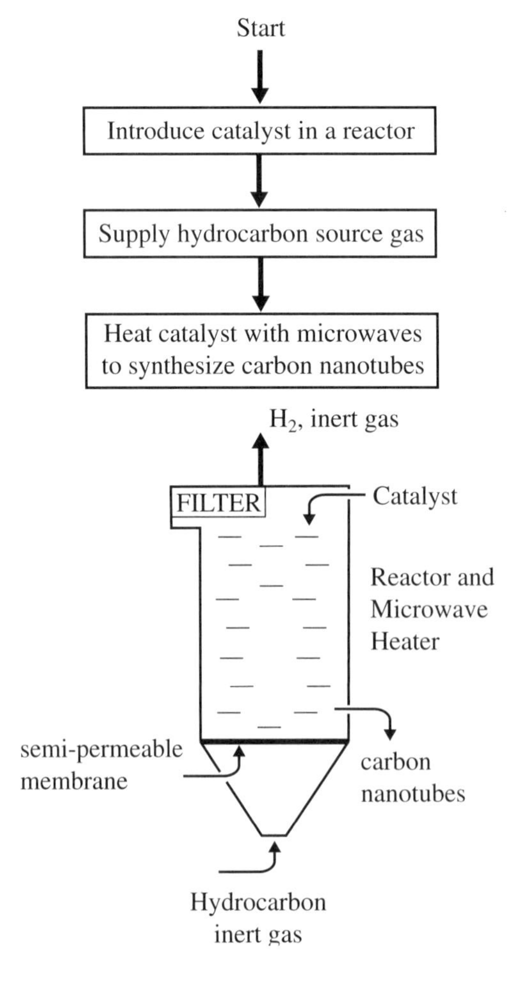

FIGURE 24-2 Process of making carbon nanotubes.

- Nanoscale materials have relatively high surface areas when compared to the same mass of material produced in a larger form, making them ideal for use in composite materials.
- It is possible to place material (at nanoscale) inside living cells, a combination of material science and biotechnology.

The nanotech uses gold, silver, carbon tubes, silica, ceramics, polymers, aerosols and many other types of materials for various applications such as in medicine, chemical or computer industries. **Figure 24-2** shows a simple process of making carbon nanotubes. The nanotubes grow at the site of a metal catalyst (such as nickel, cobalt or iron) in the reactor; the carbon-containing gas i.e. hydrocarbon inert gas is broken apart at the surface of the catalyst particle, and the carbon is transposed to the edges of the catalyst particle, where it forms the nanotubes.

24.2 NANOSIZE RETOOLING IN HEALTH CARE

The following are two examples of nanosize retooling of conventional medical devices. Current endoscopes have diameters of 3 cm, but nanotechnology endoscopes can be as small as 5 mm, the diameter of spaghetti. The resolutions can be made by as little as a few microns. Doctors can see more detailed views of intestines. Similarly, a dosimeter can detect radiation and, thereby, the cancerous cells in patients. But the nano-dosimeters are so small in diameter that several of them can be connected together as a matrix of scanners with high resolution to detect radiation.

Following is a list of a few areas of biomedical nanotechnology:

1. Nanomaterials help in diagnostic and treatment options by manufacturing new drugs and their delivery systems. X-ray photoelectron spectroscopy and ion scattering spectroscopy will allow us to understand the composition and atomic bonding in nanomaterials.
2. Nanobioprobes evaluate tumors and deliver localized drugs in radiation treatments.
3. Nanobiosensors can be implanted in the body to monitor extreme health problems.
4. Viewing at nanoscale involves imaging individual atoms and molecules. Scanning electron microscopes and scanning tunneling microscopes are being developed for imaging purposes.

24.3 ANTI-CANCER NANOPARTICLES

To halt the growth of cancer cells, nanoparticles are injected into the patient to gain entry among the cancerous cells. These nanoparticles are therapeutic agents made outside of the body. The molecular assembly of nanoparticles then can be injected into a targeted disease tissue.

24.4 MICROFLUIDICS RESEARCH

Polymer-based microfabrication processes have been applied to a number of biomedical microsystems under development at the national security laboratory Lawrence Livermore National Laboratory, in Livermore, California. The technology is to enable the fabrication of thin, compliant devices with conducting lines for medical implants and hybrid microfluidic systems. Applications include biological sample preparation modules, microsyringes,

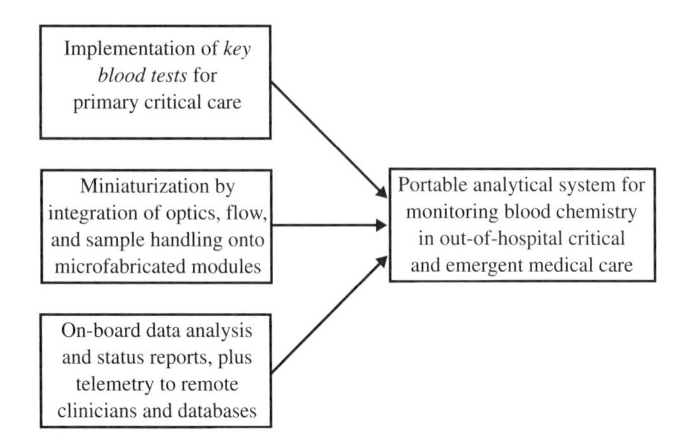

FIGURE 24-3 Microfabricated modules in blood chemistry monitoring.

electrode arrays for retinal implants, and microfluidic systems with integrated electronics. The approach enables the integration of flow channels, reservoirs, glass and silicon microfluidic chips, PC boards and electronics, and commercially available micropumps and valves into microfluidic systems.

Lawrence Livermore National Laboratory is developing instrumentation for collecting, processing, and identifying fluid-based biological pathogens in the forms of proteins, viruses, and bacteria. The goal of this microfluidic module is to input a fluid sample containing background particulates in order to potentially target compounds and deliver a processed sample for detection.

The metal features are embedded within a thin (50-micron) substrate. The advantages of the polymer-based microfluidic technology include biocompatibility, stretchability, oxygen permeability, and low water absorption. **Figure 24-3** shows the process of portable blood chemistry monitoring using microfabricated modules.

24.5 REGENERATIVE MEDICINE AND TISSUE ENGINEERING

Tissue engineering is currently used in several areas of medicine such as corneal tissue engineering, blood vessel tissue engineering, liver tissue engineering, cartilage tissue engineering, and bone tissue engineering. **Figure 24-4** shows an example of tissue engineering by growing modified cells in the lab and then injecting them into the body.

The National Institutes of Health (NIH) defines tissue engineering into the following categories:

1. Biomaterials, including novel biomaterials that are designed to direct the organization, growth, and differentiation of cells in the process of forming function tissue by providing both physical and chemical cues.
2. Cells, including enabling methodologies for the proliferation and differentiation of cells, acquiring the appropriate source of cells such as autologous cells, allogeneic cells, xenogeneic cells, stem cells, genetically engineered cells, and immunological manipulation.
3. Biomolecules, including angiogenic factors, growth factors, differentiation factors, and bone morphogenic proteins.

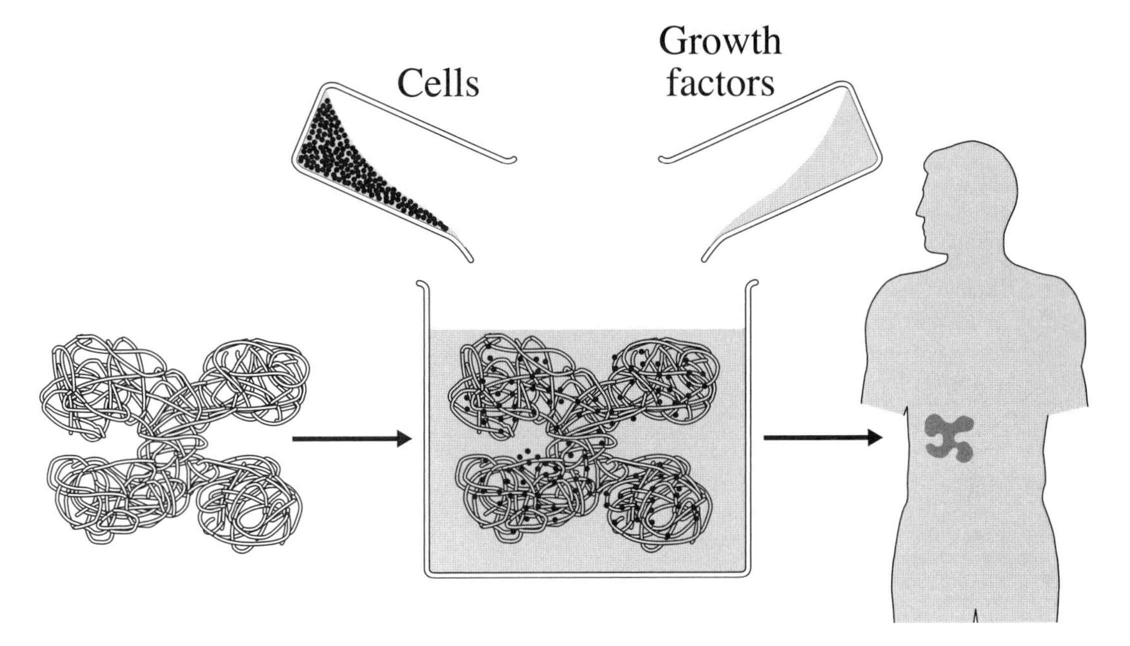

FIGURE 24-4 Nanoparticles injected into the vascular wall.

4. Engineering design aspects, including two-dimensional cell expansion, three-dimensional tissue growth, bioreactors, vascularization, cell and tissue storage, and shipping (biological packaging).
5. Biomechanical aspects of design, including properties of native tissues, identification of minimum properties required of engineered tissues, mechanical signals regulating engineered tissues, and efficacy and safety of engineered tissues.
6. Informatics to support tissue engineering, including gene and protein sequencing, gene expression analysis, protein expression and interaction analysis, quantitative cellular image analysis, quantitative tissue analysis, in silico tissue and cell modeling, digital tissue manufacturing, automated quality assurance systems, data mining tools, and clinical informatics interfaces.
7. Stem cell research, including research that involves stem cells, whether from embryonic, fetal, or adult sources, human and nonhuman. It should include research in which stem cells are isolated, derived, or cultured for purposes such as developing cell or tissue therapies, studying cellular differentiation, research to understand the factors necessary to direct cell specialization to specific pathways, and other developmental studies. It should not include transgenic studies, gene knockout studies, or the generation of chimeric animals.

Figure 24-5a and **Figure 24-5b** are images taken from the image gallery of the National Institute of Arthritis and Musculoskeletal and Skin Diseases (NIAMS). **Figure 24-5a** is a sample of tissue-engineered cartilage produced using a biodegradable nanofibrous scaffold seeded with stem cells. **Figure 24-5b** shows nanocomposite (calcium phosphate) filling in a tooth. The composite releases decay-fighting agents to buffer against acids produced by bacteria.

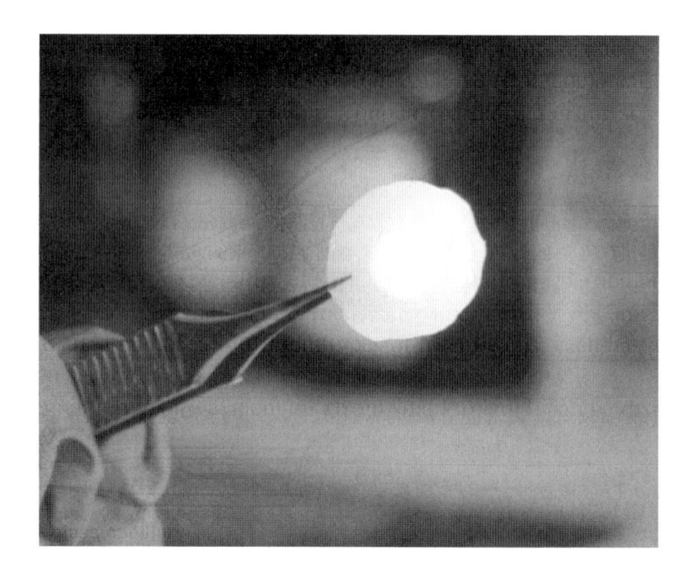

FIGURE 24-5a Tissue engineered cartilage.

Stem Cell Research

Stem cells are cells found in most, if not all, multi-cellular organisms. They are characterized by the ability to renew themselves through mitotic cell division and by differentiating into a diverse range of specialized cell types. Stem cells are important to medical science because they are able to transform into different cell types and can be used to mimic an original tissue. Embryonic stem cells are pluripotent, meaning that they can transform into many different cell types; adult stem cells are multipotent, meaning that they are less plastic and cannot transform into as many different cell types. **Figure 24-6** shows a research chemist examining human stem cells in a flask.

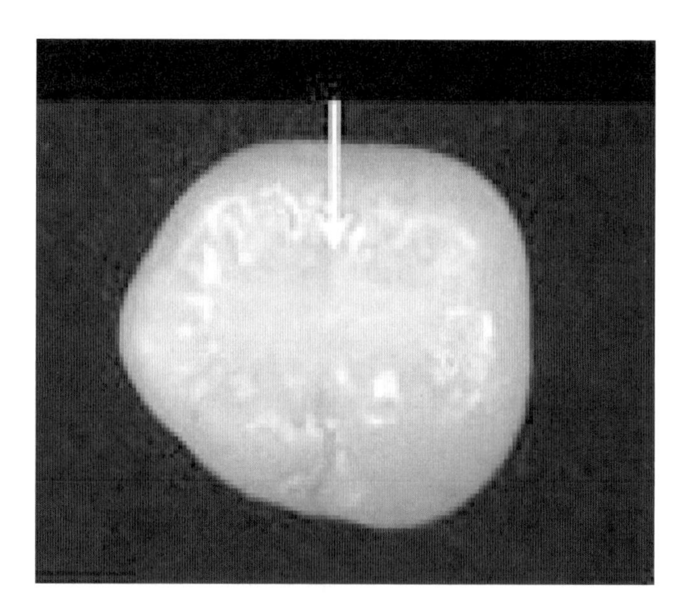

FIGURE 24-5b Nanocomposite filling in a tooth.

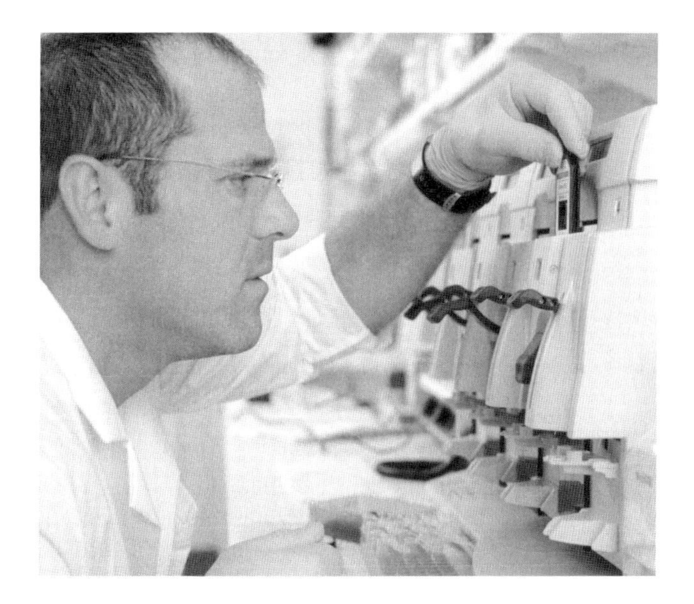

FIGURE 24-6 A chemist examines human stem cells.

Tissue engineering can be used to help many people whose own tissue no longer functions well. By using a person's own stem cells as a cell source, replacements can be designed to mimic the original tissue without stimulating an immunogenic response. Stem cell engineering and tissue engineering can be used together to design vascular grafts for those with atherosclerosis or cardiac replacements for those with heart failure.

24.6 NANOTECHNOLOGY AND TISSUE ENGINEERING ORGANIZATIONS AND COMPANIES

Several centers and laboratories contribute to the advancements in biomedical nanotechnology in the United States. Research the following companies for much more information about their contributions: Motorola Labs, Berkeley Sensor and Actuator Center, Lawrence Livermore National Laboratory, MicroFab Technologies, NASA Ames Research Center, National Cancer Institute, Johns Hopkins University, and Hitachi Ltd. Life Science Group.

In addition, the National Institutes of Health and the United States Department of Energy are involved in genome research.

SUMMARY

The concepts in nanotechnogy and tissue engineering are discussed in this chapter.

1. The term *nano* describes the size of one-thousandth of a micron. Nanoparticles are made outside of the body and then injected into the patient to encapsulate the tumor cells.
2. Polymer-based microfluidic chips can be implanted in the body to monitor the blood chemistry.
3. Tissue engineering aims to create tissue equivalents of blood vessels, nerves, cartilages, and organs for replacement of tissues damaged through either disease or trauma.

4. Stem cells are found in multicellular organisms and are able to renew themselves through cell division and differentiating into specialized cell forms.

MEDICAL TERMINOLOGY

The following is a list of medical terms mentioned in this chapter.

In vitro culture: biological process produced in a laboratory or other controlled experimental environment rather than within a living organism or natural setting.

In vivo implantation: insertion into the body to promote a biological process produced within a living organism or natural setting.

Nanoparticles: a microscopic particle measured in nanometers.

Nanorobotics: technology related to constructing and creating machines or robots close to a nanometer.

Regenerative tissue engineering: area of medicine concerned with the properties and functions of living tissue with the purpose of creating replacement organs and tissue that adds to or substitutes damaged tissue.

Stem cells: primitive, precursor cells that produce differentiated cells. Sources come from a newly formed embryo, cord blood from discarded umbilical cord, and adult tissues, such as bone marrow, muscle, and specialized areas of the brain.

QUIZ

1. Nano-scale is ________________.

   a) One-millionth of a centimeter
   b) 10–9 meter
   c) The size of a single red blood cell

2. What is the main difference between tissue engineering and stem cell engineering?

   ____

3. A major cause of tissue damage is ________________.

   a) Low blood pressure in the tissue
   b) Inadequate oxygen to the tissue cells
   c) Cells not linking up to each other

4. A microfluidic system does not include ________________.

   a) A programmable fluidic processor
   b) Silicon chips
   c) Plastic material
   d) Carbon
   e) Copper

5. Nano tubes can help in the ________________.

   a) Blood flowing in tissues
   b) Breakup of tumor cells
   c) Delivery of drugs to tissues

6. MEMS stands for ________________.

   a) Magnetic electromechanical systems
   b) Micro-electromechanical systems
   c) Memory systems
   d) None of the above

7. Which of the following wavelengths is within the visible (light) spectrum of electromagnetic radiation?

   a) 200 nanometers
   b) 1 nanometer
   c) 500 nanometers
   d) None of the above

8. Scaffolds in tissue engineering:

   a) Allow cell attachment
   b) Are non-synthetic materials
   c) Are bio-degradable
   d) None of the above

9. The three roles of a normal stem cell are:

   1. ______________________________
   2. ______________________________
   3. ______________________________

10. The meaning of biocompatibility is:

    ____

    ____

PROBLEMS

The reader may use the Internet in answering the following problems.

1. Discuss the smallest component in each of the physiological systems: circulatory, respiratory, digestive, urinary, nervous, endocrine, and reproductive, and determine their dimensions.
2. Discuss the software implementation in the programmable fluidic processors. What is it? How is it done?
3. Discuss carbon electrode arrays, glucose biosensor electrodes, and polymer-based electrodes. Compare their applications, similarities, and differences.
4. Discuss how nanoparticles are used to seek out and encapsulate tumor cells and also deliver anti-cancer drugs.
5. Compare the unique properties of adult stem cells with those of embryonic stem cells. Also, describe the limitations of stem cell research in the United States.
6. Discuss how stem cells are used to regenerate tissues and organs and how the interaction between "engineered tissues" and native tissues can be characterized.
7. Explain in vitro culture in tissue engineering. Provide a few examples of this idea.
8. Discuss biomedical polymers and their properties.
9. Describe the interior structures of a typical cell and the types of cellular measurements.
10. Describe the following topics in detail:

    a) Cell differentiation

    b) Extracellular matrix (ECM)

    c) Nanostructured titanium alloys

    d) Nanoparticles for bio-sensing and imaging

CASE STUDIES

1. The role of the Food and Drug Administration (FDA) is well established, but a case study is appropriate to focus on the FDA's role in cancer nanotechnology. In certain cancer types, nanotechnology is used for cancer prevention, diagnosis, and treatment. It is important then to research how the FDA has provided the guidelines for these types of nanotechnology applications.
2. Mary's breast cancer has not spread and she has gone through chemotherapy. Her doctor is proposing direct intervention of a targeted delivery of nanomedicine. The case study must include the following information:

   a) The difference between chemotherapy and nanomedicine

   b) The delivery process and technique

   c) The success rates of these nanotechnology deliveries

RESEARCH TOPICS

1. Micro-electromechanical systems (MEMS) may be larger than nanoscales but are used in tissue engineering. MEMS coupled with biocompatible electronic devices can be applied in the treatment of medical disorders.

   The research paper topic should look into the companies who are manufacturing MEMS and the applications of such biomechanical devices.
2. Some of the nanoparticles can be covalently linked to biological molecules and can then be applied to applications such as contrast agents in imaging, carriers in drug delivery, and scaffolds. These nanoparticles are called nanoprobes or nanoscaffolds. The research topic should focus on some specific nanoprobes and the techniques of biological covalent links.

Index

Page numbers followed by an "*f*" indicate that the entry is included in a figure.

Q

R

T

W

X

Z